TCM-Klinik Bad Kötzting

Dieter Melchart • Jingzhang Dai
Stefan Hager • Anton Staudinger
Christina Staudinger
Editors

TCM-Klinik Bad Kötzting

First German Hospital for Traditional Chinese Medicine

TCM-KLINIK BAD KÖTZTING

First German Hospital for Traditional Chinese Medicine
Special hospital for psychosomatic and psychotherapy
University Hospital at Beijing University of Chinese Medicine

Springer

OPEN ACCESS

Editors
Dieter Melchart
Faculty of Applied Healthcare Sciences
Deggendorf Institute of Technology
Deggendorf, Germany

Stefan Hager
TCM-Klinik Bad Kötzting
Bad Kötzting, Germany

Christina Staudinger
TCM-Klinik Bad Kötzting
Bad Kötzting, Germany

Jingzhang Dai
TCM-Klinik Bad Kötzting
Bad Kötzting, Germany

Anton Staudinger
TCM-Klinik Bad Kötzting
Bad Kötzting, Germany

ISBN 978-3-032-23306-6 ISBN 978-3-032-23307-3 (eBook)
https://doi.org/10.1007/978-3-032-23307-3

This work was supported by TCM Clinic Bad Kötzting.

This Springer imprint is published by the registered company Springer Nature Switzerland AG
The registered company address is: Gewerbestrasse 11, 6330 Cham, Switzerland

Foreword 1

序

中医药学是中华民族的伟大创造，是中国古代科学的瑰宝，凝聚着数千年文明智慧与生命哲学。在守护人类健康的历史进程中，中医药始终发挥着不可替代的独特作用，并以其系统思维与整体观念对世界文明进步产生了积极而深远的影响。

北京中医药大学作为中华人民共和国教育部直属唯一一所高等中医药院校，肩负传承创新中医药学术体系、推动中医药走向世界的重要使命。1991年，学校与德国施道丁尔集团联合创办德国魁茨汀中医院，开创了在海外建立中医医院的先河；2010年，医院正式挂牌为北京中医药大学魁茨汀医院，标志着中医药国际化发展迈入更加规范化、体系化的新阶段。

建院以来，北京中医药大学魁茨汀医院始终秉持严谨规范的医疗理念和高水平的专业服务，成功诊治了大量患者，逐步形成了以中医药为主体、融合西方身心医学与生活方式、独具特色且行之有效的综合诊疗模式。这一模式既坚守中医药理论精髓，又注重现代医学语境下的科学表达与实践转化，在跨文化医疗环境中展现出强大的生命力与适应性。值此建院三十五周年之际，谨致以最热烈祝贺，并向所有为医院发展默默奉献的医务工作者以及长期支持医院建设的各界人士致以最诚挚的敬意!

三十五载砥砺前行，在中德政府的共同支持下，北京中医药大学魁茨汀医院不断夯实基础，实现了稳健而持续的发展。医院先后与慕尼黑工业大学、迪根道夫应用技术大学补充医学与自然疗法中心(KoKoNat)建立了重要而长期的合作伙伴关系，在中医药临床应用与科学研究领域开展深度合作，共同取得了一批高质量研究成果。目前医院已成为中医药走向世界的典范，持续为欧洲民众健康福祉贡献力量，在中医药科学研究、医学术语规范化与国际化、跨语言文化传播等方面做出开创性与示范意义的重要贡献。

本书主要以北京中医药大学魁茨汀医院年度报告为基础，结合随访调查与数据对比分析，较为系统展现了特色病种住院诊疗效果、治疗安全性与耐受性等核心指标，同时呈现医院运行架构与患者人群特征。全书为读者全面、真实地了解该院临床实践全貌提供了客观资料与多维视角，并较为系统地梳理了双方在合作框架下取得的科学研究与学术交流成果。相信本书的出版，将为推动中医药在全球范围内的学术探讨、科学评价与持续发展注入新的理论思考与实践启示。

北京中医药大学校长

Traditional Chinese medicine is a great creation of the Chinese nation and a treasure of ancient Chinese science. It encompasses the wisdom and philosophy of life of a civilization spanning several millennia. Throughout history, TCM has played a unique and irreplaceable role in safeguarding human health. Its systemic thinking and holistic approach have had a positive and lasting influence on the progress of world civilization.

Beijing University of Chinese Medicine is the only university for traditional Chinese medicine that is directly under the jurisdiction of the People's Republic of China's Ministry of Education. The university's important mission is to preserve and innovatively develop the academic system of TCM, and to bring TCM to the world. In 1991, the university established the first TCM clinic abroad in collaboration with the Staudinger Group, marking a milestone with the opening of the Chinese Clinic in Bad Kötzting. In 2010, the clinic officially became known as the "TCM Clinic Bad Kötzting of the Beijing University of Chinese Medicine," marking a more standardized and systematized phase in the international development of TCM.

Since its foundation, the TCM Clinic Bad Kötzting has consistently adhered to rigorous standards of medical quality, offering highly professional services. It has successfully treated a large number of patients and has gradually developed an independent, effective, integrative care concept based on TCM: TCM at its core, supplemented by Western psychosomatic medicine and lifestyle medicine. This model preserves the theoretical essence of TCM, emphasizing scientifically verifiable presentation and practice-oriented implementation within the context of modern medicine. It demonstrates remarkable vitality and adaptability within an intercultural healthcare environment. On the occasion of its 35th anniversary, we would like to express our warmest congratulations and sincere thanks to all the healthcare professionals who have contributed so much to the clinic's development, as well as to all the supporters from a wide variety of fields.

Over 35 years of steady progress, the TCM Clinic Bad Kötzting—with joint support from China and Germany—has continuously consolidated its foundations and achieved stable, sustainable development. It has established long-term and significant partnerships with the Center for Complementary Medicine and Naturopathy (CoCoNat) at Deggendorf Institute of Technology (formerly Technical University of Munich), among others, deepening its cooperation in the areas of the clinical application of TCM and scientific research and achieving a series of high-quality research results. Today, the clinic is considered an exemplary model for the internationalization of TCM and continues to contribute to the health and well-being of the European population. It has also done pioneering work in fields such as scientific research into TCM, the standardization and internationalization of medical terminology, and intercultural and multilingual communication.

This book is primarily based on the TCM Clinic Bad Kötzting's annual reports and combines these with follow-up surveys and comparative data analyses. It presents key figures in a relatively systematic manner, including treatment results for selected indications in an inpatient setting and information on therapy safety and tolerability. It also outlines the organizational structure of the clinic and the characteristics of its patient population. Offering readers objective material and a multidimensional perspective, the book provides a comprehensive and realistic picture of the clinic's clinical practice. It also summarizes the research successes and academic exchange activities achieved through collaboration. We are convinced that publishing this book will provide new theoretical impetus and practical inspiration to advance international scientific discussion and evidence-based evaluation of TCM worldwide, as well as its sustainable development.

The President of the Beijing University of Chinese Medicine Zhishu Tang
Chaoyang, China

Foreword 2

To mark the 35th anniversary of the TCM-Klinik in Bad Kötzting, this book uses a clinic report 2025 to describe the concept and results of the scientific cooperation with the Competence Centre for Lifestyle Medicine and Naturopathic Treatment (CoCoNat) at the Deggendorf Institute of Technology (DIT). This scientific support from CoCoNat has been in place since 2003 and is part of a research agreement between the Beijing University of Chinese Medicine (BUCM) and the Technical University of Munich (TUM), which was contractually replaced by the Deggendorf Institute of Technology (DIT) in 2020.

CoCoNat at DIT specializes in health and lifestyle research, clinical research, and quality assurance in teaching and practicing these methods.

The results demonstrate the successful collaboration between the partners in the field of traditional Chinese medicine at the Deggendorf Institute of Technology, in conjunction with the TCM-Klinik Bad Kötzting.

They have carried out and published joint work in the fields of quality assurance, active ingredient analysis, and the safety and tolerability of TCM medicines. Clinical work has also been conducted on clinical efficacy testing and systematic literature reviews on clinical acupuncture. Current work particularly focuses on health maintenance and prevention, specifically Individual Health Management (IHM).

This book fulfills the reporting requirements agreed in the cooperation agreement between the two universities regarding the results of the research work and research objectives and provides mutual information on the status of the respective research projects.

It is hoped that this successful cooperation will continue, building on the valuable clinical results achieved so far to improve medical care in Germany.

The President of the Deggendorf Institute of Technology (DIT) Waldemar Berg
Deggendorf, Germany

Preface

This clinic report 2025 offers a comprehensive insight into the clinical and scientific work of the TCM-Klinik Bad Kötzting. The book provides an in-depth analysis of the quality of medical care at the First German Clinic for Traditional Chinese Medicine (TCM) in 2023. The presentation is complemented by a 6-month follow-up survey of patients and comparisons with previous years' results.

The TCM-Klinik Bad Kötzting, a specialist clinic in the fields of psychosomatics and psychotherapy, is celebrating its 35th anniversary. It is the oldest TCM clinic in Germany and treats almost exclusively patients with statutory health insurance. The interaction between Western medicine and Far Eastern healing arts as practiced here is unique internationally and exists nowhere else outside the People's Republic of China—even though there are other outpatient, day-care, and inpatient facilities for Traditional Chinese Medicine (TCM) outside China. The close cooperation between the Beijing University of Chinese Medicine (BUCM), the Technical University of Munich (TUM), and, since 2020, the Deggendorf Institute of Technology (DIT) has resulted in scientific support that has helped to ensure the unconditional review and quality improvement of everyday clinical work since the clinic was founded. The TCM-Klinik Bad Kötzting has been an official institution of the BUCM in Germany since 2010. It plays a pivotal role in the implementation of the applied health sciences of the DIT in clinical practice, prevention, and lifestyle medicine.

In recent decades, the clinic's scientific advisory board has been instrumental in defining and implementing various research priorities within the scope of its work. Of particular note are the pharmaceutical analysis, with the creation of a comprehensive monograph on Chinese medicinal drugs, and clinical outcome research, with the testing of a web-based documentation system called VITERIO. A plethora of topics and issues from these two areas have been discussed and published at numerous conferences in Germany and the People's Republic of China. Nevertheless, over the past 35 years, there has been an absence of success in the implementation of research projects that were planned in collaboration, for example, in the field of metabolic syndrome, depression and sleep treatment, and lifestyle-oriented prevention in the form of cross-border clinical and experimental application research. This endeavor was unsuccessful due to two primary factors. Firstly, there was a deficiency in government funding for research into Chinese medicine in Germany. Secondly, there was an absence of preliminary scientific testing for Chinese medicines, which is a prerequisite for approval by medical ethics committees.

Consequently, the editors anticipate that both countries will augment their collaborative endeavors in the scientific, political, and financial domains to achieve these objectives.

An anniversary represents a valuable opportunity to express gratitude to all those who have contributed to the success of the project. This gratitude is directed primarily toward the medical and nursing personnel at the clinic, as well as the members of the scientific advisory board. However, it is important to acknowledge the vital contributions of all the clinic's employees, the constructive support and collaboration of statutory health insurance funds, the Bavarian State Ministry of Health and Care, supervisory authorities, administrations, and local and supra-regional politicians. In addition, the important work of the company VITERIO should also be mentioned, which is responsible for the successful development of the software of the same name. The success achieved thus far would not have been possible without these collective efforts.

In this context, we would like to make a special mention and express our appreciation to the following organizations and individuals for their invaluable contributions:

The Centre for Complementary Medicine and Naturopathy (CoCoNat) at the DIT, which has served as an active scientific partner on site

The Erich Rothenfußer Foundation in Munich, which has provided CoCoNat with unwavering support

The World Federation of Chinese Medicine Societies (WFCMS), which has generously supported numerous scientific symposia

We would also like to thank the participating Bavarian and Chinese universities for their significant contribution to the administrative and scientific support of the work in general, and to the TCM-Klinik Bad Kötzting in particular.

Deggendorf, Germany — Dieter Melchart
Bad Kötzting, Germany — Jingzhang Dai
Bad Kötzting, Germany — Stefan Hager
Bad Kötzting, Germany — Anton Staudinger
Bad Kötzting, Germany — Christina Staudinger

Acknowledgments

As the corresponding author and editor, I would like to acknowledge the following individuals from the TCM-Klinik Bad Kötzting, who made substantial contributions to this work. Nevertheless, they do not fulfill the criteria for authorship.

The collection of clinical data from patients by the designated study nurses is a fundamental aspect of the research process:

The following study nurses at the TCM-Klinik are to be singled out for commendation: Kerstin Bauer, Sabrina Lummer, Christina Treimer, and Alexandra von Grotthuss. It is my privilege to acknowledge the contributions in this context of the following Chinese employees: Ma Shuhui, Siong Hang, and Zhao Jing.

The responsibility for the administration of the survey questionnaires, both prior to and following hospitalization, lies with the designated individuals:

Teresa Zemmler and Heike Heitzer have been specifically appointed to this area of data management.

I would like to express my gratitude to the following individuals for their comprehensive technical support in relation to the web-based documentation system VITERIO^R:

Representing the entire VITERIO^R company is the Managing Director, Rudolf Brunner, who has been responsible for the technical development of the software of the same name for decades. He has made a tremendous contribution and shown tireless dedication.

Finally, on behalf of all the editors, I would like to thank the book's coauthors, especially Lara Isabel Jötten, for her extensive statistical work and her overall contribution to the book.

Ethics Approval The work follows ethical standards for research involving human subjects. All scientific activities are authorized and reviewed by an Academic Exchange Agreement between the Beijing University of Chinese Medicine and Deggendorf Institute of Technology resp. Technical University of Munich. The patients gave their written consent on admission to the TCM-Klinik Bad Kötzting.

Declaration of Competing Interests

The coauthors Stefan Hager, Jingzhang Dai, and Likun Yang have had personal affiliations in the TCM-Klinik Bad Kötzting during the time of reporting. The two managing directors, Anton and Christina Staudinger, have competing interests due to their professional positions. Erich Wühr is the owner of a private publishing house that has received several commissions from the TCM clinic.

The corresponding author and editor Dieter Melchart and all other authors have had no relevant financial interests or personal affiliations in connection with the content of this manuscript.

About the Corresponding Author/Editor

From 2010 to 2015, Prof. Dr. med. Dieter Melchart held the first professorship for naturopathy and complementary medicine in Bavaria at the Klinikum rechts der Isar of the Technical University of Munich (TUM) (endowed professorship of the Erich Rothenfußer Foundation, Munich). There, he headed the "Competence Centre for Complementary Medicine and Naturopathy (CoCoNat)" at the Klinikum rechts der Isar and the associated outpatient clinic and day clinic for naturopathy and health promotion. In addition, he was titular professor at the University of Zurich, Switzerland, from 2010 to 2019, and is a visiting professor at Beijing University of Traditional Chinese Medicine. Since 2020, he has been an honorary professor of complementary medicine and individual health management (IHM) at the Faculty of Applied Health Sciences at the Deggendorf Institute of Technology (DIT), Germany, and was head of the CoCoNat until 2025.

Since 1991, he has been the chairman of the scientific advisory board of the first German clinic for traditional Chinese medicine in Bad Kötzting, Germany. His research focuses on the clinical evaluation of acupuncture, TCM medicines, and lifestyle medicine. As an adjunct professor of naturopathy, Melchart continues to lecture on naturopathy in interdisciplinary subject 12 at the Technical University of Munich and supervises doctoral theses.

Contents

The Patient Care Evaluation Programme (PEP)—An Introduction of the Scientific Concept

1

Dieter Melchart

1.1 Scientific Framework of the Patient Care Evaluation Programme (PEP) with Particular Emphasis on Traditional Chinese Medicine (TCM)

This 2025 clinic report from the TCM-Klinik Bad Kötzting, Germany's first clinic for traditional Chinese medicine, has been compiled in accordance with the scientific concept of the Programme for the Evaluation of Patient Care (PEP). The PEP evaluation programme is described in detail in this introductory chapter. The clinic is portrayed in terms of its structures, processes, and results in the 2023 operating year. The presentation of results is supplemented by a follow-up survey of patients approximately 6 months after their discharge from the clinic, with the survey continuing into 2024.

The report, which was primarily compiled by the Competence Centre for Lifestyle Medicine and Naturopathic Treatment (CoCoNat) at the Deggendorf Institute of Technology (DIT), is jointly edited and authorised in collaboration with the TCM Clinic, the Scientific Advisory Board, and the Beijing University of Chinese Medicine (BUCM).

The TCM-Klinik Bad Kötzting commenced its medical operations in 1991, marking the inaugural establishment of a German clinic specialising in traditional Chinese medicine. Patients who are referred by doctors on the basis of a hospital admission are treated as persons insured under the German statutory health insurance system. The present TCM Clinic is a specialist clinic in the field of

D. Melchart (✉)
Former Head of Competence Centre for Lifestyle Medicine and Naturopathy (CoCoNat), Faculty of Applied Healthcare Sciences, Deggendorf Institute of Technology (DIT), Deggendorf, Germany
e-mail: dieter.melchart@th-deg.de

D. Melchart et al. (eds.), *TCM-Klinik Bad Kötzting*,
https://doi.org/10.1007/978-3-032-23307-3_1

psychosomatics and psychotherapy, offering inpatient care that combines traditional Chinese medicine with a range of conventional and naturopathic/complementary therapies.

Following several decades of research, teaching, and clinical treatment, the TCM- Klinik Bad Kötzting was officially designated a University Hospital at Beijing University of Chinese Medicine (BUCM) in 2010.

In Germany, there are a number of clinical facilities that offer traditional Chinese medicine to the population, either exclusively (e.g. Klinik am Steigerwald) or partially (e.g. Kliniken Essen Mitte). These clinics primarily treat chronic (and to a lesser extent acute) patients, and the naturopathic/complementary medicine therapies offered typically encompass a wide range of procedures. It is evident that a proportion of these procedures are not scientifically recognised or are recognised to a limited extent. However, the TCM-Klinik Bad Kötzting is the only TCM clinic in Germany that has been granted authorisation to treat patients covered by German statutory health insurance with a cost coverage statement.

In the course of the scientific monitoring of the clinic, it became evident that the implementation of randomised studies for the evaluation of specific isolated procedures, which are generally applied in combination in routine clinical practice, yielded only very limited meaningful results. Moreover, such studies necessitate an inordinate level of organisational, financial, and temporal investment. While a randomised comparison of clinical facilities in this area would be desirable in principle, it is particularly difficult to implement in this case, as patients often opt for treatment in such clinics after having already undergone lengthy and unsuccessful conventional treatments. Moreover, it would be challenging to generalise the results of such studies due to the predominantly clinic-specific nature of the procedures.

Consequently, health insurance funds, patients, and referring physicians have been unable to base their decisions regarding treatment preferences, referrals, and reimbursement primarily on 'scientific findings' from randomised controlled clinical trials.

Thus, there is an imperative for the development of pragmatic and innovative concepts, with the objective of facilitating the formulation of rational decisions by doctors, patients, health insurance funds, and politicians. The present programme for the evaluation of patient care (PEP) with naturopathic/complementary medicine is therefore proposed as a possible solution.

PEP is a documentation and evaluation programme designed to record everyday care practices in outpatient and inpatient facilities. Its aim is to describe the quality of everyday clinical work in terms of its structure, processes, and outcomes, with a particular focus on complementary medicine procedures.

PEP integrates two largely separate areas: quality assurance and clinical research. Quality management aims to determine and describe the 'nature' (quality) of structures and processes, and to document and continuously improve therapy outcomes under practical conditions [1, 2]. As well as assessing individual services from a patient perspective, the focus is on the overall benefit and risk to the individual patient [1–3]. The patient-centred outcome assessment approach does not examine the objective effectiveness of an intervention; rather, it maps the application and impact of interventions in routine clinical or everyday medical practice, presenting and determining the personally perceived benefit or 'real-world effectiveness' from the patient's perspective [4]. Real-world evidence (RWE) from large, well-designed research projects is increasingly viewed as potential tools, although it is sometimes perceived as "less robust" compared to RCTs due to potential biases [5].

The aim is to contribute to outcome research in complementary medicine in the sense of ensuring the quality of results in inpatient psychosomatic complementary medical care.

This results-oriented approach is not usually limited to medically definable outcomes, but also includes health-related results of interventions, such as the influence of risk and protective factors, general health status, life satisfaction, and quality of life. Patient sovereignty also requires information on satisfaction with individual aspects of care, such as accommodation, information, and services. Patient-centred quality assurance is also supported by Section 70 of the German Social Code V (SGB V), which explicitly requires medical services to be high-quality, cost-effective, and humane.

The results of patient-centred quality assessments can be compared between different users, albeit with some limitations. However, a particular problem is that hardly any such data is available for comparison. The continuous description of the quality of the results achieved by individual service providers is an important addition to evidence from controlled clinical studies. Ideally, they should form a rational basis together to help patients and referring physicians make an informed decision about the use of defined medical services and individual providers. This comparative data should therefore primarily be generated and made accessible for patients and interested physicians.

Traditional clinical research, on the other hand, primarily attempts to investigate the effectiveness of interventions through controlled clinical trials. It also aims to increase benefits for patients. However, the following questions are increasingly coming to the fore:

- Causality of the connection between intervention and outcome?
- Generalisability and provability of the overall or individual intervention?

Nonetheless, it is often impossible to provide scientific proof of efficacy in the narrower sense for the highly diverse and variable 'therapy cocktails' used in naturopathy and complementary medicine in an inpatient setting. While testing individual components in randomised trials would be desirable, this is often not representative due to the highly clinic-specific nature of most procedures, and of limited informative value. For this reason, randomised comparative studies are not always the first step in clinical research into naturopathic treatments, as issues other than the efficacy of a single treatment method often take precedence, or the methodological design is not suitable for answering the research question. This is due to the fundamental differences between research strategies oriented towards drug research and the testing of naturopathic efficacy. Before a drug can be recommended and approved for medical use, it must undergo the standard phases of clinical testing.

Innovation therefore only enters healthcare when sufficient evidence is available from study results. In the case of naturopathic treatments and complementary medicine, the 'product' is usually already widely used in medical care and has a long tradition of use. However, there is little or no supporting evidence due to a lack of controlled study results and other research material. The fact that naturopathic treatments and other traditional healing systems are already in use means there is a need to research practical questions regarding benefits and safety, as well as a high demand for information on various aspects of application quality from patients, service providers, politicians, and the insurance industry.

Based on the above, the PEP at the TCM-Klinik Bad Kötzting will primarily address the following questions and objectives:

- What happens in clinical practice, with whom, and with what results? (*transparency*)
- Do patients benefit from the interventions? (*benefit*)
- How safe and tolerable are the interventions? (*safety*)
- Can these interventions save costs? (*costs*)
- How can the quality of the interventions be controlled, assured, and improved? (*quality assurance and optimisation*)
- Can causal effectiveness be demonstrated under controlled and randomised conditions? What is the state of evidence for the complementary healing methods used? (*experimental proof of efficacy*)

The principle of 'research transfer' from universities to the mostly non-university application of complementary medicine remains a primary research requirement to this day because, to date, there has not been, nor is there currently, enough patients or university teachers with the necessary theoretical and practical expertise available within university hospitals. In the field of complementary medicine, applied science is the most important and innovative part of clinical research.

Although this strategic approach is very successful, several legal, operational, and methodological research restrictions must be considered. In addition, considerable problems have been encountered in securing the necessary financial support from the outset. Over the past 35 years, government funding agencies have not provided sufficient funding to answer the most pressing questions about the global benefits of complex inpatient intervention services. This lack of financial support means that evaluative evidence must be and continues to be primarily provided within the standard medical care system. By contrast, traditional university clinical research, which typically involves testing the effectiveness of individual therapies and diagnostic methods using randomised, controlled trials, has considerably more financial resources and personnel available from government funding and industry.

In the case of the TCM-Klinik Bad Kötzting, the clinic itself, CoCoNat, and the Erich Rothenfußer Foundation in Munich provide all the necessary personnel, technical resources, and direct financial funds for clinical research.

1.1.1 The Utilisation of Patient-Reported Outcomes (PRO) and the Web-Based Health Portal VITERIO® for PEP

The presentation of results for all serial case studies in PEP leads to an overall assessment of medical services from the perspective of patients or clients treated at a specific clinical facility or by a specific medical provider. At the individual level, this presentation of symptoms, findings, behaviour, and feelings can be used for personal feedback. An essential feature of naturopathy and complementary medicine is promoting patients' self-awareness. The emphasis on 'salutogenesis' and 'inner healing powers' is also important in traditional Chinese medicine.

Complementary medicine and TCM focus on health promotion. They look at what causes illness and what keeps us healthy. A holistic approach to health involves considering not only the clinical picture, but also the patient's living conditions, to understand how the disease developed and what can be done to promote lasting recovery. Personal protective and risk factors are key to maintaining health. Teaching modern risk and protective factor management as a lifestyle medicine component is an important aspect of the concept and documentation.

Modern complementary medicine and TCM consider all the diagnostic and therapeutic procedures that conventional medicine currently considers necessary. However, the holistic approach of complementary medicine often leads to an anamnesis that covers the patient's biography and living circumstances in terms of family, career, and housing situation, and includes aspects of individual lifestyle, behaviour, life goal planning, and personal constitution.

This issue is addressed by means of active involvement of the individual in the documentation process through a web-based health portal developed by CoCoNat called VITERIO®. This so-called PRO (Patient-Reported Outcome) approach is supported by the VITERIO® web software.

VITERIO (the TCM health portal) has a doctor-side patient file (Provider Reported Outcomes and Findings-PROFI) and a patient-side health portal (Patient Reported Outcomes and a Measurement-Information-System-PROMI). See Fig. 1.1.

The web portal VITERIO (Fig. 1.2) is intended to increase the preventive value for patients. Medical care still primarily refrains from utilising patients' health potential, focusing on pharmacological and interventional treatment of late and consequential damage. This service is geared towards patient passivity and places a heavy burden on solidarity, resulting in high costs. The web portal's structure and concept are described elsewhere [6]. One of the improvement projects planned by CoCoNat in cooperation with the clinic is the future creation of a mobile version of the PROMI side of VITERIO.

The key components of the TCM health portal with its PROMI function are:

- Biographical medical history
- Classical system medical history
- Neurovegetative medical history

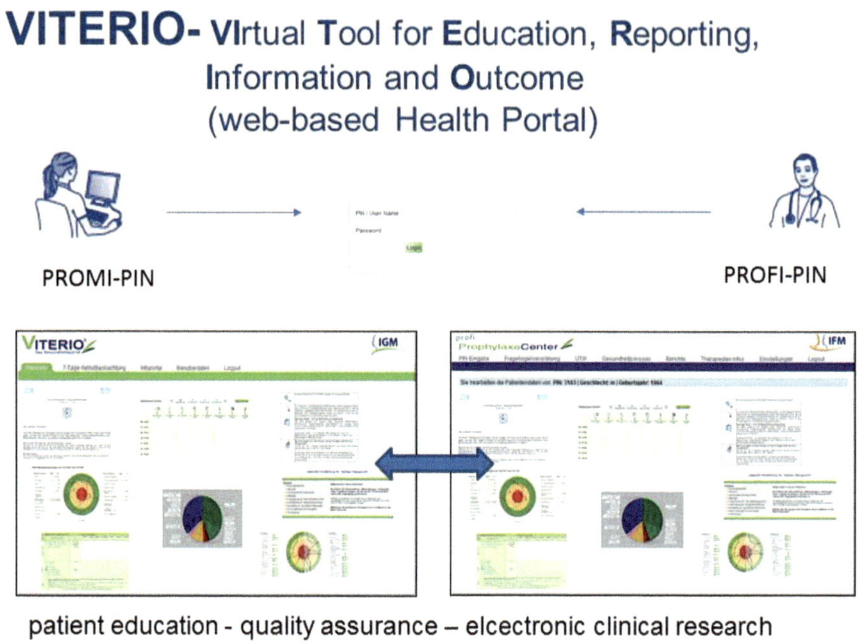

Fig. 1.1 VITERIO web portal. This is the input page for patients and doctors on the VITERIO web portal [6]

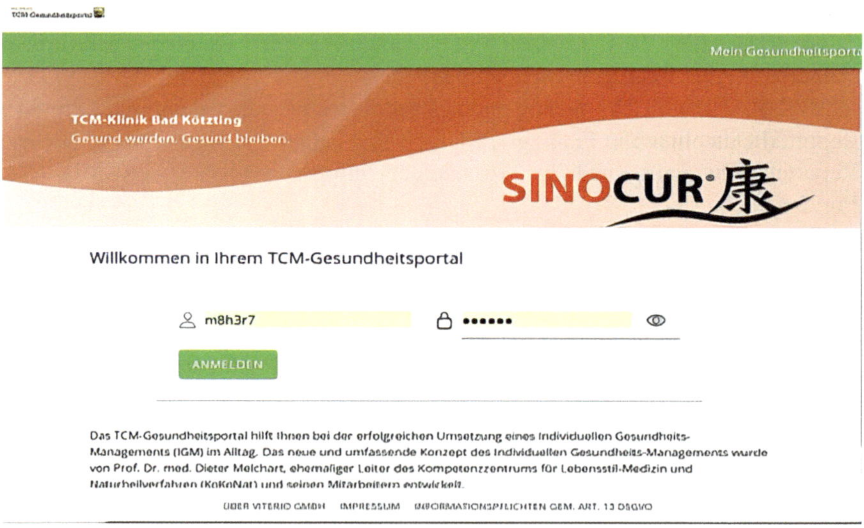

Fig. 1.2 TCM-Gesundheitsportal: tcmklinik.viterio.de

- Risk and protective factors history with traffic light display and detailed instruction in self-help techniques (Western and Chinese)
- Self-observation tools for emotion regulation and behaviour in the areas of exercise, nutrition, and stress management (steps taken, weight, five-a-day, visual analogue scale)
- Regular monitoring of symptoms and findings by the user (in particular, the ICD symptom rating and the perceived stress questionnaire)
- Support for health management through accompanying material for the individual teaching units of the education programme, and if necessary, risk-adapted training plans for post-hospital care

The basis for the individual feedback system is long-term self-monitoring of symptoms and findings, and regular self-assessment using questionnaires (assessment tools). The system is designed to enable users to reflect on and optimise their own physical and mental health behaviour and lifestyle, and to confirm or correct it [6]. The health portal thus serves not only for healthcare research and scientific evaluation of everyday behaviour and changes in findings through interventions, but also for supporting users in implementing a health-promoting lifestyle programme known as 'Individual Health Management IHM' [7–9].

The lifestyle programme employs the pedagogical approach of 'blended learning', integrating personal coaching with web-based health promotion. The portal identifies and supports individuals by means of continuous measurement of "basic physical functions", including nutrition, exercise, sleep, immunity, thermoregulation, and "basic cognitive-psychosocial skills", such as a sense of coherence, optimism, self-efficacy, and life satisfaction. This enables the portal to maintain and optimise their mental and physical health. Furthermore, the system under discussion facilitates the efforts of health coaches by means of digital recording, thereby ensuring the provision of timely feedback on data for everyone, as well as for the entire group. This facilitates the optimisation of coaching support.

The patients themselves and the therapists are informed of the various risk and protective factors in the form of a traffic light graphic (Fig. 1.3).

Certain findings and questionnaire algorithms are collected to describe physical and psychosocial health. These consist of fixed indicators and variable parameters and can be adapted to specific settings or project-related questions from studies. This standard survey is referred to as a 'health check'. The collected data can then be generated independently via various automated reports and document creation tools and made accessible to users.

With regard to Individual Health Management (IHM), the TCM-Klinik Bad Kötzting is part of a consortium consisting of the Competence Centre for Lifestyle Medicine and Naturopathic Treatment (CoCoNat) at the Faculty of Applied Health Sciences at the Deggendorf Institute of Technology (DIT); the Beijing University of Chinese Medicine (BUCM); the company Viterio®; the Erich Rothenfusser Foundation in Munich; the town of Bad Kötzting; and the IHM Campus network. The IHM Campus network involves project partners from fields such as spa

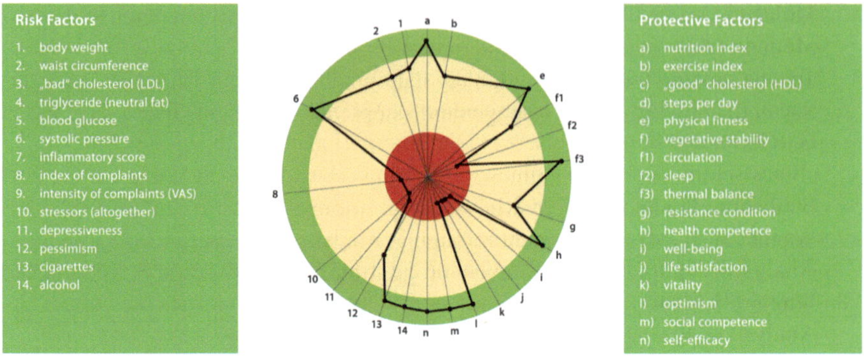

Fig. 1.3 The VITERIO health portal (Virtual Tool for Education, Reporting, Information and Outcome) with risk and protective factors displayed in a traffic light system [6]

treatment, rehabilitation, and outpatient care for a limited period. Currently, the database is exclusively managed by CoCoNat, the DIT's scientific partner, as a trust centre.

IHM is primarily intended to significantly increase preventive care for patients. Currently, medical care largely avoids utilising patients' health potential and focuses on the medicinal and interventional treatment of late and consequential damage. This form of service provision is geared towards patient passivity and places a heavy financial burden on the healthcare system. People's own health resources remain largely untapped, and service provision is geared towards patient passivity. This results in both healthy and sick people being dissuaded from taking an active role in maintaining and strengthening their health protection factors. This often results in patients developing chronic conditions. There is a lack of sufficient professional services to empower people to implement health-promoting and symptom-oriented self-help measures in their everyday lives, in both health and illness.

Patient competence and self-management remain neglected aspects of modern healthcare. The focus is on the medical expertise of specialists. Conversely, medicine and modern humans have largely lost the ability to activate self-healing powers. Consequently, the power of information and decision-making in the doctor–patient relationship is usually unilaterally shifted to the therapist. This asymmetry must be reduced by strengthening patient autonomy. The TCM clinic promotes competence and improves patient self-determination as independent treatment goals, attempting to achieve this in various ways in terms of content and technology. Key components in achieving this goal include the use of tools such as patient books, info@zepte, patient passports, health reports, and treatment protocols, as well as integrating patients into a patient-centred assessment of the quality of medical and psychosomatic services, and a post-hospitalisation lifestyle support programme.

Doctors, psychologists, and health coaches can enter their data on the PROFI-page of the VITERIO® portal. Different professional access rights apply here. The following data can be recorded:

- TCM diagnosis tool
- ICD-10 tool
- Acupuncture documentation
- Special TCM medication documentation with prescription system
- Western medication documentation
- Systematic medical history
- Electronic patient files with findings (including blood and urine laboratory results), diagnoses, medication, and medical passports.

Interfaces to statutory electronic patient files will be created here in future.

Data is available to patients and doctors. Doctors or coaches can then generate medical entries in the form of medical histories, acupuncture reports, or case report forms (CRFs).

1.1.2 Portrait of the Quality Levels of the TCM-Klinik Bad Kötzting and Time Frame of Observation

The description of quality characteristics at the TCM clinic is comprehensive in nature, incorporating all levels of quality. However, the primary emphasis is on the presentation of results, which is a key aspect of the clinic's approach. The clinic report under consideration herein delineates so-called quality profiles, with the aim of presenting the structural, process, and outcome quality of the clinic [10–16]. At the present time, there is no universally accepted form of presentation for these quality profiles.

Table 1.1 provides an overview of the various dimensions of the individual quality profiles.

The quality profiles are self-explanatory in terms of the structure, process, and results of a clinic and are intended to portray the facility characteristics, diagnostic and therapeutic processes, and clinical results for specific and unspecific diseases. The patient profile is primarily utilised by therapists during the admission process for the purpose of therapy planning. The identification of personal risk factors and the provision of health resources are imperative for the individualisation of treatment and for patient participation. A final and follow-up collection of data allows for an evaluation of changes in subjective parameters, showing the success of psychotherapy and lifestyle medicine. The evaluation and quality assurance profile shows the clinic's activities, including studies, reports, courses, and projects.

Observation Time

All patients of the clinic will be included consecutively in 2023. The observation data is recorded at the time of admission to the clinic, discharge from the clinic, and a follow-up survey approximately 6 months after discharge (see Table 1.2 for details).

Table 1.1 Quality profiles of the hospital to be portrayed in the hospital report

Structural profile	1. **General information** on the structure of the hospital 2. **Staff description** (number of medical staff; professional qualifications; employee satisfaction; continuing education and training programmes) 3. **Medical equipment** and **structural conditions** 4. **Medical concept** of the clinic (general therapy goals, general description of procedures; exemplary treatment plan and process organisation for a patient) 5. **Post-hospital care** (interface management; case management) 6. **Communication structures** (rounds, team meetings)
Patient profile	1. **Socio-biographical** and **socio-epidemiological data**: age, gender, type of health insurance, education, occupational status, etc. 2. **General medical data**: primary and secondary diagnoses (ICD 10; ICIDH), severity per diagnosis, problem assessment, degree of chronicity, intensity of primary complaint; duration of complaint, general complaints and impairments of well-being; Type and reason for admission, previous medical treatment (number and type of hospital stays; visits to the doctor within the last 12 months; days of sick leave); use of self-help techniques; standard survey: risk and protective factors; medication history and status 3. **Special medical data**: medical history and status assessment 4. **Person-oriented data**: previous experience with treatment; overall expectation of success; illness-related change in values; intervention-related change in values; subjective aetiology of illness; personal satisfaction with diet; exercise behaviour including cognitive assessment; motivation, compliance, pension application; General life satisfaction; quality of life—vitality (SF36) and functionality in everyday life; stress management; life orientation, sense of coherence (SOC) *(temporarily available for therapy decisions at the beginning and then presented as progress data in the report as a results profile)*
Intervention profile	1. Type and frequency of **therapeutic procedures** 2. Type and frequency of **diagnostic procedures** 3. Quality and appropriateness of procedures
Outcome profile	*General assessment:* 1. Overall symptom relief and general reduction in symptoms (**symptom relief**) 2. Overall assessment of the success of the intervention by the patient and the doctor with a target/actual comparison (**success assessment**) 3. Improvement in quality of life (**quality of life**) 4. Reduction in utilisation behaviour (**utilisation**) 5. Reduction of risk factors and optimisation of protective factors (**preventive value**) 6. Assessment of safety and tolerability (**complications**) 7. Patient satisfaction with the service (**patient satisfaction**) 8. Evaluation of post-hospitalisation service structure *Medical assessment:* 1. Formal medical assessments for defined tracer diagnoses (**formal assessment**)

(continued)

Table 1.1 (continued)

Evaluation and quality assurance profile	1. Quality assurance projects and/or own clinical studies within the last 12 months? 2. Continuous audit and peer review? **(Support from an external institution)** 3. Member of a data collection centre, assessment centre, evaluation network, quality circle? 4. Has a comparison with another institution been carried out within the last 2 years? (**Quality comparison, benchmarking**) 5. Is there a clinic report from the last 12 months and can you draw your own preliminary comparisons with the current data? 6. What literature evidence is available for the interventions and indications used? **(State of effectiveness)** 7. Are there any publications or study results from the reporting period? (**Publications**) 8. Have **case studies** (responders, non-responders) been documented? 9. Are **improvement projects** being planned based on the current data collection?

Table 1.2 Components and schedule for basic documentation

Schedule for basic documentation (quality of results)	Admission	Discharge	Follow-up after 6 months
Information from the patient:			
Biographical/sociographical characteristics	•		
Current complaints	•	•	•
Previous treatment	•		•
Intensity of the main complaint	•	•	•
ISR (ICD symptom rating)	•	•	•
Expected treatment outcome	•		•
Life satisfaction questionnaire	•	•	•
Documentation of risk and protective factors for health	•	•	•
Implementation of lifestyle change measures			
Satisfaction with treatment; clinic recommendation	(•)	•	•
Medication use; additional treatments	•	•	•
Undesirable therapeutic effects (UTW)		•	•
Information from the doctor and hospital staff:			
Medical history data, preliminary diagnosis	•		
Expected treatment outcome	•		
Final primary/secondary diagnoses		•	
Therapy outcome; incapacity to work		•	•
Adverse treatment effects (ATE)		•	•
Diagnostic/therapeutic services		•	•

Study Design

The study design is a one-group pretest-post-test design. This is a cross-diagnostic, indication-specific, monocentric before-and-after study on inpatient psychosomatic hospital treatment incorporating traditional Chinese medicine. The evaluation is presented in the form of quality profiles of the TCM-Klinik Bad Kötzting. The observation data is partly compared with a separate reference group from previous years. Table 1.2 provides a rough overview.

1.1.3 Methodological Aspects of the Evaluation and the Concept of Confidence-Based Medicine (CBM)

Dependence on Initial Values

From a methodological point of view, the results of 'before-and-after' comparisons are difficult to interpret. They reflect the overall effects of interventions, but do not allow definitive statements to be made about causality or the specificity of the intervention in relation to the observed effect. The respective contributions of the contextual factors involved, such as the placebo effect, chance, bias, and the natural course of the disease, to the total effect remain unknown.

An important aspect of presenting observation sequences is the difference between baseline and discharge or follow-up values. This raises the question of whether the indicators and quality criteria measured at the time of admission reflect the 'real' condition and measured value prior to the intervention phase, or what the patients actually represent now. Important indicators here are 'severity of symptoms/pain' (VAS) and quality of life (FLZ). Experience to date shows that baseline values for complaints and pain with phasic or periodic courses (e.g. migraine or episodic diseases of various origins) do not simply correspond to a theoretical averaging algorithm; rather, the information provided by patients is more oriented towards previous extreme pain situations. By contrast, patients with continuous, i.e. chronic, back pain predominantly report average values for pain and symptom severity experienced daily in the inpatient admission questionnaire. These differing findings suggest that it is necessary to offer a diagnosis-dependent representation of symptom severity in individual cases. The quality of life was found to be higher in the 'pre-value' at admission than in the admission value. This was due to positive expectations, which were slightly more common than negative ones. When comparing the two values, it was also found that the values were more stable and less dependent on diagnosis. Therefore, it is unlikely that the level of symptoms is unrealistically high or that an overestimation of the therapeutic effect will be observed.

Selection Effects of the Follow-Up Survey

Data loss or non-response to follow-up questionnaires suggests the presence of selection effects. In the case of patients without follow-up, who are rated as having experienced less therapeutic success on average at discharge, it can be assumed that these patients benefited less on average from inpatient treatment, and that the average clinical course was assessed somewhat too favourably based on the available or reported data.

It is therefore essential to establish how data loss is to be handled. Based on our experience, response rates of at least 70% can be achieved in routine clinical practice. This response rate should always be the minimum requirement. In addition, to estimate the 'true' result value, the 'last value carried forward' or 'baseline value carried forward' method should be used for the entire surveyed group in the event of data loss.

Another issue is determining follow-up times adequately. This makes it hard to know how to measure the success of naturopathic/complementary medicine. This is because these procedures require a lot of interaction, i.e. they are usually labour-intensive and often effective in the long term but are therefore also costly. Lastly, many inpatient (and sometimes outpatient) treatments are quite intense because they use a variety of different methods. The initial costs of these treatments can only be offset by long-term improvements in patients' health, lifestyle changes and a significant reduction in patients' use of medical services.

However, the results of medium- to long-term follow-ups cannot be clearly linked to the treatment that was evaluated, especially for patients who are in hospital. This is because the results of the treatment after the intervention are 'distorted' by other treatments given to patients during this time, at least when things are done as normal.

PEP Is an Example of 'Confidence-Based Medicine' (CBM)

To date, few systematic, critical, or comparative evaluations of routine care using naturopathic treatments and special therapeutic approaches have been conducted. Alongside the increased use of traditional clinical studies to improve the methodological evidence base ('evidence-based medicine') of individual complementary healing methods, greater consideration should be given to everyday, user-oriented documentation and evaluation of healthcare research. This involves recording the 'gross effects' of interventions and application concepts of individual medical service providers, based on the benefits of diagnostic and therapeutic applications as perceived by clients or patients themselves. In democratic liberal societies, citizens primarily determine which medical services they wish to use and from which provider (keyword: free choice of doctor). This requires data-supported decision-making aids. In cases of long-term chronic illness especially, the focus shifts from individual diseases to the sick person as a whole. This often highlights the limitations of decisions based exclusively on evidence-based medicine (EBM), which typically focus on specific diagnoses and procedures.

Using systematically collected healthcare data professionally could increase confidence in the quality of care provided by individual providers and complex therapy concepts and help improve targeted utilisation. Other groups of authors also refer to the supplementation of randomised study evidence with observational studies within the reality of care as 'real-world evidence' (RWE) [5, 17]. This methodological approach is currently primarily used in the pharmaceutical industry, but it is also well-suited to the entire field of routine medical care. In my opinion, this is called 'outcome research' all over the world. Of course, reliable and robust recommendations for specific therapeutic measures are usually only possible in combination with RWE and controlled randomised studies. But what if there is no evidence on which to base a clinical decision? In that case, RWE data can still provide a wealth of information on safety and tolerability, specific patient groups, and responder/non-responder analyses. So-called "quasi-experimental designs" are also used when classic experimental design is not feasible or ethical [18]. Further important developments in the RWE approach are also expected in the future with mobile e-health technologies and artificial intelligence. Increased availability of real-world data is leading to observational studies being used by regulators worldwide [19].

In short, the implementation of patient-centred quality assessments provides important information for doctors, patients, health insurance companies, and politicians to make decisions about utilisation, care management, product safety, and control. In line with the motto 'trust through quality', this can also be referred to as 'confidence-based medicine' (CBM). The present programme for the evaluation of patient care (PEP) encompasses both basic concepts and combines them. Such quality assessments can also create realistic and comprehensible quality standards in the provision of complementary medicine, supporting continuous quality improvement. The continuous integration of quality management and research into medical practice is described in more detail elsewhere [13–15, 20].

Moreover, the quality of reporting and interpretation of data from observational studies can be significantly improved by existing guidelines such as STROBE (Strengthening the Reporting of Observational Studies in Epidemiology) and RECORD (Reporting of Studies Conducted Using Observational Routinely Collected Health Data) [21, 22]. Further optimisation of statements regarding possible causal relationships in observational studies should be made by imitating randomised study designs. Current considerations on this topic are provided by the guideline entitled TARGET (The Transparent Reporting of Observational Studies Emulating a Target Trial) [23, 24].

Figure 1.4 illustrates the integration of quality management and real-world data research

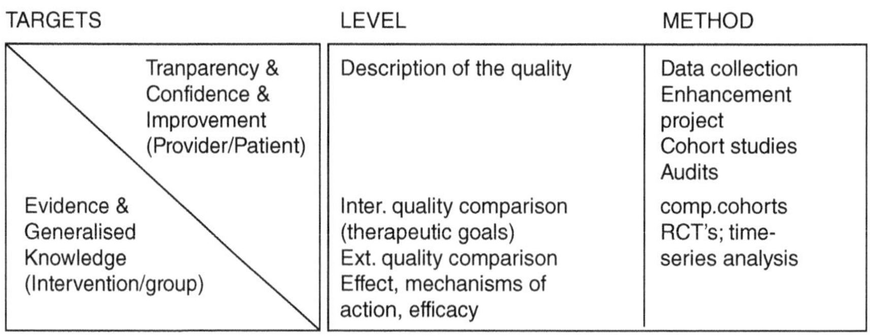

Fig. 1.4 Ongoing integration of quality management and real-world data research into medical practice—confidence vs. evidence-based medicine

1.2 The Development of PEP and the Creation of a Reference Database

The TCM-Klinik Bad Kötzting has been the subject of scientific monitoring since its inception in 1991. The clinic has been producing regular clinic reports since 1992. From 1991 to 1995, paper-based documentation was carried out, and a summary clinic report was produced. In the period between 1992 and 2000, a total of 2868 patients out of 5132 patients treated at the clinic were documented. From 1992 to 1997, comprehensive surveys were conducted, whereby all patients were documented over the course of an entire year. Due to the stable and easily comparable data from the various survey years, only partial surveys, i.e. quarterly surveys at different times of the quarter, were conducted from 1998 to 2000.

In 2001, the electronic and PC-based Medical Monitoring (MM) system of the CoCoNat at the Technical University of Munich (TUM) was tested and used for data collection and quality assurance at the clinic. The routine documentation encompassed various domains, including the patient's medical history, an evaluation of their current state, the identification of any pertinent diagnoses, and the classification of these diagnoses according to the International Classification of Diseases, Tenth Revision (ICD-10). The structure of the medical history and physical examination corresponded to a basic internal medicine survey with occasional naturopathic dimensions. Subsequently, TCM-specific documentation for acupuncture and Chinese herbal medicine therapy was developed, tested, and implemented in the software. It was determined that the software was not suitable for routine documentation due to a number of issues with its application and the export of data from the database. Consequently, a web-based documentation system known as 'E-Quality Profiling' was developed concurrently with MM from 2004 onwards, with financial support provided by the Acupuncture Model Project and the Erich Rothenfußer Foundation.

The web portal www.E-Qualityprofiling.org, subtitled EQP-ECR (Electronic Clinical Research), was conceived with the intention of providing support for all research activities in the areas of quality research and clinical trial implementation in general, and the focus areas of TCM in particular.

The documentation systems for acupuncture, TCM medication, and TCM diagnosis (pulse, tongue, diagnosis) were further developed and adapted to the quality assurance requirements of the SGBV. The EQP portal was subsequently developed into the TCM health portal, which was first used routinely in April 2008 and continues to provide scientific documentation to this day.

Subsequent to the initial 10-year documentation period, a series of comparative studies were conducted with other clinics. For instance, patients suffering from chronic headaches were consecutively recorded from spring 2001 to autumn 2002, provided that the relevant inclusion and exclusion criteria were met. This was also carried out concurrently at two other comparative clinics in the field of complementary medicine. The results of this inpatient quality comparison, in the form of a comparative series case study, were published [12]. Furthermore, diagnosis-independent comparisons of quality profiles with other inpatient facilities for complementary medicine and naturopathy were carried out and published. Subsequent controlled randomised studies were either conducted directly on site in a monocentric setting or in which the TCM-Klinik Bad Kötzting served as a trial centre in a multicentre study. One of the studies under discussion was conducted on behalf of the Federal Ministry of Education, Science, Research and Technology (BMBF), with the funding code [01KT9408/7]. The randomised clinical study was conducted to ascertain the efficacy of traditional Chinese acupuncture in comparison to subcutaneously administered sumatriptan (5-HT1 receptor agonist) and placebo drug therapy as early treatment (attack relief) for patients in the initial stage of an acute migraine attack [25].

The observation periods from 2001 to 2004 were documented in a summary clinical report and made available to the cooperation partners.

The follow-up periods, initially set at 12 months, were subsequently reduced to 6 months. The follow-up rates, defined as the proportion of patients who responded to a follow-up survey, exhibited a range between 70% and 80%. No clinic data was collected in 2003. From 2004 to 2007, the decision was taken to conduct additional quarterly surveys in lieu of the conventional annual documentation. This approach was adopted to optimise the allocation of time and human resources of employees to support a range of scientific research initiatives and dissertations. During this period, several other activities were undertaken. These included the development of new health-oriented indicators and the technical optimisation of the web-based documentation system. Since 2008, the practice of conducting comprehensive surveys of clinic data has seen a marked increase. The following tables and figures offer a comprehensive overview of all observation periods. The collated data also functions as a reference database for the presentation and comparison with the newly obtained annual data.

For reasons of clarity, only complete data from the patient questionnaires are used for the evaluation of the reference data in the results profile. Depending on the questions asked, only complete data at the time of admission and discharge or at all three survey times (admission—A, discharge—D and follow-up—F) were included in the analyses for the calculation of reference values. This procedure leads to a significant reduction in the total number of documented patients presented here.

Table 1.3 and Fig. 1.5 provide a summary of the documentation periods at the TCM-Klinik Bad Kötzting from 1992 to 2023. The table shows how many months were documented in each reporting year. The number of patients recorded is also shown. The number of questionnaires answered for quality assurance is important for evaluating the reference values. Only complete historical data from quality assurance questionnaires were available for evaluating reference data from April 2008 to December 2023. The 'ICD-10 Symptom Rating' questionnaire could only be included in the calculation of reference data from December 2014 onwards.

Table 1.3 A compilation of all documentation periods from 1992 to 2023 at the TCM-Klinik Bad Kötzting

Year	1992/93	1994	1995	1996	1997	1998	1999	2000	2001	2002	2003	2004	2005	2006	2007	2008	2009	2010	2011	2012	2013	2014	2015	2016	2017	2018	2019	2020	2021	2022	2023	Total
No. of months	19	10	8	12	12	4	3	3	11	3		16	12	12	12	9	12	12	12	12	12	12	12	12	12	12	12	9*	12	12	12	
No. of patients	1596	840	667	1036	1030	334	252	234	1007	975	1069	1117	904	809	1086	814	739	866	853	882	944	977	1030	1059	1035	1026	980	619	729	730	825	**27,065**
No. doc. patients	1553	825	640	1026	1022	330	250	234	102	205	*	345	125	160	113	797	692	848	839	882	938	977	943	1007	1010	1003	959	605	725	725	821	**20,701**
F/U 2 mon.(%)	86	87	87	85	84	-	-	-	94	-	-	-	-	-	-	-	-	-	-	-	-	-	-	-	-	-	-	-	-	-	-	
F/U 6 mon. (%)	81	76	75	78	76	80	82	84	84	69	-	73	73	71	-	73	77	78	74	67	65	-	75	83	81	82	82	79	78	69	75	
Survey period Reference data																	Quality assurance questionnaires (incl. complaint strength): April 2008 to December 2023 (only complete historical data A-D-F)															**9189**
																							ICD-10 Symptom Rating (ISR): December 2014 to December 2023 (only complete historical data A-D-F)									**6284**
F/U 12 mon.(%)	72	70	69	75	71	71	74	80	-	-	-	-	-	-	-	-	-	-	-	-	-	-	-	-	-	-	-	-	-		-	

No. of patients: the number of patients with basic documentation (n = 27,065). No. doc. Patients: the number of documented patients with available quality assurance questionnaires. F/U.: patient follow-up survey after hospital discharge. *2003/4: unsystematic documentation. *Mon.* months, *No.* number, *F/U* follow-up

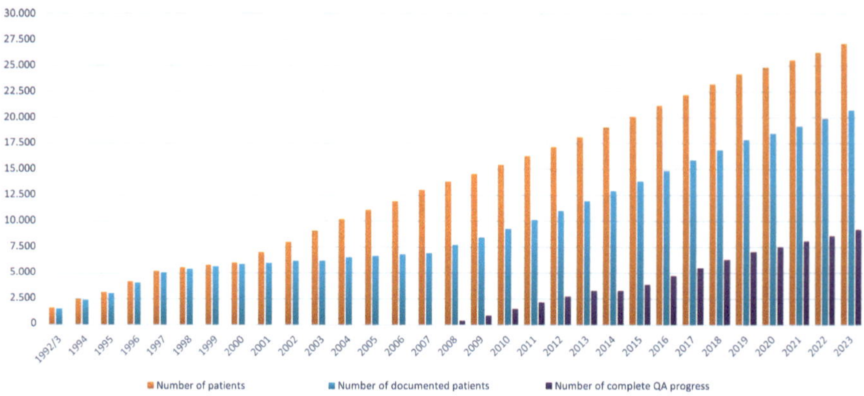

Fig. 1.5 The graphical overview of the additively summarised documented patients of the TCM-Klinik Bad Kötzting from 1992 to 2023. Light blue columns: data history based on the presence of discomfort (VAS). Violet columns show patients with a complete dataset (admission, discharge, follow-up) for the quality assurance questionnaire

1.3 Data Quality and Statistical Analysis

The flow chart 2023 shows the number of inquiries, admissions, and all available or complete data sets at all measurement points (Fig. 1.6).

Total inquiries were 1666 people. Of these, 455 patients (27.3%) were rejected by doctors as part of the hospital's internal admission procedure. A further 386 (31.9%) interested patients were lost due to refusal of payment by health insurance companies or at the applicants' own request. Ultimately, 825 patients were admitted to the clinic in 2023.

Complete data sets are available for 821 vs. 774 vs. 618 patients (99.5% vs. 93.8% vs. 74.9%) at admission, discharge, and follow-up. As the available data varies depending on the measurement, the number for the complete data set here is based on the availability of the main complaint severity (VAS) across the time points for each patient.

1.3.1 Valid and Missing Data

Table 1.4 shows all indicators recorded for the PEP, completeness, and missing data. It also displays the number of patients in the reference group.

To obtain data sets that are as complete as possible, particularly for the surveys conducted as part of quality assurance, the follow-up survey after approx. 6 months is subject to a standardised procedure, which proceeds as follows:

- 6 months after discharge, every person previously admitted to hospital receives a standardised letter asking them to complete the follow-up questionnaire for quality assurance, the ICD-10 symptom rating (ISR), and (since 2022) the protective and risk factors.

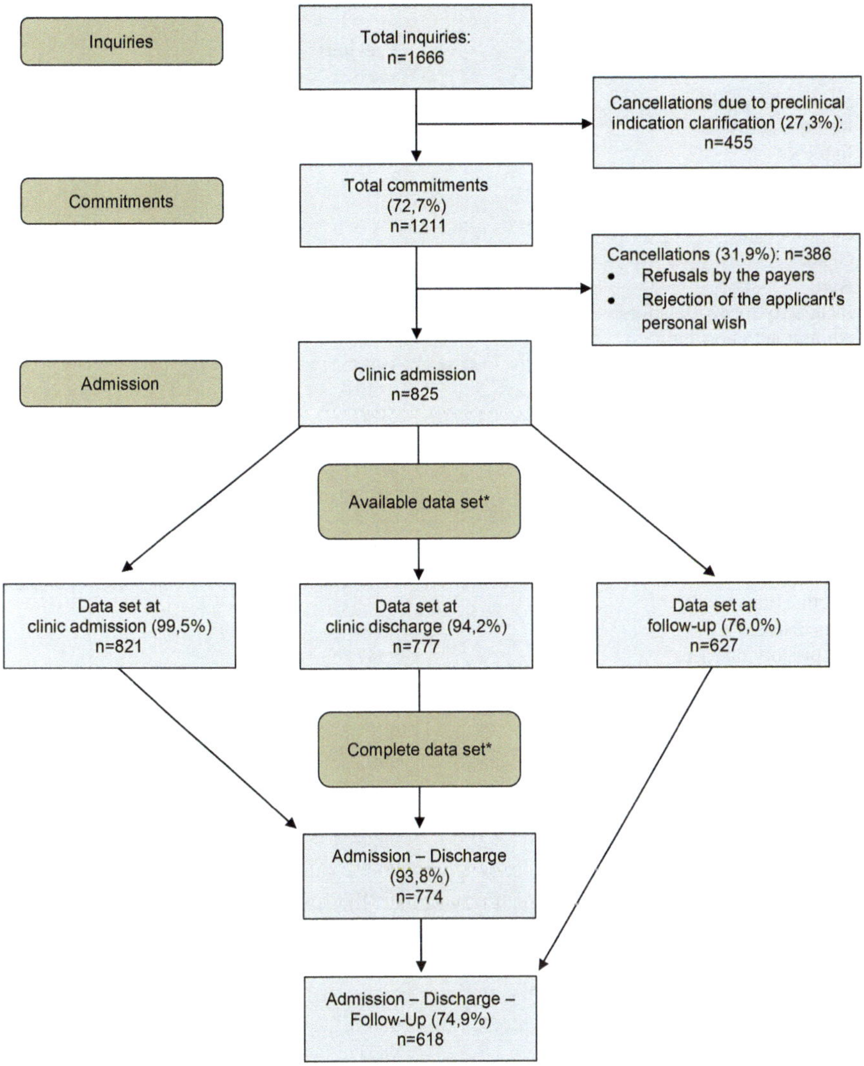

Fig. 1.6 Flow chart 2023. * The number of available or complete data sets is based on the information on the main complaint severity. Since not all patients consistently answer all questions, the available data sets per questionnaire or item may vary

Table 1.4 Valid and missing data

Structural profile	**2023 Valid**	**Missing**	**Previous years Valid**	**Remark**
Referrer statistics	839	–	–	Multiple answers possible for cost bearers due to repeated hospital stays and supplementary insurances
Inquiries	1666	–	–	
Cost unit	833	–	–	
Admission month	825	0	–	
Length of stay	825	0	–	
Gender	825	0	–	
Age	825	0	–	
Incapacity for work before admission to hospital	821	4	–	
General health	Valid	Missing	Valid	Remark
Back problems	823	2	9849	Survey period of previous year's data from Jan 2009 to Dec 2022
Joint/muscle diseases	823	2	9840	
Allergies/intolerances	823	2	9848	
Nervous/mood disorders	823	2	9840	
Gastrointestinal diseases	823	2	9965	
Thyroid disease	823	2	9855	
High blood pressure	823	2	10,006	
Vascular diseases (e.g. calcification)	823	2	9983	
Skin diseases	823	2	9826	
Respiratory diseases	823	2	9947	
Eye diseases	823	2	9828	
Liver/bile duct disease	823	2	9954	
Dental diseases	823	2	9827	
Cardiac arrhythmia	823	2	9967	
Bone diseases	823	2	9819	
Kidney/sexual diseases	823	2	9849	
Severe oral/ENT diseases	823	2	9828	
Childhood/infectious disease	823	2	9809	
Cancer	823	2	9846	
Lipometabolic disease	823	2	9829	
Anemia/other bleeding disorders.	823	2	9823	
Other metabolic diseases	823	2	9816	
Diabetes	823	2	9963	
Other cardiovascular diseases	823	2	9831	
Stroke, cerebral haemorrhage	823	2	9967	
Addiction	823	2	9830	
Illnesses in the family	823	2	9804	

(continued)

Table 1.4 (continued)

Diagnoses	Valid	Missing	Valid	Remark
ICD diagnoses	825	0	10,227	Data collection period of the previous year from April 2008 to Dec 2022
Primary and secondary diagnoses at discharge	825	0	10,227	
Frequency of psychological comorbidities	825	–	9207	
Frequency of somatic comorbidities	825	–	9658	
Main mental health diagnoses on discharge	825	0	8954	
Psychological secondary diagnoses on discharge	703	–	–	
Somatic secondary diagnoses on discharge	823	–	–	
TCM syndrome diagnoses	804	21	–	
Motivation	Valid	Missing	Valid	
Pay more attention to health	822	3	–	
Changing behaviour in everyday life	822	3	–	
Use the health portal	822	3	–	
Possession of a PC with Internet access	822	3	–	
Risk factors	**2023**		**Previous years**	
Tedium–Measure (Burnout)	Valid	Missing	Valid	Remark
Total value	823	2	11,519	Survey period of previous year's data from Jan 2009 to Dec 2022
Loss of motivation	823	2	11,520	
Exhaustion	823	2	11,521	
Discouragement	823	2	11,520	
Perceived Stress Questionnaire	Valid	Missing	Valid	Remark
Total score	822	3	6150	Data collection period of the previous year from Jan 2013 to Dec 2022
Worries	822	3	6150	
Requirements	822	3	6150	
Joy	822	3	6150	
Tension	822	3	6150	
Three-level stress test	Valid	Missing	Valid	Remark
Cognitive-emotional level	821	4	12,189	Data collection period of the previous year from April 2008 to Dec 2022
Vegetative level	821	4	12,189	
Motor level	821	4	12,189	
Stressors and burdens	Valid	Missing	Valid	Remark
Total value	822	3	12,376	Data collection period of the previous year from April 2008 to Dec 2022
Professional	822	3	12,376	
At home / in everyday life	822	3	12,376	
Financial	822	3	12,376	
Life events	822	3	12,376	

(continued)

Table 1.4 (continued)

Psycho-vegetative stability test	Valid	Missing	Valid	Remark
Psycho-vegetative individual complaints	823	2	13,266	Data collection period of the previous year from April 2008 to Dec 2022
Psycho-vegetative stability Total value	823	2	12,615	
Psycho-vegetative stability Complaint index	823	2	12,610	
General Anxiety Disorder	815	10	406	The GAD has only been in use since May 2022
Medical history (anamnesis and risk screening)	**Valid**	**Missing**	**Valid**	**Remark**
Functional questionnaire Hanover (FFbH-R)	447	–	–	FFbH-R evaluation only for back pain diagnosis
Pain Disability Index (PDI)	816	9	8900	Previous year's data from Jan 2012 to Dec 2022
CAGE test on alcohol consumption behaviour	7	–	41	
Diabetes/high blood pressure risk	817	8	8900	Previous year's data from Jan 2012 to Dec 2022
Smoking questionnaire	84	-	1538	Only activated if a patient agrees to the question 'Are you a smoker?'
Metabolic Syndrome Index	747	78	8652	Previous year's data from Jan 2009 to Dec 2022
Fatty liver	801	24	3825	Previous year's data from Jan 2018 to Dec 2022
Cardiovascular risk (ESC score)	719	6	471	The ESC has been collected since mid-2022
Risk of high blood pressure	Valid	Missing	Valid	Remark
1 year high blood pressure risk	608	8	8857	Already ill, therefore excluded: $n = 209$
2 year high blood pressure risk	608	8	8857	
4 year high blood pressure risk	608	8	8857	
Diabetes risk	Valid	Missing	Valid	Remark
Findrisk point value	775	9	8858	Already ill, therefore excluded: $n = 41$
Findrisk percentage value	775	9	8860	
Protective factors	**2023**		**Previous years**	
Life Satisfaction Questionnaire (FLZ)	valid	missing	valid	Remark
Total value	824	1	12,570	Data collection period of the previous year from April 2008 to Dec 2022
Friends/acquaintances	824	1	12,570	
Leisure/hobbies	824	1	12,570	
Health	824	1	12,570	
Income	824	1	12,570	
Profession	824	1	12,570	
Housing situation	824	1	12,570	
Family/Children	824	1	12,570	
Partnership	824	1	12,570	

(continued)

Table 1.4 (continued)

Sense of coherence (SOC)	Valid	Missing	Valid	Remark
Total value	820	5	12,482	Data collection period of the previous year from April 2008 to Dec 2022
Significance	820	5	12,482	
Understandability	820	5	12,482	
Manageability	820	5	12,482	
Well-being WHO-5	822	3	12,249	Data collection period of the previous year from April 2008 to Dec 2022
Vitality SF-36	822	3	12,248	
SWOP optimism	821	4	12,241	
SWOP self-efficacy	821	4	12,241	New survey algorithms for physical activity index since 2023 & nutrition index since 2022
SSS Social competence	799	26	12,424	
Movement index	814	11	–	
Nutrition index	821	4	718	
Psycho-vegetative stability test	Valid	Missing	Valid	Remark
Sleep	823	2	12,610	Data collection period of the previous year from April 2008 to Dec 2022
Dizziness	823	2	12,610	
Heat balance	823	2	12,610	
Perceived Sleep Quality (PSQI)	Valid	Missing	Valid	Remark
Sleep quality	814	11	722	The PSQI has been collected since mid-2021
Sleep latency	814	11	722	
Sleep duration	814	11	722	
Sleep efficiency	814	11	722	
Sleep disorders	814	11	722	
Sleeping pills	814	11	722	
Daytime sleepiness	814	11	722	
Intervention profile	**2023**		**Previous years**	
	Valid	**Missing**	**Valid**	**Remark**
TCM drug therapy	823	2	11,087	Previous years: Feb 2008 to March 2022
TCM acupuncture	819	6	6148	Jan 2015 to March 2022
Range of services and utilisation	133,916		–	Pure frequency listing without allocation to patients
Result profile	**2023**		**Previous years**	
QA questionnaire on admission	Valid	Missing	Valid	Remark
Main complaint	821	4	11,862	Data collection period of the previous year from April 2008 to Dec 2022
Psychotherapy	821	4	11,865	
Illness	820	5	11,863	

(continued)

Table 1.4 (continued)

QA questionnaire on discharge	Valid	Missing	Valid	Remark
Change in health status A–D	774	51	11,145	Data collection period of the previous year from April 2008 to Dec 2022; only complete historical data (A–E) *The question about AE was answered with "yes" by 414 of the 825 patients; specific NW were reported by 414 patients. specified
Change in complaint	777	48	11,218	
Benefits of the forms of therapy	777	48	10,783	
Change Influenceability of the Complaint history	774	51	11,151	
Treatment result	777	48	11,211	
ZSH overall success and side effects	774	51	11,215	
Side effects/adverse events (AE)	774	51	–	
QA questionnaire for follow-up	Valid	Missing	Valid	Remark
Change in health status A-F	625	200	7898	Data collection period of the previous year from April 2008 to Dec 2022
Change in complaint	625	200	7961	
Benefits of the forms of therapy	625	200	7527	
Change Influenceability of the Complaint history	623	202	7891	
Treatment result	623	202	7934	
Visits to the doctor	624	201	6926	
Hospitalisation	624	201	6926	
Current in Psychotherapy	624	201	6926	
Incapacity for work and disability of Daily activities before admission to hospital	821	4	725	
Incapacity to work/ impairment of everyday life activity after discharge from hospital (follow-up)	623	202	465	
Taking medication	625	200	7243	
QS complaint severity: Main complaint	Valid	Missing	Valid	Remark
Main weight strength A	821	4	11,862	Data collection period of the previous year from April 2008 to Dec 2022
Main weight strength D	777	48	11,216	
Main weight F	627	198	8934	
Expected discharge value at A	821	4	11,864	
Main weight strength A–D	777	48	11,155	
Main weight strength A–F	627	198	8815	
Main weight strength A–D–F	618	207	8571	
Expected discharge value A—actual discharge value Discharge value E	777	48	11,155	

(continued)

Table 1.4 (continued)

QS complaint strength: second complaint	Valid	Missing	Valid	Remark
Second complaint severity A	821	4	11,155	Data collection period of the previous year from April 2008 to Dec 2022
Second severity of complaint D	767	58	10,557	
Second complaint severity F	610	215	7288	
Expected discharge value at A	821	4	11,383	
Second complaint severity A–D	767	58	10,260	
Second complaint severity A–F	610	215	7079	
Second complaint severity A–D–F	595	230	6667	
Expected discharge value A—actual discharge value D	767	58	10,259	
ICD-10 symptom rating ISR	Valid	Missing	Valid	Remark
ISR all dimensions A	824	1	11,032	Data collection period of the previous year from Dec 2014 to Dec 2022; only complete historical data
ISR all dimensions D	778	47	–	
ISR all dimensions F	608	217	–	
ISR all dimensions A–D	778	47	5681	
ISR all dimensions A–F	608	217	–	
ISR all dimensions A–D–F	603	222	5681	
ISR suicidality (single item) A	824	1	11,036	
ISR load levels A–D–F	603	217	5681	
Routine laboratory and liver value screening	**2023**		**Previous years**	
Routine laboratory	Valid	Missing	Valid	Remark
Cholesterol A–D	779	46	11,219	Data collection period of the previous year from April 2008 to Dec 2022; only complete historical data
LDL A–D	780	45	11,219	
HDL A–D	780	45	11,219	
Chol/HDL A–D	779	46	11,219	
LDL/HDL A–D	780	45	11,219	
Triglycerides A–D	780	45	11,219	
Glucose i.S. A–D	780	45	11,219	
Sodium A–D	782	43	8856	
Calcium A–D	782	43	8856	
Iron A–D	782	43	8856	
Potassium A–D	782	43	8856	
Uric acid A–D	781	44	8864	
Creatinine A–D	781	44	8864	
Erythrocytes A–D	779	46	8766	
Leucocytes A–D	779	46	8766	
Platelets A–D	779	46	8766	
Haematocrit A–D	779	46	8766	
Haemoglobin A–D	779	46	8766	
HbE (MCH) A–D	779	46	8766	
MCHC A–D	779	46	8766	
MCV A–D	779	46	8766	
GOT A–D	786	39	11,380	
ALT A–D	787	38	11,383	
Gamma-GT A–D	788	37	11,384	
AP A–D	783	42	4687	

(continued)

Table 1.4 (continued)

Liver value screening	Valid	Missing	Valid	Remark
ALT on admission—in the further course	792	33	11,383	Data collection period of the previous year from April 2008 to Dec 2022
AP on admission—in the further course	739	86	4687	
Vital screening	Valid	Missing	Valid	Remark
Pulse A–D	795	35	11,312	Data collection period of the previous year from April 2008 to Dec 2022; only complete historical data
RR systolic A–D	795	35	11,499	
RR diastolic A–D	795	35	11,499	
Weight A–D	801	29	11,532	
Weight (BMI >25) A–D	393	–	5770	
BMI A–D	798	32	11,364	
Abdominal circumference A–D	790	40	11,452	

- 2 weeks after this letter, a 1st reminder (by post/email) will be sent to those patients who have not yet completed the questionnaires.
- 4 weeks after the standard letter, a second reminder is sent to those patients who have still not completed the questionnaires. The 2nd reminder is usually sent by post and contains the questionnaires to be completed in paper form.

This procedure is documented as part of follow-up survey statistics, so that the number of reminder letters sent in each month, including the resulting participation in the follow-up survey, can be clearly shown in Table 1.5.

1.3.2 Statistical Procedures

The statistical analysis was performed using R-Studio version 2023.12.0, a statistical programming language. The following descriptive statistics were calculated: frequency count and distribution; mean (mw); median; minimum and maximum values; lower and upper confidence intervals (CIs); range; and standard deviation (SD). The significance or tendency of the change in mean values between measurement points was tested using a paired samples t-test. Since the t-test is relatively robust for large samples ($n > 30$), it was also used for non-parametrically distributed data [26–29]. In addition, depending on the question (e.g. the predictive significance of disease-related and sociodemographic variables), chi-square tests were used to examine possible influencing factors and group differences.

To calculate the treatment effects for mean differences at various inpatient admission, discharge, and follow-up points in time, the effect size d was calculated according to Cohen (values of 0.2, 0.5, and 0.8 indicate small, moderate, and large effects, respectively). Effect sizes are independent of the measuring instrument used and the sample size, which is why they are well-suited to comparing results from different studies. Figures and tables were introduced for greater clarity.

Table 1.5 Follow-up survey statistics as part of the Patient Evaluation Program (PEP) in 2023

Month of discharge	Standard cover letter (post/e-mail)	Filled out after 1st reminder		filled out on paper after 2nd reminder/ after dispatch of the Qnr	Filled out in %	Number of sheets—F/U
		Paper	Online			
January 23[a]	34 (4/30)	2	15	5	65%	22
February	72 (6/66)	5	41	14	83%	60
March	84 (8/76)	6	34	17	68%	57
April	68 (2/66)	2	34	18	79%	54
May	64 (8/56)	6	29	10	70%	45
June	73 (8/65)	7	44	9	82%	60
July	63 (12/51)	8	30	10	76%	48
August	71 (5/66)	4	36	15	77%	55
September	66 (3/63)	3	30	17	76%	50
October	63 (7/56)	7	30	8	71%	45
November	52 (2/50)	1	27	8	69%	36
December	67 (3/64)	3	30	12	67%	45
January 24	52 (7/45)	5	29	9	83%	43
Total	795 (71/724)	57	394	146	**75%**	**597**
	795	597				

[a]Not included in the calculations, as most of the patients discharged in January 2023 were already admitted in December of the previous year (2022) and are therefore attributable to the 2022 reporting year

References

1. Berger A. Why doesn't audit work? BMJ. 1998;316(7135):875–6. https://doi.org/10.1136/bmj.316.7135.875. PMID: 9552829; PMCID: PMC1112807.
2. Black N. Why we need observational studies to evaluate the effectiveness of health care. BMJ. 1996;312(7040):1215–8. https://doi.org/10.1136/bmj.312.7040.1215. PMID: 8634569; PMCID: PMC2350940.
3. Greenfield S, Kaplan SH, Silliman RA, Sullivan L, Manning W, D'Agostino R, Singer DE, Nathan DM. The uses of outcomes research for medical effectiveness, quality of care, and reimbursement in type II diabetes. Diabetes Care. 1994;17(Suppl 1):32–9. PMID: 8088221.
4. Long AF. Key issues in outcomes measurement. Int J STD AIDS. 1997;8(11):663–7. https://doi.org/10.1258/0956462971919020. PMID: 9363539.
5. Kaufmann NC, Pereira PL. Real-world evidence: better than nothing or the future? A perspective on clinical evidence generation in interventional oncology. Cardiovasc Intervent Radiol. 2025; https://doi.org/10.1007/s00270-025-04179-4. Epub ahead of print. PMID: 40999075.
6. Melchart D, Eustachi A, Gronwald S, Wühr E, Wifling K, Bachmeier BE. Introduction of a web portal for an Individual Health Management and observational health data sciences. Patient Relat Outcome Meas. 2018;9:183–96. https://doi.org/10.2147/PROM.S157410. PMID: 29950912; PMCID: PMC6016587.
7. Melchart D, Eustachi A, Wellenhofer-Li Y, Doerfler W, Bohnes E. Individual health management—a comprehensive lifestyle counselling programme for health promotion, disease prevention and patient education. Forsch Komplementmed. 2016;23:30–5.
8. Melchart D, Bachmeier BE. The comprehensive lifestyle intervention program "Individual Health Management" (IHM)—an exemplar for complementary medicine. J Transl Sci. 2018;4(3):1–3. https://doi.org/10.15761/JTS.1000221.

9. Bachmeier BE, Wühr E, Wifling K, Melchart D. Participant satisfaction with a comprehensive lifestyle counselling Program for health promotion, disease prevention and patient education. Health Edu Care. 2019;4:1–8. https://doi.org/10.15761/HEC.1000153.
10. Melchart D. Kontinuierliche Integration von Qualitätsmanagement in die ärztliche Praxis. In: Melchart, Brenke, Dobos, Gaisbauer, Saller, editors. Naturheilverfahren Leitfaden für die ärztliche Aus-, Fort- und Weiterbildung. Schattauer Verlag; 2002. p. 616–31.
11. Melchart D, Wessel A, Wunderlich S. Qualitätsprofil einer Rehabilitationsfachklinik für Naturheilverfahren—Teil 1: Struktur, Qualitätssicherung und Interventionen [Quality profile of a CAM rehabilitation clinic--Part 1: Structure, quality assurance and interventions]. Forsch Komplementmed. 2007;14(5):281–8. https://doi.org/10.1159/000107698. German. Epub 2007 Oct 25. PMID: 17971669.
12. Melchart D, Wessel A, Brand R, Hager S, Weidenhammer W. Profiling quality of care for patients with chronic headache in three different German hospitals—a case study. BMC Health Serv Res. 2008;16(8):13. https://doi.org/10.1186/1472-6963-8-13. PMID: 18199321; PMCID: PMC2262884.
13. Melchart D, Staudinger A, editors. TCM-Klinik Bad Kötzting 20 Jahre wissenschaftliche Evaluation der Traditionellen Chinesischen Medizin und Klinikbericht 2011. Bad Kötzting: Verlag systemische Medizin; 2011.
14. Weidenhammer W, Melchart D. Quality profiling at the TCM hospital bad Kötzting—examples from an ongoing systematic patient documentation. Forsch Komplementmed. 2016;23(Suppl 2):8–15. https://doi.org/10.1159/000445009. Epub 2016 May 30. PMID: 27272539.
15. Melchart D, Dai J. Chinesisch-Deutsches Zentrum für Traditionelle Chinesische Medizin (Bad Kötzting) Klinikbericht 2017/8. China Press of Traditional Chinese Medicine, Beijing. 1. Auflage; 2020. ISBN 978-7-5132-6130-2.
16. Melchart D, Dai J, Staudinger A. Evaluation der Patientenversorgung in der Chinesischen Medizin. Verlag systemische Medizin, Bad Kötzting. 1. Auflage; 2021. ISBN 978-3-86401-037-8.
17. Khosla S, White R, Medina J, Ouwens M, Emmas C, Koder T, Male G, Leonard S. Real world evidence (RWE)—a disruptive innovation or the quiet evolution of medical evidence generation? F1000Research. 2018;25(7):111. https://doi.org/10.12688/f1000research.13585.2. PMID: 30026923; PMCID: PMC6039945.
18. Capili B, Anastasi JK. An introduction to types of quasi-experimental designs. Am J Nurs. 2024;124(11):50–2. https://doi.org/10.1097/01.NAJ.0001081740.74815.20. Epub 2024 Oct 24. PMID: 39446515; PMCID: PMC11741180.
19. Blacketer C, Schuemie MJ, Moinat M, Voss EA, Camprubi M, Rijnbeek PR, Ryan PB. Advancing real-world evidence through a Federated Health Data Network (EHDEN): descriptive study. J Med Internet Res. 2025;27:e74119. https://doi.org/10.2196/74119. PMID: 40774333; PMCID: PMC12331365.
20. Haug C. Confidence-based medicine. Tidsskr Nor Laegeforen. 2011;131(23):2329. https://doi.org/10.4045/tidsskr.11.23E1. English, Norwegian. PMID: 22139095.
21. von Elm E, Altman DG, Egger M, Pocock SJ, Gøtzsche PC, Vandenbroucke JP, STROBE Initiative. Strengthening the Reporting of Observational Studies in Epidemiology (STROBE) statement: guidelines for reporting observational studies. BMJ. 2007;335:806–8. https://doi.org/10.1136/bmj.39335.541782.AD.
22. Benchimol EI, Smeeth L, Guttmann A, RECORD Working Committee, et al. The REporting of studies Conducted using Observational Routinely-collected health Data (RECORD) statement. PLoS Med. 2015;12:e1001885. https://doi.org/10.1371/journal.pmed.1001885.
23. Cashin AG, Hansford HJ, Hernán MA, Swanson SA, Lee H, Jones MD, Dahabreh IJ, Dickerman BA, Egger M, Garcia-Albeniz X, Golub RM, Islam N, Lodi S, Moreno-Betancur M, Pearson SA, Schneeweiss S, Sharp MK, Sterne JAC, Stuart EA, McAuley JH. Transparent reporting of observational studies emulating a target trial: the TARGET Statement. BMJ. 2025;3(390):e087179. https://doi.org/10.1136/bmj-2025-087179. PMID: 40903028.
24. Hansford HJ, Cashin AG, Jones MD, Swanson SA, Islam N, Douglas SRG, et al. Reporting of observational studies explicitly aiming to emulate randomized trials: a systematic review. JAMA

Netw Open. 2023;6(9):e2336023. https://doi.org/10.1001/jamanetworkopen.2023.36023. PMID:37755828.
25. Melchart D, Thormaehlen J, Hager S, Liao J, Linde K, Weidenhammer W. Acupuncture versus placebo versus sumatriptan for early treatment of migraine attacks: a randomized controlled trial. J Intern Med. 2003;253(2):181–8. https://doi.org/10.1046/j.1365-2796.2003.01081.x. PMID: 12542558.
26. Pagano RR. Understanding statistics in the behavioural sciences. 9th ed. Belmont: Thomson Wadsworth; 2010.
27. Rasch D, Guiard V. The robustness of parametric statistical methods. Psychol Sci. 2004;46:175–208.
28. Stone ER. t test, paired samples. In: Salkind NJ, editor. Encyclopedia of research design. Los Angeles: SAGE; 2010. p. 1560–5.
29. Wilcox RR. Introduction to robust estimation and hypothesis testing. In: Statistical modelling and decision science. 3rd ed. Amsterdam/Boston: Academic; 2012.

Structural Profile of the TCM-Klinik Bad Kötzting

2

Anton Staudinger, Stefan Hager, Jingzhang Dai, Likun Yang, Christina Staudinger, Erich Wühr, and Dieter Melchart

2.1 General Information on the Structure of the Clinic

This structural profile of the hospital is a revised and updated version of an article by A. Staudinger, S. Hager, V. Fischer, E. Wühr and D. Melchart. The original paper was published in the book "Evaluation der Patientenversorgung in der Chinesischen Medizin" (2021, Verlag Systemische Medizin) edited by Melchart D, Dai Y, Staudinger A. [1]. Some of the text below can also be found in a special edition of the publication to mark the clinic's 25(th) anniversary, published by Karger in 2016 [2].

Address
TCM-Klinik Bad Kötzting
First German Clinic for Traditional Chinese Medicine GmbH
Specialist Clinic for Psychosomatics and Psychotherapy
Ludwigstr. 2
D-93444 Bad Kötzting
Internet: www.tcm.info
Email: klinik@tcm.info
Institution code: 260 930 857

A. Staudinger · S. Hager · J. Dai · L. Yang · C. Staudinger
TCM-Klinik Bad Kötzting, Bad Kötzting, Germany
e-mail: a.staudinger@tcm.info; st.hager@tcm.info; l.yang@tcm.info; c.staudinger@tcm.info

E. Wühr
Member of the Faculty of Applied Healthcare Sciences, Deggendorf Institute of Technology (DIT), Deggendorf, Germany
e-mail: erich.wuehr@th-deg.de

D. Melchart (✉)
Former Head of Competence Centre for Lifestyle Medicine and Naturopathy (CoCoNat), Member of the Faculty of Applied Healthcare Sciences, Deggendorf Institute of Technology (DIT), Deggendorf, Germany
e-mail: dieter.melchart@th-deg.de

D. Melchart et al. (eds.), *TCM-Klinik Bad Kötzting*,
https://doi.org/10.1007/978-3-032-23307-3_2

Location of the Clinic, Accessibility, Catchment Area

The TCM-Klinik Bad Kötzting is centrally located in the town of Bad Kötzting, in the district of Cham. It is approximately 250 m from the train station and bus terminal, making it easily accessible. Sufficient parking spaces are available. The outpatient clinic of the TCM-Klinik Bad Kötzting is located in SINOCUR, between the railway station and the hospital.

SINOCUR is the new health and prevention centre, which houses not only the outpatient clinic of the TCM-Klinik Bad Kötzting, but also the health and guest services of the town of Bad Kötzting, the IHM® prevention centre with Kneipp training and teaching kitchen, and the conference and training centre with lecture hall, seminar rooms and gym.

Bad Kötzting is connected to the national rail network via the district town of Cham.

There are good connections to the national road network via the B85, B20 and B16 federal highways to the Straubing, Deggendorf and Schwandorf motorway junctions. A private helipad is also available.

Infrastructure of the TCM-Klinik Bad Kötzting

The TCM-Klinik Bad Kötzting, Germany's first clinic for traditional Chinese medicine, was founded in 1991 and is a state-approved hospital. What makes our clinic special is the combination of psychosomatic medicine, lifestyle medicine and traditional Chinese medicine [1, 2].

The medical concept requires a high level of expertise and multi-professionalism from the team of doctors and therapists. The German team of doctors has specialist qualifications in psychosomatic, psychiatric, internal medicine and naturopathic medicine.

All Chinese doctors and professors come directly from Beijing University of Chinese Medicine and its affiliated university hospitals. They are responsible for TCM therapy.

In 2008, the TCM-Klinik Bad Kötzting was awarded the "International Award of Contribution to Chinese Medicine 2008", the most prestigious award in the field of Chinese medicine, by the State Administration of TCM (Ministry of Health in China) and the World Federation of Chinese Medicine Societies. In the same year, the clinic was awarded first prize in the "Food for Health" competition in the hospitals category by the Bavarian State Ministry of the Environment and Health. In 2010, the clinic was officially designated as the University Hospital at Beijing University of Chinese Medicine. In December 2018, the TCM-Klinik Bad Kötzting was included in a Chinese funding project and became the Chinese German TCM Centre. The cooperation partners in this project are the Beijing University of Chinese Medicine and the Deggendorf Institute of Technology (DIT). The Technical University of Munich was a cooperation partner until 2019.

The TCM-Klinik Bad Kötzting has a capacity of 81 beds in 25 double rooms, 29 single rooms and 1 suite. Approximately 1500–2000 inpatient requests are processed each year. The maximum number of patients that can be treated as inpatients is approximately 1000 per year.

Existing Care Contracts
In August 1991, the TCM-Klinik Bad Kötzting concluded a care contract for inpatient hospital treatment with the Working Group of Bavarian Health Insurance Associations. Under this agreement, the clinic provided therapeutic services as a "special therapy facility" (Section 2 of the German Social Code, Book V) in the form of hospital treatment in accordance with Section 39 of the German Social Code, Book V. This agreement was not subject to the provisions of Sections 107 ff. of the German Social Code, Book V. Since 2010, a care agreement has been in place in accordance with Sections 108 No. 3/109 SGB V, according to which the clinic provides acute inpatient treatment (§ 39 (1) SGB V) for insured persons of the member health insurance funds of the health insurance associations in the field of psychosomatic medicine and psychotherapy in a total of 70 contract beds if outpatient, pre- and post-inpatient or semi-inpatient medical treatment is not sufficient. In addition, services in traditional Chinese medicine are also provided in accordance with the clinic's concept. Since 2016, the number of contract beds has increased from 70 to 75.

The services provided by the TCM-Klinik Bad Kötzting correspond to the service catalogue of the statutory health insurance (GKV). They are also—insofar as they are complementary services of traditional Chinese medicine (TCM)—hospital treatment (§ 39 SGB V) and thus legally privileged in accordance with the recognition of services of special therapeutic directions (§ 2 (1) sentence 2 SGB V). The services provided by TCM are included as the subject matter of the contract in the care contract concluded in 2010 between the statutory health insurance funds and the TCM-Klinik Bad Kötzting and are listed as planned TCM services in Section 1 (1) sentence 2 of the care contract. This also results in a statutory obligation on the part of the health insurance funds to reimburse costs in accordance with Section 109 (4) sentence 3 SGB V. Nevertheless, a declaration of cost coverage from the responsible health insurance fund is required.

In view of this, when assessing their obligation to cover the costs for an insured person who applies for admission to the TCM-Klinik Bad Kötzting, health insurance funds are bound by the content of the care agreement, the legality of covering the costs of TCM treatment and the necessity of prior approval of costs.

Admission takes place after hospital treatment has been prescribed by registered doctors in accordance with Section 39 of the German Social Code, Book V (SGB V) or by transfer from acute hospitals after registration by telephone or in writing.

Existing Scientific Collaborations and Clinic Advisory Board
The special focus of the clinic and the associated responsibility for providing the best possible care for patients requires a large number of regional and superregional collaborations. Cooperation agreements exist between the TCM-Klinik Bad

Kötzting and the TCM University of Beijing, and between the TCM-Klinik Bad Kötzting and the universities participating in the Scientific Advisory Board of the TCM-Klinik Bad Kötzting. In particular, these include agreements between Beijing University of Chinese Medicine and Deggendorf Institute of Technology (DIT).

The Hospital is scientifically supported by a clinic advisory board. This board consists of the following individuals:

- Prof. Dr. med. Dieter Melchart, Honorary Professor of Individual Health Management (IHM) and Complementary Medicine at the DIT. Former Head of CoCoNat at the DIT. Chairman of the Clinic Advisory Board
- Prof. Dr. med. Michael Frey, Head of the Master's programme in Mental Health and Head of CoCoNat (Competence Centre for Lifestyle Medicine and Naturopathy) at the DIT
- TCM University of Beijing, PR China, represented by the President
- TCM-Klinik Bad Kötzting, First German Clinic for Traditional Chinese Medicine GmbH, represented by the Managing Director Dipl. Kfm. Anton Staudinger
- Prof. Dr. med. dent. Erich Wühr, Honorary Professor for Health Promotion, Deputy Head of CoCoNat at DIT
- Prof. Dr. Rudolf Bauer, former Head of the Institute of Pharmaceutical Sciences, Department of Pharmacognosy at the University of Graz, Austria
- Dr. med. Stefan Hager, Medical Director of the TCM-Klinik Bad Kötzting
- Dr Filipiak, Medical Director of Psychosomatics, TCM-Klinik Bad Kötzting
- Prof. Yang Likun, Medical Director of Traditional Chinese Medicine (TCM) at the TCM-Klinik Bad Kötzting
- Prof. Dai Jingzhang, TCM University of Beijing/PR China/TCM-Klinik Bad Kötzting; former Director of the TCM-Klinik Bad Kötzting

Technical Equipment

The clinic's technical equipment includes laboratory, sonography, ergometry, ECG, spirometry, monitoring monitor and defibrillator (AED). Advanced sonographic, endoscopic, radiological and laboratory diagnostics as well as advanced cardiological, angiological and neurological-psychiatric diagnostics are provided through cooperation with a laboratory association (24-h on-call service), registered specialists (in all disciplines) and the Sana clinics in the district of Cham.

The emergency equipment includes:

- Defibrillator (automated external defibrillator, AED) (Cardiac Science Powerheart AED G3).
- Modern monitoring monitor with units for measuring or recording ECG or heart rate, oxygen saturation and blood pressure (maintenance in accordance with QM manual).
- Two emergency kits (Weinmann, Bayern type) with all the necessary equipment for treating emergency situations in accordance with the recommendations of the American Heart Association and leading professional associations (maintenance in accordance with the QM manual).
- Mobile oxygen cylinder with suction unit—this is also subject to the above inspection.

All medical devices are also tested in the specified monitoring cycles in accordance with the Medical Devices Act. The testing intervals and contents are specified and documented in the QM manual, among other places. The aforementioned devices and an emergency kit are centrally located in the immediate vicinity of the nurses' station on Ward 1A on the first floor and are designed as a mobile unit. The ECG room contains a mobile standard ECG device and a second emergency kit (the contents of both emergency kits are identical). It is also located in the immediate vicinity of the laboratory, which offers the possibility of immediate emergency diagnostics (e.g. rapid troponin test, blood sugar measurement). The ECG room offers sufficient space for emergency interventions (e.g. CPR or intubation) and the handover of the patient to the emergency services.

The generally extensive specialist medical/psychological findings available are incorporated into the diagnostic decision and considered. This avoids multiple examinations, which reduces the burden on the individual patient and also reduces the financial burden on the entire healthcare system.

The diagnostic and therapeutic processes are recorded in the clinic's web-based health portal using the VITERIO system [3, 4]. There are important interfaces between the VITERIO health portal and the ITR company's computer-based clinic communication system.

Facilities

The TCM-Klinik Bad Kötzting has a capacity of 81 beds in 25 double rooms, 29 single rooms and 1 suite (2 bedrooms, 1 living area, 1 bathroom). The patient rooms are equipped as standard with a hospital bed, sitting area, wardrobe, wet room (with toilet and bathtub or shower), television and lockable safe. All rooms are connected to the nurses' station via a bell system or telephone system (also for external calls). Some rooms have a balcony and a refrigerator.

The rooms and corridors are fitted with anti-allergenic carpeting. Wards 1A and 1B have disabled-friendly care rooms and, for reasons of hospital hygiene, are fitted with rubber flooring so that patients with special care needs can also be cared for. All rooms, corridors and other common areas are cleaned daily by the hospital's cleaning staff. The relevant hospital hygiene guidelines, considering occupational health and safety, are posted in all affected areas and in the QM manual.

In addition to the patient rooms, the clinic has the following facilities:

- In the basement: 1 Chinese herbal medicine department with pharmacy, kitchen for preparing decoctions and storage area, 1 kitchen area including cold storage and storage rooms, 1 office for the head chef, 1 boiler room, 1 laundry room, 1 staff changing room, 1 staff shower 1 patient dining room with terrace and garden access, 1 group therapy room, 1 patient lounge, which is also used for joint leisure activities, 2 staff lounges with cooking facilities, terrace and garden access, 1 waste collection room, goods reception area, 1 lift room, 1 storage room, sanitary facilities

- On the ground floor above 2 reception rooms, the larger of which is also used as a group therapy room, 1 emergency therapy room with ECG and emergency unit (also referred to as the ECG room in the concept), 1 laboratory, 2 Tuina therapy rooms, 5 acupuncture rooms, 1 treatment room for passive (individual) Qigong, 1 treatment room for physiotherapy, offices for Chinese doctors and interpreters, 1 doctor's room, 3 treatment rooms for psychologists, 1 data entry room with 3 workstations for patients for computer-assisted medical history taking, 1 managing director's office, 1 chief physician's office, 1 senior physician's office, 1 managing director's office, 1 secretarial office, 1 reception, 1 administration area, 1 accounting department, 1 planning office, 1 admissions office, 1 server room, storage rooms, sanitary facilities
- On the first floor above 5 doctors' rooms, 2 nurses' stations, 1 nurses' lounge, 1 kitchenette, 1 unclean work room, 1 work room for house cleaning, 1 room with lockable cupboards for storing medicines and infusions, 2 refrigerators, 1 room with cupboards for medical consumables, 1 exhibition area for traditional Chinese medicine, sanitary facilities
- On the second floor, 1 Qigong Hall, which is also used as a group therapy room, seminar and lecture room, exercise room for Qigong and PMR according to Jacobson, and in the evenings as a "room of silence", 2 workrooms for house cleaning, 1 storage room, sanitary facilities
- On the third floor, there are 5 treatment rooms for psychologists, 2 work rooms for house cleaning, 1 storage room
- On the fourth floor, there is 1 office for nursing management, 2 offices for accounting, 1 office for quality management, 1 office for scheduling, 1 office for billing, 4 staff changing rooms, 2 staff showers, 1 work room for house cleaning, 1 on-call doctor's room, 1 storage room, sanitary facilities.

2.2 Staff Description

Number of Medical Staff and Qualifications

The medical, therapeutic and nursing staff are listed below:

- 3 chief physicians
- 1 senior physician
- 13 doctors
- 12 psychologists
- 1 physiotherapist
- 2 dieticians
- 3 specialist therapists
- 1 pharmaceutical technical assistant
- 35 nursing staff

The permanent medical on-call service is provided by assistant doctors, while the background service is provided by chief physicians or their representatives.

The Chinese TCM doctors, most of whom are qualified, hold management, senior physician and lecturer positions at the Beijing University of Chinese Medicine (BUCM) and are on leave from their positions for a period of 1–2 years to work at the TCM-Klinik in Bad Kötzting. The Chinese TCM doctors have completed a 5-year university degree and a subsequent specialisation of at least 2 years in their chosen field (Chinese herbal medicine, acupuncture, tuina therapy, qigong). In addition to studying TCM, Chinese university education covers the content of Western or "conventional medicine" at least at the level of German specialist training in general medicine. Tuina doctors in China also perform orthopaedic and surgical procedures. At the time of their employment at the TCM-Klinik in Bad Kötzting, the Chinese doctors have many years of clinical experience with patients. The Chinese doctors are authorised to practise medicine in Germany under delegation and supervision. Furthermore, Chinese doctors are involved in training German doctors in the subjects of Chinese drug therapy and acupuncture and give lectures on TCM-specific topics at conferences. The cooperation with the BUCM ensures the highest internationally recognised therapeutic and scientific standards in the field of traditional Chinese medicine.

The nursing staff currently consists of 23 registered nurses (3-year training), 5 nursing assistants, 3 medical assistants, 1 pharmaceutical commercial assistant, 1 ward assistant and 1 office clerk. The nursing staff works in a 3-shift system, with at least two nurses on duty at night. A Chinese nurse works full-time on the day shift as a scientific assistant to the Chinese doctors.

The non-medical team also includes a physiotherapist with special treatment focuses, two dieticians, three specialist therapists, a pharmaceutical technical assistant, three Chinese interpreters and two Chinese herbal medicine specialists (pharmacists from BUCM).

In addition to physiotherapy, lymphatic drainage, manual therapy and remedial gymnastics, the special therapy Matrix Rhythm Therapy according to Dr Randoll is also used.

The dieticians' responsibilities include group lectures on nutrition and lifestyle based on the principles of both Western and Chinese dietetics. These group lectures are offered daily with systematically changing content. In addition, individual consultations are held with patients on the recommended diet for the relevant clinical pictures (according to Chinese syndrome diagnosis). Patients receive corresponding written information material.

The Chinese medicinal herb specialists have completed university training as pharmacists in China and work in the university hospital pharmacy. The preparation of individual decoctions at the TCM-Klinik Bad Kötzting is discussed and determined between the Chinese doctor and the hospital pharmacist.

Further Training and Supervision

We believe that continuous training and supervision are the foundation of quality. Internal supervision and case discussions are as much a matter of course as training courses on specialist topics. These are organised regularly and documented in our QM system. The focus is particularly on imparting an understanding of psychosomatic illness and health, and the corresponding therapeutic treatment approaches. All doctors, therapists and nursing staff participate in these training courses. The results of the Patient Evaluation Programme (PEP) are communicated to employees at training events. In the outpatient area, core team meetings are held approximately every 14 days to discuss outpatient and inpatient lifestyle issues within the framework of the IHM. A key feature of these meetings is the implementation of a 'journal club' focusing on the most important current studies in the fields of TCM, psychosomatics, and lifestyle medicine.

2.3 Medical Concept of the Hospital

2.3.1 General Aspects and Overview

At its core, treatment at our clinic involves complex psychotherapeutic or psychosomatic-psychotherapeutic treatment. We see our core competence in specialising in the treatment and therapy of people with multimorbid clinical pictures, in particular the occurrence of acute mental illnesses against the background of a (mostly chronic) underlying somatic disease, e.g. in the neurological, internal medicine or orthopaedic field.

The severity and acuteness of illnesses within the scope of psychosomatic medicine require inpatient hospital treatment with intensive medical and nursing care and monitoring. In most cases, this acute hospital treatment is necessary in accordance with Section 39 of the German Social Code, Book V (SGB V), because all outpatient, day-care and home care measures have already been exhausted.

The aim is to promote the patient's recovery through a structured medical-psychotherapeutic and lifestyle-medicine process to such an extent that the patient can continue to be treated on an outpatient or semi-inpatient basis. The duration of treatment is therefore based on the individual requirements of the respective clinical picture and the associated symptoms at the level of damage.

Our patients' inpatient stay ends as soon as the severity of their psychosomatic symptoms (ICD 10) has demonstrably improved, there has been an improvement in their bodily functions or damage, and outpatient or semi-inpatient measures are once again effective. This assessment is made by both the doctors and therapists and the patient.

In addition to our TCM health portal, we use elements of PsyBaDo (psychosomatic basic documentation), a standardised survey of psychopathological findings by the Working Group for Methodology and Documentation in Psychiatry (AMDP), and the BSS or GAF scale for severity assessment as diagnostic tools.

During the initial consultations with the specialist or psychologist, it must be clarified whether the treatment can be carried out on an outpatient basis or whether it should be carried out on an inpatient basis.

Inpatient treatment may be necessary for more severe, chronic mental health problems, also in order to break a social vicious circle in the patient's current living conditions and remove them from their normal environment, as otherwise there would be no prospect of change.

In hospital treatment of an acute or subacute medical condition requiring treatment, the therapy setting and frequency of therapy are crucial, with the option of 24-h medical, psychological and nursing interventions. This cannot be guaranteed on an outpatient or day-care basis if interventions or care are required during the night and at weekends.

The inpatient treatment setting facilitates the development of a shared psychosomatic understanding with the patient concerned. The presentation of the connections between psycho-emotional conflicts and an associated acute deterioration of somatic symptoms is an essential part of therapeutic interventions in the acute clinic.

The following therapies are used:

- Psychotherapeutic interventions are served in individual and group therapy sessions based on the principles of behavioural therapy.

Following psychological testing, these are modified on an individual basis in accordance with personality structure, age, factors triggering and perpetuating the illness, and underlying family, psychosocial and professional circumstances.

- Lifestyle medicine interventions are principally initiated with an emphasis on the dissemination of relaxation techniques, drawing primarily from the discipline of Qigong. Additionally, training is provided to support the adoption of routine exercise regimens.

The aim is to achieve successful self-regulation of the inner psychological and psycho-vegetative state of arousal. The medium-term goals of lifestyle medicine are to teach systematic self-awareness of one's own behaviour and mental attitudes towards one's own everyday demands, behaviour and somatic risks with the help of the health portal. It has been demonstrated that this can initiate the process of self-reflection and cognitive re-evaluation, thus helping to avoid potential health risks.

- Traditional Chinese medicine is practised with acupuncture, TCM-drug-therapy, Tuina-Manipulation, TCM-diet and Qigong. The application of treatment methods is depending on the TCM-diagnostic.
- Western somatic medicine as much as necessary.

The treatment goals are to be developed individually and are not determined "a priori". In most cases, the goal is psycho-vegetative stability, or the processing and integration of cognitively split-off, dysfunctional behaviours, or de-somatisation (instead of regressive re-somatisation, according to A. Mitscherlich [5]).

In addition to the criteria already mentioned in the concept, inpatient treatment is also necessary if outpatient therapy is not available or reasonably accessible, or if the therapy process is suspended, or if distancing and removal from the pathogenic social environment is medically indicated. The improvement of interpersonal interaction patterns through self-help strategies is developed in the form of group therapy programmes.

2.3.2 Multimodal Concept and Description of Procedures

Our clinic concept combines "the best of both worlds"—Chinese and Western medicine. It is based on four pillars (Fig. 2.1).

At the hospital, patients are usually treated with the millennia-old healing methods of traditional Chinese medicine and the necessary "conventional medicine"/psychosomatic therapies in the sense of a polymodal integrative concept. In addition to individually tailored psychosomatic treatment (individual psychotherapy, group therapy, lectures, psychoeducation) and lifestyle medicine (exercise, nutrition, creation of a risk protection factor profile using the internet-based TCM health portal), it also includes comprehensive holistic diagnostics, Chinese herbal medicine, acupuncture, moxibustion, Chinese medical massage technique (TUINA therapy), Chinese medical energetic acupuncture treatment (QIGONG individual therapy), concentrative breathing and movement therapy (QIGONG group therapy) and a balanced diet (nutrition).

2.3.2.1 Psychosomatic Medicine

The psychological concept of the TCM-Klinik Bad Kötzting is based on behavioural therapy with a focus on the targeted control of emotions. Patients are taught that this is also of great importance from a traditional Chinese medical perspective, as Chinese medicine believes that excessive emotions lead to functional disorders (Qi flow disorders) and somatic symptoms (Qi and blood flow disorders), which are significant factors in the development of disease.

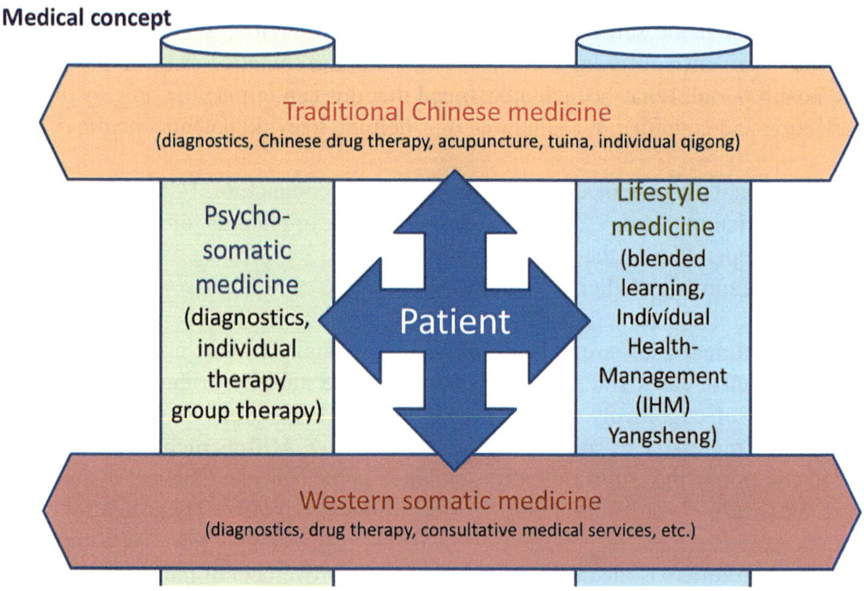

Fig. 2.1 Multimodal medical concept of the TCM-Klinik Bad Kötzting

On the second day of the inpatient stay, the attending psychologist conducts the initial psychological interview, which determines the psychological ICD diagnosis, which also defines the severity of the depressive mood. During this interview, the psychologists also address the topic of life satisfaction, which is presented to the patient in an understandable illustration based on the data they entered in the TCM health portal.

The aim is also to deepen a sustainable psychotherapeutic working alliance, to collect psychopathological findings (e.g. affective disorders) and to develop a diagnosis-related disorder model (Fig. 2.2). The psychopathological process or problem and symptom burden is defined based on the patient's life history, medical history and psychosomatic test results. The multimodal therapy concept encompasses behaviour, feelings, physical sensations, imagination and attitudes.

With the help of the health portal, patients receive step-by-step support in developing self-awareness and self-monitoring skills through psychosomatic testing. If desired, they can also receive medium to long-term support in achieving their individual goals in everyday life after their hospital stay.

The therapy goals are set individually and agreed upon with the patient. These include, for example:

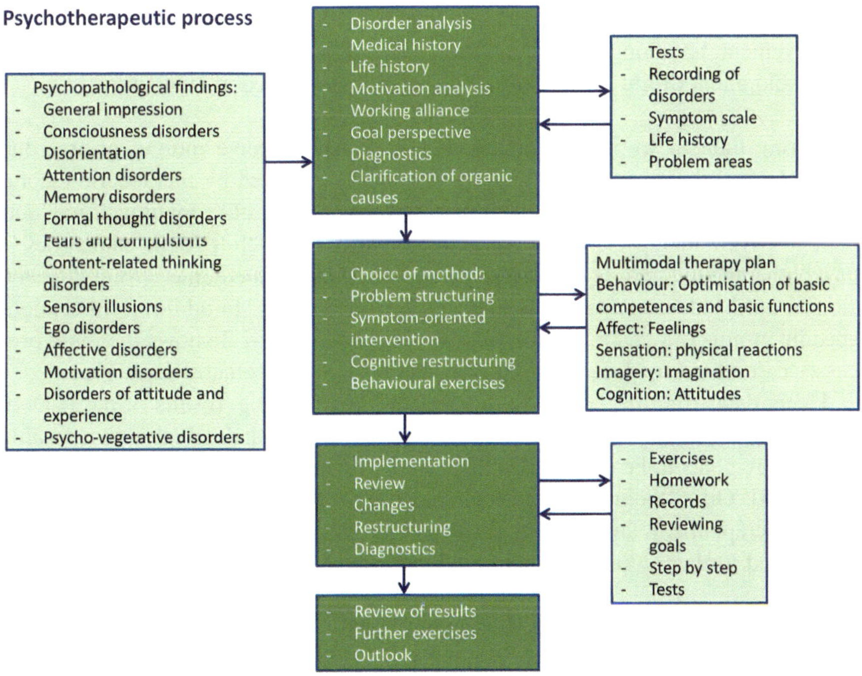

Fig. 2.2 Psychotherapeutic processes at the TCM-Kötzting in Bad Kötzting

- Promoting a more competent perception and identification of feelings and bodily inner states
- Promoting an understanding of one's own personality structure
- Acquisition of self-regulation skills
- Expanding relaxation and stress reduction abilities
- Improving relationship skills
- Strengthening self-esteem
- Strengthening the experience of self-efficacy
- Taking responsibility for physical and mental health, caring for a healthier body, nutrition, physical performance and relaxation skills
- Reduction of avoidance behaviour
- Improving body awareness
- Promoting an active, self-determined lifestyle, also in the sense of a psychoeducational approach
- Promoting health-promoting behaviours
- Building motivation for therapy for further outpatient psychotherapeutic treatment
- Processing stressful or traumatic events in the patient's life history
- Reducing stress-inducing thought patterns and avoiding self-critical or self-hostile cognitions
- Psychoeducation regarding specific deficits or symptom areas (e.g. sleep, pain, movement, breathing, nutrition, anxiety, depression)
- Development of life goals, action plans and aftercare recommendations

During their 4- to 5-week inpatient stay, patients receive individual or group psychological therapy at least three times a week, followed by therapeutic recommendations, including recommendations regarding the possible continuation of outpatient psychotherapy. During their inpatient stay, each patient undergoes a psychotherapeutic and psycho-educational, i.e. lifestyle medicine, group concept, carried out by doctors, psychologists and health coaches. In addition, indication-specific groups (e.g. pain, depression) are offered. Figure 2.3 shows the main processes carried out by doctors and therapists in the psychosomatic department.

Using data from the TCM health portal VITERIOR (e.g. results of the ICD-10 Symptom Rating Questionnaire), a comparison of target and actual data regarding the therapy goals to be achieved is discussed with the patient in the final consultation [3, 4]. Other therapeutic aspects are also presented to the patient. If further psychotherapeutic treatment is indicated, a motivational discussion is held with the patient and further outpatient treatment is initiated.

2.3.2.2 Traditional Chinese Medicine (TCM)

Traditional Chinese medicine does not have a uniform theory that is universally applicable to all existing schools. The following ideas are the result of a consensus process at the TCM-Klinik in Bad Kötzting. The aim of the doctor working with traditional Chinese medicine is to understand the patient in his or her mental and spiritual dimension. For TCM, the psyche and soma are an inseparable unit. Physical

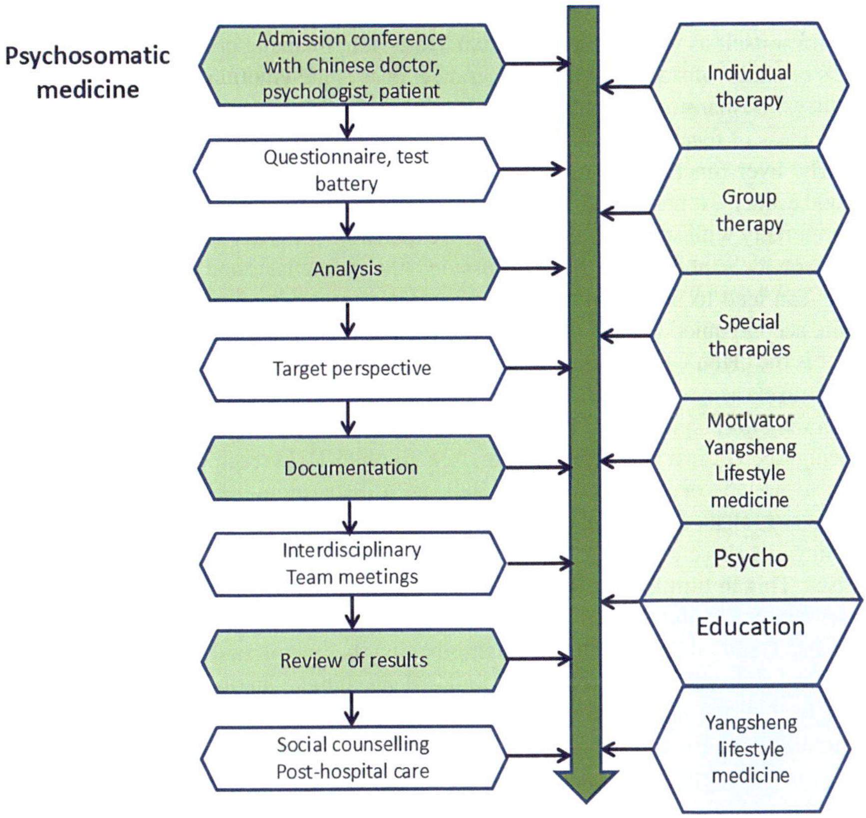

Fig. 2.3 Process profile of clinical procedures at the TCM-Klinik Bad Kötzting

symptoms and emotions, external factors and life events are equally interconnected and influence each other. Psychosomatics in traditional Chinese medicine must differentiate and name these interactions as syndromes and identify the causes of psycho-emotional illnesses.

According to TCM, organs not only fulfil a material function in terms of chemical and physical processes but also have an "energetic" function in that they move the life energy in a certain direction. This results in movement and transformation on both a substantial and energetic level. Organs are regarded as carriers of emotional and mental functions. Each organ system has complex tasks and its own soul-spirit aspect. On a material level, the kidneys are said to have the task of "converting water and purifying the blood". Among other things, the kidney function circle (kidney shen) is said to carry the "fire of life (mingmen), which warms the body, maintains all processes in the body and keeps the person upright". The soul-spirit aspect "Zhi" applies to this functional circuit. This part of the soul is associated with willpower, stamina and steadfastness. If the kidneys become diseased, somatic problems with urination or oedema may occur, accompanied by exhaustion and obesity.

On a psychological level, disharmony in the kidney functional circuit is said to manifest itself as weak willpower, sexual aversion, financial problems, inner numbness or a lack of stamina and perseverance. Fear is the emotion associated with the kidneys. Disharmony therefore means excessive fear or—the opposite—a lack of awareness of fear, i.e. recklessness.

The liver function cycle (liver-gan) is said to "bring qi upwards and distribute blood evenly". It has a close connection to the uterus. The liver function cycle reacts emotionally with struggle, assertiveness, expansion, progress and self-realisation. If a person feels inhibited in their expression, "the qi stagnates and so does the blood". This can lead to migraines, digestive problems, high blood pressure or menstrual pain, accompanied by frustration, irritability and aggression. The soul aspect of the liver is the "Hun". Hun is the "vehicle with which our consciousness travels and our soul travels as a whole". The organ is said to represent "contact" and communicates with the entire spiritual world. This gives rise to visions and plans. This happens during sleep or in a very relaxed state. According to TCM teachings, disturbed sleep due to dreams or even nightmares indicate a disharmony of the liver. The same applies to chaotic emotions, stress and tension. The soul communicates through feelings. If these cannot be integrated or if the soul cannot express itself, tension arises. This in turn hinders clear vision, because the liver function cycle is associated with inner and outer vision. That is why visions and the "ability to plan" and "realise goals" are also included. Strengthening the liver is said to strengthen assertiveness and willpower. According to TCM teachings, "harmonising the liver" is said to improve emotional turmoil and emotional complaints such as aggression, irritability and frustration (harmonisation of disturbed hormone functions?). Anger is the negative emotion associated with the liver function cycle. A pattern of disharmony manifests itself through excessive anger or an inability to feel or express it.

The lung function cycle (lung-fei) has the task of absorbing oxygen and enriching the blood with it. The lungs are said to be "in contact with the heavens" and bring inspiration and awareness of the "connections of the cosmos". At the same time, they house the "Po" part of the soul, which is responsible for maintaining bodily functions and body awareness. They are the point of contact between the cosmos and the body. If there is disharmony in the lungs, this should manifest itself in susceptibility to colds, allergies and lung diseases. However, there may also be a tendency towards melancholy, a lack of social skills and loneliness, or a "feeling of not being right in one's body" and a "tendency to bump into things everywhere, both physically and figuratively". According to TCM, the person does not see the meaning and value behind the visible manifestations. Sadness is the emotion associated with the lungs. Disharmony is said to manifest itself in inappropriate sadness or an inability to feel grief.

In TCM the spleen function circle (spleen-Pi) refers to the digestive function and corresponds to the pancreas and small intestine. It "absorbs food pulp, converts it and helps nourish the body". It absorbs things from outside and turns them into something of its own. The spleen is associated with the mental aspect "Yi". Yi is responsible for the thinking function. All information that flows into us from outside should be organised, digested and integrated into our own system through thinking.

A disturbance in the function of the spleen can manifest itself on a physical level through digestive problems, sluggishness and fatigue. On an emotional/mental level, there may be a tendency to go round in circles, not to come to a conclusion, to keep mulling over the same problems without being able to solve them. Brooding, circular thoughts, concentration problems, bad habits, the feeling of not making progress and of "getting bogged down" are all part of the spleen function cycle. So is the tendency to worry unnecessarily, mainly about oneself but also about one's loved ones. Worry is the emotion associated with the spleen.

The heart function circuit (heart-Xin) is associated with the fire element and is referred to as the emperor in Chinese medicine. It "rules without doing anything" simply by its existence. On a physical level, the heart distributes blood. Blood carries all information within it. It is said to be "connected to our genes, our ancestors, and what we have made of all our collected impressions, food, water and radiation". According to TCM teachings, it is connected to the air we breathe—in other words, to the outside world and the universe. The heart "connects all of this". The heart's task is to "connect and communicate". The soul aspect of the heart is the "Shen". Shen is "that which radiates from us and illuminates the world". Shen is "our inner light". Disharmony on the physical level manifests itself "through heart disease, blood circulation disorders or even non-organic heart pain". On the emotional/mental level, this manifests itself through an unclear mind, restlessness, sleep disorders, an inability to relax and communication problems. Problems such as talking too much or too little, "being unable to connect with other people" or a "constant search for connections and communication", as well as "being unable to be alone" are expressions of this disharmony. The emotion associated with the heart is joy. Joy here refers to exaltation, i.e. "exuberance". "Being beside oneself with joy and excitement" indicates a disharmony of the heart, but the "inability to feel joy" also represents a disturbance.

With these examples, TCM aims to illustrate how closely organs, their functions and the emotional and mental aspects of human existence are linked. TCM doctors do not recognise the separation of body, mind and soul as is customary in the West. Emotional disharmony, psychosomatic or mental illnesses are not treated separately, but together with the body. In most cases, emotional problems are accompanied by physical ailments and vice versa. When illnesses are treated with TCM, the conceptual aim is to change both the physical and "energetic state" as well as the emotional state in a holistic sense.

TCM Drug Therapy

Chinese drug therapy is the oldest and most important therapy in traditional Chinese medicine. It mainly uses herbal substances, but also minerals and, in rare cases, animal components. These are usually administered to the patient in the form of decoctions (medicinal "boils") as extracts. The decoction is produced by a concentrated decoction of approx. 10–12 solid medicinal substances with water. The daily amount of decoction is approx. 150–200 ml and is prescribed in the form of thermos flasks to be drunk as a "medicinal tea". In addition to decoctions, drops, creams or partial baths are also used. TCM medicines are adapted to the changing physical situation in accordance with Chinese diagnostics and the course of therapy. The drugs used are prescribed by experienced TCM professors at Beijing University of Chinese Medicine (BUCM) and manufactured by Chinese medicinal herb specialists who have completed university training as pharmacists in China.

Acupuncture and Moxibustion

Acupuncture is a healing method that dates back thousands of years and is the best known of all Chinese healing methods in the West. Fine acupuncture needles are used to prick points that, according to Chinese belief, lie on so-called meridians ("energy channels") in a differentiated manner. According to traditional belief, acupuncture can remove so-called "energy blockages" that are responsible for functional disorders or pain. Moxibustion is a special form of acupuncture. This involves burning pressed herbs in the form of cigars or attached to acupuncture needles to apply local heat to specific acupuncture points to achieve healing. Acupuncture treatments also include other therapeutic methods such as micro-bloodletting, cupping, electrostimulation of the inserted needles and laser acupuncture. People who cannot tolerate needles for various reasons are treated with modern laser acupuncture at the clinic. In addition, other special forms of acupuncture that work via so-called microsystems, such as ear acupuncture, skull acupuncture or mouth acupuncture according to Dr J. Gleditsch, can also be used [6].

Acupuncture is intended to reduce general stress levels and contribute to relaxation and inner peace. This is intended to have a positive effect on emotionality and facilitate the start of psychotherapeutic treatment. TCM doctors regard acupuncture as a method that clears the mind, promotes serenity, regulates appetite and facilitates concentration.

Tuina Therapy

This form of therapy is a special, differentiated massage treatment that is applied by doctors with 5–7 years of training in traditional Chinese medicine with a special focus on orthopaedics. These doctors are also active in the field of orthopaedic surgery in China, among other places. Like acupuncturists, the Tuina doctors at the TCM Hospital focus on the body's meridians. They postulate that by treating different points and areas of the body, they can directly influence functional disorders within the body. Tuina therapy incorporates elements of connective tissue massage, reflexology, acupressure, periosteal massage, chiropractic therapy and manual therapy.

Qigong Therapy

Qigong is a Chinese umbrella term for a variety of ancient exercises for maintaining health. Although the term Qigong only became established in China a few decades ago, its history goes back much further. Qi exercises are part of the term "YangSheng" (nourishing or cultivating life), which comprehensively represents an art of living. Qigong loosely translates as "gaining control of life energy". "Qi" is the term for life energy and "Gong" means "work" or "success through perseverance and practice". As Qi is a dynamic principle, the most important tasks in Qigong are to allow Qi to flow freely, to expel used Qi and to absorb fresh Qi. The exercises can be performed in soft, flowing movements while standing, walking, sitting or lying down.

Passive qigong is a medical treatment performed by a qigong doctor in the form of an "energetic massage" that is applied along the energy channels using weaker or stronger stimulation stimuli by means of finger pressure.

Active qigong (qi = life energy/gong = practice) is a form of concentrated, meditative breathing and movement therapy that is primarily used for disease prevention and has a certain similarity in its effects to Western relaxation techniques (autogenic training, progressive muscle relaxation).

As part of the inpatient therapy concept at the TCM clinic, patients perform 25 min of Qigong exercises twice a day under the guidance of a Qigong master. In addition, 18 easy-to-learn Qigong exercises are broadcast twice a day on the television in the room for practice purposes. These involve performing prescribed movement exercises with a focus on breathing and simultaneous visualisation of images from nature. The purpose of these exercises is to harmonise bodily functions and achieve deep relaxation. At regular intervals, silent Qigong is practised as a concentrative, i.e. meditative form, with a strong introspective component to achieve even deeper relaxation.

Chinese Dietetics

Like Chinese herbs, foods can also be classified according to taste, temperature behaviour, site of action and direction of action, as well as strength. This enables a highly differentiated nutritional therapy with specific disease-related dietary recommendations. In Chinese poetry there is a saying "Is he a cook or a doctor? Is this a pharmacy or a kitchen?"—makes it clear that in China, food is also considered and used as medicine to maintain and restore health. For example, warm or even hot foods (e.g. ginger or cinnamon) are used for so-called "cold illnesses", while cooling foods (e.g. peppermint) are used for "heat illnesses". This way of thinking is also reflected in European herbal medicine. As nutritional therapy is very individual, it can only be implemented daily in a few exceptional cases within the framework of the clinic concept. It is easier for patients to implement individual recommendations from TCM doctors in everyday clinical practice if they only must avoid certain foods. In addition, special hospital diets and light meals are offered individually to patients according to their medical condition—such as diabetic diets, vegetarian diets, etc.

The medical concept provides for the majority of the clinic's patients to be given a wholesome diet that is largely acceptable in terms of taste. The principles and practice of wholesome nutrition are explained to clinic visitors in weekly lectures by dieticians and head chefs. The long-term goal is to change patients' eating habits towards a wholesome diet. Figure 2.4 provides an overview of the main areas of focus and tasks of the Chinese doctors and therapists.

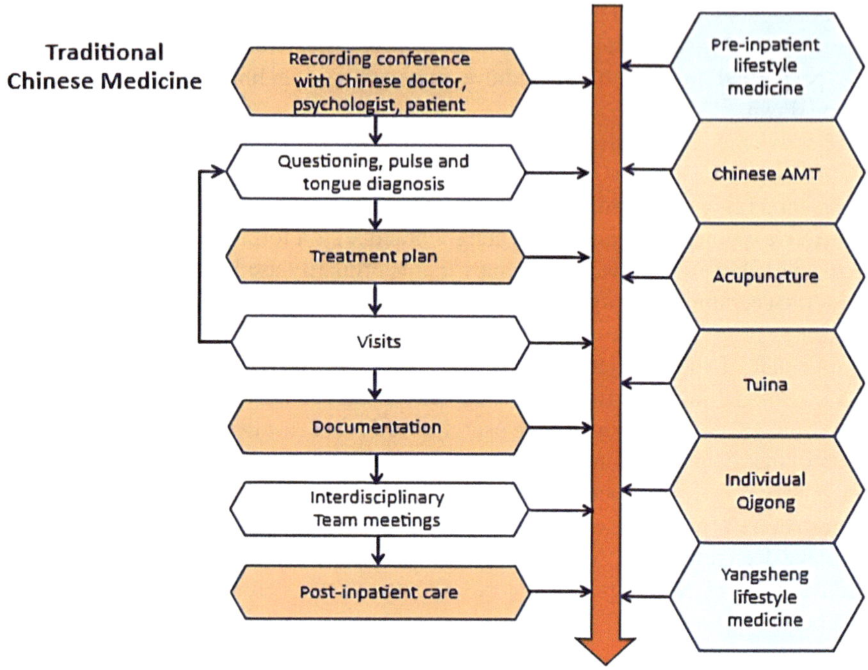

Fig. 2.4 Focus areas and tasks of the TCM-treatment team

TCM Diagnosis and Therapy Process

The Chinese doctor documents all symptoms, including a neuro-vegetative medical history (symptoms), and supplements this with a TCM-specific tongue and pulse diagnosis (signs). Based on this information, he or she makes an "energetic diagnosis", e.g. of a pain syndrome with depression, in accordance with the theories of traditional Chinese medicine (qi, blood, Yin/Yang, 6-layer model, etc.). The TCM doctor divides symptoms and signs into different categories and names them using corresponding Chinese therapeutic terms (e.g. congestion in the meridians, liver qi stagnation, blood stasis and dampness). Based on this diagnosis, he establishes a therapeutic principle to treat the identified patterns of disturbance. The doctor then prescribes a high-dose Chinese herbal remedy tailored to the symptoms. This consists of approximately 10–15 Chinese herbs and is to be taken in two doses daily.

In a further step, the medical colleague responsible for acupuncture also receives this written anamnesis data. Once the acupuncture points relevant to the diagnosis have been determined, the needles are inserted. The patient usually receives three medical acupuncture sessions per week. Since most patients also complain of pain in the muscles, joints and back, they also receive two sessions of manual therapy per week (Chinese medical Tuina massage/energetic individual Qigong treatment).

As a counterpart to Western relaxation methods, patients learn 18 exercises from a Tai Chi Qigong training programme. They perform these exercises in the morning and evening under intensive guidance.

Patients also learn the "healing sounds" of TCM and a 3-1-2 programme developed in China (3 = self-acupressure of main acupuncture points, 1 = deep abdominal breathing, 2 = squats) for self-administered therapy in the spirit of prevention.

2.3.2.3 Lifestyle Medicine

The lifestyle medicine concept of the TCM-Klinik Bad Kötzting focuses on psychoeducation and sustainability through self-awareness, self-reflection and self-efficacy. This is to be achieved through psychological consultations, lifestyle medicine lectures and exercises, as well as through self-observation and self-assessment of feelings, attitudes and behaviours in everyday life with the help of the personal health portal VITERIO®. This systematic self-observation is used to encourage patients to engage in comprehensive self-reflection and self-awareness. The aim is to identify individual chronic stimuli and stresses (mental stress, exposure to wind/cold, poor diet and posture, poor sleep hygiene) and to have them cognitively restructured or, if possible, eliminated by the patient themselves.

Patients who have been suffering from chronic complaints for a long time and often believe that they have been "fully diagnosed" by conventional medicine and, in many cases, have "exhausted all treatment options" are usually admitted to the TCM-Klinik Bad Kötzting. In principle, treatment using traditional Chinese medicine methods is also suitable for acute illnesses and for the prevention of disease.

Through the systematic assessment of basic psychosomatic-cognitive skills such as self-efficacy, optimism, sense of coherence (according to Antonovsky) and resilience, as well as the measurement of basic physiological functions such as exercise, nutrition, breathing, circulation and sleep, chronic risk factors can be uncovered and weakened protective factors of mental and physical health identified. This allows lifestyle-related chronicity factors to be reduced in the long term through targeted lifestyle medicine training, and dysfunctional behaviour and self-assessment patterns to be changed and optimised.

Health (being healthy, becoming healthy, staying healthy) is primarily the responsibility of everyone. The therapist resp. coach acts only as an advisor and companion. Learning a preventive and health-promoting lifestyle is supported by a comprehensive range of tools. These include keeping diaries (pain, joy, exercise, nutrition, etc.), conducting a structured daily review in which defined events of the day are emotionally evaluated retrospectively, feelings are consciously named and rated according to their intensity on a visual analogue scale from 0 to 100.

In principle, lifestyle training covers four of the six core components of a patient training measure in accordance with the "Joint Recommendations for the Promotion and Implementation of Patient Training in SGBV (2022): raising awareness of body perception, teaching self-management skills for dealing with stress, communicating needs and learning to say no; acquiring social skills and mobilising social support (e.g. through group contact; role-playing in person and online; self-monitoring)" [7].

This should contribute to optimising treatment outcomes and improving patients' social participation, motivation for therapy and quality of life.

Academic and clinical interest in the relationship between health behaviour, lifestyle factors, mental health and psychological well-being is reinforced by current clinical evidence [8–10]. A systematic review and meta-analysis by Amiri et al. (2024) examined the effect of lifestyle interventions on depression, anxiety and stress in randomised controlled trials [8]. The results showed that a healthy lifestyle improves mental health and significantly reduces stress, with the effects being particularly pronounced in patients with depressive symptoms and in women.

Lifestyle changes such as increased exercise, a healthier diet and improved sleep quality can effectively reduce stress by lowering cortisol levels and increasing endorphin release [9, 10]. Furthermore, findings suggest that psychological factors such as increased mindfulness and improved sleep quality may have a positive influence. Recent research shows that sleep disorders are associated with cognitive impairments such as memory lapses and attention deficits, which act as mediators between insomnia and emotional disorders such as anxiety and depression [11].

Lifestyle-based interventions as part of disease self-management are already recommended by international working groups and commissions [12, 13] as a fundamental component of mental health care in clinical practice for adults with major depression, whereby other evidence-based therapies can be added or used in combination. This means that intensive lifestyle intervention (ILI) is recognised and required internationally in the training of this target group, as well as in general mental healthcare. Figure 2.5 illustrates the processes involved in lifestyle medicine.

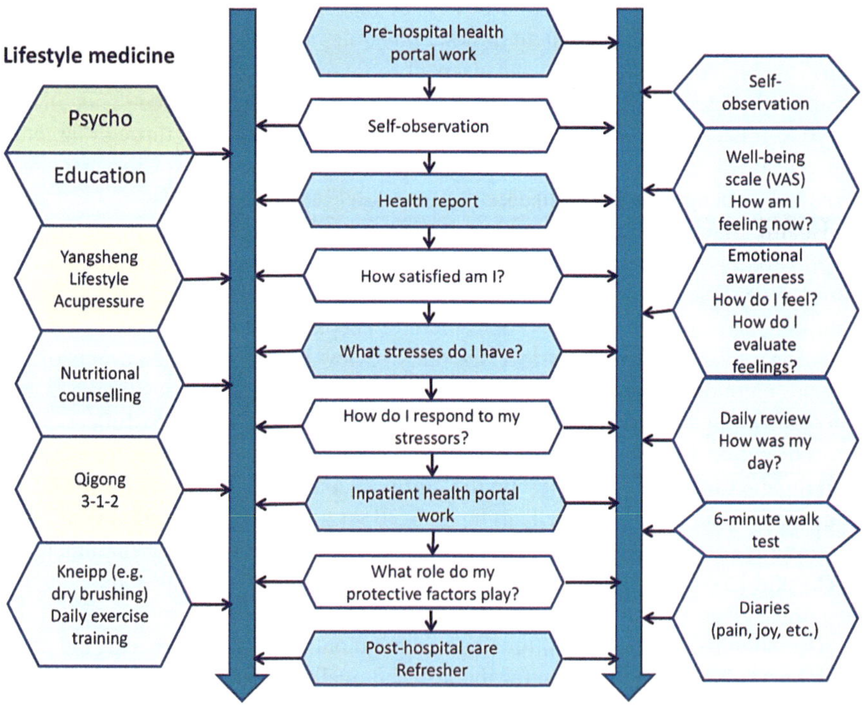

Fig. 2.5 Processes of lifestyle medicine at the TCM-Klinik Bad Kötzting

With their treatment approval for inpatient or outpatient care, each patient receives individual access to the TCM health portal VITERIO®. All patients at the TCM-Klinik Bad Kötzting have free access to the TCM health portal for "self-data entry" for up to 6 months.

The TCM health portal provides support with important questions:

- How can I improve my health?
- Which measures have which effects?
- How and when can I carry out health-promoting activities myself?
- The following functions are available on the health portal:
  - Training planner for implementing a health-promoting lifestyle in everyday life
  - Diary for documenting your health-promoting activities
  - Graphical progress charts that track important parameters and their development over the long term
  - Information and instructions for designing a healthy lifestyle

The aim is to implement a healthy lifestyle in everyday life and to improve the situation of those affected in the long term.

The concept is based on Individual Health Management (IGM®), which was developed by Prof. Dr. med. Dieter Melchart over many years of research [14]. As part of Bad Kötzting's development as a prevention region, these comprehensive options and services are also offered to all citizens as well as holidaymakers and spa guests. IHM has also been successfully tested regionally in the form of municipal and workplace health promotion.

IHM = IGM is offered at the SINOCUR prevention centre via the TCM outpatient clinic and/or by the town of Bad Kötzting in various forms, ranging from a 2-h health investment to a 12-month IGM® lifestyle programme at SINOCUR. This intensive IHM® lifestyle programme was evaluated over several years as part of a pilot project with AOK Bayern and is currently available as patient training recognised by health insurance companies in accordance with § 43 SGB V for the area of obesity [15]. For the indication of stress-related depression, the clinic has applied for recognition as a supplementary rehabilitation service to the Bavarian Medical Service.

2.3.2.4 Western Somatic Medicine

The range of therapeutic services in the field of conventional medicine extends from medically necessary drug therapies, which are usually continued or, if needed, reduced step by step, to physiotherapy and comprehensive psychotherapy. Multimodal pain therapy includes infusion therapy, neural chiropractic therapy, inhalations, bath treatments, wraps, relaxation techniques (including progressive muscle relaxation according to Jacobsen) and lectures as well as group and individual discussions. In addition, Western nutritional counselling is provided, which is combined with TCM principles.

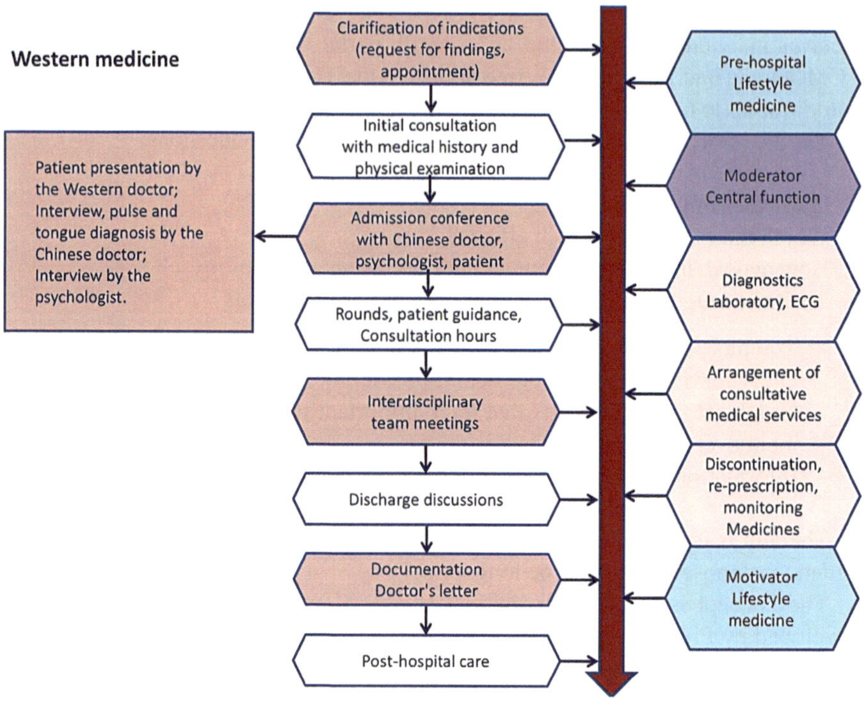

Fig. 2.6 Process of Western medicine at the TCM-Klinik Bad Kötzting

Careful Western medical diagnostics are a prerequisite for implementing the clinic's multimodal medical concept. Repeated case history taking and the continued administration of analgesic and psychotherapeutic medication necessitate close somatic monitoring and care of patient. The essential processes of somatic physicians are shown in Fig. 2.6.

2.3.3 Treatment Spectrum—Indications and Contraindications

The treatment concept is suitable for patients with acute, chronic and functional somatic disorders who suffer primarily from somatic complaints and psychological stress such as anxiety and depression. Pain relief, regaining quality of life and developing and maintaining health are the core concerns and expectations that people have when they come to the TCM Clinic. Depending on the type, severity, duration and complexity of the symptoms, inpatient treatment is advisable and promising for the following conditions (*indications*):

- Functional and somatoform pain conditions
- Chronic fatigue syndrome and burnout
- Depression, anxiety and adjustment disorders
- Diseases of the musculoskeletal system (Achillodynia, knee and hip pain, etc.)

- Polyneuropathies
- Migraine, tension headaches, trigeminal neuralgia, phantom pain and vertigo
- Chronic sleep disorders
- Fibromyalgia
- Respiratory disorders (e.g. bronchial asthma, bronchitis and sinusitis)
- Gastrointestinal disorders (e.g. irritable bowel syndrome, Crohn's disease, gastritis)
- Functional cardiovascular disorders (artificial hypotension, tachycardia)
- Neurodermatitis, urticaria, eczema and psoriasis

Before admission to hospital, all patients are examined by an interdisciplinary team about their existing findings and symptoms, and the indication for admission is decided after weighing up the probable individual success of the therapy. For this purpose, patients fill out special questionnaires to record their symptoms.

The following are considered *contraindications* for inpatient admission:

- Psychosis and severe personality disorders
- Eating disorders, including obesity
- Patients who pose a danger to themselves or others
- Severe neurotic disorders and stress disorders
- Severe affective disorders
- Dementia and organic brain psychosis syndromes
- Addictions
- Manic disorders
- Infectious diseases
- Conditions requiring intensive care
- Diseases with acute surgical indications

This list is for guidance purposes only. If you have symptoms or illnesses that are not listed, we recommend making an individual enquiry. Not all patients with a listed symptom can be successfully treated. The likelihood of successful treatment depends on various factors, such as constitution, age and previous medication. If treatment is unsuccessful, we will of course refer the patients concerned to possible alternatives.

Patients with cognitive and emotional insight and self-reflection abilities comparable to the average population and sufficient self-care are treated in a targeted manner. Patients with moderate intellectual disability, delusional and psychotic patients, and patients with forensic personality disorders should be excluded. Also excluded are physically and/or mentally disabled people. 'Effective treatment' encompasses a therapeutic outcome in the areas of social, cognitive, emotional and behavioural modification, which can be verified as ego-congruent according to the person's self-image and which can be observed objectively (using psychological testing methods if necessary). Figure 2.7 shows the process of approving or rejecting inpatient treatment or recommending outpatient treatment in the so-called "logbook". If there is a contraindication, the requesting patient receives a rejection.

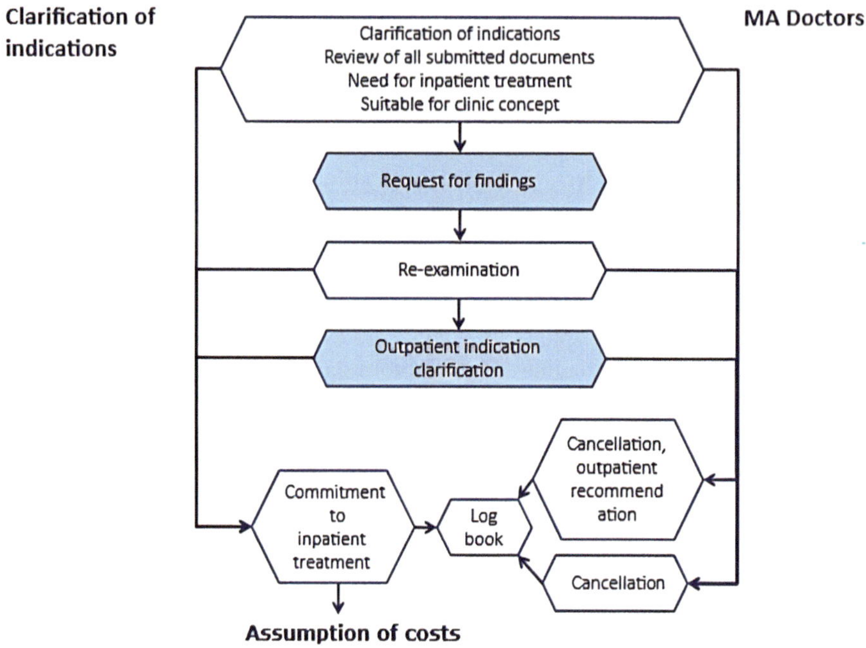

Fig. 2.7 Process for clarifying indications at the TCM-Klinik Bad Kötzting

If there is no need for inpatient hospital treatment, outpatient treatment may be recommended. If inpatient treatment is approved and a prescription for hospital treatment is issued by the referring doctor, the patient contacts their health insurance company and obtains a written declaration of cost coverage, if this has not already been done. If medically necessary inpatient hospital treatment is required, all statutory health insurance companies cover the treatment costs at the TCM-Klinik Bad Kötzting. If optional services are to be used, the patient should also obtain a declaration of cost coverage from their supplementary insurance in advance.

Due to the TCM Clinic usually being fully occupied, there is a waiting period for most patients. During this time, patients are asked to complete questionnaires on the health portal, which are used for inpatient treatment and scientific monitoring. If patients are unable or unwilling to complete these questionnaires electronically, they will be provided with paper copies as an alternative. Patients are advised of their obligation to cooperate with the treatment. If the questionnaires have not been completed or have not been completed in full by the time of admission, this will be done by the first individual psychotherapy session at the latest.

2.3.4 Communication Structures—Case Conference, Transfer of Information

All newly admitted patients are usually presented to the assigned psychologist on the same day during a case conference attended by German and Chinese doctors. This also gives the psychologist a good overview of the somatic aspects of the patient's illness.

During their inpatient stay, patients are consulted both in individual visits (German doctor, Chinese doctor and interpreter) and in team visits (German and Chinese doctors together), and interdisciplinary team meetings and chart reviews are held regularly. During the Chinese German chief physician visit, the therapy strategy for the following week is determined and any necessary changes to the treatment are discussed and decided upon.

The Chinese doctors in the acupuncture, tuina therapy and qigong treatment units are informed by their Chinese colleagues about the progress of treatment and any changes to therapy. Similarly, the German doctors share new relevant findings (laboratory values, consultations) and planned "conventional" or naturopathic treatments (e.g. increase, decrease or resumption of "conventional" medication, complementary neural therapies, etc.) with their Chinese colleagues.

The lifestyle lectures are organised and delivered by IHM coaches in the lecture hall of the SINOCURE prevention centre, which is part of the TCM-Klinik Bad Kötzting outpatient unit. They are designed and supervised by professors from the Faculty of Applied Health Sciences at the Deggendorf Institute of Technology (DIT), represented by the CoCoNat Institute. Core team meetings are held approximately every 14 days to discuss all essential aspects of the IHM lifestyle programme and to inform participants about the most important new releases of relevant publications through a so-called 'journal club'.

2.3.5 The Outpatient Clinic

The costs of outpatient treatment and examinations at the TCM-Klinik in Bad Kötzting are not covered by statutory health insurance funds. These are calculated according to the German Scale of Medical Fees (GOÄ), depending on the time and examination required. The outpatient clinic of the TCM Hospital is in SINOCUR. SINOCUR is a health resort housing not only the TCM outpatient clinic, but also the town of Bad Kötzting's health resort and guest services, the IGM® prevention centre with a teaching kitchen and Kneipp training facilities, and a conference and training centre with a lecture hall, seminar rooms and a gym. It was designed by a consortium comprising the TCM-Klinik Bad Kötzting, the town of Bad Kötzting, the Competence Centre for Lifestyle Medicine and Naturopathy (CoCoNat) and the Rothenfußer Foundation in Munich.

An additional outpatient branch of the TCM-Klinik Bad Kötzting has been established in the Hotel Sonnenhof in Lam. Guests and patients can now combine a holiday in the Bavarian Forest with outpatient treatment at the TCM Hospital or hotel.

References

1. Staudinger S, Hager V, Fischer E. Wühr and D. Melchart. In: Melchart D, Dai J, Staudinger A, editors. Evaluation der Patientenversorgung in der Chinesischen Medizin. Bad Kötzting: Verlag Systemische Medizin; 2022. p. 22–66.
2. Hager S, Dai J, Fischer V, Lüthke F, Staudinger A. East meets West: synergy through diversity. Forsch Komplementmed. 2016;23(Suppl 2):3–7. https://doi.org/10.1159/000444766. Epub 2016 May 30. PMID: 27272152.
3. Melchart D, Eustachi A, Gronwald S, Wühr E, Wifling K. Bachmeier BE Introduction of a web portal for an Individual Health Management and observational health data sciences. Patient Relat Outcome Meas. 2018;9:183–96. https://doi.org/10.2147/PROM.S157410. eCollection 2018.
4. Viterio GmbH. VITERIO website. https://www.viterio-gmbh.de/. Accessed 11 Oct 2025.
5. Dörre S. Epistemologische Neupositionierungen. Alexander Mitscherlich zwischen „naturwissenschaftlicher Methodik", Psychoanalyse und Psychosomatischer Medizin [Shifts in Epistemological Position. Alexander Mitscherlich's Plea for Psychosomatic Medicine]. NTM. 2021;29(4):417–46. German. https://doi.org/10.1007/s00048-021-00318-3. Epub 2021 Nov 10. PMID: 34757447; PMCID: PMC8608775.
6. Schmid-Schwap M, Simma-Kletschka I, Stockner A, Sengstbratl M, Gleditsch J, Kundi M, Piehslinger E. Oral acupuncture in the therapy of craniomandibular dysfunction syndrome—a randomized controlled trial. Wien Klin Wochenschr. 2006;118(1–2):36–42. https://doi.org/10.1007/s00508-005-0501-1. PMID: 16489524.
7. Joint recommendations for the promotion and implementation of patient education based on Section 43(1)(2) of the German Social Code, Book V (SGB V) dated 8 February 2017, as amended on 1 February 2022. https://www.gkv-spitzenverband.de/media/dokumente/krankenversicherung_1/rehabilitation/patientenschulung/2022_03_16_GE_Patientenschulung_Allgemeiner_Teil.pdf. Accessed 11 Oct 2025.
8. Amiri S, Mahmood N, Javaid SF, Khan MA. The effect of lifestyle interventions on anxiety, depression and stress: a systematic review and meta-analysis of randomised clinical trials. Healthcare (Basel). 2024;12(22):2263. https://doi.org/10.3390/healthcare12222263. PMID: 39595461; PMCID: PMC11594078.
9. Yadav RK, Magan D, Mehta N, Sharma R, Mahapatra SC. Efficacy of a short-term yoga-based lifestyle intervention in reducing stress and inflammation: preliminary results. J Altern Complement Med. 2012;18:662–7.
10. Daubenmier JJ, Weidner G, Sumner MD, Mendell N, Merritt-Worden T, Studley J, Ornish D. The contribution of changes in diet, exercise, and stress management to changes in coronary risk in women and men in the multisite cardiac lifestyle intervention programme. Ann Behav Med. 2007;33:57–68.
11. Akpoveta ED, Okpete UE, Byeon H. Sleep disorders and mental health: understanding the cognitive connection. World J Psychiatry. 2025;15(6):105362. https://doi.org/10.5498/wjp.v15.i6.105362. PMID: 40574781; PMCID: PMC12188900.
12. Marx W, Manger SH, Blencowe M, Murray G, Ho FY, Lawn S, Blumenthal JA, Schuch F, Stubbs B, Ruusunen A, Desyibelew HD, Dinan TG, Jacka F, Ravindran A, Berk M, O'Neil A. Clinical guidelines for the use of lifestyle-based mental health care in major depressive disorder: World Federation of Societies for Biological Psychiatry (WFSBP) and Australasian Society of Lifestyle Medicine (ASLM) taskforce. World J Biol Psychiatry. 2023;24(5):333–86. https://doi.org/10.1080/15622975.2022.2112074. Epub 2022 Oct 6. PMID: 36202135; PMCID: PMC10972571.

13. Teasdale SB, Machaczek KK, Marx W, Eaton M, Chapman J, Milton A, Oyeyemi AL, Pelupessy DC, Schuch FB, Gatera G, Ahmed HU, Diatri H, Jidda IM, Gutiérrez-Peláez M, ElShazly M, Fugu MA, Grinko N, Indu PS, Oo SS, Balasubramanian S, et al. Implementing lifestyle interventions in mental health care: third report of the Lancet Psychiatry Physical Health Commission. Lancet Psychiatry. 2025;12(9):700–22. https://doi.org/10.1016/S2215-0366(25)00170-1.
14. Melchart D, Bachmeier BE. Comprehensive lifestyle intervention program "Individual Health Management" (IHM)—an exemplar for complementary medicine. J Transl Sci. 2018;4(3):1–3. https://doi.org/10.15761/JTS.1000221.
15. Melchart D, Löw P, Wühr E, Kehl V, Weidenhammer W. Effects of a tailored lifestyle self-management intervention (TALENT) study on weight reduction: a randomized controlled trial. Diabetes Metab Syndr Obes. 2017;10:235–45. https://doi.org/10.2147/DMSO.S135572. eCollection 2017.

Patient Profile

3

Dieter Melchart and Lara Isabel Jötten

3.1 General Information

Overview

- Referring physicians, catchment areas, health insurance
- Pre-inpatient indication checks (acceptances and rejections)
- Number of inpatients per month and length of stay
- Age and gender distribution
- Self-disclosure of previous illnesses (personal medical history data)
- Duration of complaints in years, progression of complaints, intensity of main complaints
- Diagnoses (Western/Chinese): psychological and somatic
- Previous use of psycho-medical services and sick leave (sick days)
- Subjective assessment of self-efficacy and psycho-social changes
- Subjective causation of illness
- Expectations of the TCM treatment
- Subjective assessment of the current state of health
- Self-motivation and willingness to change
- Anthropometric data/blood pressure

D. Melchart (✉) · L. I. Jötten
Former Head of Competence Centre for Lifestyle Medicine and Naturopathy (CoCoNat), Faculty of Applied Healthcare Sciences, Deggendorf Institute of Technology (DIT), Competence Centre for Lifestyle Medicine and Naturopathy, Bad Kötzting, Germany
e-mail: dieter.melchart@th-deg.de; lara.joetten@th-deg.de

D. Melchart et al. (eds.), *TCM-Klinik Bad Kötzting*,
https://doi.org/10.1007/978-3-032-23307-3_3

3.1.1 Referring Physicians, Catchment Area, Health Insurance, Indication Check, Inpatients Per Month, Length of Stay, Age and Gender Distribution

A comprehensive description of the patient profile initially includes general information about the referring doctors, the catchment areas of the patients admitted in 2023 and their health insurance companies.

Table 3.1 shows that around 76% of patients in the reporting year were referred to the TCM-Klinik Bad Kötzting by general practitioners, internists and psychiatrists. The vast majority of referring doctors are conventional medical practitioners and not alternative therapists. As some referring physicians may have several specialties, multiple answers are possible. A total of 1666 people requested admission to the clinic during the reporting period (Tables 3.1 and 3.2). After a comprehensive pre-inpatient medical assessment, 1211 patients (72.7%) received approval for inpatient admission.

Table 3.3 provides information on the various reasons that led to inpatient inquiries being rejected as well as general criteria for an inpatient commitment.

The most common reason for exclusion from inpatient treatment in 2023 was unrealistic treatment goals that were not further justified by the assessing physicians.

Of the 1211 inpatient commitments, only 825 patients were admitted to the TCM-Klinik Bad Kötzting. The discrepancy is mainly due to refusals by health insurance companies or—in individual cases—spontaneous rejection of the applicant's personal wish for admission. The clinic was thus 78% occupied in 2023

Table 3.1 Referring physicians in 2023; sorted in descending order of frequency

Referring physician	2023 Number of physicians	Referring physician	2023 Number of physicians
General medicine	440	Palliative medicine	6
Internist Cardiology	114	Diabetologist	6
Psychiatry/ Psychotherapy	79	No briefing	4
Neurology and psychiatry	47	Gynecology	3
Naturopathy	18	Trauma surgery	2
Psychosomatics	13	Hematology	2
Homeopathy	12	Chirotherapy	2
Orthopedist	11	Rheumatology	2
Acupuncture	10	Surgery	2
Sports medicine	10	Neurology	2
Anesthesiologist	10	Physical and rehabilitative medicine	1
General practitioner	9	Nephrology	1
Emergency medicine	8		
Internal medicine	8	Gastroenterology	1
Neurologist	7	Cardiology	1
Pain therapy	7	Spa/spa doctor	1
		Total	**839**[a]

[a]Multiple entries due to specialist and additional designations of the referring physicians

Table 3.2 Requests and rejections due to preclinical indication clarification in 2023

	n	%
Total inquiries	**1666**	100
Stationary commitments	1211	72.7
Outpatient commitments	–	–
Total commitments	1211[a]	–
Cancellation 1 (stationary cancellation)	146	32.1
Cancellation 2a (inpatient cancellation, but outpatient recommendation)	94	20.7
Refusal 2b (no outpatient recommendation, as not psychiatric, but physical causes)	22	4.8
Cancellation 2c (no outpatient recommendation, as not required)	9	2.0
Outstanding requests for findings	138	30.3
Documents returned to patient (without examination)	46	10.1
Total cancellations	**455**	**100**

[a]These included 260 insured persons AOK Bayern and 293 insured persons from TKK

Table 3.3 List of the various reasons that led to an inpatient rejection (top); sorted in descending frequency and various criteria for an inpatient commitment (bottom); without frequency designation

14 possible reasons for rejection	***n* of patients**
Unrealistic therapy goals	50
Presumed resistance to therapy	32
Severe affective disorder	12
Extreme food intolerances/allergies	9
Eating disorders	8
Addictive disorders	5
Psychoses and severe personality disorders	4
Severe neurotic disorders and stress	4
severe obesity	3
Dementia and organic brain psychosyndromes	2
Without somatic complaints	1
Manias	1
Danger to yourself and others	1
Ongoing pension proceedings	0
18 Criteria for stationary commitment	
Outpatient, day-care, home-care measures exhausted	
Acute deterioration due to critical life events	
Lack of effectiveness or standstill of previous therapies	
Structured intervention is intended to provide further care (e.g. due to lack of insight into the illness, etc.)	
Incompatibility of a classic psychotherapeutic medication treatment	
Condition threatens to deteriorate if no other measures are taken	
Previous successful treatment at the TCM clinic	
Removal from the home environment is necessary	
Particularly high level of suffering (acute symptomatology)	
The clinical picture of a chronic disease worsens significantly	
Inpatient treatment of concomitant diseases	
Impending chronification despite ongoing outpatient treatment	
The ability to work is at risk	
Multimorbidity with further diagnostic and therapeutic co-treatment	
Severe symptoms require intensive intervention	
Intensive conflict management is necessary on an inpatient basis	
Massive restrictions in everyday life	
High mental and/or physical instability	

(with 81 available beds and an average stay of 4 weeks). The overall bed occupancy rate in 2019 (before coronavirus) was 77.2% of all hospital beds in Bavaria. In 2022, the hospital had an occupancy of 730 patients.

The TCM clinic is one of the contract hospitals in Bavaria with a care contract with the state associations of health insurance companies and is listed in the Bavarian Hospital Plan 2023. 94% of the patients documented in 2023 are insured by a statutory health insurance fund, the majority by TKK (27.7%), AOK Bayern (24.2%) and Barmer (5.3%). A further 5.2% are covered by private or subsidized insurance. Only 0.5% are self-paying patients (Table 3.4). The majority of patients come from statutory health insurance funds due to the existing care contract, which stipulates that private patients should be limited to less than 10%.

Table 3.4 Types of insurance for inpatients in 2023; sorted in descending order of frequency

Health insurance	*n*	%	Health insurance	*n*	%
Techniker Krankenkasse	231	27.7	BKK Pronova	3	0.4
AOK Bayern	202	24.2	BKK R+V/West	3	0.4
BARMER	44	5.3	SBK/West	3	0.4
Private/aid	43	5.2	BG ETEM Nuremberg	2	0.2
DAK	34	4.1	BKK BAHN/West	2	0.2
Siemens company health insurance	19	2.3	BKK Deutsche Bank/West	2	0.2
AOK Saxony	18	2.2	BKK Energie/West	2	0.2
BKK Faber-Castell & Partner	18	2.2	BKK Gildemeister Seidensticker	2	0.2
Mobile health insurance	16	1.9	BKK SBH	2	0.2
AOK Baden-Württemberg	15	1.8	BKK Verkehrsbau Union	2	0.2
KKH	14	1.7	BKK Werra-Meissner	2	0.2
BKK Securvita/West	13	1.6	AOK Berlin	1	0.1
IKK classic	12	1.4	AOK Lower Saxony	1	0.1
mhplus BKK Königswinter	12	1.4	Companion	1	0.1
BKK Audi	10	1.2	BG for SVLFG BG benefits	1	0.1
AOK Westfalen-Lippe Detmold	9	1.1	BGHW	1	0.1
HKK	7	0.8	BKK Bertelsmann/East	1	0.1
BKK BMW/West	6	0.7	BKK Die Continentale/West	1	0.1
BKK 24/West	5	0.6	BKK Linde/West	1	0.1
BKK Bosch/West	5	0.6	BKK NOVITAS/West	1	0.1
LKK North Rhine-Westphalia	5	0.6	BKK Pfalz/ West	1	0.1
AOK Rheinland	4	0.5	BKK PwC	1	0.1
AOK Saxony-Anhalt	4	0.5	BKK Salus/West	1	0.1
BKK Akzo Nobel Bavaria	4	0.5	BKK Scheufelen	1	0.1
BKK atlas ahlmann	4	0.5	BKK Technoform	1	0.1
BKK KRONES	4	0.5	BKK VDN/West	1	0.1
BKK ProVita/West	4	0.5	BKK VOR ORT/West	1	0.1
BKK VerbundPlus	4	0.5	BKK Würth/West	1	0.1
HEK	4	0.5	BKK ZF & Partner/West	1	0.1
Self-payer	4	0.5	THE BERGISCHE KK	1	0.1
AOK Hessen	3	0.4	Military welfare Hamburg	1	0.1
AOK Rhineland-Palatinate	3	0.4	IKK Saxony	1	0.1
BIG Health, West	3	0.4	Miners' insurance	1	0.1
BKK Debeka/West	3	0.4			
Total health insurance				**786**	**94.4**
Private/aid				**43**	**5.2**
Self-payer				**4**	**0.5**
Total[a]				**833**	**100**

[a]Multiple answers possible due to repeated hospital stays and supplementary insurance

Demographic Characteristics

The basis for the description of the patient profile for the reporting period 2023 is based on all inpatients documented with an admission date between 1 January and 31 December 2023. The starting point for the evaluation by CoCoNat is the VITERIO® documentation system. The annual list of inpatients is synchronized with the list from the ITR clinic documentation system.

The list for the year 2023 contains 825 entries. A detailed inspection of the data showed that 6 patients each had 2 inpatient stays in 2023. For the following analysis, the last stay with complete data records was considered. Of the 825 patients available for analysis, two had no data entries for the questionnaires (inpatient stay was only 1 day).

Figure 3.1 shows the number of patients admitted each month. As in previous years, there was a decrease in the number of admissions in December, which can be attributed to the holidays and family time at Christmas.

The average length of hospital stay in 2023 is 27 days (SD = 2.4). The distribution in Fig. 3.2 shows that most patients stay in hospital for 27 days ($n = 310$, 37.6%) or 28 days ($n = 388$, 47.0%). Only a few patients stayed in hospital for significantly less than 4 weeks. The longest stay was 35 days and two people left the clinic after only 1 day.

The length of hospital stay varies only slightly over the year (Table 3.5). The median varies between 27 and 28 days. On average, 69 patients are admitted to the clinic each month.

79.4% of patients are female and the average age across both genders is 55.1 years (SD = 11.6). The feminization of complementary medicine is typical for Germany, with women making up the majority of consumers in this field. The mean age of men and women differs only slightly. The frequency distribution in the individual age groups also differs only marginally when comparing the two genders. The lowest proportion of patients is represented in the two age groups up to 40 years and over 70 years. Patients aged between 51 and 60 are the most common (Table 3.6).

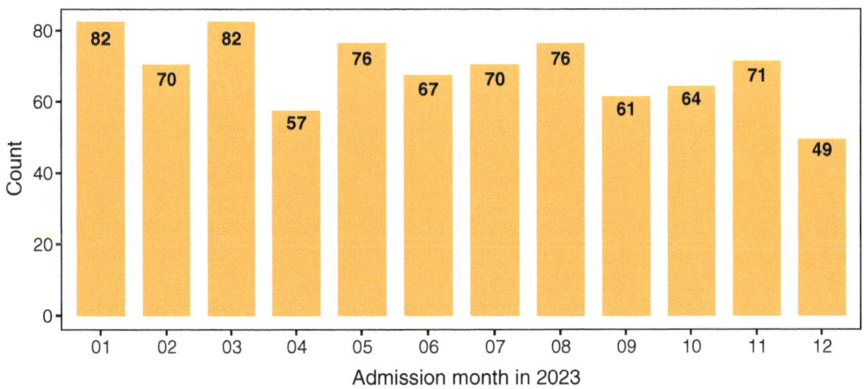

Fig. 3.1 Patients admitted as inpatients per month in 2023 ($n = 825$)

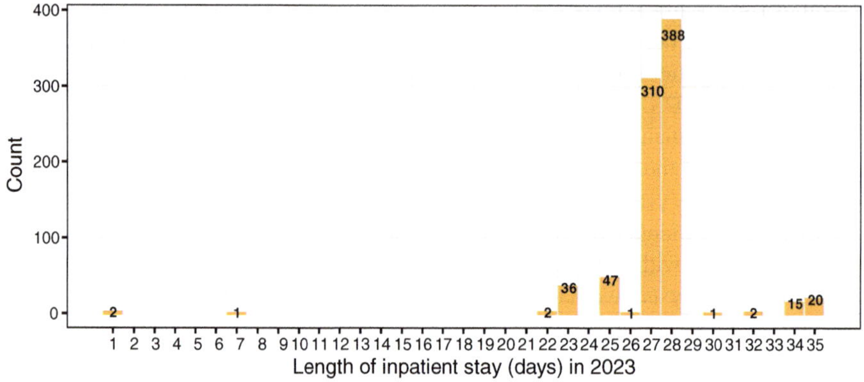

Fig. 3.2 Length of inpatient stay in days of patients in 2023 ($n = 825$)

Table 3.5 The number of patients and the median length of stay broken down by month in 2023 ($n = 825$) compared to previous years; M = mean, SD = standard deviation

	2023				Previous years			
Month	*n*	Median	M	SD	*n*	Median	M	SD
1	82	28.0	27.4	1.2	1129	27	25.3	5.1
2	70	27.0	27.4	1.8	991	27	25.3	6.0
3	82	28.0	28.7	3.2	1081	27	25.5	5.1
4	57	27.0	27.5	2.2	1070	27	26.1	10.7
5	76	27.0	28.1	2.6	1040	27	25.3	4.8
6	67	28.0	27.3	1.3	964	27	25.6	4.7
7	70	27.5	27.2	1.7	1095	27	25.6	4.1
8	76	27.0	26.9	2.7	1176	27	25.3	5.2
9	61	27.0	27.3	1.8	1141	27	25.4	4.8
10	64	28.0	27.1	1.4	1147	27	25.7	4.3
11	71	28.0	26.5	4.6	1032	27	25.8	7.9
12	49	27.0	27.2	1.0	516	27	25.8	8.4
Total	**825**	**28.0**	**27.4**	**2.4**	**12,382**	**27**	**25.5**	**6.1**

Table 3.6 The age structure of inpatients in 2023 ($n = 825$) and previous years ($n = 13250$), broken down by gender and age group

	2023						Previous years					
	Male		Female		Total		Male		Female		Total	
Age distribution	*n*	%	*n*	%	*n*	%	*n*	%	*n*	%	*n*	%
Up to 30 years	9	5.3	17	2.6	26	3.2	171	4.9	452	4.6	623	4.7
31–40 years	17	10.0	55	8.4	72	8.7	258	7.4	745	7.6	1003	7.6
41–50 years	23	13.5	100	15.2	123	14.9	708	20.3	2194	22.5	2902	21.9
51–60 years	70	41.2	301	46.0	371	45.0	112	31.9	3215	36.0	4624	34.9
61–70 years	38	22.4	127	19.4	165	20.0	740	21.2	1835	18.8	2575	19.4
over 70 years	13	7.6	55	8.4	68	8.2	502	14.4	1021	10.5	1523	11.5
Total	**170**	**100**	**655**	**100**	**825**	**100**	**3491**	**100**	**9759**	**100**	**13,250**	**100**
Age M (SD)	**54.6 (12.6)**		**55.2 (11.3)**		**55.1 (11.6)**		**55.6 (13.6)**		**54.4 (12.7)**		**54.7 (12.9)**	

Table 3.7 Incapacity of patients to work in 2023 and previous years due to their main complaint

In the past 6 months, have you had to leave the hospital because of your sickness from time to time?

Incapacity for work (IFW)		2023 In the past 6 months before admission $n = 821$		2022 In the past 6 months before admission $n = 725$		Previous years In the past 6 months before admission $n = 11915$	
		n	%	*n*	%	*n*	%
	Not gainfully employed	305	37.1	218	30.1	4402	36,9
	Employed	**516**	**62.9**	507	69.9	7513	63.1
Of which[a]	Yes, with IFW	**432**	**83.7**	**400**	**78.9**	**5677**	**75.6**
	Up to 1 month	196	50.8	185	50.8	3064	57.7
	Up to 2 months	27	7.0	28	7.7	626	11.8
	Up to 3 months	20	5.2	20	5.5	334	6.3
	Up to 4 months	22	5.7	29	8.0	339	6.4
	Up to 5 months	5	1.3	14	3.8	170	3.2
	Up to and over 6 months	116	30.1	88	24.2	779	14.7
	Total	**386**	**100**	***364***	***100***	**5312**	**100**
	Missing information on days	46	10.7	*36*	*9.0*	365	6.4
IFW days	Median	30.0		30.0		26.0	
	Mean value (SD)	76.39 (74.17)		73.91 (69.63)		56.52 (62.09)	
	Total of IFW days	29488		26905		300598	

[a]All data that exceeded a sick leave period of 6 months were changed to 183 days

Despite the considerable impairments caused by mental disorders, mental illnesses often go unrecognized or are only diagnosed and treated years after they first occur. In the meantime, the symptoms often become chronic, leading to increased absences from work or early retirement.

Of the 821 patients who stated that they were unable to work due to their main complaint, just under 63% were employed (Table 3.7). The majority of the 516 people in employment, namely 83.7%, stated that they had been unable to work in the past 6 months. Of these, almost half of the patients were unable to work for between 2 and 6 months.

3.1.2 Self-Reported Medical History

To optimize the admission medical examination at the clinic, patients fill in a general medical history questionnaire before they are admitted to the clinic or at the latest during the first few days of their stay.

There is also an option to answer "not known". If this question is answered in the affirmative, two additional questions on medication use and possible activity limitations are activated. Data from a total of 823 patients are available for the evaluation of this personal history in 2023. As can be seen in Table 3.8, the presence of a back

Table 3.8 General health (medical history) of patients in 2023 (n = 823); sorted in descending frequency of the disease present

	2023					
	Yes		No		Unknown	
Disease	*n*	%	*n*	%	*n*	%
Back problems	588	71.4	169	20.5	66	8.0
Allergies/intolerances	498	60.5	205	24.9	120	14.6
Joint/muscle diseases	452	54.9	240	29.2	131	15.9
Nervous/mood disorders	360	43.7	300	36.5	163	19.8
Gastrointestinal diseases	323	39.2	327	39.6	173	21.0
Thyroid diseases	284	34.5	356	43.3	183	22.2
High blood pressure (arterial hypertension)	228	27.7	426	51.8	169	20.5
Vascular diseases	219	26.6	382	46.4	222	27.0
Skin diseases	219	26.6	448	54.4	156	19.0
Eye diseases	199	24.2	462	56.1	162	19.7
Respiratory diseases	183	22.2	450	54.7	190	23.1
Cardiac arrhythmia	133	16.2	464	56.4	226	27.5
Liver and biliary diseases	130	15.8	475	57.7	218	26.5
Dental diseases	125	15.2	536	65.1	162	19.7
Kidney/sexual diseases	104	12.6	516	62.7	203	24.7
Severe oral & ENT diseases	103	12.5	545	66.2	175	21.3
Bone diseases	97	11.8	507	61.6	219	26.6
Infectious diseases	86	10.4	542	65.9	195	23.7
Cancer	84	10.2	590	71.7	149	18.1
Lipometabolic disease	74	9.0	473	57.5	276	33.5
Anaemia/other blood disorders	65	7.9	541	65.7	217	26.4
Other cardiovascular diseases	62	7.5	511	62.1	250	30.4
Other metabolic diseases	61	7.4	490	59.5	272	33.0
Diabetes mellitus	47	5.7	583	70.8	193	23.5
Addictive disorders	32	3.9	681	82.7	110	13.4
Stroke or cerebral haemorrhage	32	3.9	630	76.5	161	19.6
Illnesses in the family	602	73.1	157	19.1	64	7.8

condition is the most reported condition, with 71.4% of patients reporting this, followed by allergies or intolerances (60.5%) and joint/muscle disorders (54.9%). The greatest uncertainty (not known) about whether patients had the condition in question was for possible metabolic and cardiovascular diseases. For both lipo-metabolic diseases and other metabolic diseases, almost 33% of patients chose "not known". For other cardiovascular diseases, the figure was 30%. According to the self-reported medical history, 27.7% of all patients actively suffer from arterial hypertension and 5.7% from known diabetes mellitus.

Table 3.9 shows the additional questions on medication use and possible limitations in daily activities in the presence of a disease. Due to predominant back problems, 71.4% of all patients have limitations in their daily activities. Of these, 32.5% treat their back problems with medication. A similar picture emerges for the reported joint and muscle disorders, which are associated with activity limitations in 78.3% of respondents and are treated with medication in 39.4% of patients. Activity limitations are also documented for bone diseases (55.7%), nervous and mood disorders

(72.8%), respiratory diseases (61.7%) and oral and ENT (ear, nose and throat) diseases (62.1%). Medication use is most frequent among patients with high blood pressure (85.1%), thyroid disorders (70.4%) and diabetes mellitus (63.8%). The spectrum of diseases recorded by the self-report in 2023 largely corresponds to that of the patients at the TCM-Klinik Bad Kötzting in previous years from 2009 to 2022 (→ Table 3.9).

Table 3.9 General health in 2023 (n = 823) and previous years (fluctuating number per item, n ˜ 10,000); percentages for medication use and activity restrictions in relation to the number of people with the disease; sorted in descending order of frequency of the disease present in 2023

	2023						Previous years (2009–2022)					
	Yes		No		Unknown		Yes		No		Unknown	
Disease	*n*	%	*n*	%	*n*	%	*n*	%	*n*	%	*n*	%
Back problems	588	71.4	169	20.5	66	8.0	7114	72.2	2300	23.4	435	4.4
If yes, medication?	191	32.5	384	65.3	13	2.2	2573	36.5	4367	62.0	105	1.5
If yes, activity restricted?	420	71.4	154	26.2	14	2.4	4851	69.1	2070	29.5	100	1.4
Allergies/intolerances	498	60.5	205	24.9	120	14.6	5348	54.3	3303	33.5	1197	12.2
If yes, medication?	89	17.9	400	80.3	9	1.8	1073	20.3	4127	78.2	80	1.5
If yes, activity restricted?	149	29.9	333	66.9	16	3.2	1551	29.6	3567	68.0	124	2.4
Joint/muscle diseases	452	54.9	240	29.2	131	15.9	5473	55.6	3273	33.3	1094	11.1
If yes, medication?	178	39.4	266	58.8	8	1.8	2439	45.1	2894	53.5	79	1.5
If yes, activity restricted?	354	78.3	93	20.6	5	1.1	4097	76.0	1212	22.5	85	1.6
Nervous/mood disorders	360	43.7	300	36.5	163	9.8	3730	37.9	4663	47.4	1447	14.7
If yes, medication?	200	55.6	157	43.6	3	0.8	1897	51.3	1759	47.6	39	1.1
If yes, activity restricted?	262	72.8	89	24.7	9	2.5	2248	61.3	1333	36.3	87	2.4
Gastrointestinal diseases	323	39.2	327	39.6	173	21.0	3699	37.1	4806	48.2	1460	14.7
If yes, medication?	124	38.4	193	59.8	6	1.9	1674	45.6	1945	53.0	50	1.4
If yes, activity restricted?	168	52.0	143	44.3	12	3.7	1552	42.6	1997	54.8	96	2.6
Thyroid disease	284	34.5	356	43.3	183	22.2	3342	33.9	4894	49.7	1619	16.4
If yes, medication?	200	70.4	76	26.8	8	2.8	2338	70.4	953	28.7	30	0.9
If yes, activity restricted?	59	20.8	203	71.5	22	7.7	505	15.4	2595	79.0	186	5.7
High blood pressure (arterial hypertension)	228	27.7	426	51.8	169	20.5	2931	29.3	5669	56.7	1406	14.1
If yes, medication?	194	85.1	29	12.7	5	2.2	2434	83.4	463	15.9	23	0.8
If yes, activity restricted?	85	37.3	126	55.3	17	7.5	800	27.6	1967	67.9	130	4.5
Vascular diseases	219	26.6	382	46.4	222	27.0	2648	26.5	5337	53.5	1998	20.0
If yes, medication?	53	24.2	158	72.1	8	3.7	554	21.1	2010	76.7	56	2.1
If yes, activity restricted?	71	32.4	132	60.3	16	7.3	653	25.0	1870	71.5	94	3.6

(continued)

Table 3.9 (continued)

Disease	2023						Previous years (2009–2022)					
	Yes		No		Unknown		Yes		No		Unknown	
	n	%	*n*	%	*n*	%	*n*	%	*n*	%	*n*	%
Skin diseases	219	26.6	448	54.4	156	19.0	2491	25.4	6111	62.2	1224	12.5
If yes, medication?	51	23.3	158	72.1	10	4.6	627	25.5	1785	72.6	46	1.9
If yes, activity restricted?	55	25.1	151	68.9	13	5.9	666	27.2	1731	70.7	50	2.0
Eye diseases	199	24.2	462	56.1	162	19.7	2193	22.3	6120	62.3	1515	15.4
If yes, medication?	57	28.6	135	67.8	7	3.5	617	28.4	1519	70.0	33	1.5
If yes, activity restricted?	88	44.2	104	52.3	7	3.5	728	33.8	1368	63.6	56	2.6
Respiratory diseases	183	22.2	450	54.7	190	23.1	2294	23.1	6145	61.8	1508	15.2
If yes, medication?	85	46.4	90	49.2	8	4.4	1054	46.3	1181	51.9	42	1.8
If yes, activity restricted?	113	61.7	62	33.9	8	4.4	1187	52.3	1019	44.9	64	2.8
Cardiac arrhythmia	133	16.2	464	56.4	226	27.5	1645	16.5	6360	63.8	1962	19.7
If yes, medication?	38	28.6	92	69.2	3	2.3	508	31.2	1080	66.3	41	2.5
If yes, activity restricted?	48	36.1	79	59.4	6	4.5	408	25.2	1152	71.1	60	3.7
Liver/bile duct disease	130	15.8	475	57.7	218	26.5	1532	15.4	6428	64.6	1994	20.0
If yes, medication?	27	20.8	99	76.2	4	3.1	199	13.1	1295	85.3	25	1.6
If yes, activity restricted?	32	24.6	91	70.0	7	5.4	286	18.9	1183	78.2	43	2.8
Dental diseases	125	15.2	536	65.1	162	19.7	1515	15.4	6918	70.4	1394	14.2
If yes, medication?	6	4.8	114	91.2	5	4.0	71	4.8	1379	92.4	42	2.8
If yes, activity restricted?	27	21.6	92	73.6	6	4.8	294	19.8	1137	76.7	51	3.4
Kidney/sexual diseases	104	12.6	516	62.7	203	24.7	1324	13.4	6802	69.1	1723	17.5
If yes, medication?	21	20.2	78	75.0	5	4.8	245	18.7	1038	79.2	27	2.1
If yes, activity restricted?	33	31.7	66	63.5	5	4.8	277	21.4	967	74.8	49	3.8
Severe oral/ENT disease	103	12.5	545	66.2	175	21.3	1336	13.6	7123	72.5	1369	13.9
If yes, medication?	33	32.0	65	63.1	5	4.9	289	24.5	866	73.5	24	2.0
If yes, activity restricted?	64	62.1	34	33.0	5	4.9	641	48.9	642	49.0	27	2.1
Bone diseases	97	11.8	507	61.6	219	26.6	1307	13.3	6496	66.2	2016	20.5
If yes, medication?	38	39.2	55	56.7	4	4.1	585	45.5	683	53.1	19	1.5
If yes, activity restricted?	54	55.7	39	40.2	4	4.1	790	61.6	470	36.7	22	1.7
Infectious disease	86	10.4	542	65.9	195	23.7	1313	13.4	6770	69.0	1726	17.6
If yes, medication?	20	23.3	64	74.4	2	2.3	219	17.1	1030	80.5	30	2.3
If yes, activity restricted?	38	44.2	46	53.5	2	2.3	352	27.6	883	69.3	39	3.1
Cancer	84	10.2	590	71.7	149	18.1	814	8.3	7638	77.6	1394	14.2
If yes, medication?	17	20.2	66	78.6	1	1.2	131	16.4	653	81.5	17	2.1
If yes, activity restricted?	31	36.9	52	61.9	1	1.2	253	31.7	520	65.2	25	3.1

(continued)

Table 3.9 (continued)

Disease	2023						Previous years (2009–2022)					
	Yes		No		Unknown		Yes		No		Unknown	
	n	%	*n*	%	*n*	%	*n*	%	*n*	%	*n*	%
Lipometabolic disease	74	9.0	473	57.5	276	33.5	934	9.5	6375	64.9	2520	25.6
If yes, medication?	33	44.6	38	51.4	3	4.1	348	37.7	548	59.4	26	2.8
If yes, activity restricted?	19	25.7	52	70.3	3	4.1	147	16.2	710	78.1	52	5.7
Anaemia/other bleeding disorders	65	7.9	541	65.7	217	26.4	831	8.5	7128	72.6	1864	19.0
If yes, medication?	13	20.0	49	75.4	3	4.6	231	28.3	573	70.2	12	1.5
If yes, activity restricted?	16	24.6	44	67.7	5	7.7	221	27.4	566	70.0	21	2.6
Other cardiovascular diseases	62	7.5	511	62.1	250	30.4	787	8.0	6920	70.4	2124	21.6
If yes, medication?	29	46.8	31	50.0	2	3.2	371	48.1	381	49.4	20	2.6
If yes, activity restricted?	34	54.8	25	40.3	3	4.8	334	43.4	404	52.5	31	4.0
Other metabolic diseases	61	7.4	490	59.5	272	33.0	673	6.9	6631	67.6	2512	25.6
If yes, medication?	21	34.4	37	60.7	3	4.9	263	39.7	385	58.1	15	2.3
If yes, activity restricted?	33	54.1	27	44.3	1	1.6	233	35.4	402	61.0	24	3.6
Diabetes	47	5.7	583	70.8	193	23.5	559	5.6	7780	78.1	1624	16.3
If yes, medication?	30	63.8	15	31.9	2	4.3	353	63.7	190	34.3	11	2.0
If yes, activity restricted?	15	31.9	27	57.4	5	10.6	91	16.7	421	77.4	32	5.9
Stroke, cerebral haemorrhage	32	3.9	630	76.5	161	19.6	316	3.2	8473	85.0	1178	11.8
If yes, medication?	16	50.0	14	43.8	2	6.2	164	52.6	142	45.5	6	1.6
If yes, activity restricted?	10	31.2	22	68.8	–	–	143	45.8	158	50.6	11	3.5
Addiction	32	3.9	681	82.7	110	13.4	330	3.4	8639	87.9	861	8.8
If yes, medication?	1	3.1	31	96.9	–	–	26	8.0	293	90.4	5	1.5
If yes, activity restricted?	7	21.9	25	78.1	–	–	72	22.5	240	75.0	8	2.5
Illnesses in the family	602	73.1	157	19.1	64	7.8	6686	68.2	2418	24.7	700	7.4

3.1.3 Duration of Complaints, Progression of Complaints, Medical-Psychological Utilization and Intensity of the Main Complaints

The questions specifically asked on admission to the clinic are summarized in Tables 3.10, 3.11, 3.12, 3.13, 3.14, and 3.15. Regarding the main complaints (a maximum of two main complaints could be named), patients stated that they had been suffering from them for an average of 10 years (SD = 11.0). The median duration of the main symptoms was approximately 6 years. In 43% of the patients, the symptoms have been present for 10–20 years. This indicates a long duration of chronic symptoms for many patients. Regardless of the length of the complaint, most patients (86.2%) reported that the main complaint had changed since the onset

Table 3.10 Information on the main complaint on admission to hospital, in 2023 ($n = 821$) and in previous years (fluctuating number per item; $n \approx 11865$)

		2023		Previous years	
Main complaint	Years. M (SD)	10.3 (11.0)	Median 6.0	10.6 (11.1)	Median 7.0
		n	%	*n*	%
Main complaint since	Up to 1 year	69	8.4	1622	14.3
	1 to 3 years	169	20.6	2081	18.3
	3 to 6 years	157	19.1	1918	16.9
	6 to 10 years	73	8.9	1963	17.3
	10 to 20 years	169	20.6	2149	18.9
	Over 20 years	184	22.4	1636	14.4
Change since the onset of the disease	Yes	708	86.2	10248	86.4
	No	113	13.8	1618	13.6
If so, how	Stronger	415	58.6	6241	60.9
	Weaker	62	8.8	805	7.9
	Alternating	231	32.6	3198	31.2
Visits to the doctor in the past year	None	32	3.9	455	3.8
	1–3	221	26.9	2466	20.8
	4–10	382	46.5	5076	42.8
	11–25	134	16.3	2464	20.8
	>25	39	4.8	1224	10.3
	I don't know	13	1.6	180	1.5
If yes	Without success	398	50.4	5674	49.8
	Partial success	385	48.8	5479	48.1
	Good success	6	0.8	248	2.2
Hospital visits last year	None	672	81.9	8630	72.8
	1–7 days	74	9.0	1259	10.6
	8–14 days	37	4.5	863	7.3
	3–4 weeks	20	2.4	572	4.8
	> 4 weeks	18	2.2	512	4.3
	I don't know	0	0.0	26	0.2
If yes	Without success	69	46.3	3085	64.5
	Partial success	71	47.7	1416	29.6
	Good success	9	6.0	281	5.9

of the disease. Furthermore, 58.6% stated that the main complaint had worsened over time.

Many patients visited a doctor for outpatient treatment several times in the past year (67.6% had more than three visits). Most visits were unsuccessful or only partially successful. 18.1% of patients reported being admitted to hospital for the treatment of their main complaint in the past year (Table 3.10).

Overall, 71.9% of patients reported having received psychotherapy at least once, and 37.8% of these were undergoing acute treatment at the time of the survey (Table 3.11). Slightly less than half of the patients who had received psychotherapy (43.8%) underwent between 26 and 160 h of therapy. Furthermore, 66.7% of patients either remained with one psychotherapist or changed therapist only once (Table 3.11).

Most patients (75.8%) consider stress or work and stressful life events (72.0%) to be the subjective cause of their symptoms. Heredity (45.8%) and fate (33.2%) were considered slightly less significant. However, only 28.2% of patients

Table 3.11 QS questionnaire, information on the use of psychotherapy on admission to hospital in 2023 (n = 821), and previous years (n = 11865)

		2023		Previous years	
		n	%	*n*	%
Already undergoing psychotherapy?	Yes	590	71.9	6965	58.7
	No	231	28.1	4900	42.3
If yes,	Up to 5	48	8.1	1042	15.0
Total **psychotherapy hours** to date	6–25	167	28.3	2092	30.1
	26–160	259	43.8	2839	40.9
	161–300	69	11.7	641	9.2
	> 300 h	48	8.1	333	4.8
If yes, treated by how many	1	212	36.1	2976	43.5
Psychotherapists/psychiatrists	2	180	30.6	1995	29.2
	3–5	162	27.6	1606	23.5
	6–10	29	4.9	212	3.1
	>10	5	0.9	54	0.8
Currently undergoing psychotherapy?	Yes	310	37.8	3436	29.0
	No	511	62.2	8429	71.0

Table 3.12 QS questionnaire, information on cause of illness on admission to hospital in 2023 (n = 820), and previous years (n = 11863)

		2023		Previous years	
		n	%	*n*	%
Subjective causes for the disease:	Stress/workload	618	75.8	8432	71.1
(multiple answers possible)	Life events	590	72.0	7458	62.9
	Heredity	375	45.8	5323	44.9
	Fate	272	33.2	4091	34.5
	Environment	291	35.5	3869	32.6
	Lifestyle	231	28.2	2986	25.2
	Third-party fault	129	15.7	1791	15.1
	Other	217	26.5	2410	20.3
Number of persons in the **social environment**	None	29	3.5	386	3.3
	1	90	11.0	1703	14.4
	2–3	397	48.5	4935	41.6
	4–6	221	27.0	3300	27.8
	>6	82	10.0	1540	13.0

recognize their own lifestyle as the cause of the disease (Table 3.12). Most patients can be assumed to have a sufficient social environment.

Most patients express a strong belief that treatment at the TCM clinic will help them. Specifically, 62.2% of patients are certain that they can be helped, while 33.6% consider this possible. Only very few patients express a sceptical attitude in this regard (Table 3.13). These figures were also confirmed in previous years' clinic surveys (63.3%/32.9%).

Above all, patients rate their self-esteem (70.3%) and their relationship with their own body (69.9%) as having deteriorated because of the illness. Patients describe a lesser influence of the disease on their assertiveness (54.7% worse/very worse) and on how others perceive them (37.3% worse/very worse). However, these two characteristics remain unaffected for 37.9% (assertiveness) and 56.8% (appreciation) of patients, respectively (Table 3.14).

Table 3.13 Information on the change caused by the disease on admission to hospital in 2023 (n = 819), previous years (n = 11864), and expectations of TCM treatment

		2023 (n = 819)		Previous years[a] (n = 11864)	
Changes due to the disease (A–D):		n	%	n	%
A self-esteem	Very deteriorated	177	21.6	1286	18.2
	Deteriorated	399	48.7	3479	49.3
	Equal	209	25.5	2010	28.5
	Slightly improved	26	3.2	198	2.8
	Very improved	8	1.0	80	1.1
B Relationship to the own body	Very deteriorated	173	21.1	1201	17.0
	Deteriorated	400	48.8	3457	49.0
	Equal	156	19.0	1580	22.4
	Slightly improved	69	8.4	600	8.5
	Very improved	21	2.6	215	3.0
C Assertiveness	Very deteriorated	100	12.2	680	9.6
	Deteriorated	348	42.5	2782	39.4
	Equal	310	37.9	2980	42.3
	Slightly improved	43	5.3	484	6.9
	Very improved	18	2.2	127	1.8
D Appreciation by others	Very deteriorated	53	6.5	391	5.5
	Deteriorated	252	30.8	1852	26.3
	Equal	465	56.8	4381	62.1
	Slightly improved	34	4.2	334	4.7
	Very improved	15	1.8	95	1.3
Belief in help	Yes, for sure	509	62.2	4460	63.3
	Yes, maybe	275	33.6	2321	32.9
	I don't know	28	3.4	220	3.1
	Sceptical	6	0.7	43	0.6
	No	0	0.0	3	0.0

[a]Data from previous years since 2015

Table 3.14 Subjective assessment of current state of health on admission to hospital in 2023 (n = 818) and previous years (n = 11,858)

	On admission in 2023 (n = 818)		For previous years (n = 11,858)	
State of health	n	%	n	%
Excellent	1	0.1	26	0.2
Very good	8	1.0	101	0.9
Good	72	8.8	1462	12.3
Less good	428	52.3	6236	52.6
Bad	309	37.8	4033	34.0
Total	**818**	**100**	**11858**	**100**

On a numerical scale from 0 to 100 (VAS), the intensity of the two main complaints was rated between 68 and 72 points, with a median of 70 (Table 3.15 and Fig. 3.3). These values are slightly higher than the intensity assessments of complaints from around 11,000 patients at the TCM clinic in previous years. Examining the expected discharge values of the patients (29/ or 28/100), the high and unrealistic expectations of TCM effectiveness are confirmed once again, as reflected in previous years' figures.

Table 3.15 Cross-section of average complaint severity and expectations (scaled from 0 to 100) at admission in 2023 and previous years; *M* mean, *SD* standard deviation, *Md* median

	2023				Previous years			
Main complaint strength VAS 1	*n*	**M**	**SD**	**Md**	*n*	**M**	**SD**	**Md**
Admission (recorded value)	821	71.16	18.95	70.00	11,862	66.56	19.26	70.00
Expected discharge value on admission	821	29.32	18.15	30.00	11,864	24.72	17.03	20.00
Secondary complaint strength VAS 2	*n*	**M**	**SD**	**Md**	*n*	**M**	**SD**	**Md**
Admission (recorded value)	821	68.49	21.24	70.00	11,384	59.20	22.91	60.00
Expected discharge value on admission	821	27.69	19.16	20.00	11,383	22.67	17.47	20.00

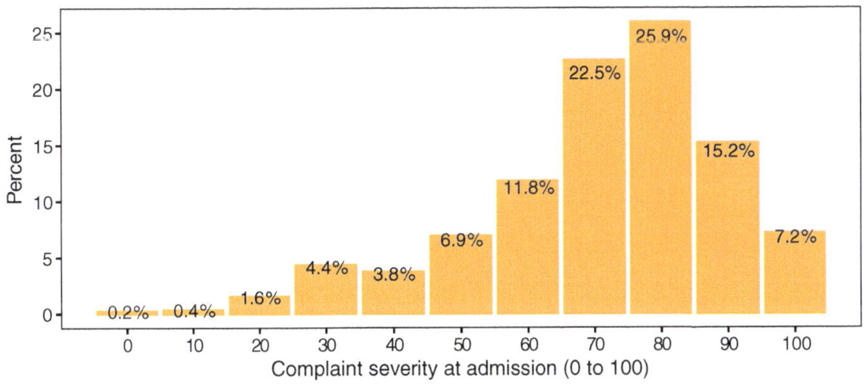

Fig. 3.3 Distribution of the VAS assessments of the main complaint severity (0–100) at hospital admission 2023 ($n = 821$)

3.2 Diagnoses

3.2.1 ICD-10 Diagnoses at the Time of Discharge

Western diagnoses are coded and electronically documented by the doctors at the TCM clinic according to the ICD classification (ICD-10). The individual diagnoses are assigned to different groups according to the ICD-10 chapters, resulting in a total of 21 areas. A distinction is made between the primary mental diagnosis and possibly one or more secondary mental or somatic diagnoses. For the reporting period 2023, diagnoses at the time of discharge can be identified for a total of 825 patients. For previous years, all diagnoses recorded during inpatient stays were included (between 40 days prior and 14 days after discharge). Where differentiation was possible, only discharge diagnoses were used.

Primary and secondary diagnoses are documented for a total of 825 patients. As mentioned above, each of the 825 patients has at least one secondary diagnosis in addition to the primary diagnosis. On average, 8.6 diagnoses (primary and secondary) were documented per patient. This results in more than 7000 coded and documented diagnoses.

The distinction between primary and secondary diagnoses is less important for the medical indication spectrum of the TCM clinic. Rather, it is more relevant to consider the whole range of diagnoses against the background of the predominantly chronically ill and multimorbid patients. From this perspective, group M (diseases of the musculoskeletal system) is just as common as the diseases in chapter F (Figs. 3.4 and 3.5).

If only the mental health diagnoses of the ICD-10-F chapter are considered when examining the primary and secondary diagnoses, somatoform disorders (F45) dominate with 42.0%, followed by recurrent depressive disorders (F33; 20.5%), non-organic sleep disorders (F51; 10.9%), depressive episodes (F32; 7.0%) and reactions to severe stress and adjustment disorders (F43; 6.2%; Fig. 3.6).

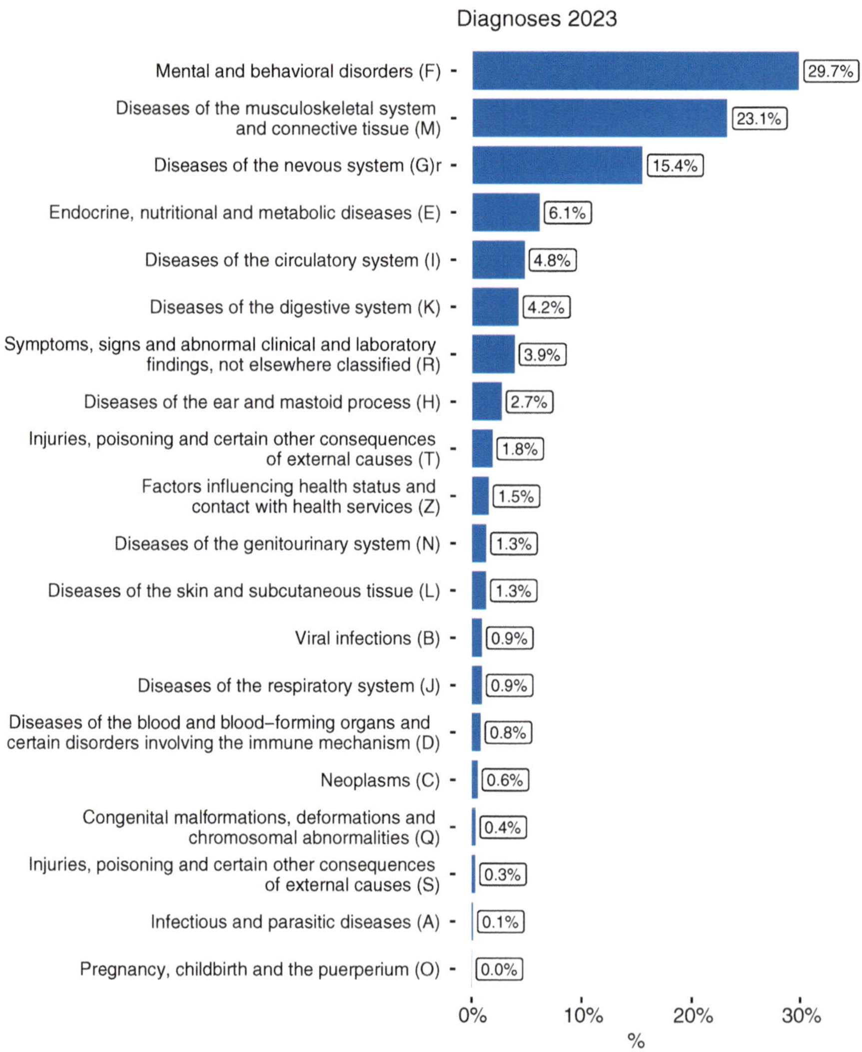

Fig. 3.4 Distribution of all documented primary and secondary diagnoses by ICD chapter code in 2023 ($n = 825$; 7082 diagnoses)

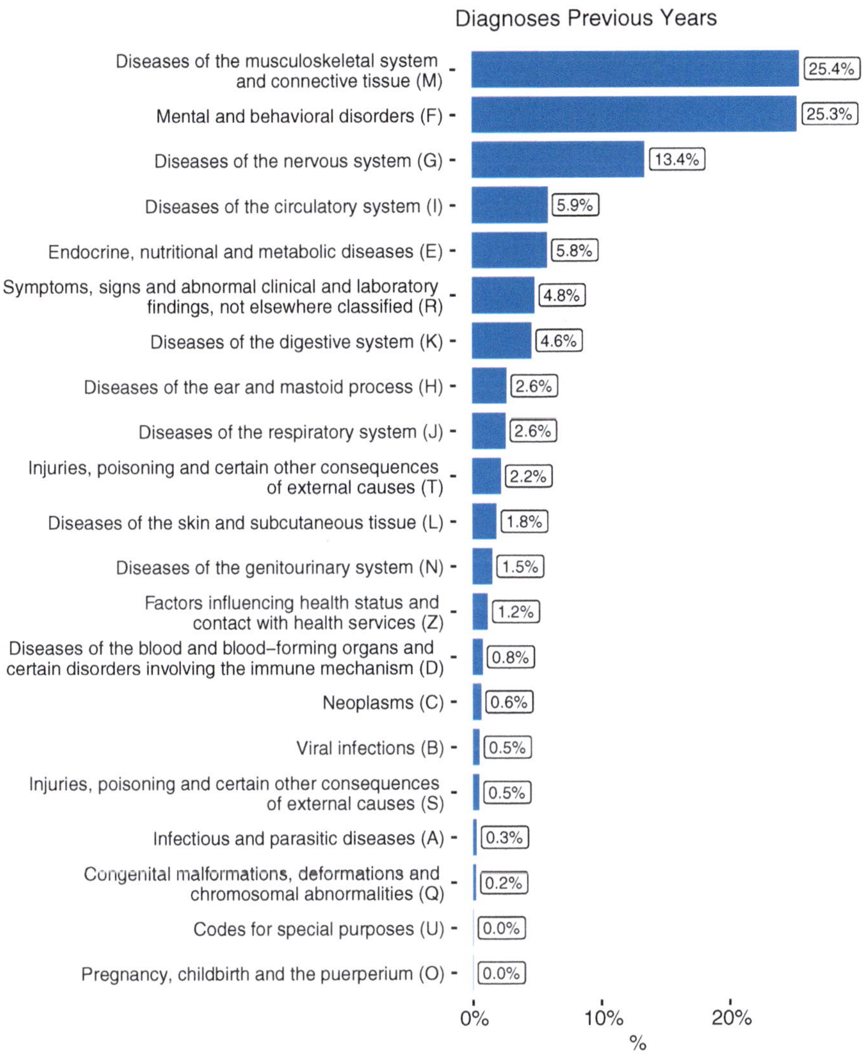

Fig. 3.5 Distribution of all documented principal and secondary diagnoses to the higher-level ICD chapters for the previous years (n = 10,227, 64804 diagnoses)

Compared to previous years, there was a significant increase in the ICD-10 category for depressive patients (F33/F32: 27.5% vs. 22.5%; Figs. 3.6 and 3.7). A detailed overview of all diagnoses documented in 2023 can be found in Tables 3.68 and 3.69 in the Appendix. In addition to the frequency distribution of each primary and secondary diagnosis, the percentage of patients affected is also shown. For the sake of clarity, the ICD-10 diagnoses are sorted by frequency (Appendix Table 3.68) and by organ system of the ICD nomenclature (Appendix Table 3.69).

As the majority of patients in 2023 have more than one diagnosis documented, Table 3.16 shows the frequency of diagnoses per patient, divided into mental

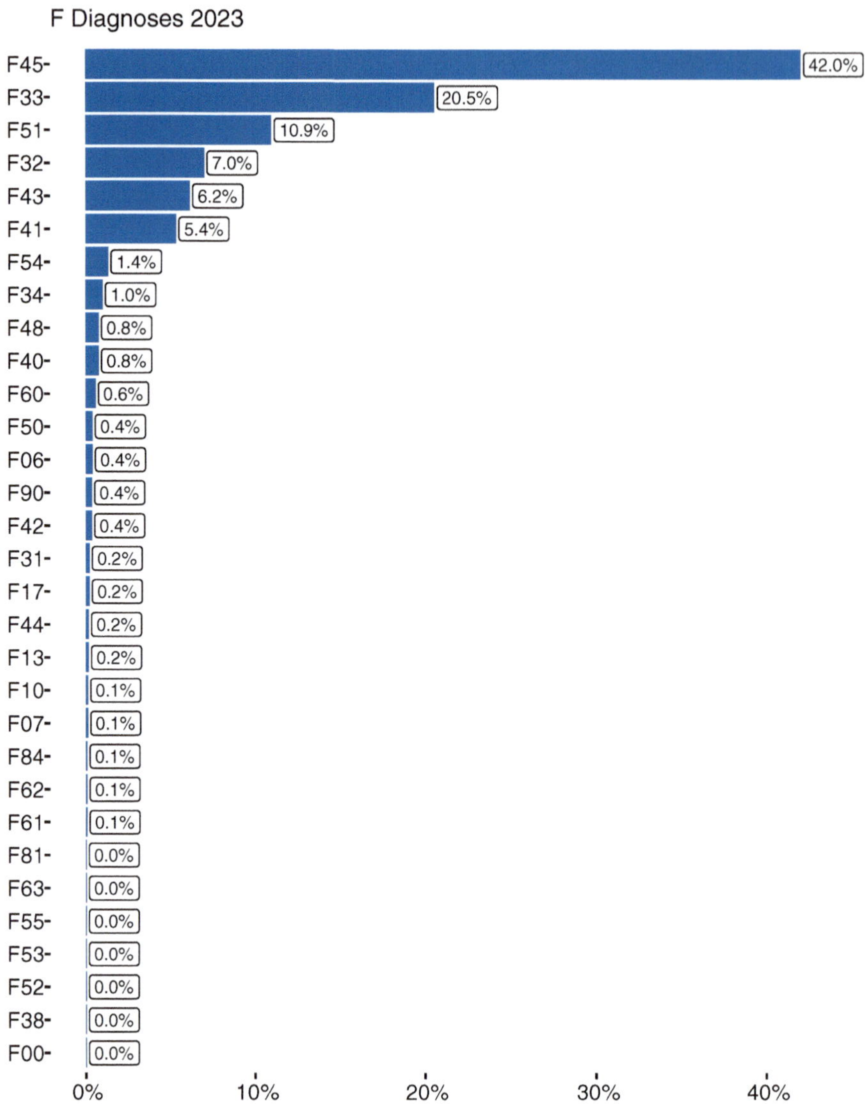

Fig. 3.6 Distribution of all primary and secondary mental health diagnoses (F diagnoses) of patients in 2023 (n = 825; 2106 diagnoses)

diagnoses (1st mental diagnosis, 2nd mental diagnosis, etc.) and somatic diagnoses (1st somatic diagnosis, 2nd mental diagnosis, etc.).

This shows that, in terms of co-morbidity, different diagnoses are often present at the same time. Patients in 2023 are most often diagnosed with between two and three mental health diagnoses. For 54.7% of all patients with somatic diagnoses, six or more somatic diagnoses were documented (Table 3.16). To illustrate these results, the frequency of mental and somatic diagnoses are also compared in a bar chart (Fig. 3.8).

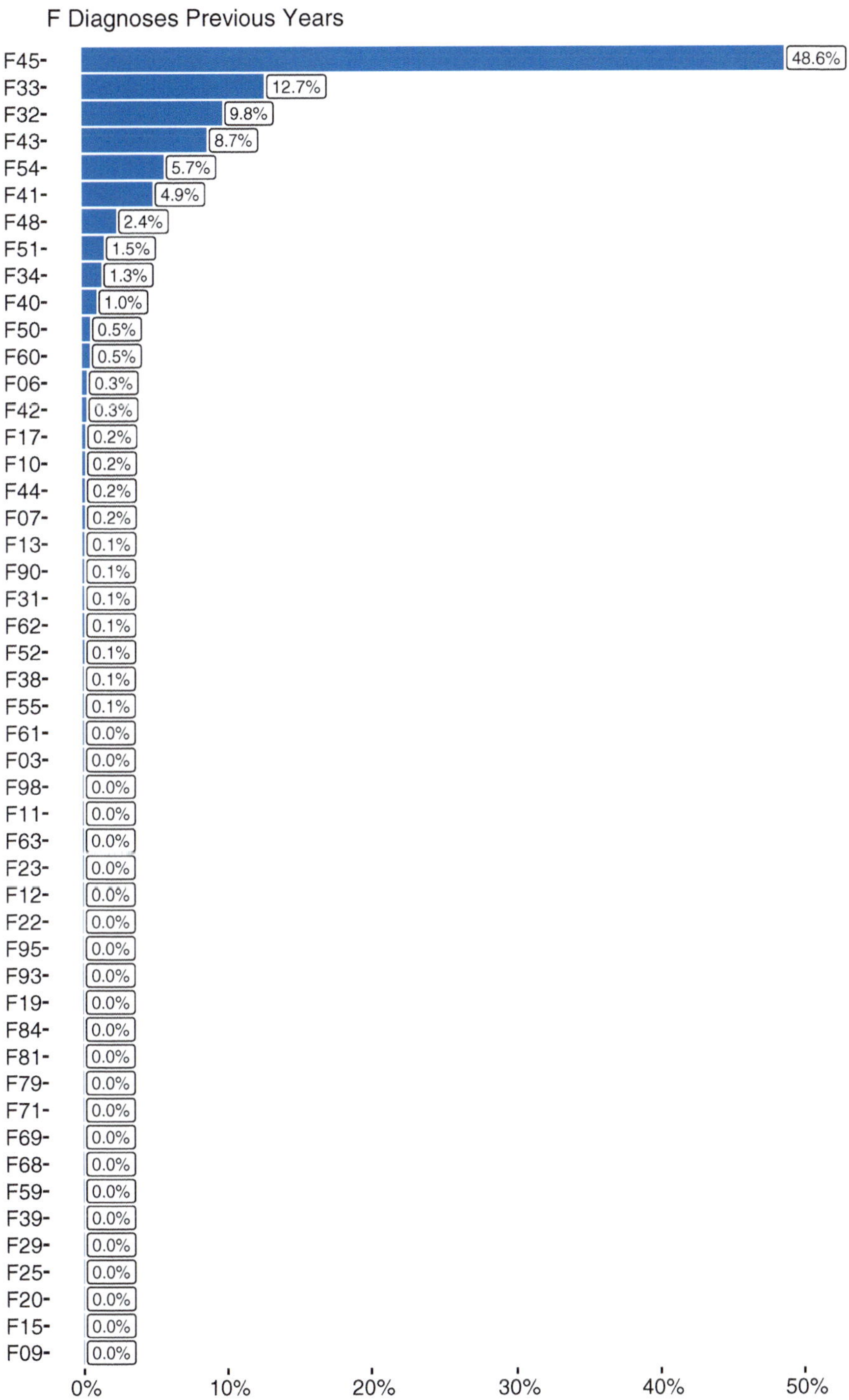

Fig. 3.7 Distribution of the 15 most common main and secondary mental health diagnoses (F diagnoses) in previous years (n = 9207; 16375 diagnoses)

Table 3.16 Frequency of comorbidities broken down by mental and somatic diagnoses of patients in 2023 ($n = 825$) and previous years ($n = 9207/9658$)

	2023				Previous years			
	Mental diagnoses		Somatic diagnoses		Mental diagnoses		Somatic diagnoses	
Frequency	*n*	%	*n*	%	*n*	%	*n*	%
1 diagnosis	125	15.2	6	0.7	4633	50.3	747	7.7
2 diagnoses	328	39.8	35	4.2	3093	33.6	1482	15.3
3 diagnoses	227	27.5	88	10.7	907	9.9	1733	17.9
4 diagnoses	89	10.8	139	16.8	323	3.5	1472	15.2
5 diagnoses	52	6.3	106	12.8	124	1.4	1124	11.6
=6 diagnoses	4	0.5	451	54.7	127	1.4	3100	32.1
Total	**825**	**100**	**825**	**100**	**9207**	**100**	**9658**	**100**

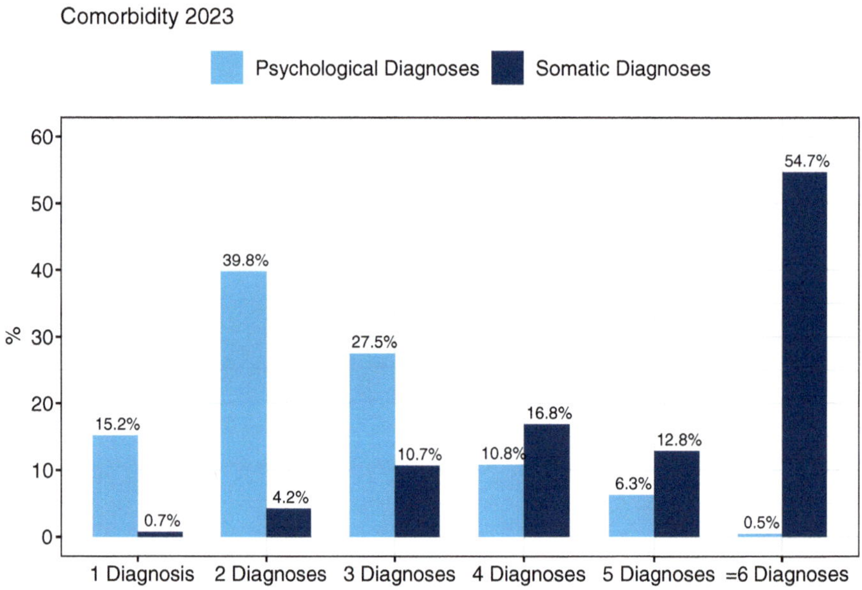

Fig. 3.8 Percentage distribution of the frequency of diagnoses, broken down into psychological ($n = 824$) and somatic ($n = 825$) Diagnoses of patients in 2023

3.2.1.1 Main Diagnoses at the Time of Discharge

The leading group of diagnoses for the main mental health diagnosis are those in ICD Chapter F (mental and behavioural disorders). All patients can be assigned to this group. Within the F category, based on the three-digit ICD codes, most patients fall into the group of somatoform disorders F45 (62.3%), followed by recurrent depressive disorders F33 (25.1%). Next in frequency are depressive episodes F32 (7.3%). There are no clear differences between men and women in the spectrum of main diagnoses (Table 3.17).

Table 3.17 Primary diagnoses (ICD-10 chapter) of patients in 2023 ($n = 825$); separated by gender and sorted by ICD-10 code; for each patient, the last recorded primary F diagnosis was used

		2023					
ICD- 10		Male		Female		Total	
Code	Main diagnosis (ICD-10 chapter) 2023	*n*	%	*n*	%	*n*	%
F31	Bipolar affective disorder	2	1.2	0	–	2	0.2
F32	**Depressive episode**	11	6.5	49	7.5	**60**	**7.3**
F33	**Recurrent depressive disorder**	47	27.6	160	24.4	**207**	**25.1**
F34	Persistent affective disorders	0	–	1	0.2	1	0.1
F40	Phobic disorders	0	–	1	0.2	1	0.1
F41	Other anxiety disorders	0	–	13	2.0	13	1.6
F43	Reactions to severe stress and adaptation faults	3	1.8	15	2.3	18	2.2
F44	Dissociative disorders [conversion disorders]	0	–	1	0.2	1	0.1
F45	**Somatoform disorders**	105	61.8	409	62.4	**514**	**62.3**
F48	Other neurotic disorders	2	1.2	6	0.9	8	1.0
Total		**170**	**100**	**655**	**100**	**825**	**100**

Furthermore, the diagnosis is coded using a more detailed system, which provides two additional digits for further specification after the 3-digit coding. This classification shows that the most documented diagnosis is F45.41 "Chronic pain disorder with somatic and psychological factors", which is reported by 47.9% of patients (Table 3.18). This is followed by recurrent depressive disorder with a current moderate episode in 23.3% of all patients (Table 3.18).

If the mental disorders are categorized as affective disorders, neurotic stress and somatoform disorders or behavioural disorders with physical manifestations, 1/3 of all patients fall into the category of affective disorders and 2/3 of patients into the category of neurotic or somatoform disorders (Table 3.19). Compared with the figures for previous years, there has been a significant increase in affective disorders (32.8% vs. 18.4%).

3.2.1.2 Secondary Diagnoses at the Time of Discharge

The secondary diagnoses recorded are presented below. Table 3.20 describes the mental diagnoses documented as secondary diagnoses in more detail. The 1281 mental diagnoses presented are attributable to a total of 700 patients, meaning that 581 diagnoses are multiple comorbid F-diagnoses. The dominant diagnoses in 2023 were non-organic insomnia (F51.0), chronic pain disorder (F45.41) and recurrent depressive disorder with moderate episode (F33.1).

At least one additional somatic secondary diagnosis was documented for 825 patients. Table 3.21 shows the total of 4976 somatic diagnoses in descending frequency, including only diagnoses that were documented at least three times.

Table 3.18 Main diagnoses (ICD-10 code) of patients in 2023 (n = 825) and previous years (n = 8954, 11010 diagnoses); each sorted in descending frequency of the year 2023 (only ICD codes of the year 2023 are shown)

	2023		Previous years	
ICD-10	*n*	%	*n*	%
F45.41	395	47.9	4427	40.2
F33.1	192	23.3	917	8.3
F32.1	52	6.3	586	5.3
F45.32	38	4.6	238	2.2
F45.40	25	3.0	587	5.3
F45.38	21	2.5	84	0.8
F33.2	12	1.5	18	0.2
F45.37	10	1.2	53	0.5
F43.2	9	1.1	721	6.5
F48.0	8	1.0	212	1.9
F41.1	7	0.8	66	0.6
F43.1	6	0.7	61	0.6
F45.33	6	0.7	71	0.6
F41.2	5	0.6	196	1.8
F45.31	5	0.6	80	0.7
F32.0	4	0.5	154	1.4
F32.2	4	0.5	13	0.1
F33.0	3	0.4	134	1.2
F43.8	3	0.4	94	0.9
F45.0	3	0.4	175	1.6
F45.34	3	0.4	22	0.2
F45.9	2	0.2	56	0.5
F45.1	2	0.2	208	1.9
F31.3	1	0.1	3	0.0
F31.4	1	0.1	1	0.0
F33.4	1	0.1	29	0.3
F34.1	1	0.1	67	0.6
F40.2	1	0.1	10	0.1
F41.0	1	0.1	69	0.6
F44.4	1	0.1	5	0.0
F45.30	1	0.1	24	0.2
F45.39	1	0.1	24	0.2
F45.8	1	0.1	69	0.6

Back pain (M54) is the dominant somatic condition, accounting for 10% of all somatic secondary diagnoses, followed by

- G93 Other diseases of the brain
- M79 Other diseases of soft tissue, not elsewhere classified
- G47 Sleep disorders
- I10 Essential (primary) hypertension
- G44 Other headache syndromes
- H93 Other diseases of the ear, not elsewhere classified
- G43 Other diseases of the brain
- K58 Irritable bowel system
- E03 Other hypothyroidism

Table 3.19 Primary mental health diagnoses (ICD-10 code) in 2023 ($n = 825$) and previous years ($n = 9224$, 11405 diagnoses); sorted by ICD-10 category

		2023		Previous years	
ICD-10 categories diagnoses	Psychological diagnoses	*n*	%	*n*	%
Affective disorders	**F31** Bipolar affective disorder	2	0.2	5	0.0
	F32 Depressive episode	60	7.3	832	7.6
	F33 Recurrent depressive episode	207	25.1	1118	10.2
	F34 Persistent affective disorders	1	0.1	72	0.7
	F38 Other affective disorders	0	0.0	3	0.0
	F39 Unspecified affective disorders	0	0.0	1	0.0
	Total	**270**	**32.8**	**2031**	**18.4**
Neurotic. Stress and somatoform disorders Malfunctions	**F40** Phobic disorders	1	0.1	37	0.3
	F41 Other anxiety disorders	13	1.6	367	3.3
	F42 Specific (isolated) phobias	0	0.0	9	0.1
	F43 Reactions to severe stress and adjustment disorders	18	2.2	935	8.5
	F44 Dissociative disorders	1	0.1	13	0.1
	F45 Somatoform disorders	514	62.3	6347	57.6
	F48 Other neurotic disorders	8	1.0	219	2.0
	Total	**555**	**67.3**	**7927**	**72.0**
Behavioural abnormalities with physical disruptions and factors	**F50** Eating disorders	0	0.0	19	0.2
	F51 Non-organic sleep disorders	0	0.0	83	0.8
	F52 Sexual dysfunction not caused by an organic disorder or illness	0	0.0	1	0.0
	F54 Psychological factors or behavioural factors in other places classified diseases	0	0.0	852	7.7
	F59 Unspecified behavioural abnormalities with physical disruptions and factors	0	0.0	1	0.0
	Total	**0**	**0.0**	**956**	**8.7**
Other	F00-F09, F10-F19, F20-F29, F60-F69, F70-F79, F80-89, F90 F99	0	0.0	96	0.9
Total		**825**	**100**	**11010**	**100**

3.2.2 Diagnoses According to TCM

For 804 of the 825 patients at the TCM clinic in 2023, a diagnosis was documented according to the TCM system and stored in the database. The same is true for pulse and tongue diagnoses. The complex TCM diagnoses are difficult to translate into simple coding. The resulting coding frequency of TCM diagnoses, which reflects more of a trend, is shown in Table 3.22. The coding system was developed in the hospital.

Despite these challenges, work is underway to develop a suitable classification scheme that enables quantitative evaluation while accounting for the complexity of TCM diagnoses. The inclusion of the new ICD-11 classification for TCM syndrome diagnoses (26 Supplementary Chapters of Traditional Medicine Conditions—Module I) is under discussion.

Table 3.20 Psychological secondary diagnoses 2023 (n = 700 of 825; 1281 diagnoses); sorted in descending frequency

ICD-10	*n*	%	ICD-10	*n*	%	ICD-10	*n*	%	ICD-10	*n*	%
F51.0	220	17.2	F06.7	9	0.7	F60.31	3	0.2	F42.8	1	0.1
F45.41	180	14.1	F33.4	9	0.7	F13.1	2	0.2	F42.9	1	0.1
F33.1	160	12.5	F48.0	9	0.7	F41.8	2	0.2	F43.0	1	0.1
F45.32	58	4.5	F45.30	7	0.5	F42.0	2	0.2	F44.6	1	0.1
F33.0	51	4.0	F45.8	7	0.5	F51.1	2	0.2	F44.7	1	0.1
F43.8	48	3.7	F90.0	7	0.5	F60.5	2	0.2	F44.88	1	0.1
F32.1	47	3.7	F40.01	6	0.5	F61	2	0.2	F45.9	1	0.1
F32.0	40	3.1	F40.2	6	0.5	F84.5	2	0.2	F50.1	1	0.1
F45.38	35	2.7	F45.33	6	0.5	F00.1	1	0.1	F50.3	1	0.1
F41.0	34	2.7	F43.9	5	0.4	F07.0	1	0.1	F51.8	1	0.1
F43.1	31	2.4	F60.6	5	0.4	F07.2	1	0.1	F52.2	1	0.1
F54	29	2.3	F17.1	4	0.3	F07.9	1	0.1	F53.0	1	0.1
F43.2	27	2.1	F33.2	4	0.3	F13.2	1	0.1	F60.7	1	0.1
F45.31	27	2.1	F42.1	4	0.3	F13.3	1	0.1	F60.8	1	0.1
F41.2	24	1.9	F50.9	4	0.3	F17.2	1	0.1	F60.9	1	0.1
F34.1	21	1.6	F51.9	4	0.3	F31.3	1	0.1	F62.0	1	0.1
F41.1	20	1.6	F10.1	3	0.2	F31.6	1	0.1	F62.88	1	0.1
F41.9	17	1.3	F40.1	3	0.2	F31.9	1	0.1	F63.3	1	0.1
F45.40	13	1.0	F41.3	3	0.2	F32.2	1	0.1	F81.0	1	0.1
F45.0	11	0.9	F45.34	3	0.2	F33.8	1	0.1	F90.9	1	0.1
F45.1	11	0.9	F50.8	3	0.2	F38.1	1	0.1			
F45.37	11	0.9	F51.5	3	0.2	F40.8	1	0.1			

Table 3.21 Somatic secondary diagnoses (ICD-10 chapter) of patients in 2023 (n = 825; 4976 diagnoses); sorted in descending frequency; % refer to all documented somatic diagnoses

ICD- 10	*n*	% of all somat. Diagn.	ICD- 10	*n*	% of all somat. Diagn.	ICD- 10	*n*	% of all somat. Diagn.	ICD- 10	*n*	% of all somat. Diagn.
M54	496	10.0	I25	17	0.3	K10	7	0.1	R25	4	0.1
G93	410	8.2	M35	17	0.3	N80	7	0.1	R26	4	0.1
M79	266	5.3	J30	16	0.3	G40	6	0.1	R32	4	0.1
G47	236	4.7	M20	16	0.3	G53	6	0.1	R43	4	0.1
I10	201	4.0	K59	15	0.3	G63	6	0.1	R49	4	0.1
G44	146	2.9	N39	15	0.3	H35	6	0.1	R61	4	0.1
H93	110	2.2	N95	15	0.3	H53	6	0.1	T88	4	0.1
G43	106	2.1	Z96	15	0.3	I44	6	0.1	Z90	4	0.1
K58	104	2.1	H91	14	0.3	K76	6	0.1	Z95	4	0.1
E03	92	1.8	I89	14	0.3	Z92	6	0.1	B00	3	0.1
M53	88	1.8	M48	14	0.3	I11	5	0.1	B27	3	0.1
E66	86	1.7	R06	14	0.3	K64	5	0.1	C34	3	0.1
M25	85	1.7	Z73	14	0.3	L80	5	0.1	D47	3	0.1
T73	79	1.6	C50	13	0.3	M05	5	0.1	D64	3	0.1
E06	67	1.3	E88	13	0.3	M10	5	0.1	D75	3	0.1
M51	56	1.1	E89	13	0.3	M70	5	0.1	D89	3	0.1
E78	55	1.1	G56	13	0.3	M72	5	0.1	E07	3	0.1
G62	51	1.0	H81	13	0.3	M85	5	0.1	E28	3	0.1
M17	47	0.9	K07	13	0.3	R07	5	0.1	E74	3	0.1
M42	46	0.9	K50	13	0.3	R11	5	0.1	E83	3	0.1
M15	45	0.9	M06	13	0.3	R55	5	0.1	G04	3	0.1

(continued)

Table 3.21 (continued)

ICD-10	*n*	% of all somat. Diagn.	ICD-10	*n*	% of all somat. Diagn.	ICD-10	*n*	% of all somat. Diagn.	ICD-10	*n*	% of all somat. Diagn.
M19	45	0.9	D50	12	0.2	R63	5	0.1	G24	3	0.1
R52	44	0.9	M23	12	0.2	B99	4	0.1	G51	3	0.1
B34	40	0.8	M43	12	0.2	E27	4	0.1	G55	3	0.1
T78	39	0.8	H40	11	0.2	E55	4	0.1	G83	3	0.1
E11	35	0.7	I73	11	0.2	E80	4	0.1	H10	3	0.1
R10	35	0.7	J44	11	0.2	G35	4	0.1	H26	3	0.1
R42	34	0.7	E73	10	0.2	G45	4	0.1	H52	3	0.1
M16	32	0.6	I83	10	0.2	G54	4	0.1	H54	3	0.1
M75	32	0.6	Q66	10	0.2	G57	4	0.1	I26	3	0.1
M47	30	0.6	R20	10	0.2	G60	4	0.1	I67	3	0.1
K21	29	0.6	D68	9	0.2	G90	4	0.1	J06	3	0.1
K29	29	0.6	I48	9	0.2	I20	4	0.1	J34	3	0.1
L40	29	0.6	K57	9	0.2	I34	4	0.1	K30	3	0.1
Z98	29	0.6	M76	9	0.2	I63	4	0.1	K74	3	0.1
G25	28	0.6	N18	9	0.2	I69	4	0.1	K80	3	0.1
L20	28	0.6	N30	9	0.2	I70	4	0.1	M22	3	0.1
M18	25	0.5	A69	8	0.2	K90	4	0.1	M24	3	0.1
M62	25	0.5	B02	8	0.2	K91	4	0.1	M65	3	0.1
M81	25	0.5	E79	8	0.2	L30	4	0.1	M84	3	0.1
J32	24	0.5	K52	8	0.2	L50	4	0.1	M94	3	0.1
M77	24	0.5	M07	8	0.2	L70	4	0.1	N19	3	0.1
R51	24	0.5	M21	8	0.2	M13	4	0.1	N83	3	0.1
M41	23	0.5	M32	8	0.2	M71	4	0.1	Q44	3	0.1
G50	22	0.4	M40	8	0.2	M80	4	0.1	R14	3	0.1
K51	22	0.4	M45	8	0.2	M93	4	0.1	R27	3	0.1
M99	22	0.4	N40	8	0.2	M96	4	0.1	R45	3	0.1
Z88	21	0.4	R12	8	0.2	N32	4	0.1	S22	3	0.1
E04	19	0.4	I47	7	0.1	Q65	4	0.1	S83	3	0.1
R53	19	0.4	I49	7	0.1	R00	4	0.1	T65	3	0.1
M50	18	0.4	I87	7	0.1	R05	4	0.1	Z85	3	0.1

Table 3.23 shows the 15 most common combinations of TCM diagnoses. The combination of Liver-Qi stagnation, Spleen-Qi weakness and stasis in general is the most common at 3.6%, followed by the combination of stasis in general and dampness (3.2%).

According to traditional Chinese medicine (TCM) teachings, long-lasting or suppressed anger and frustration can block the flow of liver Qi. Disruptions to the smooth flow of this life energy can lead to emotional and physical issues, such as a feeling of tightness in the chest. It is the most common syndrome pattern in patients suffering from depressive symptoms. This is consistent with ICD-10 Western diagnoses.

Table 3.22 Frequency of documented TCM syndrome diagnoses in the 2023 reporting year (n = 804; 2284 TCM diagnoses); sorted in descending frequency

Code	TCM syndrome diagnoses	n
175	Stasis in general	630
208	Liver Qi stagnation	312
491	Spleen Qi deficiency	224
91	Moisture	143
513	Moisture (wetness) stagnation	134
266	Kidney Qi deficiency	102
506	Spleen-kidney-Qi deficiency	85
569	Slime wetness	73
224	Liver and kidney yin deficiency	54
430	Humidity (wetness)-cold	53
564	Slime	40
353	Liver-stomach disharmony	37
50	Heart-spleen Qi deficiency	36
307	Humidity (wetness)-heat	30
516	Lung-spleen Qi deficiency	30
109	Qi stagnation	29
170	Blood deficiency	20
289	Lung Qi deficiency	17
216	Liver yin weakness	16
273	Kidney yin deficiency	16
38	Heart-blood deficiency	15
102	Qi Yin deficiency	14
107	Liver-spleen disharmony	12
226	Qi weakness	12
200	Yin weakness	11
124	Cold-humidity stagnation	9
427	Wind-chill	9
557	Bi-syndrome	8
220	Rising liver yang	7
121	Liver Qi attacks the stomach	6
230	Wind-heat	6
52	Bubble-wetness (moisture)-heat	5
182	Heart-kidney disharmony	5
218	Cold blood stasis	5
228	Liver-blood deficiency	5
271	Liver fire	5
362	Gastrointestinal wetness heat	5
576	Kidney yang deficiency	5
36	Heart yin deficiency	4
119	Stomach Qi deficiency	4
344	Wind	4
94	Outbreak of internal wind of the liver	3
212	Gallbladder heat	3
267	Heat (endogenous)	3
309	Lack of bodily fluids	3
372	Lung-kidney-yin deficiency	3
396	Spleen yang weakness	3
496	Kidney essence deficiency	3
101	Heat in the colon	2
233	Liver fire rises	2

(continued)

Table 3.22 (continued)

Code	TCM syndrome diagnoses	n
391	Qi blood deficiency	2
608	Wind-dryness	2
11	Attack of wind-chill on the lungs	1
32	Intestinal dryness-constipation	1
40	Moisture and heat in the liver and gallbladder	1
48	Gallbladder deficiency	1
234	Heart is attacked by slime fire	1
293	Heart-blood stasis	1
297	Heart fire rises	1
329	Heart Qi deficiency	1
349	Cold (cold syndrome)	1
351	Cold in the colon	1
355	Gastrointestinal disharmony	1
360	Stomach heat (fire)	1
363	Stomach Qi rises	1
373	Stomach Yin deficiency	1
395	Spleen cannot control the blood	1
490	Spleen-stomach disharmony	1
530	Mucus moisture in the lungs	1
566	Mucus heat in the lungs	1
Total		**2284**

Table 3.23 The most frequent combinations of TCM syndrome diagnoses in the 2023 reporting year ($n = 804$; 2284 TCM diagnoses); sorted in descending frequency

Diagnosis combinations	n	%
Liver Qi stagnation, spleen Qi deficiency, stasis in general	29	3.6
Stasis in general, moisture	26	3.2
Moisture (wetness)-stagnation, stasis in general	20	2.5
Liver Qi stagnation, spleen Qi deficiency stasis in general, dampness	20	2.5
Spleen-kidney-Qi deficiency, stasis in general	16	2.0
Spleen-kidney-Qi deficiency, liver-Qi stagnation, stasis in general	15	1.9
Stasis in general, moisture (wetness)-stagnation	14	1.7
Liver Qi stagnation, stasis in general	13	1.6
Liver Qi stagnation, spleen Qi deficiency	12	1.5
Liver and kidney yin deficiency	11	1.4
Liver Qi stagnation, spleen Qi weakness, dampness (wetness) stagnation, stasis in general	11	1.4
Liver Qi stagnation, kidney Qi deficiency, stasis in general, dampness	10	1.2
Liver and kidney yin deficiency, stasis in general	9	1.1
Mucus wetness, stasis in general	9	1.1
Stasis in general, mucus	9	1.1

3.2.3 Self-Motivation and Willingness to Change

The questionnaire on motivation (Table 3.24) measures personal readiness to make lasting changes to one's own health behaviour and willingness to work with an Internet-based health promotion service. It is striking that only 56% of respondents are completely certain that they want to use a health portal to implement a lifestyle programme. This figure is even lower for men than for women. The results of the questionnaire on self-motivation are shown in Table 3.25 and Fig. 3.9.

Table 3.24 Questionnaire on self-motivation and willingness to change

	No	Yes, partly	Yes, absolute
In future, I want to pay much more attention to my health	1	2	3
I am prepared to maintain or improve my health by changing my everyday behaviour (in terms of diet, exercise or relaxation)	1	2	3
I am prepared to implement an internet-based health portal for the implementation of a lifestyle programme	1	2	3
I have a PC with Internet access at home	1	2	3

Table 3.25 Scatter values of the questionnaire on self-motivation and willingness to change at admission in 2023 ($n = 822$)

Self-motivation 2023		No		Yes, partially		Yes, absolutely		Total			
	Gender	*n*	%	*n*	%	*n*	%	*n*	M	SD	Md
Pay attention to health	Males	3	1.8	37	21.9	129	76.3	169	2.75	0.48	3
	Fem.	6	0.9	106	16.2	541	82.8	653	2.82	0.41	3
	Total	9	1.1	143	17.4	670	81.5	822	2.80	0.42	3
Change behaviour	Males	2	1.2	40	23.7	127	75.1	169	2.74	0.47	3
	Fem.	3	0.5	83	12.7	567	86.8	653	2.86	0.36	3
	Total	5	0.6	123	15.0	694	84.4	822	2.84	0.39	3
Use the health portal	Males	19	11.2	68	40.2	82	48.5	169	2.37	0.68	2
	Fem.	64	9.8	211	32.3	378	57.9	653	2.48	0.67	3
	Total	83	10.1	279	33.9	460	56.0	822	2.46	0.67	3
Internet access	Males	21	12.4	13	7.7	135	79.9	169	2.68	0.69	3
	Fem.	46	7.0	81	12.4	526	80.6	653	2.74	0.58	3
	Total	67	8.2	94	11.4	661	80.4	822	2.72	0.60	3

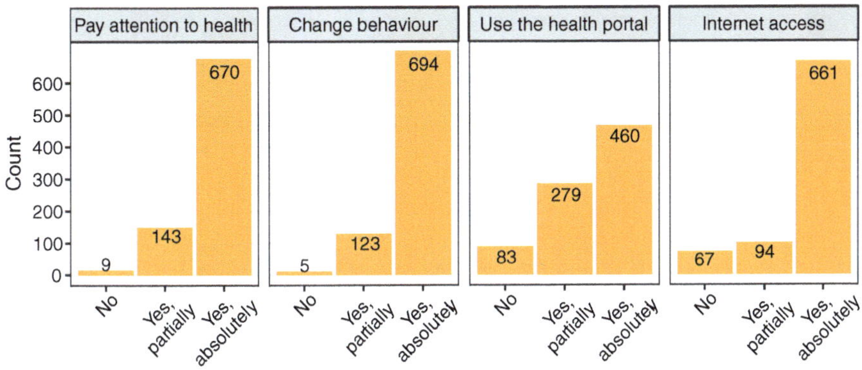

Fig. 3.9 Distribution of responses on self-motivation and willingness to change at admission in 2023 ($n = 822$)

3.2.4 Anthropometric Data

The 2023 clientele shows an average anthropometric distribution pattern (Table 3.26). Compared with the reference values of previous years, the slight increase in blood pressure/hypertension (HT) values is noteworthy (systolic: 33.2% vs. 18.7%; diastolic: 29.1% vs.13.6%).

Table 3.26 Anthropometric data for the 2023 cohort and previous years

Weight classes	**For hospital admission in 2023**						**Previous years**					
	Male $n = 169$		**Female** $n = 650$		**Total** $n = 819$		**Male** $n = 3390$		**Female** $n = 9608$		**Total** $n = 13{,}000$	
	n	%	*n*	%	*n*	%	*n*	%	*n*	%	*n*	%
<55 kg	1	0.6	80	12.3	81	9.9	35	1.0	1265	13.2	1300	10.0
56–60 kg	4	2.4	89	13.7	93	11.4	61	1.8	1328	13.8	1389	10.7
61–65 kg	8	4.7	86	13.2	94	11.5	141	4.2	1547	16.1	1688	13.0
66–70 kg	13	7.7	91	14.0	104	12.7	254	7.5	1413	14.7	1667	12.8
71–75 kg	18	10.7	77	11.8	95	11.6	377	11.1	1116	11.6	1495	11.5
76–80 kg	21	12.4	57	8.8	78	9.5	430	12.7	805	8.4	1235	9.5
81–85 kg	20	11.8	48	7.4	68	8.3	505	14.9	671	7.0	1179	9.0
86–90 kg	23	13.6	35	5.4	58	7.1	420	12.4	479	5.0	899	6.9
91–95 kg	18	10.7	30	4.6	48	5.9	368	10.9	344	3.6	712	5.5
96–100 kg	7	4.1	22	3.4	29	3.5	249	7.3	252	2.6	501	3.9
>100 kg	36	21.3	35	5.4	71	8.7	550	16.2	388	4.0	938	7.2
BMI	**Male** $n = 170$		**Female** $n = 647$		**Total** $n = 817$		**Male** $n = 3383$		**Female** $n = 9579$		**Total** $n = 12{,}963$	
	n	%	*n*	%	*n*	%	*n*	%	*n*	%	*n*	%
Underweight	3	1.8	30	4.6	33	4.0	54	1.6	365	3.8	419	3.2
Normal weight	63	37.1	313	48.4	376	46.0	1134	33.5	4848	50.6	5983	46.2
Overweight	71	41.8	176	27.2	247	30.2	1452	42.9	2611	27.3	4063	31.3
Grade I obesity	25	14.7	91	14.1	116	14.2	567	16.8	1188	12.4	1755	13.5
Grade II obesity	8	4.7	27	4.2	35	4.3	126	3.7	410	4.3	536	4.1
Grade III obesity	–	–	10	1.5	10	1.2	50	1.5	157	1.6	207	1.6
Blood pressure (BP)	**Male** $n = 170$		**Female** $n = 650$		**Total** $n = 820$		**Male** $n = 3392$		**Female** $n = 9595$		**Total** $n = 12{,}989$	
Systolic BP	*n*	%	*n*	%	*n*	%	*n*	%	*n*	%	*n*	%
Optimal	27	15.9	167	25.7	194	23.7	1109	32.7	4479	46.7	5589	43.0
Normal	38	22.4	158	24.3	196	23.9	868	25.6	2009	20.9	2877	22.1
High-normal	39	22.9	118	18.2	157	19.1	649	19.1	1437	15.0	2086	16.1
Grade 1 HT	44	25.9	131	20.2	175	21.3	614	18.1	1335	13.9	1950	15.0
Grade 2 HT	15	8.8	68	10.5	83	10.1	132	3.9	271	2.8	403	3.1

Grade 3 HT	7	4.1	8	1.2	15	1.8	20	0.6	64	0.7	84	0.6
	M	**SD**	**M**	**SD**	**M**	**SD**	**M**	**SD**	**M**	**SD**	**M**	**SD**
Total	136.5	19.2	132.0	19.4	132.9	19.5	126.2	17.8	121.1	19.5	122.5	19.2
Diastolic BP	***n***	**%**	***n***	**%**	***n***	**%**	***n***	**%**	***n***	**%**	***n***	**%**
Optimal	44	25.9	232	35.7	276	33.7	1533	45.2	5510	57.4	7044	54.2
Normal	47	27.6	136	20.9	183	22.3	871	25.7	2109	22.0	2980	22.9
High-normal	27	15.9	96	14.8	123	15.0	385	11.4	804	8.4	1189	9.2
Grade 1 HT	35	20.6	152	23.4	187	22.8	479	14.1	929	9.7	1409	10.8
Grade 2 HT	12	7.1	27	4.2	39	4.8	100	2.9	192	2.0	292	2.2
Grade 3 HT	5	2.9	7	1.1	12	1.5	24	0.7	51	0.5	75	0.6
	M	**SD**	**M**	**SD**	**M**	**SD**	**M**	**SD**	**M**	**SD**	**M**	**SD**
Total	84.8	11.8	82.5	10.5	83.0	10.8	79.3	10.6	76.3	10.9	77.1	10.9

3.3 Description of Health Risk and Protective Factors of Health

To further describe the clinic's patient profile, various risk and protective factors relating to mental and somatic health are outlined. This data is routinely collected to support a comprehensive lifestyle programme that optimizes bio-psycho-social health, as part of the psychosomatic clinic's care, and to help patients adjust to a new lifestyle after hospitalization. The Individual Health Management (IHM-IGM®) concept of the THD CoCoNat is firmly integrated into the TCM-Klinik Bad Kötzting's comprehensive therapy concept. Upon admission, patients complete a health check in the VITERIO® health portal, which provides an initial assessment of their mental and physical health, forming the basis for therapeutic and lifestyle medicine interventions. Several questionnaires are used to record various protective and risk factors for health, the results of which are presented in this section. For the initial measurement, all patient profile records documented up to 3 months before and no more than 7 days after the admission date are used. According to the IHM assessment, these indicators provide an important component of a comprehensive picture of risk and protective factors of psychosocial resources for mental health, as well as basic physical health functions.

The mental health of patients is presented below using an IHM resource profile, an IHM stress profile, and existing mental stress.

Overview

- Psychosocial basic skills for the mental health
- IHM stress profile
- Mental stress
- Physiological basic functions of physical health
- Risks to physical health

3.3.1 Psychosocial Basic Skills (IHM Resource Profile) for the Mental Health

Overview

- Life satisfaction (FLZ)
- Health literacy (SOC-13)
- Well-being and vitality (WHO-5)
- Self-efficacy, optimism, pessimism (SWOP)
- Social support (SSS)

The psychosocial IHM resource profile is recorded using the following questionnaires: Life Satisfaction (FLZ; [1]), Sense of Coherence (SOC; [2]), Wellbeing

(WHO-5-Wellbeing; [3]), Vitality (sub-dimension of the SF36; [4]), SWOP (Self-Efficacy, Optimism, (Pessimism); [5]), and Social Support Survey (SSS; [6]).

Apart from the SOC health literacy scores, the individual measurements can all be divided into three categories using standardization data. According to the health traffic light of the Individual Health Management (IHM), this results in three areas for the presentation, which indicate desirable, improvable or critical characteristics (Table 3.27).

The values are read out for the clinic's patients in a health report. Figure 3.10 shows an overview of the distribution of psychosocial protective factors within the three categories of the health traffic light for the current reporting year. Table 3.28 also shows the scatter values for the basic psychosocial skills.

The Psychosocial Basic Skills show that, upon admission to the clinic, vitality (SF-36 sub score) is noticeably impaired in 82% of all patients. Life satisfaction and well-being are also significantly reduced, at 56.3% and 60.7% respectively. Self-efficacy and social support are within the normal range for half of the patients admitted—values that are surprising at first glance (51.8% and 50.2%).

3.3.1.1 Life Satisfaction (FLZ)

The starting point for determining the current situation is the description of individual life satisfaction (surveyed using the "Questionnaire on Life Satisfaction"

Table 3.27 Resource profile of threshold values

Resource profile Threshold values	*Green* desirable	*Yellow* could be improved	*Red* critical
Life satisfaction (FLZ total)	=61	30–60	=29
Sense of Coherence (SOC-13)	=65	52–64	=51
Well-being (WHO-5)	=51	29–50	=28
Vitality (SF-36)	=64	45–63	=44
Optimism (SWOP)	=6	4–5	=3
Self-efficacy (SWOP)	=13	10–12	=9
Social competence Total (SSS)	=56	31–55	=30

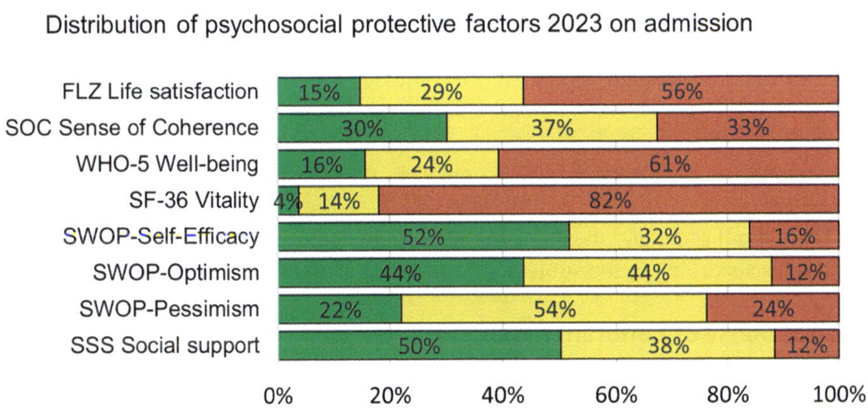

Fig. 3.10 Distribution of psychosocial protective factors in 2023 on admission

Table 3.28 Cognitive-psychosocial protective factors; measures of dispersion and frequency distribution within the three categories of the health traffic light for 2023

	Admission								
				Green		Yellow		Red	
Protective factors	*n*	M	SD	*n*	%	*n*	%	*n*	%
FLZ-Total	824	24.15	34.92	121	14.7	239	29.0	464	56.3
Total SOC	820	57.60	12.42	248	30.2	305	37.2	267	32.6
SOC meaningfulness	820	19.04	4.16	–	–	–	–	–	–
SOC comprehensability	820	21.32	5.67	–	–	–	–	–	–
SOC-manageability	820	17.23	4.73	–	–	–	–	–	–
WHO-5 Well-being	822	28.78	19.35	128	15.6	195	23.7	499	60.7
Vitality SF-36	822	27.78	17.78	31	3.8	117	14.2	674	82.0
SWOP optimism	821	5.02	1.46	358	43.6	363	44.2	100	12.2
SWOP-Self-efficacy	821	12.44	3.01	425	51.8	264	32.2	132	16.1
SWOP pessimism	821	4.45	1.41	181	22.0	445	54.2	195	23.8
SSS-Total	799	53.15	17.08	401	50.2	305	38.2	93	11.6
SSS emot./inform.	799	17.69	5.58	0	0.0	700	87.6	99	12.4
SSS social interaction	799	10.49	3.79	202	25.3	463	57.9	134	16.8
SSS material	799	11.37	4.54	329	41.2	329	41.2	141	17.6
SSS affective	799	8.71	3.17	311	38.9	386	48.3	102	12.8
Number of people	822	3.70	2.45	–	–	–	–	–	–

Table 3.29 Life satisfaction—threshold values

Threshold values Life satisfaction	*Green* Desirable	*Yellow* Could be improved	*Red* Critical
FLZ total value	**=61**	**30–60**	**=29**
FLZ friends/acquaintances	=9	3–8	=2
FLZ Leisure/hobbies	=7	1–6	=0
FLZ Health	=9	2–8	=1
FLZ Income/Finances	=8	1–7	=0
FLZ Profession/Work	=6	0–5	=-1
FLZ Housing situation	=9	3–8	=2
FLZ Family/Children	=10	3–9	=2
FLZ Partnership/Sexuality	=8	1–7	=0

FLZ [1]), both overall and differentiated by various life. For this purpose, eight areas of life are specified, which are first assessed according to *how important* they are perceived to be. The respondents are then asked *how satisfied* they currently feel in these areas. From this, an individual measurement of life satisfaction can be determined for each patient, which considers the different weighting of the individual areas.

The overall score and the eight sub-scores are determined and divided into three categories according to the subjectively assessed level of satisfaction (Table 3.29).

3.3.1.2 Sense of Coherence (SOC-13)

The "Sense of Coherence" questionnaire is about the extent of health literacy. SOC refers to a general attitude towards life, expressing the extent to which one has an enduring, dynamic sense of confidence that one's internal and external environments are predictable, and that things will turn out as one reasonably expects. It describes the ability to react flexibly to stressful events and is therefore considered an important characteristic for strengthening and maintaining health.

This version of the questionnaire contains 13 questions [2]. It was originally developed in English more than 20 years ago and later translated into German. It has been used in numerous international studies, providing comparative values for patients with different illnesses and healthy individuals. The questionnaire offers the possibility of calculating partial scores for the dimensions of "comprehensibility", "manageability" and "meaningfulness". Each dimension includes four questions, each of which can be answered on a scale from one to seven. This results in a total score ranging from 4 to 91 points.

High SOC values act as resilience factors and indicate a low psychopathological status or vice versa. Table 3.30 provides an overview of how the total score is distributed across the three categories of the health traffic light system.

3.3.1.3 Well-Being Questionnaire (WHO-5)

The WHO-5-well-being questionnaire was developed by researchers in cooperation with the World Health Organization (WHO) [3]. This five-question test is designed to determine whether further clarification of a possible depression is needed. This should be done if a significantly poorer state of health below the threshold value becomes apparent when answering the five questions.

If the score is below the threshold of 13 points, a further medical examination should be carried out. The questionnaire can also be used as a short test for the extent of well-being. Changes of three or more points are considered clinically significant.

The answers are coded from 0 = "at no time" to 5 = "all the time". Values from 0 to 25 can be calculated from the sum of the coded answers. The total value is additionally multiplied by four to obtain a value of the state of mind from 0 to 100. Values of approximately 70 points are used for the general population [3].

Scores below 50 are an indication of poor well-being. Significantly lower scores may indicate the development of depression (Table 3.31).

Table 3.30 Health literacy—threshold values

Threshold values Health literacy	*Green* Desirable	*Yellow* Could be improved	*Red* Critical
Overall health literacy	>64	52–64	<52

Table 3.31 Well-being—threshold values

Threshold values Well-being	*Green* Desirable	*Yellow* Could be improved	*Red* Critical
Well-being (WHO-5)	>50	29–50	<29

3.3.1.4 Vitality Questionnaire (SF-36)

The extent of vitality is also surveyed as a relevant sub-dimension when describing health-related quality of life. The scale with four questions is based on the German version of the SF-36 Health Survey [4]. The questionnaire was developed in the United States about 20 years ago and has since been used worldwide in many languages. The test results obtained in individual cases can be compared with the values of groups with various illnesses and with a group of almost 3000 healthy people in the German population.

Each of the four items can be answered on a scale from 1 to 6. After the first two questions have been reversed as part of the evaluation, the total sum of the items can then be calculated.

The following formula is used to convert the total sum into a standardized scale from 1 to 100:

$$\left(\left(\text{total sum}-4\right)/20\right)*100$$

Table 3.32 provides the threshold values for the vitality index across the three categories of the health traffic light system.

3.3.1.5 Self-Efficacy, Optimism, Pessimism (SWOP)

This is a questionnaire to measure self-efficacy, optimism and pessimism [5]. Self-efficacy refers to a person's expectation of being able to master stressful situations through appropriate action. It refers to confidence in one's own ability to achieve a goal, for example, even if obstacles arise. This attitude has a lot to do with the optimistic basic attitude of being able to cope well with life in general. Conversely, we speak of a rather pessimistic or sceptical basic attitude. To calculate the "measured values" of these three components of self-efficacy, optimism and pessimism, nine questions must be answered: five for self-efficacy and two each for optimism and pessimism. The questionnaire has proven its worth in numerous studies. The points achieved are evaluated in comparison with the results previously obtained by other patients. It is not yet possible to classify the results regarding healthy people. Each answer is given a value from 1 to 4 and the result is the sum of the respective sub-scores (self-efficacy, optimism, pessimism). Higher values represent a higher level of the evaluated sub-score (Tables 3.32 and 3.33).

3.3.1.6 Social Support Questionnaire (SSS)

The SSS serves as a self-assessment procedure, which measures the extent of subjectively perceived social support. The clinic uses the modified version of the questionnaire with an adapted factor structure [6] (original version: Social Support Scale SSS [7]). The questionnaire asks about the frequency of being able to rely on people

Table 3.32 Vitality—threshold values

Threshold values Vitality	*Green* Desirable	*Yellow* Could be improved	*Red* Critical
Vitality (SF-36)	>63	45–63	<45

Table 3.33 SWOP—threshold values

Threshold values SWOP	*Green* Desirable	*Yellow* Could be improved	*Red* Critical
Self-efficacy	=13	10–12	=9
Optimism	=6	4–5	=3
Pessimism	=3	4–5	=6

Table 3.34 Social support—threshold values

Threshold values Social support	*Green* Desirable	*Yellow* Could be improved	*Red* Critical
Total social competence	=56	31–55	=30
Emotional/informational factor	=25	24–11	=10
Social interaction	=14	7–13	=6
Material factor	=14	7–13	=6
Affective factor	=11	5–10	=4

around you when you need help and support with problems and stress. This involves practical help, emotional support and understanding as well as so-called cognitive support. A measure of the extent of social support is determined from the answers to the 19 specified questions. The questionnaire has proven its worth in numerous studies. Each answer is given a value from 0 to 4, these are added together, resulting in a possible total score of between 0 and 76. Table 3.34 presents the distribution of values across the three categories of the health traffic light system.

3.3.2 IHM Stress Profile

Overview

- Tedium scale (burnout)
- Perceived Stress Questionnaire (PSQ)
- 3-Level Stress Test
- Psycho-vegetative complaints (somatic stress disorders)
- Stressors and burdens

The following questionnaires are used to assess the IHM stress profile of mental health: Tedium test [8], Perceived Stress Questionnaire (PSQ [9]), 3-Level Stress Test (3-LST [10]), the psycho-vegetative complaints (self-developed questionnaire) and stressors and burdens (self-developed questionnaire). In principle, the coherence value (SOC) described above can also be regarded as a stress parameter. Apart from the 3-Level Stress Test, the individual measured values can also all be divided into three categories with the help of standardization data (Table 3.35).

Figure 3.11 and Table 3.36 show an overview of the distribution of the IHM stress profile within the three categories of the health traffic light system for the 2023 reporting year.

Table 3.35 Stress profile—threshold values

Stress profile threshold values	*Green* Desirable	*Yellow* Could be improved	*Red* Critical
Tedium scale (burnout)	=3.2	3.21–4.5	>4.5
Perceived Stress Questionnaire (PSQ)	=41.5	51.51–58.50	=58.5
3-Level Stress Test (3-LST)	–	–	–
Vegetative Stability Complaint Index	Based on the number of answers in the severity category		
Stressors and burdens	If no area is yellow or red	If at least one area is yellow and no area is red	If at least 1 area is red

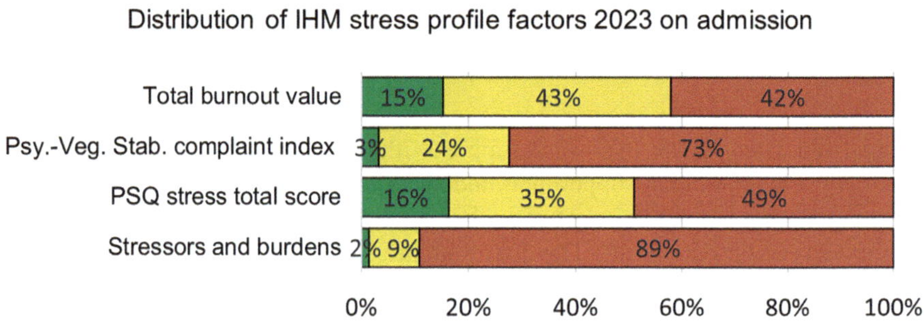

Fig. 3.11 Distribution of IHM stress profile factors on admission

Table 3.36 IHM stress profile: measures of dispersion and frequency distribution within the three categories of the health traffic light

	Admission								
				Green		Yellow		Red	
	n	M	SD	*n*	%	*n*	%	*n*	%
Tedium scale	823	4.24	0.94	126	15.3	351	42.6	346	42.0
PSQ	822	57.63	18.07	135	16.4	284	34.5	403	49.0
3-LST cognitive	821	22.91	10.13	–	–	–	–	–	–
3-LST vegetative	821	19.43	7.79	–	–	–	–	–	–
3-LST motoric	821	27.76	8.79	–	–	–	–	–	–
Vegetative Stability Complaint	823	0.31	0.53	27	3.3	199	24.2	597	72.5
Stressors and burdens	822	1.88	0.37	12	1.5	77	9.4	733	89.2

3.3.2.1 Tedium Scale (Burnout)

The Tedium Scale (tedium = annoyance) questionnaire is used to assess the development of burnout syndrome. 21 questions with predefined response levels are evaluated and presented in the form of an overall score on a scale of 1 (= lowest) to 7 (= highest) points [8].

The final value is known as the "*annoyance value*". The assessment is based on the number of points calculated:

- 2–3.2 points: Currently no recognizable risk of burnout (green)
- 3.2–4.5 points: Pre-burnout syndrome with critical stress load (yellow)
- from 4.5 points: Clear signs of burnout (red)

3.3.2.2 Perceived Stress Questionnaire (PSQ)

The "Perceived Stress Questionnaire (PSQ)" is used in to assess the extent of self-perceived stress. The survey focuses on the subjective assessment of the stress reaction and the less objectifiable stress factors. The questionnaire consists of 20 statements, each of which can be answered using four response options ("almost never", "sometimes", "often" and "most of the time") [9].

In addition to the overall score, four sub-scores can form: Worry, Tension, Demands and Joy. The total score and the sub-scores are on a uniform scale from 0 to 100, but the "Joy" factor is reversed, i.e. a lower score contributes to a higher total stress score.

These preliminary "norm limits" were derived from the values of healthy adults for the PSQ total score (Table 3.37):

3.3.2.3 Three-Level Stress Test

People react very differently to stressful situations. This questionnaire is about describing how you react to stress [10]. This usually affects the weakest points of body and soul. The three most important levels on which stress reactions can occur are queried in the form of 24 statements. The reaction on the "cognitive/affective" level includes thinking, perception and feelings. It ranges from uncertainty and nervousness to strong feelings of anxiety. The reaction at the "vegetative" level refers to changes in the cardiovascular system, digestion, breathing and sleep-wake behaviour. The reaction at the "motor" level is a tensing of the muscles, e.g. tension in the shoulder and neck area, in the face or teeth grinding.

The evaluation of the answers provides a measured value for each of the three areas (a), (b) and (c) in the form of the sum score of all associated items. The decisive factor for the meaning of the test is at which level the numerically highest score lies, i.e. in which area the susceptibility to stress is greatest. The absolute level of the scores is not taken into account any further. The 3-level stress test is taken on admission and at follow-up.

The three stress levels:

- Sum A: cognitive/affective level
- Sum B: vegetative level
- Sum C: motor level

Table 3.37 PSQ—threshold values

Threshold values PSQ	*Green* Inconspicuous	*Yellow* Increased	*Red* Significantly increased
PSQ total value	=41.5	51.51–58.50	=58.5

3.3.2.4 Psycho-Vegetative Complaints (Functional Somatic Disorders)

This questionnaire (developed in-house) asks about a range of symptoms, findings and complaints that cover both physical symptoms and mental health. A total of 42 complaints and symptoms are given as a question profile (Table 3.38). The frequency or severity of the complaints/symptoms experienced "recently" must be assessed. The totality of all 42 symptoms describes the regularity of the psycho-neuro-vegetative organization and is regarded as a complaint index or stress factors and risks. The individual complaints can be assigned to different functional and organ systems as categories. The questionnaire was developed by Prof. D. Melchart and is intended for recording the numerous different complaints of patients with functional somatic disorders. These individual symptoms are often reported by clients of complementary medicine and naturopathy.

Table 3.38 Questionnaire on psycho-vegetative complaints and functional somatic disorder

How severe or how frequently have the following symptoms occurred for you recently?		No/ never	Somewhat/ rarely	Fairly/ often	Strongly/ frequently
01	General fatigue				
02	Difficulty concentrating				
03	Tremors (eyelid, tongue, mouth, hands)				
04	Difficulty falling asleep				
05	Restless sleep				
06	Muscle weakness in the legs				
07	Reduced reaction time				
08	Rapid fatigue				
09	Chills/freezing				
10	Susceptibility to infections				
11	Sadness				
12	Shortness of breath				
13	Poor tolerance to heat or cold				
14	Frequent urination				
15	No memory of dreams				
16	Feeling unrefreshed after waking up				
17	Abdominal pressure/ bloating				
18	Memory disturbances				
19	Delayed rewarming after cold exposure				
20	Irritability				
21	Head or facial pain				
22	Irregular heartbeat				
23	Dry mouth				
24	Intense thirst				

(continued)

Table 3.38 (continued)

How severe or how frequently have the following symptoms occurred for you recently?		No/ never	Somewhat/ rarely	Fairly/ often	Strongly/ frequently
25	Dizziness when standing up or bending over				
26	Restlessness				
27	Dizziness when looking down				
28	Sensation of heat				
29	Heart and chest pain				
30	Skin rashes/changes				
31	Skin itching				
32	Joint discomfort				
33	Excessive sweating				
34	Dizziness when getting up in the morning				
35	Allergic reactions (including asthma attacks)				
36	Mood swings				
37	Indecisiveness				
38	Anxiety				
39	Reduced sexual desire				
40	Cold hands/feet				
41	Back discomfort				
42	Hypersensitivity to cold and wind				

Based on the number of answers in the severity category (0 = no/never, 1 = somewhat/rarely, 2 = fairly/often and 3 = strongly/very often), an overall complaint index is formed. Depending on the severity and frequency of the symptoms, a qualitative assignment is made to an overall symptom index. This can lie between the following categories that also form the three categories of the health traffic light system:

- 0 = high somatic functional stress disorder
- 1 = moderate somatic functional stress disorder
- 2 = no relevant somatic functional stress disorder

The index 0 is assigned if the answer "strongly/very frequently" occurs more than twice, or if the answer "fairly/often" occurs more than 16 times. The index 1 is given if "strongly/frequently" occurs once or twice, or if "fairly/often" occurs between eight and 16 times. The index 2 is assigned if none of the above criteria are met (Table 3.39).

3.3.2.5 Questionnaire on Stressors and Burdens

This questionnaire, developed by CoCoNat, is designed to assess stressors and burdens. The answers provide information on the presence and frequency of stress in the domestic, professional and financial spheres, as well as on the occurrence of major life events in the last 12 months. The questionnaire is administered on admission and at follow-up. Table 3.40 shows the individual items of the questionnaire and their response options.

Table 3.39 Complaint Index—threshold values

Index	Traffic light	Index assignment based on the frequency of response categories
0	Red	"strongly/very frequently" = 3 times OR "fairly/often" = 17 times
1	Yellow	"strongly/frequently" = 1 time OR "fairly/often" = 8 times
2	Green	none of the above conditions are met (default category green)

Table 3.40 Questionnaire on stressors and burdens

For each of the following stressors and burdens, please indicate whether you have been affected by them in the past 12 months. Multiple answers possible				
1. Occupational stress	**Never**	**Sometimes**	**More often**	**Always**
Double burden of work and household	0	1	2	3
Poor working atmosphere	0	1	2	3
Shift work	0	1	2	3
Unemployment	0	1	2	3
Becoming self-employed	0	1	2	3
Trouble with the supervisor	0	1	2	3
Promotion	0	1	2	3
Change of workplace	0	1	2	3
Work overtime	0	1	2	3
On the road a lot/business trips	0	1	2	3
Trouble with colleagues	0	1	2	3
2. At home / in everyday life	**Never**	**Sometimes**	**More often**	**Always**
Arguing with your partner	0	1	2	3
House construction	0	1	2	3
Education of the children	0	1	2	3
Noisy residential area	0	1	2	3
Difficulties with parents/parents-in-law	0	1	2	3
Illness/stay in hospital	0	1	2	3
Relocation	0	1	2	3
Social obligations	0	1	2	3
Vacation preparation/holiday preparation	0	1	2	3
Weekend/leisure hustle and bustle	0	1	2	3
3. Financial burdens	**None/ mild**	**Moderate**	**Severe**	
Mortgages/ Loans	0	1	2	
Legal disputes	0	1	2	
4. Major life events	**None**	**One**	**More than 1**	
Accident	0	1	2	
Bereavement in the family	0	1	2	
Separation/divorce from partner	0	1	2	
Family disputes	0	1	2	
Bankruptcy	0	1	2	
Loss of the job	0	1	2	
Violence	0	1	2	

Table 3.41 Stressors—threshold values

	Red	*Yellow*	*Green*
Stressors level	Striking	Could be improved	Desirable
Total	If at least 1 area is "red"	If at least 1 area is "yellow" and none is red"	If none if the other applies
Professional	If at least 1 question with "more often" or "always" was answered	If at least 1 question with "sometimes" and none with "more often" or "always" was answered	If none if the other applies
Domestic	If at least 1 question with "more often" or "always" was answered	If at least one question was answered with "sometimes" and none with "more often" or "always"	If none if the other applies
Financial	If at least 1 question was answered with "severe"	If at least 1 question was answered with "moderate" and none with "severe"	If none if the other applies
Major life events	If at least 2 events have occurred	If one event has occurred	If none if the other applies

The corresponding categorization of the values in the context of the health traffic light is as shown in Table 3.41.

3.3.3 Mental Stress and Burden

Overview
- ICD symptom rating (ISR)
- WHO-5 well-being (depression)
- Generalized Anxiety Disorder Scale

Individual mental stress is important for a comprehensive description of mental health. The questionnaires of the ICD-10 Symptom Rating (ISR [11]) with specific additional questions, the WHO-5 Well-being Depression [3, 12] and the Generalized Anxiety Disorder (GAD [13]) questionnaire are used for this purpose.

Figure 3.12 and Table 3.42 show an overview of the distribution of the IHM stress profile within the three categories of the health traffic light system for the 2023 reporting year.

For the mental stress and burden profile, the yellow and red categories are subdivided further to allow for more detailed specification of the clinical indication. Overall, 63% of patients exhibit moderate to severe symptoms of mental health issues. The 5-WHO index shows that 36% of patients exhibit symptoms of major depression, while 25% exhibit symptoms of minor depression. The Generalized Anxiety Disorder Scale-7 (GAD-7) questionnaire indicates elevated anxiety levels in 54% of respondents.

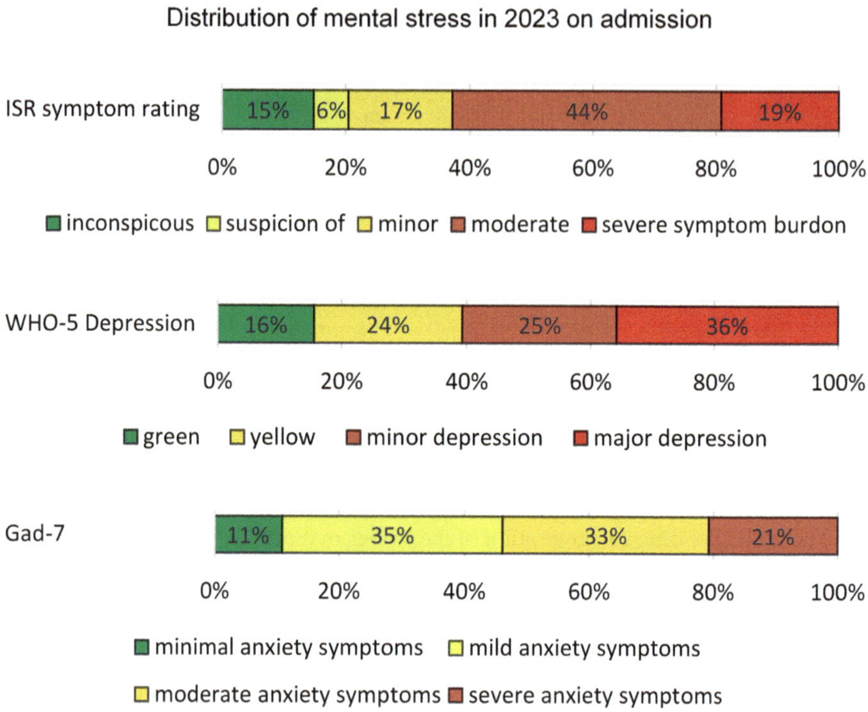

Fig. 3.12 Distribution of IHM mental stress profile factors

Table 3.42 IHM stress profile: measures of dispersion and frequency distribution within the categories of the health traffic light for 2023

Mental stress and burdens	Admission												
				Green		Yellow 1		Yellow 2		Red 1		Red 2	
	n	M	SD	*n*	%	*n*	%	*n*	%	*n*	%	*n*	%
ISR	824	1.14	0.59	123	14.9	46	5.6	138	16.7	360	43.7	157	19.1
WHO-5 Depression	822	28.78	19.35	128	15.6	195	23.7	–	–	205	24.9	294	35.8
GAD-7	815	10.36	4.81	89	10.9	287	35.2	270	33.1	169	20.7	–	–

3.3.3.1 ICD Symptom Rating (ISR)

For the TCM-Klinik Bad Kötzting as a specialist hospital for psychosomatics, it is of particular importance to record psychopathological syndromes as a relevant outcome variable and to measure their change after treatment. A patient questionnaire, developed in 2008 by the Institute for Quality Development in Psychotherapy and Psychosomatics, Munich (IQP), and used in numerous psychosomatic specialist clinics in Bavaria, serves this purpose [11]. The questionnaire is based on the globally established consensus of the ICD-10. As an "ICD-10 Symptom Rating" (ISR), the questionnaire instrument comprises 29 items, which are divided into 5 individual scales and an additional scale:

- Depressive syndrome (4 items)
- Anxiety syndrome (4 items)
- Obsessive-compulsive syndrome (3 items)
- Somatoform syndrome (3 items)
- Eating disorder syndrome (3 items)
- Supplementary items (12 items)

The total score includes all individual scales with a single weighting and the additional scale with a double weighting. All sub-scores and the total score are mapped on a scale from 0 "strongly disagree" to 4 "strongly agree". The ICD-10 Symptom Rating ISR enables a comprehensive evaluation of the status and development of psychological symptoms (also under psychotherapeutic treatment) and can depict the process and outcome quality. The instrument is also used to assess severity.

The ISR was presented to patients at the beginning and end of their inpatient stay and around 6 months after discharge in the VITERIO® health portal.

Burden Levels of the Individual ISR Dimensions

Due to the standardized evaluation of the ISR, it is possible to transform the numerical scale values into stress levels, which facilitate the interpretation of the measured values. It is important to note that both the subscale scores and the total value of the ISR are based on different threshold values. The designation of the individual burden levels and the corresponding threshold values for each score are summarized in Table 3.43).

3.3.3.2 WHO-5 Well-Being (Depression)

As mentioned in Sect. 3.3.1.3, the questionnaire was developed by researchers in cooperation with the World Health Organization (WHO) [3]. Five questions are used to determine whether there is a need for a more detailed clarification of a possible depression. This should be considered if the answers to the five questions indicate a significantly reduced well-being below the threshold value. If the score is below the threshold of 13 points, a further medical examination should be carried out. The questionnaire can also be used as a short test for the extent of well-being (see Sect. 3.3.1.3). The answers are coded from 0 = "at no time" to 5 = "all the time". Values from 0 to 25 can be calculated from the sum of the coded responses.

The total value is multiplied by 4 to give a mood score ranging from 0 to 100, which is then categorized using the traffic light system (Table 3.44). A cut-off score

Table 3.43 ISR—threshold values

	Green	Yellow	Yellow	Red	Red
Disorder syndrome (DS)	No indication	Possible burden	Mild burden	Moderate burden	Severe burden
Depressive DS	<0.75	0.75–0.99	1.0–1.99	2.0–2.99	=3.0
Anxiety DS	<0.75	0.75–0.99	1.0–1.99	2.0–2.99	=3.0
Compulsive-Obsessive DS	<0.67	0.67–0.99	1.0–1.99	2.0–2.99	=3.0
Somatoform DS	<0.33	0.33–0.749	0.75–1.249	1.25–2.669	=2.67
Eating DS	<0.33	0.33–0.669	0.67–1.499	1.5–2.669	=2.75
Total score	**<0.5**	**0.5–0.599**	**0.6–0.899**	**0.9–1.699**	**=1.7**

Table 3.44 Depression (WHO-5)—threshold values

Threshold values Depression/well-being	*Green* Desirable	*Yellow* Improvable	*Red* Minor depression	*Red* Major depression
Depression (WHO-5)	>50	32–50	20 to <32	<20

Table 3.45 GAD-7—threshold values

Threshold values GAD-7	*Red* Severe anxiety symptoms	*Yellow* Moderate anxiety symptoms	*Yellow* Low anxiety symptoms	*Green* Minimal anxiety symptoms
GAD-7 values	15–21	10–14	5–9	0–4

of >50 indicates good well-being and no symptoms of depression. Among WHO-5 studies on depression, the work of Krieger et al. investigated the Hamilton Depression Scale (HAM-D) and the Hamilton Anxiety Scale (HAM-A) alongside the WHO-5 [12]. A HAM-D score of 18, indicating the level of depression at which treatment is needed (major depression), corresponded to a WHO-5 score of 20; an HAM-D score of 13 (minor depression) corresponded to a WHO-5 score of 32.

3.3.3.3 Generalized Anxiety Disorder Scale-7 (GAD-7) Questionnaire

The Generalized Anxiety Disorder Scale-7 (GAD-7) has been in use since May 2022 and is a brief instrument for assessing generalized anxiety disorder. It is administered over the course of admission, discharge and follow-up. The GAD-7 scale has a high diagnostic validity with low processing effort and can be used for the diagnosis, screening and measurement of the severity as well as for the follow-up measurement of generalized anxiety disorder.

The 7 items of the GAD-7 ask about the most important diagnostic criteria of generalized anxiety disorder according to the DSM-IV and ICD-10 criteria [13].

The severity of the anxiety symptoms can divide into different levels of severity: minimal, mild, moderate or severe.

- With a cut-off of =10 points, a generalized anxiety disorder is *possible*
- With a cut-off =15 points, this is *likely*

The corresponding categorization of the values in the context of the health traffic light system are shown in Table 3.45.

3.3.4 Physiological Resource Profile (Basic Functions of Physical Health)

Overview

- IHM Movement Index
- IHM Nutrition Index
- Psycho-vegetative stability (circulation, heat balance, sleep)
- Pittsburgh Sleep Quality Index (PSQI)

To depict physical health, the physiological resource profile of the patients is now presented with the IHM movement and nutrition index, the psycho-vegetative stability with circulation, heat balance and sleep, as well as the comprehensive Pittsburgh Sleep Quality Index (PSQI).

For the evaluation of the results, the results are also divided into areas of the health traffic light system, which are categorized in Table 3.46.

An overview of the distribution within the physiological protective factors of patients on admission in 2023 is illustrated in Fig. 3.13. Table 3.47 shows an overview of the distribution values of all physiological resources. The distribution pattern of basic physiological functions relating to nutrition, exercise, vegetative stability and sleep quality shows that 76% of all patients have significant problems falling asleep and staying asleep. This is confirmed by the Pittsburgh Sleep Quality Index, which shows that 50% have poor sleep and 38% have restricted sleep. Neurovegetative regulation is noticeable in terms of cardiovascular stability and thermoregulation in 43% and 50% of all patients, respectively. In addition, 47% of respondents report insufficient daily exercise. In contrast, only 19% of respondents say they have a poor diet.

Table 3.46 Physiological resource profile—threshold values

Threshold values	*Green* Desirable	*Yellow* Improvable	*Red* Critical
IHM-Nutrition Index	=11	8–10	=7
IHM-Movement Index	=6	4–5	=3
Vegetative Stability Sleep	=2	3–5	=6
Vegetative Stability Dizziness/Circulation	=1	2–3	=4
Vegetative Stability Thermoregulation	=2	3–5	=6
PSQI total value	=5	6–10	=11

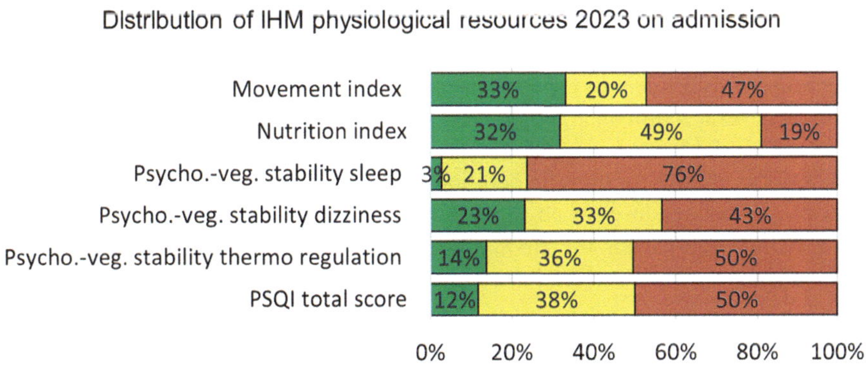

Fig. 3.13 Body-oriented protective factors—frequency of patients in the desirable (green), improvable (yellow) and critical (red) range in 2023

Table 3.47 Physiological resource profile: measures of dispersion and frequency distribution within the three categories of the health traffic light for 2023

	Admission								
				Green		Yellow		Red	
Resource profile	*n*	M	SD	*n*	%	*n*	%	*n*	%
IHM-Nutrition Index	821	9.45	2.13	262	31.9	404	49.2	155	18.9
IHM-Movement Index	814	3.90	2.74	270	33.2	161	19.8	383	47.1
Psycho-vegetative stability: sleep	823	7.06	2.21	23	2.8	173	21.0	627	76.2
Psycho-vegetative stability Dizziness/ circulation	823	3.36	2.23	192	23.3	275	33.4	356	43.3
Psycho-vegetative stability Thermoregulation	823	5.61	2.79	114	13.9	294	35.7	415	50.4
PSQI total value	814	10.45	3.99	96	11.8	312	38.3	406	49.9

3.3.4.1 IHM Movement Index

The IHM Movement Index—revised in 2023—is composed of information on everyday physical activity, overall activity level (mainly at work) and average daily sitting behaviour. The index was developed by Prof. Melchart, CoCoNat, Munich. The benchmarks are based on the WHO's international activity recommendations for endurance-oriented exercise for adults published at the end of 2020 with regard to achieving additional health benefits. It is made up of four questions, which are distributed across three questionnaires. Two of these questions relate to moderate physical activity in everyday life and in leisure time. One question relates to general physical activity levels, and one relates to average daily sitting behaviour.

Questionnaire A on Moderate Exercise in Everyday Life and Leisure Time

The determination of moderate exercise in everyday life and leisure time is based on a point algorithm in which the frequency, duration and intensity of exercise are queried and offset against each other in MET-min [14] (Table 3.48).

Questionnaire B on General Physical Activity Level—Mainly at Work

The activity level refers to the PAL factor and is collected as part of the questionnaire on general health data, blood pressure and diabetes risk (Table 3.49).

The PAL factor (measurable activity level) describes the amount of energy required for physical activity in addition to the basal metabolic rate. It is used to classify the average level of physical activity. An appropriate score is awarded for each answer option. For the answer option "physically demanding work", eight working hours are assumed and therefore six points are awarded.

Questionnaire C on Average Daily Sitting Behaviour

In addition, the assessment of daily sitting behaviour serves as another way of obtaining the most comprehensive possible picture of physical activity behaviour. The average daily sitting time during the week is assessed in accordance with the Marshall Sitting Questionnaire [15] (Table 3.50). If the sum of the minutes is less than 240 (i.e. less than 4 h), one point is awarded, otherwise zero points.

Table 3.48 Physical activity index (IHM Movement Index)—questionnaire on moderate physical activity in everyday life and leisure time

Question 1: Moderate exercise in everyday life and leisure time	**Min. × MET × Days**	**MET-Min. per week**	**Point-value**
How many minutes per day do you engage in light physical activity, such as brisk walking?			
At least 30 min a day	30 × 4 × 7	>600	3
5 times a week for 30 min a day	30 × 4 × 5	600	2
Less than 5 times a week 30 min daily	<150 min	<600	1
Predominantly sedentary, hardly any daily movement	<150 min	<600	0
Question 2: Intensive exercise in everyday life and leisure time	**Min/week × MET**	**MET-Min. per week**	**Point-value**
I don't do any sport	<75 × 8	<600	0
I do at least 75 min per week of intensive running, mountain hiking, fast swimming or other intensive sports that make me sweat	>75 × 8	˜600	3
I do more than 75 min up to a maximum of 150 min per week of intensive running, mountain hiking, fast swimming or other intense sports that make me sweat	>75 × 8 <150 × 8	600–1200	4
I do more than 150 min of intensive sport per week	>150 × 8	>1200	6

Table 3.49 Physical activity index—questionnaire on activity level

Question 3: General activity level (PAL query)	Coding	Point value
Please select the physical activity that suits you best on average		
Exclusively sitting/lying down	0	0
Sedentary, hardly any physical activity	1	0
Sitting, temporarily walking/standing	2	0
Predominantly standing/walking	3	1
Physically demanding work	4	6

Overall Movement Index

Table 3.51 summarizes the value ranges used for calculating points for each question. For the evaluation of the partial results of the questionnaires A–C and the achievable points (0–10 points), the classification is made into the known areas of the health traffic light system, which are categorized as shown in Table 3.52.

3.3.4.2 IHM Nutrition Index

The content of the revised nutrition index, which has been in use since the start of 2022, comprises the 10 rules for wholefood nutrition proposed by the German Nutrition Society (DGE) [16]. The questions are divided into different question blocks or dimensions, which conceptually align with the 10 guidelines of the DGE (Table 3.53).

Table 3.50 Movement index—questionnaire on daily sitting behaviour (minutes per day)

Question 4: Average daily sitting behaviour	min/d
How many minutes do you spend sitting …	
… while commuting to work or running errands etc., for example in a car, bus, or train?	
… during work?	
… on television?	
… during recreational computer or other electronic media use?	
… during other free time (e.g. reading, movies, meeting friends?)	

Table 3.51 Value ranges for calculating the movement index

Questionnaire	Minimum value	Maximum value
A: Moderate exercise in MET-min per week	0	3
A: Intensive exercise in MET-min per week	0	6
B: Activity level (PAL factor)	0	6
C: Daily sitting behaviour	0	1
Movement index (total value)	**0**	**10**

Table 3.52 Movement index—threshold values

Threshold values Movement index	*Green* desirable	*Yellow* improvable	*Red* critical
IHM Movement index	=6 (max 16 points)	4–5 points	=3

Table 3.53 Questionnaire for the nutrition index

1. Enjoy food diversity	**Point value**	
Do you follow a varied diet?	Yes	No
Does your diet include plant-based foods such as vegetables, fruit, grains and cereals as well as potatoes, vegetable oils and nuts?	1	0
Do you supplement your diet with animal-based food?		
Is your diet supplemented by animal-based foods such as milk, dairy products, fish, meat and eggs?	1	0
2. Vegetables and fruit—"take 5 a day"		
How many portions of fruit and vegetables do you eat at least once a day? (1 portion corresponds to about a handful of fruit and vegetables)		
1–2 portions of fruit	1	
3–4 portions of vegetables	1	
5 or more portions of fruit and vegetables	2	
Not daily	0	
3. Choose whole grain		
How often in the last week have you eaten wholemeal bread, brown bread, wholegrain pasta or wholegrain rice?		
Not at all	0	
1–2 times a week	0	
3–4 times a week	0	
5–6 times per week	1	
Daily	2	

(continued)

Table 3.53 (continued)

4. Supplement the selection with animal-based foods		
How often did you eat fish or seafood last week?		
Not at all	0	
1–2 times per week	1	
3–4 times a week	1	
5–6 times per week	0	
Daily	0	
How often did you eat meat (pork, beef, poultry, sausage) last week?		
Not at all	1	
1–2 times per week	1	
3–4 times a week	1	
5–6 times per week	0	
Daily	0	
How often did you eat milk, yogurt, cheese last week?		
Not at all	0	
1–2 times per week	0	
3–4 times a week	1	
5–6 times per week	1	
Daily	1	
5. Using healthy fats	**Yes**	**No**
I consciously pay attention to oils with unsaturated fatty acids	2	0
6. Cut down on sugar and salt		
7. It is best to drink water		
8. Prepare gently		
One point is given for the entire block if =1 question is answered with yes		
Which statements apply to you?	**Yes**	**No**
I avoid or use sugar-sweetened drinks or food sparingly		
I rarely, if ever, add salt to my dishes at the table		
I drink about 1.5 l of water or unsweetened drinks a day		
I do not drink alcohol regularly or frequently, e.g. in the form of beer, wine or other alcoholic beverages		
I avoid burning food when frying, grilling, baking and deep-frying		
9. Eat mindfully and enjoy	**Point value**	
How much time do you take for the main meal?		
Up to 10 min	0	
Approximately 10–20 min	0	
Approximately 20–30 min	1	
More than 30 min	2	
10. Watch your weight and stay active	**Yes**	**No**
I watch my body weight and keep moving regularly	1	0

The questionnaire was developed based on the guidelines valid at the time and is subject to ongoing revision to reflect updates in scientific knowledge and changes in official recommendations.

In total, the nutrition index can range from 0 to 15 points. The corresponding categorization of the values in the context of the health traffic light system is shown in Table 3.54.

Table 3.54 Nutrition index—threshold values

Threshold values Nutrition index	*Green* Desirable	*Yellow* Improvable	*Red* Critical
Nutrition index	=11	8–10	=7

Table 3.55 Questionnaire blocks on dizziness, sleep and heat balance

Category	Item	No/ never	Somewhat/ rarely	Quite/ often	Strong/ very frequently
Dizziness (0–9 points)					
	Dizziness when standing up or bending down	0	1	2	3
	Dizziness when looking into the depths	0	1	2	3
	Dizziness when getting up in the morning	0	1	2	3
Sleep (0–12 points)					
	Problems falling asleep	0	1	2	3
	Restless sleep	0	1	2	3
	No memory of dreams	0	1	2	3
	Feeling exhausted after getting up	0	1	2	3
Heat balance (0–12 point)					
	Shivering/ freezing	0	1	2	3
	Heat or cold is poorly tolerated	0	1	2	3
	Delayed reheating after cold	0	1	2	3
	Cold hands/feet	0	1	2	3

3.3.4.3 Psycho-Vegetative Stability (Dizziness, Heat Balance, Sleep)

For the evaluation of physical resources, it is of particular interest which complaints associated with sleep behaviour, thermoregulation and dizziness.

Sleep, heat balance and dizziness (here primarily of orthostatic origin) are interpreted as representatives of the neuro-vegetative stability of thermoregulation, cardiovascular regulation and thus as protective factors of physical health.

Dizziness, Sleep and Heat Balance

The items for assessing dizziness, sleep and heat balance are part of the psycho-vegetative complaints questionnaire (Sect. 3.3.2.4).

For the separate evaluation of the dizziness, sleep and heat balance categories, the answers are coded from 0 = "no/never" to 3 = "strongly/very often" (Table 3.55). The respective sum of the answers to the individual question blocks is used to classify the areas of the health traffic light (Table 3.56).

3.3.4.4 Pittsburgh Sleep Quality Index (PSQI) Questionnaire

The PSQI [17] has been used in VITERIO since 2021 and retrospectively surveys the frequency of sleep-disturbing events, the assessment of sleep quality, usual sleep times, sleep latency and sleep duration, the use of sleep medication and daytime

Table 3.56 Psycho-vegetative stability—threshold values

Threshold values Psycho-vegetative stability	*Green* Desirable	*Yellow* Improvable	*Red* Critical
Dizziness (0–9 points)	<2	2–3	>3
Sleep (0–12 points)	<3	3–5	>5
Heat balance (0–12 points)	<3	3–5	>5

Table 3.57 PSQI—threshold values

	Red Clear signs of a sleep disorder	*Yellow* Indications of a sleep disorders	*Green* Unimpaired sleep quality
PSQI total score	11–21	6–10	0–5

sleepiness over a period of 4 weeks. A total of 18 items is used for quantitative evaluation and assigned to seven components, each of which can have a value range from 0 to 3. The PSQI is used to assess sleep quality in sleep disorders, especially insomnia.

The total score results from the summation of the component scores and can vary from 0 to 21, with a higher score corresponding to reduced sleep quality. There is an empirically determined cut-off value (of 5) that allows classification into "good" and "poor" sleepers.

The corresponding categorization of the values in the context of the health traffic light is as shown in Table 3.57.

3.3.5 Risks to Physical Health

Overview

- Cardiovascular risk (10-year forecast)
- Diabetes/high blood pressure risk
- Development of a diabetes risk
- Development of a risk of high blood pressure
- Metabolic syndrome
- Fatty liver
- Alcohol and smoking status

To identify patients with the highest cardiovascular risk who can benefit most from a preventive lifestyle programme, the following dimensions are systematically documented as part of the physical health assessment: the 10-year overall risk of cardiovascular events (such as heart attack, stroke, or sudden cardiac death) using the SCORE2 and SCORE2-OP (Older Persons); presence and risk of diabetes mellitus and arterial hypertension; risk of metabolic syndrome and fatty liver disease; as well as smoking and alcohol consumption [18].

Table 3.58 Risks to physical health—threshold values

Threshold values	*Green*	*Yellow 1*	*Yellow 2*	*Red 1*	*Red 2*
Cardiovascular Risk (SCORE2)					
<50 years	<2.5	2.5 to <7.5	–	=7.5	–
50–69 years	<5	5 to <10	–	=10	–
=70 years	<7.5	7.5 to <15	–	=15	–
Diabetes Risk (FINDRISK)	<7	7–11	12–14	15–20	>20
High Blood Pressure Risk	–	–	–	–	–
Metabolic Syndrome Index	<3	–	–	=3	–
Fatty Liver Index	<30	30–60	–	>60	–
Alcohol Consumption	<2	–	–	=2	–
Nicotine Addiction	=2	3–5	–	6–7	>7

Given the increased risk of cardiovascular disease among psychosomatic patients, monitoring physical risk factors and early detection are important measures. People with mental illness have a life expectancy that is up to 15 years shorter [19]. This population group has cardiometabolic risks and diseases at rates 1·4–2·0 times higher than people without mental illness [19].

Table 3.58 shows an overview of the classification of the "Risk to Physical Health Profile" within the three categories of the health traffic light system.

For the diabetes risk profile, the yellow and red categories are further subdivided to allow for a more detailed specification of the clinical indication. Due to the absence of established threshold values, the parameters for high blood pressure risk are not incorporated into the traffic light classification system. Figure 3.14 and Table 3.59 present an overview of the results for the risks to physical health factors.

3.3.5.1 Questionnaire on Cardiovascular Risk

The SCORE2 ("Systematic COronary Risk Evaluation") was developed by the European Society of Cardiology (ESC) in 2021 [18]. It can be used to estimate the 10-year risk of a cardiovascular disease such as the occurrence of a cardiac event in the form of a heart attack, stroke or sudden cardiac death based on the following information:

- Gender
- Age
- Total cholesterol
- HDL cholesterol
- Systolic blood pressure
- Smoking status

In addition, the regional risk of developing cardiovascular disease, which is based on the regional incidence rates for cardiovascular disease, is considered for the calculation. The European countries were divided into four categories (low-risk, medium-risk, high-risk and very high-risk regions). Germany was classified as a medium-risk region (100 to <150 deaths per 100,000 due to cardiovascular disease) [20, 21].

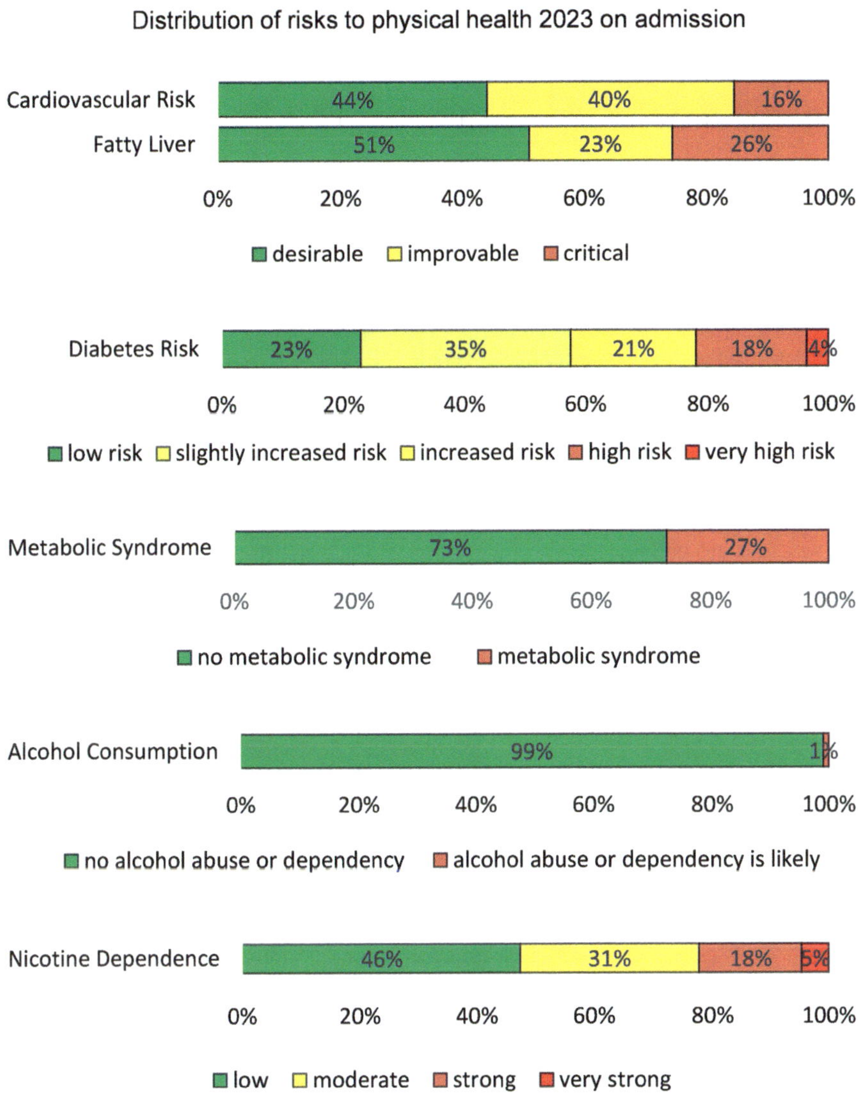

Fig. 3.14 Distribution of the "risks to physical health" profile factors

The corresponding categorization of the score-values (10-year risk in %) by the ESC in the context of the health traffic light system is as shown in Table 3.60.

3.3.5.2 Risk of Developing Diabetes (FINDRISK)

The risk assessment requires information on age, BMI, waist circumference (separated by gender), exercise and dietary habits, blood pressure and diabetes in personal history and family history of hypertension (Findrisk [22]). These are combined

Table 3.59 Risks to physical health profile: measures of dispersion and frequency distribution within the three categories of the health traffic light for 2023

Risks to physical health	Admission												
				Green		Yellow 1		Yellow 2		Red 1		Red 2	
	n	M	SD	*n*	%	*n*	%	*n*	%	*n*	%	*n*	%
SCORE2	719	6.58	5.84	316	43.9	288	40.1	–	–	115	16.0	–	–
FINDRISK	775	10.62	5.00	177	22.8	270	34.8	159	20.5	141	18.2	28	3.6
HBP Risk	608	5.60	5.85	–	–	–	–	–	–	–	–	–	–
MS Index	747	1.88	1.28	452	73.0	–	–	–	–	167	27.0	–	–
Fatty Liver	801	37.62	30.12	409	51.1	187	23.3	-	–	205	25.6	–	–
Alcohol	825			818	99.1	–	–	–	–	7	0.9	–	–
Smoking[a]	84			39	44.7	26	31.0	–	–	15	17.9	4	4.8

HPB high blood pressure, *MS* metabolic syndrome

[a]The questionnaire on nicotine dependence is only activated for patients who reported being smokers

Table 3.60 ESC—threshold values

ESC total score values in % for age	*Red*	*Yellow*	*Green*
<50 years	=7.5	2.5 to <7.5	<2.5
50–69 years	=10	5 to <10	<5
=70 years	=15	7.5 to <15	<7.5

Table 3.61 FINDRISK—threshold values

Category	Points	10-year probability of developing type 2 diabetes mellitus
Low risk	<7	<1%
Slightly increased risk	7–11	Approximately 4%
Increased risk	12–14	Approximately 17%
High risk	15–20	Approximately 33%
Very high risk	>20	Approximately 50%

into a total score, and the total score corresponds to a certain probability of developing type 2 diabetes mellitus in the next 10 years. A test result of 12 points or more is considered "increased risk".

First, this point value is determined for each patient, which can then be divided into five risk groups (i.e. the percentage probability of developing diabetes in the next 10 years). Patients with known diabetes are excluded from the analyses.

Table 3.61 summarizes the corresponding categories.

3.3.5.3 Risk of Developing High Blood Pressure

Information on age, gender, blood pressure, BMI, smoking habits and family history of hypertension is required for the risk assessment [23]. For this purpose, point values are assigned that are added to an overall score. The total score corresponds to a certain probability of developing hypertension within 1, 2 or 4 years. The test result is considered abnormal in terms of the 1-year risk if there are at least 15

Table 3.62 Calculation of the hypertension risk

Total score	1-year Risk %	2-year Risk %	4-year Risk %	Total score	1-year Risk %	2-year Risk %	4-year Risk %
-12	0.06	0.11	0.22	9	1.94	3.84	7.53
-11	0.07	0.13	0.27	10	2.29	4.53	8.86
-10	0.08	0.16	0.31	11	2.71	5.34	10.40
-9	0.09	0.19	0.37	12	3.20	6.30	12.20
-8	0.11	0.22	0.44	13	3.78	7.41	14.28
-7	0.13	0.26	0.52	14	4.46	8.72	16.68
-6	0.15	0.31	0.62	15	5.26	10.24	19.43
-5	0.18	0.37	0.73	16	6.20	12.01	22.58
-4	0.22	0.43	0.86	17	7.30	14.06	26.14
-3	0.26	0.51	1.02	18	8.58	16.43	30.16
-2	0.30	0.61	1.21	19	10.08	19.15	34.63
-1	0.36	0.72	1.43	20	11.82	22.25	39.55
0	0.43	0.85	1.69	21	13.85	25.77	44.91
1	0.50	1.01	2.00	22	16.18	29.74	50.64
2	0.60	1.19	2.37	23	18.86	34.17	56.66
3	0.71	1.41	2.80	24	21.93	39.05	62.85
4	0.84	1.67	3.31	25	25.41	44.36	69.05
5	0.99	1.97	3.90	26	29.33	50.06	75.06
6	1.17	2.33	4.61	27	33.71	56.06	80.69
7	1.39	2.75	5.43	28	38.55	62.24	85.74
8	1.64	3.25	6.40				

points. A 1-year risk >5% is considered "medium risk" and >10% is considered high risk. If the calculated "total score" of the Hypertension Risk Questionnaire [21] yields at least 15 points for the characteristics of hypertension in relatives, age, gender, blood pressure, BMI and smoking, this indicates a "medium risk" of 5–10% of developing hypertension in the next year. Two further prognosis periods are considered: developing hypertension within the next 2 years and within the next 4 years. Patients with known hypertension are not included in these analyses.

Table 3.62 gives an overview of the risk calculation.

3.3.5.4 Metabolic Syndrome

Cardiovascular diseases are still one of the most common causes of death in Western industrialized countries. This is due to the widespread unhealthy lifestyle and the resulting risk factors such as obesity, lipo-metabolic disorders, diabetes mellitus, nicotine abuse and arterial hypertension [24, 25]. The steady increase in depression and burnout is also increasingly relevant for the development and treatment of cardiovascular diseases. Regardless of the diagnosis or the reason for treatment, all patients in 2023 were screened for cardiometabolic risks in terms of metabolic syndrome. These include increased waist circumference, increased blood pressure, lipo-metabolic disorders and increased blood sugar levels. Data for this were obtained from the risk assessment questionnaires used, the documented vital parameters such as blood pressure and waist circumference, as well as current laboratory values.

From the resulting irregular data pattern, the measurements taken at comparable time points were extracted. For the baseline value, the interval was defined as ±7 days around the admission date, and for the discharge value, an interval of ±7 days up to the discharge date was also applied. In order to obtain the most valid measured values possible, the vital parameters entered by the *Health Coach* (if available) were used. On average, the valid laboratory baseline values were measured 1.4 days after admission and the discharge values 3.1 days before the day of departure. The vital signs were measured on average 1.8 days after admission and 3.1 days before discharge.

According to the definition of the *International Diabetes Federation* [24], a metabolic syndrome is present, if three of the following diagnostic criteria apply:

- Increased waist circumference (=102 men, =88 women)
- Elevated blood pressure (systolic =130/diastolic =85 mmHg) or corresponding medication
- Triglycerides increased (=150 mg/dl)
- HDL-C low (men <40/women <50 mg/dl) or appropriate medication
- Fasting glucose elevated (=100 mg/dl) or appropriate medication

Additionally, a metabolic index ranging from 0 to 5 can be calculated, with one point assigned for each criterion that is met [25].

3.3.5.5 Fatty Liver

In addition to assessing metabolic syndrome, hypertension and diabetes risk, evaluating the Fatty Liver Index (FLI) provides valuable insight into hepatic metabolic health. The following parameters are used to determine the presence of fatty liver [26]:

- Body Mass Index (BMI)
- Waist Circumference (WC)
- Triglycerides
- Gamma-Glutamyltransferase (GGT)

Based on these parameters, the following calculation is used to obtain a score ranging from 1 to 100 [26]:

$$FLI = \frac{e^{0.953*\log e(\text{triglycerides})+0.139*BMI+0.718*\log e(GGT)+0.053*WC-15.745}}{1+e^{0.953*\log e(\text{triglycerides})+0.139*BMI+0.718*\log e(GGT)+0.053*WC-15.745}} * 100$$

The result can be interpreted as shown in Table 3.63.

3.3.5.6 Alcohol and Smoking Status

Alcohol Consumption

There is an optional questionnaire for querying the risk factor alcohol. The so-called CAGE test [27] is dynamically activated if the question about regular alcohol consumption in the cardiovascular/metabolic questionnaire is answered with "more than two glasses per day". The CAGE test consists of four questions, which are listed in Table 3.64.

Table 3.63 Fatty liver—threshold values

FLI	Probability of a fatty liver disease
>60	An over 80% probability that a fatty liver disease is present
<30	A high probability that there is no fatty liver present

Table 3.64 Questionnaire on alcohol status

CAGE test	Yes	No
Have you ever felt the need to cut down your alcohol consumption?	1	0
Have you ever felt annoyed by criticism of your drinking behaviour?	1	0
Have you ever felt bad or guilty about drinking?	1	0
Have you ever needed alcohol in the morning in order to get going?	1	0

Two positive answers correspond to a 60% probability of alcohol dependence. Thus, if two or more questions are answered with "yes", alcohol abuse or alcohol dependence is likely. However, further differential diagnostic steps are required to rule out alcohol dependence. Each of the dichotomous items is scored with one point if answered affirmatively.

It should be noted that the results regarding alcohol consumption do not allow firm conclusions about whether the prevalence of conspicuous alcohol consumption truly reflects reality or whether this sensitive topic may have led to response bias, for example, due to social desirability.

Out of the 821 patients who answered the questionnaire, eight reported a consumption of more than two glasses of alcohol per day. Seven of these eight patients showed a high probability of alcohol dependence according to the CAGE test. Thus, 0.9% of the patients in 2023 reported a conspicuous alcohol consumption, meaning that at least two of the four CAGE test questions were answered with "yes" (Table 3.65).

Nicotine Consumption

The nicotine consumption ("Are you a smoker?") asked in the diabetes/hypertension risk questionnaire leads to the activation of an additional test procedure if answered with "Yes"—the smoking questionnaire. This is used to assess existing nicotine behaviour or an existing nicotine addiction. Questions about smoking behaviour are asked, weighted and given a score that reflects the level of nicotine dependence. The questionnaire used for this is the Fagerström Test for Nicotine Dependence (FTNA [28]), which is a refined version of the Fagerström Tolerance Questionnaire [29] and assesses nicotine-relevant addiction criteria. The self-assessment scale is an economical way of diagnosing and grading nicotine dependence, e.g. for determining the indications for addiction therapy. The procedure consists of six items. Addiction severity is determined directly based on the total score, which ranges from 0 to 10 (Table 3.66).

Table 3.65 Frequency distribution of alcohol consumption behaviour; broken down by gender in 2023

	2023						Previous years					
	Men $n = 170$		Women $n = 651$		Total $n = 821$		Men $n = 3491$		Women $n = 9759$		Total $n = 13{,}266$	
Alcohol consumption	*n*	%	*n*	%	*n*	%	*n*	%	*n*	%	*n*	%
Conspicuous (=2 Yes-Answers)	4	2.4	3	0.5	7	0.9	24	0.7	17	0.2	41	0.3

Table 3.66 Nicotine addiction—threshold values

Threshold values Nicotine addiction	*Green*	*Yellow*	*Red*	*Red*
Level of dependency	Low	Moderate	High	Very high
Score	=2	3–5	6–7	=8

Table 3.67 Frequency distribution of nicotine consumption behaviour; separated by gender in 2023 and previous years

	2023						Previous years					
	Men $n = 16$		Women $n = 68$		Total $n = 84$		Men $n = 483$		Women $n = 1055$		Total $n = 1538$	
Nicotine dependence	*n*	%	*n*	%	*n*	%	*n*	%	*n*	%	*n*	%
Low	6	37.5	33	48.5	39	46.4	216	44.7	550	52.1	766	49.8
Medium strong	5	31.2	21	30.9	26	31.0	188	38.9	379	35.9	567	36.9
Strong	5	31.2	10	14.7	15	17.9	65	13.5	105	10.0	170	11.1
Very strong	0	0.0	4	5.9	4	4.8	14	2.9	21	2.0	35	2.3

Of the 84 patients who completed the smoking questionnaire, slightly less than half (46.4%) reported a low level of nicotine dependence, while nearly one-third (31.0%) indicated a moderate level of dependence. In percentage terms, men were more likely to exhibit higher levels of nicotine dependence (moderate to severe; Table 3.67).

The latest recommendations from leading international medical associations demonstrate how important it is to identify protective and risk factors for health.

In 2022, the AHA published Life's Essential 8, a set of guidelines for health promotion and the prevention of cardiovascular disease [30]. The components of Life's Essential 8 include diet (updated), physical activity, nicotine exposure (updated), sleep health (new), body mass index, blood lipids (updated), blood glucose (updated) and blood pressure. This is due to a constant interplay of brain-mind-heart-body connections, which can have both positive and negative effects on the cardiovascular system.

A recent study examined the relationship between various lifestyle factors and the incidence and mortality rates of non-communicable diseases (NCDs), such as cancer, cardiovascular disease (CVD) and type 2 diabetes (T2D), in 2025 [31]. Lifestyle scores that considered both smoking and BMI showed the strongest overall associations. Healthy lifestyle scores, in terms of protective health factors and a low chronic disease risk index, performed best in predicting NCDs [31].

Appendix

Table 3.68 Frequency of all diagnoses (n = 7031) in 2023 (without differentiation between primary and secondary diagnosis); 3-digit coding; sorted according to the frequency

ICD-10	n	% of diag.	% of pat.	ICD-10	n	% of diag.	% of pat.	ICD-10	n	% of diag.	% of pat.
F45	900	12.5	109.1	F54	29	0.4	3.5	E89	13	0.2	1.6
M54	500	6.9	60.6	K21	29	0.4	3.5	G56	13	0.2	1.6
F33	441	6.1	53.5	K29	29	0.4	3.5	K07	13	0.2	1.6
G93	414	5.7	50.2	G25	28	0.4	3.4	K50	13	0.2	1.6
M79	268	3.7	32.5	L20	28	0.4	3.4	M06	13	0.2	1.6
G47	258	3.6	31.3	M18	26	0.4	3.2	D50	12	0.2	1.5
F51	238	3.3	28.8	M62	26	0.4	3.2	M23	12	0.2	1.5
I10	201	2.8	24.4	M81	25	0.3	3.0	M43	12	0.2	1.5
F32	149	2.1	18.1	R51	25	0.3	3.0	H40	11	0.2	1.3
G44	146	2.0	17.7	J32	24	0.3	2.9	I73	11	0.2	1.3
F43	138	1.9	16.7	M77	24	0.3	2.9	J44	11	0.2	1.3
F41	116	1.6	14.1	M41	23	0.3	2.8	E73	10	0.1	1.2
H93	110	1.5	13.3	F34	22	0.3	2.7	F06	10	0.1	1.2
G43	109	1.5	13.2	G50	22	0.3	2.7	I83	10	0.1	1.2
K58	106	1.5	12.8	K51	22	0.3	2.7	Q66	10	0.1	1.2
E03	94	1.3	11.4	M99	22	0.3	2.7	R20	10	0.1	1.2
M53	90	1.2	10.9	Z88	21	0.3	2.5	B02	9	0.1	1.1
E66	87	1.2	10.5	E04	19	0.3	2.3	D68	9	0.1	1.1
M25	85	1.2	10.3	R53	19	0.3	2.3	F50	9	0.1	1.1
T73	80	1.1	9.7	M50	18	0.2	2.2	F90	9	0.1	1.1
E06	68	0.9	8.2	F40	17	0.2	2.1	I48	9	0.1	1.1
M51	57	0.8	6.9	F48	17	0.2	2.1	K57	9	0.1	1.1
E78	55	0.8	6.7	I25	17	0.2	2.1	M76	9	0.1	1.1
G62	52	0.7	6.3	M35	17	0.2	2.1	N18	9	0.1	1.1
M17	47	0.7	5.7	J30	16	0.2	1.9	N30	9	0.1	1.1
M15	46	0.6	5.6	M20	16	0.2	1.9	A69	8	0.1	1.0
M19	46	0.6	5.6	K59	15	0.2	1.8	E79	8	0.1	1.0
M42	46	0.6	5.6	N39	15	0.2	1.8	F42	8	0.1	1.0
R52	45	0.6	5.5	N95	15	0.2	1.8	K52	8	0.1	1.0
B34	40	0.6	4.8	R06	15	0.2	1.8	M07	8	0.1	1.0
E11	40	0.6	4.8	Z96	15	0.2	1.8	M21	8	0.1	1.0
T78	39	0.5	4.7	F60	14	0.2	1.7	M32	8	0.1	1.0
R10	35	0.5	4.2	H81	14	0.2	1.7	M40	8	0.1	1.0
R42	34	0.5	4.1	H91	14	0.2	1.7	M45	8	0.1	1.0
M16	33	0.5	4.0	I89	14	0.2	1.7	N40	8	0.1	1.0
M75	32	0.4	3.9	M48	14	0.2	1.7	R12	8	0.1	1.0
L40	30	0.4	3.6	Z73	14	0.2	1.7	G53	7	0.1	0.8
M47	30	0.4	3.6	C50	13	0.2	1.6	I47	7	0.1	0.8
Z98	30	0.4	3.6	E88	13	0.2	1.6	I49	7	0.1	0.8
I87	7	0.1	0.8	K91	4	0.1	0.5	J06	3	0.0	0.4
K10	7	0.1	0.8	L30	4	0.1	0.5	K30	3	0.0	0.4
N80	7	0.1	0.8	L50	4	0.1	0.5	K63	3	0.0	0.4
G40	6	0.1	0.7	L70	4	0.1	0.5	K74	3	0.0	0.4
G63	6	0.1	0.7	M13	4	0.1	0.5	K80	3	0.0	0.4
H35	6	0.1	0.7	M71	4	0.1	0.5	L71	3	0.0	0.4
H53	6	0.1	0.7	M80	4	0.1	0.5	M08	3	0.0	0.4
I44	6	0.1	0.7	M93	4	0.1	0.5	M22	3	0.0	0.4
K76	6	0.1	0.7	M96	4	0.1	0.5	M24	3	0.0	0.4

(continued)

Table 3.68 (continued)

ICD-10	*n*	% of diag.	% of pat.	ICD-10	*n*	% of diag.	% of pat.	ICD-10	*n*	% of diag.	% of pat.
M05	6	0.1	0.7	N32	4	0.1	0.5	M65	3	0.0	0.4
Z92	6	0.1	0.7	Q65	4	0.1	0.5	M67	3	0.0	0.4
E80	5	0.1	0.6	R00	4	0.1	0.5	M84	3	0.0	0.4
F17	5	0.1	0.6	R05	4	0.1	0.5	M94	3	0.0	0.4
F31	5	0.1	0.6	R25	4	0.1	0.5	N19	3	0.0	0.4
I11	5	0.1	0.6	R26	4	0.1	0.5	N83	3	0.0	0.4
J34	5	0.1	0.6	R32	4	0.1	0.5	Q44	3	0.0	0.4
K64	5	0.1	0.6	R43	4	0.1	0.5	R14	3	0.0	0.4
L80	5	0.1	0.6	R49	4	0.1	0.5	R27	3	0.0	0.4
M10	5	0.1	0.6	R61	4	0.1	0.5	R45	3	0.0	0.4
M70	5	0.1	0.6	T88	4	0.1	0.5	S22	3	0.0	0.4
M72	5	0.1	0.6	Z90	4	0.1	0.5	S83	3	0.0	0.4
M85	5	0.1	0.6	Z95	4	0.1	0.5	T65	3	0.0	0.4
R07	5	0.1	0.6	B00	3	0.0	0.4	Z85	3	0.0	0.4
R11	5	0.1	0.6	B27	3	0.0	0.4	B18	2	0.0	0.2
R55	5	0.1	0.6	C34	3	0.0	0.4	C18	2	0.0	0.2
R63	5	0.1	0.6	D47	3	0.0	0.4	C19	2	0.0	0.2
B99	4	0.1	0.5	D75	3	0.0	0.4	C56	2	0.0	0.2
D64	4	0.1	0.5	D89	3	0.0	0.4	C73	2	0.0	0.2
E27	4	0.1	0.5	E07	3	0.0	0.4	D05	2	0.0	0.2
E55	4	0.1	0.5	E28	3	0.0	0.4	D21	2	0.0	0.2
F13	4	0.1	0.5	E74	3	0.0	0.4	D35	2	0.0	0.2
F44	4	0.1	0.5	E83	3	0.0	0.4	D51	2	0.0	0.2
G35	4	0.1	0.5	F07	3	0.0	0.4	D56	2	0.0	0.2
G45	4	0.1	0.5	F10	3	0.0	0.4	D69	2	0.0	0.2
G54	4	0.1	0.5	G04	3	0.0	0.4	E05	2	0.0	0.2
G55	4	0.1	0.5	G24	3	0.0	0.4	E10	2	0.0	0.2
G57	4	0.1	0.5	G51	3	0.0	0.4	E24	2	0.0	0.2
G60	4	0.1	0.5	G83	3	0.0	0.4	E87	2	0.0	0.2
G90	4	0.1	0.5	H10	3	0.0	0.4	F61	2	0.0	0.2
I20	4	0.1	0.5	H26	3	0.0	0.4	F62	2	0.0	0.2
I34	4	0.1	0.5	H52	3	0.0	0.4	F63	2	0.0	0.2
I63	4	0.1	0.5	H54	3	0.0	0.4	F84	2	0.0	0.2
I69	4	0.1	0.5	H90	3	0.0	0.4	G20	2	0.0	0.2
I70	4	0.1	0.5	I26	3	0.0	0.4	G30	2	0.0	0.2
K90	4	0.1	0.5	I67	3	0.0	0.4	G58	2	0.0	0.2
G61	2	0.0	0.2	A03	1	0.0	0.1	F55	1	0.0	0.1
G71	2	0.0	0.2	A09	1	0.0	0.1	F81	1	0.0	0.1
G81	2	0.0	0.2	B15	1	0.0	0.1	G21	1	0.0	0.1
G82	2	0.0	0.2	B35	1	0.0	0.1	G31	1	0.0	0.1
H04	2	0.0	0.2	B44	1	0.0	0.1	G37	1	0.0	0.1
H20	2	0.0	0.2	B66	1	0.0	0.1	G70	1	0.0	0.1
H30	2	0.0	0.2	B96	1	0.0	0.1	G72	1	0.0	0.1
I15	2	0.0	0.2	B98	1	0.0	0.1	G91	1	0.0	0.1
I71	2	0.0	0.2	C00	1	0.0	0.1	H00	1	0.0	0.1
I95	2	0.0	0.2	C09	1	0.0	0.1	H15	1	0.0	0.1
J20	2	0.0	0.2	C16	1	0.0	0.1	H25	1	0.0	0.1
J33	2	0.0	0.2	C17	1	0.0	0.1	H34	1	0.0	0.1
K12	2	0.0	0.2	C20	1	0.0	0.1	H49	1	0.0	0.1

(continued)

Table 3.68 (continued)

ICD-10	*n*	% of diag.	% of pat.	ICD-10	*n*	% of diag.	% of pat.	ICD-10	*n*	% of diag.	% of pat.
K14	2	0.0	0.2	C21	1	0.0	0.1	H50	1	0.0	0.1
K31	2	0.0	0.2	C43	1	0.0	0.1	H57	1	0.0	0.1
K44	2	0.0	0.2	C49	1	0.0	0.1	H60	1	0.0	0.1
K70	2	0.0	0.2	C54	1	0.0	0.1	H69	1	0.0	0.1
K92	2	0.0	0.2	C61	1	0.0	0.1	H83	1	0.0	0.1
L43	2	0.0	0.2	C68	1	0.0	0.1	H92	1	0.0	0.1
L63	2	0.0	0.2	C81	1	0.0	0.1	I07	1	0.0	0.1
L92	2	0.0	0.2	C84	1	0.0	0.1	I12	1	0.0	0.1
M31	2	0.0	0.2	C85	1	0.0	0.1	I21	1	0.0	0.1
M34	2	0.0	0.2	C92	1	0.0	0.1	I30	1	0.0	0.1
M89	2	0.0	0.2	D12	1	0.0	0.1	I31	1	0.0	0.1
N20	2	0.0	0.2	D14	1	0.0	0.1	I35	1	0.0	0.1
N28	2	0.0	0.2	D16	1	0.0	0.1	I51	1	0.0	0.1
N91	2	0.0	0.2	D18	1	0.0	0.1	I60	1	0.0	0.1
N94	2	0.0	0.2	D32	1	0.0	0.1	I65	1	0.0	0.1
N99	2	0.0	0.2	D33	1	0.0	0.1	I66	1	0.0	0.1
Q61	2	0.0	0.2	D45	1	0.0	0.1	I78	1	0.0	0.1
Q79	2	0.0	0.2	D46	1	0.0	0.1	I80	1	0.0	0.1
R15	2	0.0	0.2	D52	1	0.0	0.1	I99	1	0.0	0.1
R29	2	0.0	0.2	D59	1	0.0	0.1	J09	1	0.0	0.1
R39	2	0.0	0.2	D70	1	0.0	0.1	J31	1	0.0	0.1
R41	2	0.0	0.2	D82	1	0.0	0.1	J38	1	0.0	0.1
R60	2	0.0	0.2	D86	1	0.0	0.1	J45	1	0.0	0.1
R64	2	0.0	0.2	E29	1	0.0	0.1	K04	1	0.0	0.1
R94	2	0.0	0.2	E34	1	0.0	0.1	K11	1	0.0	0.1
S06	2	0.0	0.2	E60	1	0.0	0.1	K13	1	0.0	0.1
S52	2	0.0	0.2	E61	1	0.0	0.1	K22	1	0.0	0.1
S80	2	0.0	0.2	E72	1	0.0	0.1	K38	1	0.0	0.1
S82	2	0.0	0.2	F00	1	0.0	0.1	K42	1	0.0	0.1
S92	2	0.0	0.2	F38	1	0.0	0.1	K60	1	0.0	0.1
T63	2	0.0	0.2	F52	1	0.0	0.1	K66	1	0.0	0.1
Z45	2	0.0	0.2	F53	1	0.0	0.1	K71	1	0.0	0.1
L12	1	0.0	0.1	N90	1	0.0	0.1	S62	1	0.0	0.1
L42	1	0.0	0.1	N93	1	0.0	0.1	S70	1	0.0	0.1
L52	1	0.0	0.1	O87	1	0.0	0.1	S86	1	0.0	0.1
L65	1	0.0	0.1	Q76	1	0.0	0.1	S90	1	0.0	0.1
L66	1	0.0	0.1	Q87	1	0.0	0.1	S91	1	0.0	0.1
L73	1	0.0	0.1	Q96	1	0.0	0.1	S93	1	0.0	0.1
L90	1	0.0	0.1	Q99	1	0.0	0.1	T07	1	0.0	0.1
L94	1	0.0	0.1	R09	1	0.0	0.1	T79	1	0.0	0.1
L97	1	0.0	0.1	R21	1	0.0	0.1	T84	1	0.0	0.1
M02	1	0.0	0.1	R31	1	0.0	0.1	T87	1	0.0	0.1
M11	1	0.0	0.1	R40	1	0.0	0.1	Z54	1	0.0	0.1
M12	1	0.0	0.1	R46	1	0.0	0.1	Z56	1	0.0	0.1
M66	1	0.0	0.1	R47	1	0.0	0.1	Z63	1	0.0	0.1
M95	1	0.0	0.1	R50	1	0.0	0.1	Z72	1	0.0	0.1
N03	1	0.0	0.1	R73	1	0.0	0.1	Z83	1	0.0	0.1
N11	1	0.0	0.1	R74	1	0.0	0.1	Z86	1	0.0	0.1
N31	1	0.0	0.1	R80	1	0.0	0.1	Z87	1	0.0	0.1

(continued)

Table 3.68 (continued)

ICD-10	*n*	% of diag.	% of pat.	ICD-10	*n*	% of diag.	% of pat.	ICD-10	*n*	% of diag.	% of pat.
N34	1	0.0	0.1	R90	1	0.0	0.1	Z91	1	0.0	0.1
N36	1	0.0	0.1	R91	1	0.0	0.1	Z99	1	0.0	0.1
N76	1	0.0	0.1	S30	1	0.0	0.1				
N81	1	0.0	0.1	S43	1	0.0	0.1				

Table 3.69 Frequency of all diagnoses (*n* = 7031) in 2023 (without differentiation between primary and secondary diagnosis); 3-digit coding; sorted according to ICD-10 nomenclature

ICD-10	*n*	% of diag.	% of pat.	ICD-10	*n*	% of diag.	% of pat.	ICD-10	*n*	% of diag.	% of pat.
A03	1	0.0	0.1	D33	1	0.0	0.1	E89	13	0.2	1.6
A09	1	0.0	0.1	D35	2	0.0	0.2	F00	1	0.0	0.1
A69	8	0.1	1.0	D45	1	0.0	0.1	F06	10	0.1	1.2
B00	3	0.0	0.4	D46	1	0.0	0.1	F07	3	0.0	0.4
B02	9	0.1	1.1	D47	3	0.0	0.4	F10	3	0.0	0.4
B15	1	0.0	0.1	D50	12	0.2	1.5	F13	4	0.1	0.5
B18	2	0.0	0.2	D51	2	0.0	0.2	F17	5	0.1	0.6
B27	3	0.0	0.4	D52	1	0.0	0.1	F31	5	0.1	0.6
B34	40	0.6	4.8	D56	2	0.0	0.2	F32	149	2.1	18.1
B35	1	0.0	0.1	D59	1	0.0	0.1	F33	441	6.1	53.5
B44	1	0.0	0.1	D64	4	0.1	0.5	F34	22	0.3	2.7
B66	1	0.0	0.1	D68	9	0.1	1.1	F38	1	0.0	0.1
B96	1	0.0	0.1	D69	2	0.0	0.2	F40	17	0.2	2.1
B98	1	0.0	0.1	D70	1	0.0	0.1	F41	116	1.6	14.1
B99	4	0.1	0.5	D75	3	0.0	0.4	F42	8	0.1	1.0
C00	1	0.0	0.1	D82	1	0.0	0.1	F43	138	1.9	16.7
C09	1	0.0	0.1	D86	1	0.0	0.1	F44	4	0.1	0.5
C16	1	0.0	0.1	D89	3	0.0	0.4	F45	900	12.5	109.1
C17	1	0.0	0.1	E03	94	1.3	11.4	F48	17	0.2	2.1
C18	2	0.0	0.2	E04	19	0.3	2.3	F50	9	0.1	1.1
C19	2	0.0	0.2	E05	2	0.0	0.2	F51	238	3.3	28.8
C20	1	0.0	0.1	E06	68	0.9	8.2	F52	1	0.0	0.1
C21	1	0.0	0.1	E07	3	0.0	0.4	F53	1	0.0	0.1
C34	3	0.0	0.4	E10	2	0.0	0.2	F54	29	0.4	3.5
C43	1	0.0	0.1	E11	40	0.6	4.8	F55	1	0.0	0.1
C49	1	0.0	0.1	E24	2	0.0	0.2	F60	14	0.2	1.7
C50	13	0.2	1.6	E27	4	0.1	0.5	F61	2	0.0	0.2
C54	1	0.0	0.1	E28	3	0.0	0.4	F62	2	0.0	0.2
C56	2	0.0	0.2	E29	1	0.0	0.1	F63	2	0.0	0.2
C61	1	0.0	0.1	E34	1	0.0	0.1	F81	1	0.0	0.1
C68	1	0.0	0.1	E55	4	0.1	0.5	F84	2	0.0	0.2
C73	2	0.0	0.2	E60	1	0.0	0.1	F90	9	0.1	1.1
C81	1	0.0	0.1	E61	1	0.0	0.1	G04	3	0.0	0.4
C84	1	0.0	0.1	E66	87	1.2	10.5	G20	2	0.0	0.2
C85	1	0.0	0.1	E72	1	0.0	0.1	G21	1	0.0	0.1
C92	1	0.0	0.1	E73	10	0.1	1.2	G24	3	0.0	0.4
D05	2	0.0	0.2	E74	3	0.0	0.4	G25	28	0.4	3.4
D12	1	0.0	0.1	E78	55	0.8	6.7	G30	2	0.0	0.2
D14	1	0.0	0.1	E79	8	0.1	1.0	G31	1	0.0	0.1

(continued)

Table 3.69 (continued)

ICD-10	*n*	% of diag.	% of pat.	ICD-10	*n*	% of diag.	% of pat.	ICD-10	*n*	% of diag.	% of pat.
D16	1	0.0	0.1	E80	5	0.1	0.6	G35	4	0.1	0.5
D18	1	0.0	0.1	E83	3	0.0	0.4	G37	1	0.0	0.1
D21	2	0.0	0.2	E87	2	0.0	0.2	G40	6	0.1	0.7
D32	1	0.0	0.1	E88	13	0.2	1.6	G43	109	1.5	13.2
G44	146	2.0	17.7	H90	3	0.0	0.4	J34	5	0.1	0.6
G45	4	0.1	0.5	H91	14	0.2	1.7	J38	1	0.0	0.1
G47	258	3.6	31.3	H92	1	0.0	0.1	J44	11	0.2	1.3
G50	22	0.3	2.7	H93	110	1.5	13.3	J45	1	0.0	0.1
G51	3	0.0	0.4	I07	1	0.0	0.1	K04	1	0.0	0.1
G53	7	0.1	0.8	I10	201	2.8	24.4	K07	13	0.2	1.6
G54	4	0.1	0.5	I11	5	0.1	0.6	K10	7	0.1	0.8
G55	4	0.1	0.5	I12	1	0.0	0.1	K11	1	0.0	0.1
G56	13	0.2	1.6	I15	2	0.0	0.2	K12	2	0.0	0.2
G57	4	0.1	0.5	I20	4	0.1	0.5	K13	1	0.0	0.1
G58	2	0.0	0.2	I21	1	0.0	0.1	K14	2	0.0	0.2
G60	4	0.1	0.5	I25	17	0.2	2.1	K21	29	0.4	3.5
G61	2	0.0	0.2	I26	3	0.0	0.4	K22	1	0.0	0.1
G62	52	0.7	6.3	I30	1	0.0	0.1	K29	29	0.4	3.5
G63	6	0.1	0.7	I31	1	0.0	0.1	K30	3	0.0	0.4
G70	1	0.0	0.1	I34	4	0.1	0.5	K31	2	0.0	0.2
G71	2	0.0	0.2	I35	1	0.0	0.1	K38	1	0.0	0.1
G72	1	0.0	0.1	I44	6	0.1	0.7	K42	1	0.0	0.1
G81	2	0.0	0.2	I47	7	0.1	0.8	K44	2	0.0	0.2
G82	2	0.0	0.2	I48	9	0.1	1.1	K50	13	0.2	1.6
G83	3	0.0	0.4	I49	7	0.1	0.8	K51	22	0.3	2.7
G90	4	0.1	0.5	I51	1	0.0	0.1	K52	8	0.1	1.0
G91	1	0.0	0.1	I60	1	0.0	0.1	K57	9	0.1	1.1
G93	414	5.7	50.2	I63	4	0.1	0.5	K58	106	1.5	12.8
H00	1	0.0	0.1	I65	1	0.0	0.1	K59	15	0.2	1.8
H04	2	0.0	0.2	I66	1	0.0	0.1	K60	1	0.0	0.1
H10	3	0.0	0.4	I67	3	0.0	0.4	K63	3	0.0	0.4
H15	1	0.0	0.1	I69	4	0.1	0.5	K64	5	0.1	0.6
H20	2	0.0	0.2	I70	4	0.1	0.5	K66	1	0.0	0.1
H25	1	0.0	0.1	I71	2	0.0	0.2	K70	2	0.0	0.2
H26	3	0.0	0.4	I73	11	0.2	1.3	K71	1	0.0	0.1
H30	2	0.0	0.2	I78	1	0.0	0.1	K74	3	0.0	0.4
H34	1	0.0	0.1	I80	1	0.0	0.1	K76	6	0.1	0.7
H35	6	0.1	0.7	I83	10	0.1	1.2	K80	3	0.0	0.4
H40	11	0.2	1.3	I87	7	0.1	0.8	K90	4	0.1	0.5
H49	1	0.0	0.1	I89	14	0.2	1.7	K91	4	0.1	0.5
H50	1	0.0	0.1	I95	2	0.0	0.2	K92	2	0.0	0.2
H52	3	0.0	0.4	I99	1	0.0	0.1	L12	1	0.0	0.1
H53	6	0.1	0.7	J06	3	0.0	0.4	L20	28	0.4	3.4
H54	3	0.0	0.4	J09	1	0.0	0.1	L30	4	0.1	0.5
H57	1	0.0	0.1	J20	2	0.0	0.2	L40	30	0.4	3.6
H60	1	0.0	0.1	J30	16	0.2	1.9	L42	1	0.0	0.1
H69	1	0.0	0.1	J31	1	0.0	0.1	L43	2	0.0	0.2
H81	14	0.2	1.7	J32	24	0.3	2.9	L50	4	0.1	0.5
H83	1	0.0	0.1	J33	2	0.0	0.2	L52	1	0.0	0.1

(continued)

Table 3.69 (continued)

ICD-10	*n*	% of diag.	% of pat.	ICD-10	*n*	% of diag.	% of pat.	ICD-10	*n*	% of diag.	% of pat.
L63	2	0.0	0.2	M54	500	6.9	60.6	O87	1	0.0	0.1
L65	1	0.0	0.1	M62	26	0.4	3.2	Q44	3	0.0	0.4
L66	1	0.0	0.1	M65	3	0.0	0.4	Q61	2	0.0	0.2
L70	4	0.1	0.5	M66	1	0.0	0.1	Q65	4	0.1	0.5
L71	3	0.0	0.4	M67	3	0.0	0.4	Q66	10	0.1	1.2
L73	1	0.0	0.1	M70	5	0.1	0.6	Q76	1	0.0	0.1
L80	5	0.1	0.6	M71	4	0.1	0.5	Q79	2	0.0	0.2
L90	1	0.0	0.1	M72	5	0.1	0.6	Q87	1	0.0	0.1
L92	2	0.0	0.2	M75	32	0.4	3.9	Q96	1	0.0	0.1
L94	1	0.0	0.1	M76	9	0.1	1.1	Q99	1	0.0	0.1
L97	1	0.0	0.1	M77	24	0.3	2.9	R00	4	0.1	0.5
M02	1	0.0	0.1	M79	268	3.7	32.5	R05	4	0.1	0.5
M05	6	0.1	0.7	M80	4	0.1	0.5	R06	15	0.2	1.8
M06	13	0.2	1.6	M81	25	0.3	3.0	R07	5	0.1	0.6
M07	8	0.1	1.0	M84	3	0.0	0.4	R09	1	0.0	0.1
M08	3	0.0	0.4	M85	5	0.1	0.6	R10	35	0.5	4.2
M10	5	0.1	0.6	M89	2	0.0	0.2	R11	5	0.1	0.6
M11	1	0.0	0.1	M93	4	0.1	0.5	R12	8	0.1	1.0
M12	1	0.0	0.1	M94	3	0.0	0.4	R14	3	0.0	0.4
M13	4	0.1	0.5	M95	1	0.0	0.1	R15	2	0.0	0.2
M15	46	0.6	5.6	M96	4	0.1	0.5	R20	10	0.1	1.2
M16	33	0.5	4.0	M99	22	0.3	2.7	R21	1	0.0	0.1
M17	47	0.7	5.7	N03	1	0.0	0.1	R25	4	0.1	0.5
M18	26	0.4	3.2	N11	1	0.0	0.1	R26	4	0.1	0.5
M19	46	0.6	5.6	N18	9	0.1	1.1	R27	3	0.0	0.4
M20	16	0.2	1.9	N19	3	0.0	0.4	R29	2	0.0	0.2
M21	8	0.1	1.0	N20	2	0.0	0.2	R31	1	0.0	0.1
M22	3	0.0	0.4	N28	2	0.0	0.2	R32	4	0.1	0.5
M23	12	0.2	1.5	N30	9	0.1	1.1	R39	2	0.0	0.2
M24	3	0.0	0.4	N31	1	0.0	0.1	R40	1	0.0	0.1
M25	85	1.2	10.3	N32	4	0.1	0.5	R41	2	0.0	0.2
M31	2	0.0	0.2	N34	1	0.0	0.1	R42	34	0.5	4.1
M32	8	0.1	1.0	N36	1	0.0	0.1	R43	4	0.1	0.5
M34	2	0.0	0.2	N39	15	0.2	1.8	R45	3	0.0	0.4
M35	17	0.2	2.1	N40	8	0.1	1.0	R46	1	0.0	0.1
M40	8	0.1	1.0	N76	1	0.0	0.1	R47	1	0.0	0.1
M41	23	0.3	2.8	N80	7	0.1	0.8	R49	4	0.1	0.5
M42	46	0.6	5.6	N81	1	0.0	0.1	R50	1	0.0	0.1
M43	12	0.2	1.5	N83	3	0.0	0.4	R51	25	0.3	3.0
M45	8	0.1	1.0	N90	1	0.0	0.1	R52	45	0.6	5.5
M47	30	0.4	3.6	N91	2	0.0	0.2	R53	19	0.3	2.3
M48	14	0.2	1.7	N93	1	0.0	0.1	R55	5	0.1	0.6
M50	18	0.2	2.2	N94	2	0.0	0.2	R60	2	0.0	0.2
M51	57	0.8	6.9	N95	15	0.2	1.8	R61	4	0.1	0.5
M53	90	1.2	10.9	N99	2	0.0	0.2	R63	5	0.1	0.6
R64	2	0.0	0.2	S86	1	0.0	0.1	Z63	1	0.0	0.1
R73	1	0.0	0.1	S90	1	0.0	0.1	Z72	1	0.0	0.1
R74	1	0.0	0.1	S91	1	0.0	0.1	Z73	14	0.2	1.7
R80	1	0.0	0.1	S92	2	0.0	0.2	Z83	1	0.0	0.1

(continued)

Table 3.69 (continued)

ICD-10	*n*	% of diag.	% of pat.	ICD-10	*n*	% of diag.	% of pat.	ICD-10	*n*	% of diag.	% of pat.
R90	1	0.0	0.1	S93	1	0.0	0.1	Z85	3	0.0	0.4
R91	1	0.0	0.1	T07	1	0.0	0.1	Z86	1	0.0	0.1
R94	2	0.0	0.2	T63	2	0.0	0.2	Z87	1	0.0	0.1
S06	2	0.0	0.2	T65	3	0.0	0.4	Z88	21	0.3	2.5
S22	3	0.0	0.4	T73	80	1.1	9.7	Z90	4	0.1	0.5
S30	1	0.0	0.1	T78	39	0.5	4.7	Z91	1	0.0	0.1
S43	1	0.0	0.1	T79	1	0.0	0.1	Z92	6	0.1	0.7
S52	2	0.0	0.2	T84	1	0.0	0.1	Z95	4	0.1	0.5
S62	1	0.0	0.1	T87	1	0.0	0.1	Z96	15	0.2	1.8
S70	1	0.0	0.1	T88	4	0.1	0.5	Z98	30	0.4	3.6
S80	2	0.0	0.2	Z45	2	0.0	0.2	Z99	1	0.0	0.1
S82	2	0.0	0.2	Z54	1	0.0	0.1				
S83	3	0.0	0.4	Z56	1	0.0	0.1				

References

1. Henrich G, Herschbach P. Questions on Life Satisfaction (FLZM). Eur J Psychol Assess. 2000;16:150–9. https://doi.org/10.1027/1015-5759.16.3.150.
2. Antonovsky A. The structure and properties of the Sense of Coherence Scale. Soc Sci Med. 1993;36:725–33. https://doi.org/10.1016/0277-9536(93)90033-Z.
3. Topp CW, Østergaard SD, Søndergaard S, Bech P. The WHO-5 Well-Being Index: a systematic review of the literature. Psychother Psychosom. 2015;84(3):167–76. https://doi.org/10.1159/000376585.
4. Bullinger M, Kirchberger I. SF-36 Health Status Questionnaire: manual. Göttingen: Hogrefe; 1998.
5. Scholler G, Fliege H, Klapp BF. Questionnaire on self-efficacy, optimism and pessimism: restructuring, item selection and validation of an instrument in studies of clinical samples. Psychother Psychosom Med Psychol. 1999;49(8):275–83.
6. Zanini DS, Peixoto EM, Nakano TC. The Social Support Scale (MOS-SSS): standardizing with item references. Trends Psychol. 2018;26(1):401–12. https://doi.org/10.9788/TP2018.1-15En.
7. Sherbourne CD, Stewart AL. The MOS Social Support Survey. Soc Sci Med. 1991;32(6):705–14. https://doi.org/10.1016/0277-9536(91)90150-B.
8. Pines A, Aronson E, Kafry D. Burnout: from tedium to personal growth. New York: Free Press; 1981.
9. Fliege H, Rose M, Arck P, Walter OB, Kocalevent RD, Weber C, Klapp BF. The Perceived Stress Questionnaire (PSQ) reconsidered: validation and reference values from different clinical and healthy adult samples. Psychosom Med. 2005;67(1):78–88. https://doi.org/10.1097/01.psy.0000151491.80178.78.
10. Linneweh K. Stressmanagement: Der erfolgreiche Umgang mit sich selbst [Dealing successfully with yourself]. Stuttgart: Deutscher Sparkassenverlag; 1998.
11. Tritt K, von Heymann F, Zaudig M, Zacharias I, Söllner W, Loew T. Development of the questionnaire "ICD-10-Symptom-Rating" (ISR). Z Psychosom Med Psychother. 2008;54:420–9. https://doi.org/10.13109/zptm.2008.54.4.409.
12. Krieger T, Zimmermann J, Huffziger S, Ubl B, Diener C, Kuehner C, Grosse Holtforth M. Measuring depression with a well-being index: further evidence for the validity of the WHO Well-Being Index (WHO-5) as a measure of the severity of depression. J Affect Disord. 2014;156:240–4. https://doi.org/10.1016/j.jad.2013.12.015.

13. Spitzer RL, Kroenke K, Williams JB, Löwe B. A brief measure for assessing generalized anxiety disorder: the GAD-7. Arch Intern Med. 2006;166(10):1092–7. https://doi.org/10.1001/archinte.166.10.1092.
14. Frey I, Berg A, Gratwohl D, Keul J. Freiburg Physical Activity Questionnaire—development, testing and application. Soz Präventivmed. 1999;44:55–64. https://doi.org/10.1007/BF01667127.
15. Marshall AL, Miller YD, Burton NW, Brown WJ. Measuring total and domain-specific sitting: a study of reliability and validity. Med Sci Sports Exerc. 2010;42(5):1094–102. https://doi.org/10.1249/MSS.0b013e3181c5ec18.
16. Deutsche Gesellschaft für Ernährung e. V. 10 Regeln der DGE für eine vollwertige Ernährung [Internet]. Bonn: DGE; [cited 2022 Sep 25]. Available from: https://www.dge.de/10regeln
17. Buysse DJ, Reynolds CF, Monk TH, Berman SR, Kupfer DJ. The Pittsburgh Sleep Quality Index: a new instrument for psychiatric practice and research. Psychiatry Res. 1989;28:193–213.
18. Visseren FLJ, Mach F, Smulders YM, Carballo D, Koskinas KC, Bäck M, et al. 2021 ESC Guidelines on cardiovascular disease prevention in clinical practice. Eur Heart J. 2021;42(34):3227–337. https://doi.org/10.1093/eurheartj/ehab484.
19. Teasdale SB, Machaczek KK, Marx W, Eaton M, Chapman J, Milton A, Oyeyemi AL, Pelupessy DC, Schuch FB, Gatera G, Ahmed HU, Diatri H, Jidda IM, Gutiérrez-Peláez M, Elshazly M, Fugu MA, Grinko N, Indu PS, Oo SS, Balasubramanian S, Deenik J, Vancampfort D, Stubbs B, Matthews E, Ward PB, Curtis J, Hassan L, Cortese S, Gilbody S, Lancet Psychiatry Physical Health Commission Consortium, Firth J, Rosenbaum S. Implementing lifestyle interventions in mental health care: third report of the Lancet Psychiatry Physical Health Commission. Lancet Psychiatry. 2025;12(9):700–22. https://doi.org/10.1016/S2215-0366(25)00170-1.
20. Levi F, Chatenoud L, Bertuccio P, Lucchini F, Negri E, La Vecchia C. Mortality from cardiovascular and cerebrovascular diseases in Europe and other areas of the world: an update. Eur J Cardiovasc Prev Rehabil. 2009;16(3):333–50.
21. Nichols M, Townsend N, Scarborough P, Rayner M. Cardiovascular disease in Europe 2014: epidemiological update. Eur Heart J. 2014;35(42):2950–9. https://doi.org/10.1093/eurheartj/ehu299.
22. Lindström J, Tuomilehto J. The Diabetes Risk Score: a practical tool to predict type 2 diabetes risk. Diabetes Care. 2003;26(3):725–31. https://doi.org/10.2337/diacare.26.3.725.
23. Parikh NI, Pencina MJ, Wang TJ, Benjamin EJ, Lanier KJ, Levy D, et al. A risk score for predicting near-term incidence of hypertension: the Framingham Heart Study. Ann Intern Med. 2008;148:102–10. https://doi.org/10.7326/0003-4819-148-2-200801150-00005.
24. Alberti KGMM, Eckel RH, Grundy SM, Zimmet PZ, Cleeman JI, Donato KA, et al. Harmonizing the metabolic syndrome: a joint interim statement. Circulation. 2009;120(16):1640–5. https://doi.org/10.1161/CIRCULATIONAHA.109.192644.
25. Jin H, Benyshek DC. The metabolic syndrome index: a novel, comprehensive method for evaluating the efficacy of diabetes prevention programs. J Diabetes Mellitus. 2013;3(2):96–9. https://doi.org/10.4236/jdm.2013.32014.
26. Bedogni G, Bellentani S, Miglioli L, Masutti F, Passalacqua M, Castiglione A, Tiribelli C. The Fatty Liver Index: a simple and accurate predictor of hepatic steatosis in the general population. BMC Gastroenterol. 2006;6:33. https://doi.org/10.1186/1471-230X-6-33.
27. Ewing JA. Detecting alcoholism: the CAGE questionnaire. JAMA. 1984;252(14):1905–7. https://doi.org/10.1001/jama.252.14.1905.
28. Heatherton TF, Kozlowski LT, Frecker RC, Fagerström KO. The Fagerström Test for Nicotine Dependence: a revision of the Fagerström Tolerance Questionnaire. Br J Addict. 1991;86(9):1119–27. https://doi.org/10.1111/j.1360-0443.1991.tb01879.x.
29. Fagerström KO. Measuring degree of physical dependence to tobacco smoking with reference to individualization of treatment. Addict Behav. 1978;3(3–4):235–41. https://doi.org/10.1016/0306-4603(78)90024-2.

30. Lloyd-Jones DM, Allen NB, Anderson CAM, Black T, Brewer LC, Foraker RE, Grandner MA, Lavretsky H, Perak AM, Sharma G, Rosamond W, American Heart Association. Life's Essential 8: updating and enhancing the American Heart Association's Construct of Cardiovascular Health: a presidential advisory from the American Heart Association. Circulation. 2022;146(5):e18–43. https://doi.org/10.1161/CIR.0000000000001078. Epub 2022 Jun 29. PMID: 35766027 ; PMCID: PMC10503546.
31. Ding J, Schöttker B, Brenner H, Hoffmeister M. Thirteen simple lifestyle scores and risk of cancer, cardiovascular disease, diabetes, and mortality: prospective cohort study in the UK Biobank. Int J Cancer. 2025;157(12):2495–505. https://doi.org/10.1002/ijc.70064.

Intervention Profile

4

Dieter Melchart, Jingzhang Dai, and Lara Isabel Jötten

4.1 TCM Drug Therapy (CHM = Chinese Herbal Medicine)

At the traditional Chinese medicine (TCM) clinic, each TCM prescription is documented and stored electronically on a case-by-case basis within the VITERIO® web portal (Fig. 4.1). Any changes to the prescription, such as alterations to the composition of the individual drugs and/or the dosage, are recorded as new prescriptions. During the inpatient stay in 2023 (and in previous years from 2008 to 2022), a total of 31,836 (55,387) individual drugs were prescribed, which can be assigned to 216 (264) different substances. A total of 2570 (42,606) prescriptions were written for the 822 (10,278) patients who were documented as receiving TCM therapy. Based on this data, an average of 3.0 (4.0) prescriptions per person can be determined, each containing an average of 13.0 (13.0) TCM. In relation to the number of grams per prescription, this results in an average quantity of 8.5 (6) grams per TCM. TCMs are administered daily to individual patients in their rooms in the form of decoctions kept warm in thermos flasks at midday and in the evening. In the reporting year 2023, 22 substances were not assigned to any mode of action. These substances were prescribed a total of 990 times (3.1%).

Each individual TCM is assigned a specific therapeutic effect. In the TCM clinic, this is based on the publication Materia Medica of Chinese Drug Therapy. Volume 2 is part of the Practice of Chinese Drug Therapy series [1]. These active principles are coded and can therefore be statistically evaluated in terms of their frequency. The coding system was developed in-house and is integrated into the VITERIO®

D. Melchart (✉) · L. I. Jötten
Faculty of Applied Healthcare Sciences, Deggendorf Institute of Technology (DIT), Competence Centre for Lifestyle Medicine and Naturopathy, Deggendorf, Germany
e-mail: dieter.melchart@th-deg.de; lara.joetten@th-deg.de

J. Dai
TCM-Klinik Bad Kötzting, Bad Kötzting, Germany

Beijing University of Chinese Medicine (BUCM), Beijing, People's Republic of China

D. Melchart et al. (eds.), *TCM-Klinik Bad Kötzting*,
https://doi.org/10.1007/978-3-032-23307-3_4

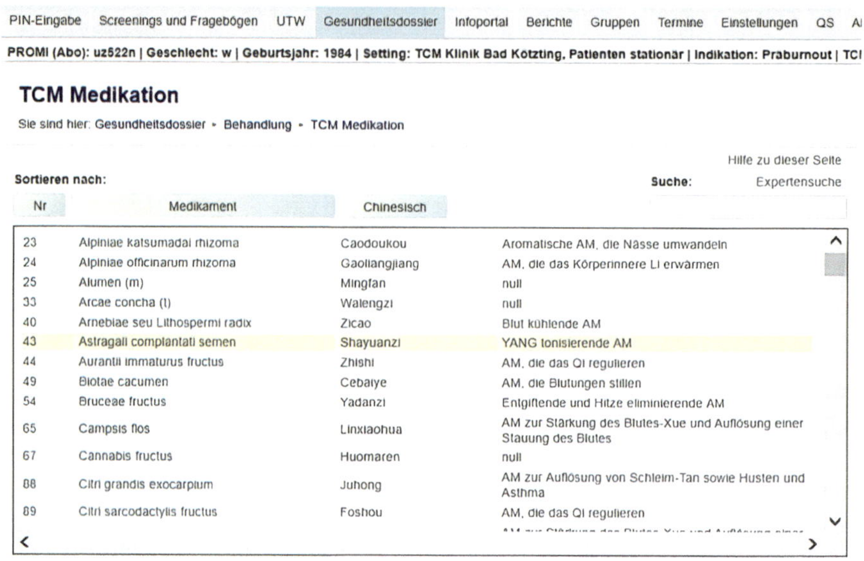

Fig. 4.1 Prescription of TCMs in web portal VITERIO®

web portal. TCMs are prescribed by compiling individual drugs via the portal, which automatically generates the required documentation and manufacturing recipes.

The active principle for strengthening the blood (Xue) and dissolving blood congestion was used most frequently (Fig. 4.2). Given the focus on 'blood stasis' and 'life qi stagnation' in Chap. 3, which presents a range of TCM syndrome diagnoses, it is logical to use medicinal interventions designed to 'dissolve blood stasis' and 'tonify qi'.

Table 4.1 refers to all prescriptions during inpatient stay in the reporting year and contains the corresponding substances sorted according to their prescription frequency. Astragali radix and Angelicae sinensis radix are the most commonly prescribed drugs.

The appendix contains a further Table 4.6 showing the same TCMs and their prescription frequency for the 2023 observation period but in alphabetical order.

For a better overview, the most frequently prescribed TCMs are presented in Fig. 4.2. In addition to all prescribed TCMs in the reporting year, the first drug prescriptions in 2023 are compared with those from previous years in Table 4.2 and Fig. 4.3.

According to TCM teachings, TCM such as Angelicae sinensis radix, Astragali radix and Paeoniae rubra radix are suitable for strengthening the blood (Xue) and dissolving blood stasis. In this combination, they also have a tonic effect on blood Qi [2, 3]. Chinese teachings say *Angelicae sinensis radix (Dang Gui)* is "warm" and "spicy and sweet". It is said to "tonify and move blood". The drug is therefore used to treat blood deficiency and pale complexion, dizziness, palpitations, abdominal

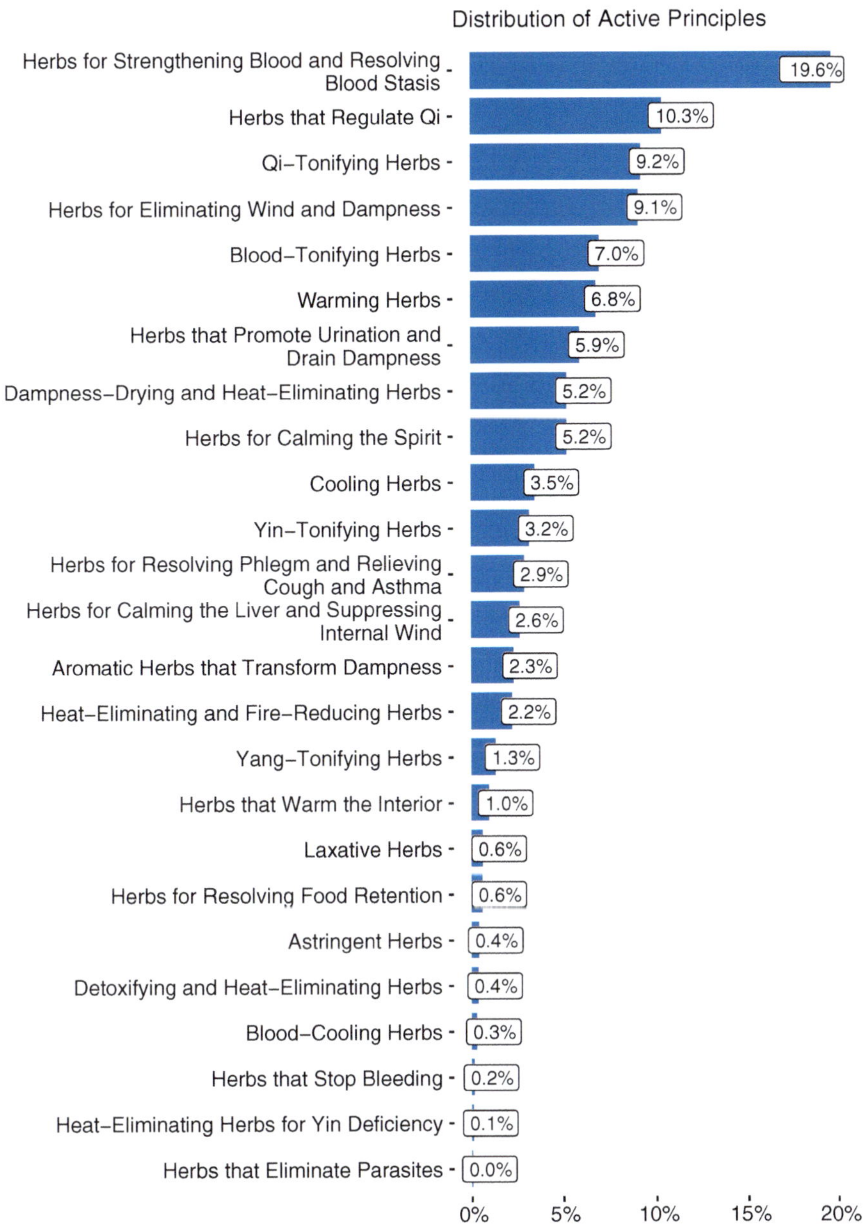

Fig. 4.2 Active principles of the prescribed TCMs (percentages in relation to the documented active principles in 2023 ($n = 30{,}846$)

Table 4.1 TCMs (percentages in relation to all prescriptions/prescribed substances in the reporting year 2023); sorted in descending frequency ($n = 31{,}836$)

TCM remedy (Latin)	*n*	%	TCM remedy (Latin)	*n*	%
Astragali radix	1322	4.2	Rehmanniae radix	220	0.7
Angelicae sinensis radix	1257	3.9	Codonopsis pilosulae radix	219	0.7
Paeoniae rubra radix	1222	3.8	Cassiae semen	218	0.7
Achyranthis bidentatae radix	1159	3.6	Citri sarcodactylis fructus	217	0.7
Spatholobi caulis	1102	3.5	Eucommiae cortex	212	0.7
Cinnamomi ramulus	1065	3.3	Trichosanthis fructus	202	0.6
Dipsaci radix	1039	3.3	Tribuli fructus	201	0.6
Poria (Stücke)	1013	3.2	Notopterygii rhizoma seu radix	198	0.6
Atractylodis macrocephalae rhizoma	961	3.0	Bombyx batryticatus (t)	195	0.6
Mori ramulus	943	3.0	Ledebouriellae radix	191	0.6
Bambusae caulis in taeniam	838	2.6	Rhei radix et rhizoma	184	0.6
Polygalae radix	801	2.5	Angelicae pubescentis radix	181	0.6
Curcumae longae rhizoma	784	2.5	Sappan lignum	171	0.5
Curcumae radix	742	2.3	Lycii fructus	169	0.5
Ligustri lucidi fructus	688	2.2	Meliae toosendan fructus	161	0.5
Aurantii fructus	655	2.1	Sinomenii caulis	159	0.5
Atractylodis rhizoma	598	1.9	Ostreae concha (m)	157	0.5
Loranthi ramulus	512	1.6	Zingiberis rhizoma	144	0.5
Sparganii tuber (rhizoma)	493	1.5	Uncariae cum uncis ramulus	142	0.4
Paeoniae alba radix	490	1.5	Mori radicis cortex	136	0.4
Albiziae cortex	476	1.5	Gentianae macrophyllae rhizoma	135	0.4
Angelicae dahuricae radix	475	1.5	Rehmanniae praeparatae rhizoma	130	0.4
Bupleuri radix	462	1.5	Ziziphi spinosae semen	111	0.3
Pinelliae praeparatae rhizoma	428	1.3	Lycopi herba	105	0.3
Magnoliae officinalis cortex	408	1.3	Prunellae spica	105	0.3
Ligustici chuanxiong rhizoma	377	1.2	Cuscutae semen	99	0.3
Puerariae radix	315	1.0	Dioscoreae rhizoma	96	0.3
Phellodendri cortex	312	1.0	Persicae semen	86	0.3
Chaenomelis fructus	303	1.0	Polygoni multiflori caulis	86	0.3
Anemarrhenae rhizoma	300	0.9	Biotae semen	85	0.3
Cyperi rhizoma	299	0.9	Citri reticulatae viride pericarpium	84	0.3
Coicis semen	279	0.9	Coptidis rhizoma	84	0.3
Scutellariae radix	277	0.9	Draconis os (t)	84	0.3
Liquidambaris fructus	274	0.9	Corydalis rhizoma	78	0.2
Salviae miltiorrhizae radix	247	0.8	Armeniacae amarum semen	75	0.2
Citri reticulatae pericarpium	233	0.7	Peucedani radix	74	0.2
Glycyrrhizae radix	225	0.7	Artemisiae argyi folium	73	0.2
Moutan radicis cortex	73	0.2	Sanguisorbae radix	35	0.1
Alismatis rhizoma	71	0.2	Pyrrosiae folium	34	0.1
Oryzae germinatus fructus	70	0.2	Leonuri fructus	33	0.1
Schisandrae fructus	70	0.2	Platycodi radix	31	0.1
Amomi cardamomi semen	69	0.2	Allii macrostemi bulbus	30	0.1
Menthae herba	69	0.2	Ecliptae herba	30	0.1
Chrysanthemi flos	68	0.2	Haliotidis concha (m)	30	0.1
Citri reticulatae semen	68	0.2	Ligustici rhizoma	29	0.1
Litchi semen	64	0.2	Cinnamomi cortex	25	0.1
Kochiae fructus	63	0.2	Imperatae rhizoma	25	0.1
Ophiopogonis radix	62	0.2	Lycii radicis cortex	25	0.1

(continued)

Table 4.1 (continued)

TCM remedy (Latin)	*n*	%	TCM remedy (Latin)	*n*	%
Sarcandrae herba	62	0.2	Myrrha	23	0.1
Arcae concha (t)	59	0.2	Pseudostellariae radix	23	0.1
Magnoliae flos	58	0.2	Xanthii fructus	23	0.1
Taraxaci herba	57	0.2	Fritillariae thunbergii bulbus	22	0.1
Carthami flos	56	0.2	Euryales semen	20	0.1
Luffae fructus retinervus	56	0.2	Hordei germinatus fructus	20	0.1
Margaritifera usta concha (t)	55	0.2	Polygoni multiflori radix	20	0.1
Scrophulariae radix	53	0.2	Psoraleae fructus (semen)	20	0.1
Perillae caulis	52	0.2	Arctii fructus	19	0.1
Corni fructus	49	0.2	Epimedii herba	19	0.1
Trichosanthis pericarpium	48	0.2	Artemisiae scopariae herba	18	0.1
Asari herba	47	0.1	Leonuri herba	18	0.1
Aurantii immaturus fructus	47	0.1	Cimicifugae rhizoma	17	0.1
Viticis fructus	46	0.1	Glehniae radix	17	0.1
Gardeniae fructus	45	0.1	Sophorae flavescentis radix	17	0.1
Amomi fructus	43	0.1	Forsythiae fructus	16	0.1
Crataegi fructus	43	0.1	Gigeriae galli endothelium corneum(t)	16	0.1
Foeniculi fructus	42	0.1	Arecae pericarpium	15	0.0
Ostreae concha (bearbeitet) (m)	42	0.1	Schizonepetae herba	15	0.0
Phaseolis semen	41	0.1	Sesami nigrum semen	15	0.0
Polyporus	41	0.1	Testudinis plastrum (t)	15	0.0
Trichosanthis radix	41	0.1	Asparagi radix	14	0.0
Mori folium	40	0.1	Dolichoris album semen	14	0.0
Olibanum	38	0.1	Lonicerae flos	14	0.0
Siegesbeckiae herba	38	0.1	Plantaginis herba	14	0.0
Perillae fructus	37	0.1	Plantaginis semen	13	0.0
Curculiginis rhizoma	36	0.1	Dictamni radicis cortex	12	0.0
Massa medicata fermentata	35	0.1	Fraxini cortex	12	0.0
Phragmitis rhizoma	35	0.1	Perillae folium	12	0.0
Citri grandis exocarpium	11	0.0	Talci pulvis (m)	4	0.0
Morindae officinalis radix	11	0.0	Zedoariae rhizoma	4	0.0
Periploca radicis cortex	10	0.0	Belamcandae rhizoma	3	0.0
Polygoni avicularis herba	10	0.0	Eriocauli flos	3	0.0
Verbenae herba	10	0.0	Ginkgo semen	3	0.0
Biotae cacumen	9	0.0	Homalomenae rhizoma	3	0.0
Eriobotryae folium	9	0.0	Indigo naturalis	3	0.0
Lysimachiae herba	9	0.0	Scutellariae barbatae herba	3	0.0
Mantidis OÃ¶theca	9	0.0	Sinapis albae semen	3	0.0
Polygonati rhizoma	9	0.0	Sojae praeparatum semen	3	0.0
Cannabis fructus	8	0.0	152 Physalis calyx seu fructus	2	0.0
Clematidis radix	8	0.0	Alpiniae officinarum rhizoma	2	0.0
Ephedrae herba	8	0.0	Cassiae folium(=Sennae folium)	2	0.0
Gypsum fibrosum (m)	8	0.0	Cephalanoploris herba	2	0.0
Astragali complantati semen	7	0.0	Isatidis radix	2	0.0
Polygonati odorati rhizoma	7	0.0	Lophateri herba	2	0.0
Rosae laevigatae fructus	7	0.0	Lycopodii herba	2	0.0
Aconiti lateralis praeparata radix	6	0.0	Tetrapanacis medulla	2	0.0
Alpiniae oxyphyllae fructus	6	0.0	Trachelospermi caulis	2	0.0
Artemisiae herba	6	0.0	Vaccariae semen	2	0.0

(continued)

Table 4.1 (continued)

TCM remedy (Latin)	*n*	%	TCM remedy (Latin)	*n*	%
Farfarae flos	6	0.0	Canarii fructus	1	0.0
Haematitum (m)	6	0.0	Cicadae periostracum (t)	1	0.0
Lepidii seu Descurainiae semen	6	0.0	Citri fructus	1	0.0
Sophorae immaturus flos	6	0.0	Ginseng radix	1	0.0
Drynariae rhizoma	5	0.0	Lonicerae caulis	1	0.0
Inulae flos	5	0.0	Portulacae herba	1	0.0
Smilacis glabrae rhizoma	5	0.0	Raphani semen	1	0.0
Asteris radix	4	0.0	Realgar (m)	1	0.0
Celosiae semen	4	0.0	Stellariae radix	1	0.0
Equiseti hiemalis herba	4	0.0	Stemonae radix	1	0.0
Evodiae fructus	4	0.0	Typhae pollen	1	0.0

pain due to cold emptiness, pain and numbness due to wind-dampness and amenorrhea, among other things [2]. *Astragali radix (Huang Qi)* has warming properties and a sweet taste. It is used to "support qi" and "strengthen the surface, eliminate toxins and promote urination". It is therefore used to treat qi and blood deficiencies, pale complexions, water retention and weakness. It can also be used to treat reduced appetite, increased sweating, diabetes mellitus with proteinuria and excessive thirst caused by internal heat [2, 3].

The comparison in Table 4.2 of the year 2023 with previous years shows that the frequency of prescription of Bupleuri radix has significantly decreased from 53.4% to 19.7% of the patients in 2023. Other changes of more than 10% are printed in bold. Further information on the evidence for individual drugs or combinations of drugs for depression, sleep or pain can be found in the chapter on the clinic's evaluation and quality assurance profile.

Table 4.2 Extract of the TCMs most frequently prescribed as part of the first prescription in 2023 (patients $n = 822$) compared to previous years (patients $n = 9695$); sorted in descending frequency of the year 2023

	2023			Previous years		
TCM remedy (Latin)	*n*	% of all drugs	% of all patients	*n*	% of all drugs	% of all patients
Angelicae sinensis radix	**438**	**4.4**	**53.3**	**3969**	**2.8**	**40.9**
Astragali radix	423	4.3	51.5	4539	3.2	46.8
Paeoniae rubra radix	377	3.8	45.9	4902	3.4	50.6
Achyranthis bidentatae radix	360	3.6	43.8	5234	3.7	54.0
Spatholobi caulis	358	3.6	43.6	3932	2.7	40.6
Cinnamomi ramulus	338	3.4	41.1	3507	2.5	36.2
Dipsaci radix	333	3.4	40.5	3050	2.1	31.5
Mori ramulus	304	3.1	37.0	3586	2.5	37.0
Polygalae radix	**289**	**2.9**	**35.2**	**1617**	**1.1**	**16.7**
Curcumae longae rhizoma	281	2.8	34.2	3308	2.3	34.1
Atractylodis macrocephalae rhizoma	256	2.6	31.1	2930	2.0	30.2
Poria (pieces)	252	2.5	30.7	3744	2.6	38.6
Bambusae caulis in taeniam	247	2.5	30.0	2486	1.7	25.6
Curcumae radix	227	2.3	27.6	3385	2.4	34.9
Ligustri lucidi fructus	215	2.2	26.2	2575	1.8	26.6
Loranthi ramulus	**210**	**2.1**	**25.5**	**4256**	**3.0**	**43.9**
Paeoniae alba radix	207	2.1	25.2	3161	2.2	32.6
Atractylodis rhizoma	201	2.0	24.5	1995	1.4	20.6
Ligustici chuanxiong rhizoma	175	1.8	21.3	1717	1.2	17.7
Albiziae cortex	174	1.8	21.2	1069	0.7	11.0
Bupleuri radix	**162**	**1.6**	**19.7**	**5176**	**3.6**	**53.4**
Aurantii fructus	161	1.6	19.6	2590	1.8	26.7
Sparganii tuber (rhizoma)	156	1.6	19.0	2270	1.6	23.4
Angelicae dahuricae radix	154	1.6	18.7	1506	1.1	15.5

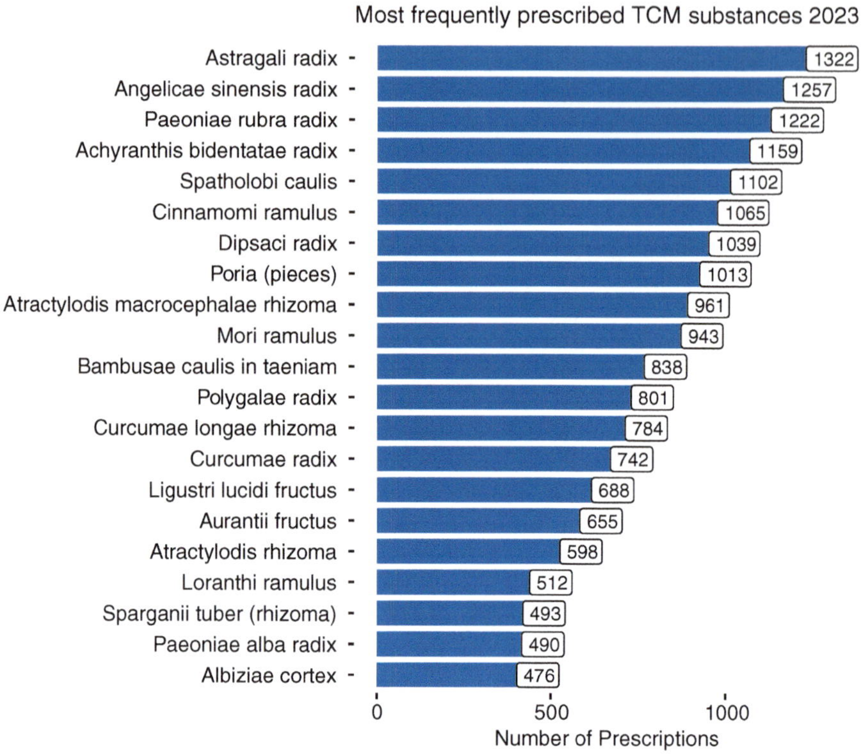

Fig. 4.3 Number of most frequently prescribed TCMs in 2023

4.2 TCM Acupuncture

At the TCM-Klinik Bad Kötzting, each individual TCM acupuncture session performed is documented and stored electronically. In 2023 (previous years 2008–2022), a total of 7946 (56,564) acupuncture sessions took place, spread over a total of 819 (6148) documented patients. From this, it can be determined that each patient was treated with acupuncture an average of 10 (8) times during their inpatient stay at the clinic. Considering the total of 83,955 (454,365) documented acupuncture points, which can be assigned to 309 (386) differently located acupuncture points, an average of 11 (8) acupuncture points per treatment can be determined (Fig. 4.4).

Table 4.3 refers to all acupuncture treatments carried out in the respective reporting year and contains the different acupuncture points sorted according to their frequency of application. Table 4.7 in the appendix lists the acupuncture points in alphabetical order. For better comparability, Table 4.4 lists the most frequently prescribed acupuncture points in the 2023 reporting year and compares them with the frequency of prescriptions in previous years (2008–2022).

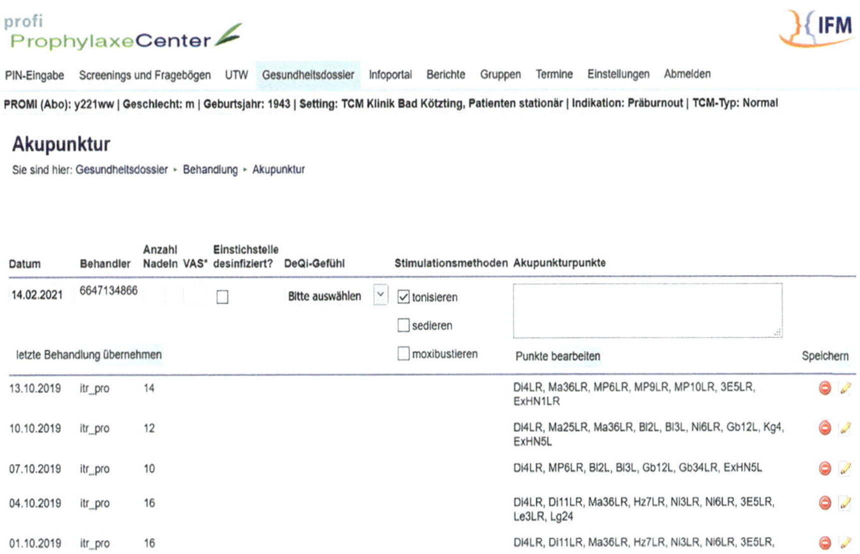

Fig. 4.4 Acupuncture documentation system in web portal VITERIO®

Table 4.3 TCM acupuncture points (percentages in relation to all acupuncture points documented in the reporting year 2023 (n = 819); sorted in descending frequency

Acupuncture point	n	%	Acupuncture point	n	%	Acupuncture point	n	%
LG20	3068	3.7	Gb41	552	0.7	Gb29	197	0.2
Ma36	2843	3.4	Tue15	521	0.6	Ma37	197	0.2
Di4	2730	3.3	ExHN5	482	0.6	Ma39	196	0.2
Ni3	2541	3.0	Gb31	455	0.5	Dü11	192	0.2
Gb20	2295	2.7	Ma44	427	0.5	Tue14	189	0.2
Le3	2267	2.7	Bl26	420	0.5	ExUE8	188	0.2
Tue11	2032	2.4	Ma38	415	0.5	Ni1	187	0.2
Kg4	1992	2.4	Kg10	406	0.5	3E17	186	0.2
Ni10	1964	2.3	Ma40	397	0.5	Hz4	170	0.2
MP6	1957	2.3	Hz7	394	0.5	Gb40	164	0.2
ExHN3	1898	2.3	LG23	383	0.5	Ma8	163	0.2
Lu8	1891	2.3	Ma35	381	0.5	Ma34	157	0.2
Le1	1798	2.1	Bl10	370	0.4	Bl15	156	0.2
Le4	1772	2.1	Hz9	366	0.4	Dü13	154	0.2
Lu11	1727	2.1	Gb43	363	0.4	Gb36	146	0.2
Kg12	1688	2.0	3E3	358	0.4	Bl27	143	0.2
Ma25	1346	1.6	Ma45	348	0.4	Bl17	142	0.2
Bl25	1270	1.5	Dü2	346	0.4	Di10	137	0.2
KS6	1243	1.5	Dü4	344	0.4	Bl2	135	0.2
Gb34	1219	1.5	Gb44	342	0.4	Kg11	128	0.2
Gb21	1204	1.4	Bl24	320	0.4	Di5	127	0.2
MP3	1192	1.4	LG3	319	0.4	KS7	126	0.2
Bl60	1184	1.4	Bl65	299	0.4	Ma7	120	0.1
Bl40	1160	1.4	Dü5	288	0.3	KS3	118	0.1
Bl23	1139	1.4	Bl18	284	0.3	3E21	110	0.1

(continued)

Table 4.3 (continued)

Acupuncture point	*n*	%	Acupuncture point	*n*	%	Acupuncture point	*n*	%
Ni6	1113	1.3	ExHN1	284	0.3	Gb7	102	0.1
ExHNS2	1104	1.3	Lu7	281	0.3	custom	102	0.1
Lu5	1076	1.3	Kg17	277	0.3	ExLE4	101	0.1
Dü3	983	1.2	Dü9	273	0.3	Kg22	101	0.1
Hz8	973	1.2	MP4	268	0.3	Ma2	100	0.1
Kg6	943	1.1	Bl57	264	0.3	Le14	96	0.1
Le2	916	1.1	Gb38	258	0.3	Bl13	95	0.1
ExB2	894	1.1	Ni7	258	0.3	Kg3	92	0.1
MP10	877	1.0	Ma26	255	0.3	Bl20	89	0.1
Le8	867	1.0	Bl28	252	0.3	Lg24	89	0.1
Gb30	821	1.0	MP5	251	0.3	Ma28	88	0.1
Lu9	765	0.9	Ma6	247	0.3	Bl12	85	0.1
Bl66	733	0.9	Hz3	234	0.3	MP2	83	0.1
Di1	683	0.8	Ma24	222	0.3	Dü1	81	0.1
Bl11	679	0.8	Lg4	220	0.3	Dü19	81	0.1
Gb8	678	0.8	MP15	208	0.2	Ni4	78	0.1
3E5	671	0.8	Di3	201	0.2	ExUE7	77	0.1
MP9	655	0.8	Dü15	201	0.2	Ma4	77	0.1
ExHN15	609	0.7	Tue20	197	0.2	ExLE5	75	0.1
Ni16	75	0.1	Lg5	20	0.0	Gb5	7	0.0
ExUE9	70	0.1	Lg6	20	0.0	KS5	7	0.0
Bl19	66	0.1	MP21	20	0.0	Le6	7	0.0
Lg14	65	0.1	Bl31	18	0.0	Bl4	6	0.0
Bl14	63	0.1	Bl56	18	0.0	Bl63	6	0.0
ExB7	59	0.1	Gb12	18	0.0	Tue16	6	0.0
Dü8	57	0.1	Ma9	18	0.0	ExHN4	6	0.0
Bl21	55	0.1	Bl22	17	0.0	Hz1	6	0.0
ExUES1	54	0.1	ExUE10	17	0.0	Lg26	6	0.0
Gb26	54	0.1	Ma32	17	0.0	Lu3	6	0.0
Bl32	53	0.1	Dü18	16	0.0	Ma33	6	0.0
Kg5	53	0.1	ExB8	16	0.0	Ni12	6	0.0
Ma41	53	0.1	Gb19	16	0.0	Bl34	5	0.0
Bl16	52	0.1	Le13	16	0.0	Tue19	5	0.0
3E1	51	0.1	Gb14	15	0.0	Gb11	5	0.0
3E6	51	0.1	Gb37	15	0.0	Gb6	5	0.0
ExLE2	51	0.1	Le11	15	0.0	Gb9	5	0.0
Bl67	48	0.1	Lg22	15	0.0	Lg16	5	0.0
3E14	47	0.1	Ni13	15	0.0	Ma23	5	0.0
Gb2	41	0.0	Dü10	14	0.0	Ma30	5	0.0
Lg13	41	0.0	Kg9	14	0.0	Ma43	5	0.0
ExCA1	37	0.0	Lu4	14	0.0	Ni14	5	0.0
Bl54	35	0.0	Bl33	13	0.0	Bl3	4	0.0
Bl1	34	0.0	MP8	13	0.0	Tue13	4	0.0
Bl36	34	0.0	ExHN2	12	0.0	ExB3	4	0.0
ExLE3	34	0.0	Kg23	12	0.0	Gb4	4	0.0
Gb1	34	0.0	Lg2	12	0.0	Lg10	4	0.0
Ma29	34	0.0	Ma27	12	0.0	Lg18	4	0.0
Ma5	32	0.0	Kg15	10	0.0	Lg7	4	0.0

(continued)

Table 4.3 (continued)

Acupuncture point	*n*	%	Acupuncture point	*n*	%	Acupuncture point	*n*	%
3E23	30	0.0	Le7	10	0.0	Lg9	4	0.0
Bl9	29	0.0	MP1	10	0.0	Ma20	4	0.0
Gb39	29	0.0	Di2	9	0.0	Bl30	3	0.0
Dü14	28	0.0	ExLE10	9	0.0	Bl8	3	0.0
Kg13	27	0.0	Gb28	9	0.0	ExHNS3	3	0.0
Bl62	26	0.0	KS8	9	0.0	ExUE4	3	0.0
Ma3	26	0.0	Le12	9	0.0	Gb32	3	0.0
Ma31	26	0.0	Ma21	9	0.0	Kg14	3	0.0
Ni17	25	0.0	3E4	8	0.0	Lg11	3	0.0
Bl7	24	0.0	Gb33	8	0.0	Lg17	3	0.0
Bl58	22	0.0	Lu6	8	0.0	Lg19	3	0.0
Lu10	22	0.0	Ma22	8	0.0	Lu2	3	0.0
Gb13	21	0.0	Ma42	8	0.0	3E11	2	0.0
Lg12	21	0.0	Bl59	7	0.0	Bl35	2	0.0
Dü6	20	0.0	Di12	7	0.0	Bl53	2	0.0
Di9	2	0.0	Ni2	2	0.0	Hz2	1	0.0
Dü12	2	0.0	Ni5	2	0.0	KS9	1	0.0
ExB5	2	0.0	3E7	1	0.0	Kg20	1	0.0
ExHN14	2	0.0	Bl38	1	0.0	Kg7	1	0.0
ExHNS5	2	0.0	Bl39	1	0.0	Kg8	1	0.0
ExLE6	2	0.0	Bl61	1	0.0	Lg21	1	0.0
Gb15	2	0.0	Di6	1	0.0	MP13	1	0.0
Gb17	2	0.0	Di8	1	0.0	MP19	1	0.0
Gb18	2	0.0	ExHN7	1	0.0	MP20	1	0.0
Gb25	2	0.0	ExHN8	1	0.0	Ma10	1	0.0
Gb3	2	0.0	ExHNS1	1	0.0	Ma15	1	0.0
KS4	2	0.0	ExLE7	1	0.0	Ma18	1	0.0
Le10	2	0.0	Gb10	1	0.0	Ni11	1	0.0
MP12	2	0.0	Gb23	1	0.0	Ni18	1	0.0
MP14	2	0.0	Gb35	1	0.0	Ni9	1	0.0
Total							**83,955**	**100**

Table 4.4 Extract of the most frequently documented TCM acupuncture points in 2023 ($n = 819$) compared to previous years ($n = 6148$); sorted in descending frequency of the year 2023

	2023		Previous years	
Acupuncture point	*n*	% of all points	*n*	% of all points
LG20	3068	3.7	7077	1.6
Ma36	2843	3.4	17,796	3.9
Di4	2730	3.3	20,614	4.5
Ni3	2541	3.0	10,425	2.3
Gb20	2295	2.7	11,177	2.5
Le3	2267	2.7	14,242	3.1
Tue11	2032	2.4	9222	2.0
Kg4	1992	2.4	7084	1.6
Ni10	1964	2.3	6985	1.5
MP6	1957	2.3	13,794	3.0
ExHN3	1898	2.3	3134	0.7
Lu8	1891	2.3	6661	1.5
Le1	1798	2.1	5895	1.3
Le4	1772	2.1	5932	1.3
Lu11	1727	2.1	5736	1.3
Kg12	1688	2.0	7819	1.7
Ma25	1346	1.6	11,305	2.5
Bl25	1270	1.5	8162	1.8
KS6	1243	1.5	2822	0.6
Gb34	1219	1.5	6474	1.4

In 2023 the three most frequently used acupuncture points at the TCM-Klinik Bad Kötzting were LG10, Ma36 and Di4 (Table 4.4). These acupuncture points were used more than 2700 times as part of treatment in 2023. When comparing the frequency of acupuncture points with findings from international literature, a consistent pattern emerges.

A recent scientific review [2], which examined 61 clinical studies worldwide, focused on acupuncture treatments for various pain conditions. These were only high-quality studies that considered STRICTA recommendations and other international standards. The following acupuncture points were used preferentially in the treatment of different localizations of pain symptoms:

- Large intestine points (mainly Di4 for low back pain and hip arthritis pain as well as for almost all other types of pain).
- Gallbladder points (mainly Gbl 30, 34 for neck, shoulder and knee pain).
- Spleen-pancreas points (MP6 Fibromyalgia, pelvic and hip pain).
- Stomach meridian (mainly Ma36 for fibromyalgia, knee and shoulder pain).

Table 4.3 shows the acupuncture points most frequently used in the clinic. Ma = ST 36 and Di = LI 4 is also ranked 2nd and 3rd in these statistics of the most frequently needled acupuncture points. This indicates that many patients at the TCM clinic in Bad Kötzting also suffer from pain.

LI 4—Hegu—is a point 'where the original qi is accessible' [4, 5]. The large intestine functional circuit is a yang meridian. Indications are portrayed as headaches and abdominal pain, toothache, nosebleeds and jaw clenching or eye pain [5]. The three yang meridians of the hand (large intestine, small intestine, triple warmer) and the foot (stomach, bladder, gallbladder) form, together with the three yin meridians of the hand (lung, heart, pericardium) and the foot (spleen, kidney, liver), the 12 main meridians in acupuncture theory. The Yang meridians are connected in the face and the Yin meridians in the thorax. The stomach and large intestine meridians, for example, run alongside the nose. The acupuncture point Stomach ST = Ma 36 (Zusanli) is indicated for stomach pain, swallowing disorders, fatigue, flatulence and diarrhoea, among other things [5].

The reason why the acupuncture point Governing Vessel = LG20 (baihui) was used so frequently may be because the point is referred to as the 'meeting point of all meridians'. GV20 is indicated by headaches, dizziness, sleep disorders and even insanity, which is also an indication for ST = Ma36 [5].

The fourth most common acupuncture point is Kidney 3, also known as 'Taixi'. It is another 'point where the primordial qi is accessible'. It is also known as 'mighty watercourse'. It is used to treat irregular menstruation, insomnia, tinnitus, impotence and lower back pain.

The gallbladder point GB20 is needled 2295 times and ranks fifth in acupuncture statistics with 2.7%. GB20 is called 'fengchi' or 'wind pond'. Indications include headaches, dizziness, eye pain, sinusitis, and neck pain and stiffness [5].

Body acupuncture is used alongside ear acupuncture, moxibustion and cupping.

The VITERIO® health portal provides therapists with an automated overview of patients' progress and therapy at the clinic. Information such as acupuncture treatments, TCMs, diagnoses and various findings are summarized and compiled into a report here (Fig. 4.5).

No	Date		
22	11.10.2023	Tongue	Teeth marks, bluish tongue colour, tongue colour spots, thin coating, whiter coating, location Rear third Coating stickier,
23	11.10.2023	Acupuncture points	Di11LR, Di14LR, Di15LR, Dü9LR, Bl60L, Ni3L, Ni4L, Gb29R, Gb30R, Gb34LR, Gb40L,
24	10 October 2023	Secondary diagnosis	F32.1
25	10.10.2023	Primary diagnosis	F45.41
26	09.10.2023	TCM	Blood stasis, dampness,
27	09.10.2023	Secondary diagnosis	F51.0
28	09.10.2023	Secondary diagnosis	M20.1
29	09.10.2023	Secondary diagnosis	M79.61
30	09.10.2023	Secondary diagnosis	S86.0
31	09.10.2023	Secondary diagnosis	U08.9
32	09.10.2023	Secondary diagnosis	G93.3
33	09.10.2023	TCM medication	Mori ramulus/Sangzhi/6 g, Cinnamomi ramulus/Guizhi/6 g, Dipsaci radix/Xuduan/6 g, Achyranthis bidentatae radix/ Niuxi/6 g, Spatholobi caulis/Jixueteng/6 g, Paeoniae rubra radix/Chishao/6 g, Curcumae longae rhizoma/Jianghuang/6 g,Bombyx batryticatus (t)/Baijiangcan/6 g, Angelicae pubescentis radix/Duhuo/3 g, Notopterygii rhizoma seu radix/Qianghuo/3 g, Bambusae caulis in taeniam/Zhuru/6 g, Albiziae cortex/Hehuanpi/6 g, Astragali radix/Huangqi/6 g, Sappan lignum/Sumu/6 g
34	16 August 2022	Secondary diagnosis	M23.39
35	16 August 2022	Secondary diagnosis	S86.0
36	16 August 2022	Primary diagnosis	U07.2
37	16 August 2022	Secondary diagnosis	U08.9
38	16 August 2022	Secondary diagnosis	G93.3
39	16 August 2022	Secondary diagnosis	G47.0
40	16 August 2022	Secondary diagnosis	M79.61
41	16 August 2022	Secondary diagnosis	M20.1
42	14 August 2022	Acupuncture points	Di4LR, Di11L, Di15L, Hz7LR, Bl34L, Bl36L, Bl60L, Le3LR, Lg20,
43	12 August 2022	Secondary diagnosis	F32.1
44	12 August 2022	Primary diagnosis	F45.41
45	10 August 2022	Acupuncture points	Di4LR, Di11L, Di15L, Hz7LR, Bl34L, Bl36L, Bl60L, Le3LR, Lg20,
46	08.08.2022	Acupuncture points	Di4LR, Di11L, Di15L, Hz7LR, Bl34L, Bl36L, Bl60L, Le3LR, Lg20,
47	04.08.2022	Consultation information@zept	Quinoa fasting day (600 kcal green)
48	04.08.2022	Consultation info@zept	Millet relief day (900 kcal green)

nd3841 2/8

Fig. 4.5 Systematic medical history in the TCM-health portal VITERIO®

4.3 Overall Spectrum of Diagnostic-Therapeutic Interventions with Prescription Frequency

As the intervention profile of the TCM-Klinik Bad Kötzting is very diverse and covers far more than the services described so far, the documented range of services will be discussed in more detail below. The individual pharmacological and non-pharmacological services recorded in 2023 via the ITR clinic programme and in the VITERIO® health portal and the associated utilization serve as the basis for these evaluations.

A total of 133,916 individual services were documented in the 43 specified service categories. Most described were Chinese medicinal therapy (CHM), followed by IHM-Yangsheng group therapy, Chinese sleeping pills, coronavirus herbal mixtures and the acupuncture treatment described earlier. Table 4.5 gives an overview of all described services at the TCM-Klinik Bad Kötzting.

The evidence base for various TCM interventions such as Chinese medicines, acupuncture, tuina and qigong is briefly described in the chapter on evidence and quality assurance profiles. No scientific studies are yet available for other procedures such as the application of Chinese medicines in the form of drops or ointments.

Table 4.5 Range of services and utilization in 2023 ($n = 133916$); sorted by therapy type and descending order of frequency without specific figures on individual prescriptions

Service/Treatment	
Chinese medication	
Chin. AMT (CHM) – individual	
Chinese medicinal therapy (new, change)	
Chin. Sleeping drops	
ACV (Corona herbal mixture)	
BST III compresses (joint pain herbal compresses)	
BST III foot bath (joint pain foot bath)	
BST III hand bath (joint pain – hand bath)	
MNT (migraine nasal tincture)	
Chin. throat tea (incl. preparation, brewing)	
Chin. anti-allergy drops	
Chin. ET Wind-Heat (ET = Cold drops)	
CM (constipation mixture)	
Chin. ET Wind-Cold (cold drops)	
Chin. Foot fungus tincture	
Chin. Nail fungus tincture	
Curd wrap	
Psychotherapy	
Psychotherapy group	
Individual psychological interview	

(continued)

Table 4.5 (continued)

Service/Treatment	
Conversation for relief	
Health applications	
Group therapy IHM-Yangsheng Qigong	
Acupuncture sessions	
Tuina massage (Tuina therapy)	
Qigong therapy	
Matrix rhythm therapy	
ECG – Electrocardiogram	
Ear acupuncture (permanent needles, exchange)	
Rubbing	
Acupuncture with cupping	
Steam Inhalation (explanation + instructions)	
Additional acupuncture	
Neural therapy	
Group therapy – Yangsheng – Special therapist	
Physiotherapy	
Visits and counselling	
Chief physician hospital visits	
Chinese hospital visits	
Visits and counselling	
General hospital visits	
Nutrition counselling	
(Free) consultation hour	
Other	
Health portal support	
Crisis intervention (psychological, medical)	
Exercise group	
Physical examination	
Qigong lecture	
Carrying out the Trop test	

Appendix

Table 4.6 TCMs (percentages in relation to all prescriptions/prescribed substances created in the reporting year 2023); sorted in alphabetical order ($n = 31836$)

TCM remedy (Latin)	*n*	%	TCM remedy (Latin)	*n*	%
152 Physalis calyx seu fructus	2	0.0	Biotae semen	85	0.3
Achyranthis bidentatae radix	1159	3.6	Bombyx batryticatus (t)	195	0.6
Aconiti lateralis praeparata radix	6	0.0	Bupleuri radix	462	1.5
Albiziae cortex	476	1.5	Canarii fructus	1	0.0
Alismatis rhizoma	71	0.2	Cannabis fructus	8	0.0
Allii macrostemi bulbus	30	0.1	Carthami flos	56	0.2
Alpiniae officinarum rhizoma	2	0.0	Cassiae folium(=Sennae folium)	2	0.0
Alpiniae oxyphyllae fructus	6	0.0	Cassiae semen	218	0.7
Amomi cardamomi semen	69	0.2	Celosiae semen	4	0.0
Amomi fructus	43	0.1	Cephalanoploris herba	2	0.0
Anemarrhenae rhizoma	300	0.9	Chaenomelis fructus	303	1.0
Angelicae dahuricae radix	475	1.5	Chrysanthemi flos	68	0.2
Angelicae pubescentis radix	181	0.6	Cicadae periostracum (t)	1	0.0
Angelicae sinensis radix	1257	3.9	Cimicifugae rhizoma	17	0.1
Arcae concha (t)	59	0.2	Cinnamomi cortex	25	0.1
Arctii fructus	19	0.1	Cinnamomi ramulus	1065	3.3
Arecae pericarpium	15	0.0	Citri fructus	1	0.0
Armeniacae amarum semen	75	0.2	Citri grandis exocarpium	11	0.0
Artemisiae argyi folium	73	0.2	Citri reticulatae pericarpium	233	0.7
Artemisiae herba	6	0.0	Citri reticulatae semen	68	0.2
Artemisiae scopariae herba	18	0.1	Citri reticulatae viride pericarpium	84	0.3
Asari herba	47	0.1	Citri sarcodactylis fructus	217	0.7
Asparagi radix	14	0.0	Clematidis radix	8	0.0
Asteris radix	4	0.0	Codonopsis pilosulae radix	219	0.7
Astragali complantati semen	7	0.0	Coicis semen	279	0.9
Astragali radix	1322	4.2	Coptidis rhizoma	84	0.3
Atractylodis macrocephalae rhizoma	961	3.0	Corni fructus	49	0.2
Atractylodis rhizoma	598	1.9	Corydalis rhizoma	78	0.2
Aurantii fructus	655	2.1	Crataegi fructus	43	0.1
Aurantii immaturus fructus	47	0.1	Curculiginis rhizoma	36	0.1
Bambusae caulis in taeniam	838	2.6	Curcumae longae rhizoma	784	2.5
Belamcandae rhizoma	3	0.0	Curcumae radix	742	2.3
Biotae cacumen	9	0.0	Cuscutae semen	99	0.3
Cyperi rhizoma	299	0.9	Leonuri fructus	33	0.1
Dictamni radicis cortex	12	0.0	Leonuri herba	18	0.1
Dioscoreae rhizoma	96	0.3	Lepidii seu Descurainiae semen	6	0.0
Dipsaci radix	1039	3.3	Ligustici chuanxiong rhizoma	377	1.2
Dolichoris album semen	14	0.0	Ligustici rhizoma	29	0.1
Draconis os (t)	84	0.3	Ligustri lucidi fructus	688	2.2
Drynariae rhizoma	5	0.0	Liquidambaris fructus	274	0.9
Ecliptae herba	30	0.1	Litchi semen	64	0.2
Ephedrae herba	8	0.0	Lonicerae caulis	1	0.0
Epimedii herba	19	0.1	Lonicerae flos	14	0.0
Equiseti hiemalis herba	4	0.0	Lophateri herba	2	0.0
Eriobotryae folium	9	0.0	Loranthi ramulus	512	1.6
Eriocauli flos	3	0.0	Luffae fructus retinervus	56	0.2
Eucommiae cortex	212	0.7	Lycii fructus	169	0.5
Euryales semen	20	0.1	Lycii radicis cortex	25	0.1

(continued)

Table 4.6 (continued)

TCM remedy (Latin)	*n*	%	TCM remedy (Latin)	*n*	%
Evodiae fructus	4	0.0	Lycopi herba	105	0.3
Farfarae flos	6	0.0	Lycopodii herba	2	0.0
Foeniculi fructus	42	0.1	Lysimachiae herba	9	0.0
Forsythiae fructus	16	0.1	Magnoliae flos	58	0.2
Fraxini cortex	12	0.0	Magnoliae officinalis cortex	408	1.3
Fritillariae thunbergii bulbus	22	0.1	Mantidis OÃ¶theca	9	0.0
Gardeniae fructus	45	0.1	Margaritifera usta concha (t)	55	0.2
Gentianae macrophyllae rhizoma	135	0.4	Massa medicata fermentata	35	0.1
Gigeriae galli endothelium corneum(t)	16	0.1	Meliae toosendan fructus	161	0.5
Ginkgo semen	3	0.0	Menthae herba	69	0.2
Ginseng radix	1	0.0	Mori folium	40	0.1
Glehniae radix	17	0.1	Mori radicis cortex	136	0.4
Glycyrrhizae radix	225	0.7	Mori ramulus	943	3.0
Gypsum fibrosum (m)	8	0.0	Morindae officinalis radix	11	0.0
Haematitum (m)	6	0.0	Moutan radicis cortex	73	0.2
Haliotidis concha (m)	30	0.1	Myrrha	23	0.1
Homalomenae rhizoma	3	0.0	Notopterygii rhizoma seu radix	198	0.6
Hordei germinatus fructus	20	0.1	Olibanum	38	0.1
Imperatae rhizoma	25	0.1	Ophiopogonis radix	62	0.2
Indigo naturalis	3	0.0	Oryzae germinatus fructus	70	0.2
Inulae flos	5	0.0	Ostreae concha (bearbeitet) (m)	42	0.1
Isatidis radix	2	0.0	Ostreae concha (m)	157	0.5
Kochiae fructus	63	0.2	Paeoniae alba radix	490	1.5
Ledebouriellae radix	191	0.6	Paeoniae rubra radix	1222	3.8
Perillae caulis	52	0.2	Sarcandrae herba	62	0.2
Perillae folium	12	0.0	Schisandrae fructus	70	0.2
Perillae fructus	37	0.1	Schizonepetae herba	15	0.0
Periploca radicis cortex	10	0.0	Scrophulariae radix	53	0.2
Persicae semen	86	0.3	Scutellariae barbatae herba	3	0.0
Peucedani radix	74	0.2	Scutellariae radix	277	0.9
Phaseolis semen	41	0.1	Sesami nigrum semen	15	0.0
Phellodendri cortex	312	1.0	Siegesbeckiae herba	38	0.1
Phragmitis rhizoma	35	0.1	Sinapis albae semen	3	0.0
Pinelliae praeparatae rhizoma	428	1.3	Sinomenii caulis	159	0.5
Plantaginis herba	14	0.0	Smilacis glabrae rhizoma	5	0.0
Plantaginis semen	13	0.0	Sojae praeparatum semen	3	0.0
Platycodi radix	31	0.1	Sophorae flavescentis radix	17	0.1
Polygalae radix	801	2.5	Sophorae immaturus flos	6	0.0
Polygonati odorati rhizoma	7	0.0	Sparganii tuber (rhizoma)	493	1.5
Polygonati rhizoma	9	0.0	Spatholobi caulis	1102	3.5
Polygoni avicularis herba	10	0.0	Stellariae radix	1	0.0
Polygoni multiflori caulis	86	0.3	Stemonae radix	1	0.0
Polygoni multiflori radix	20	0.1	Talci pulvis (m)	4	0.0
Polyporus	41	0.1	Taraxaci herba	57	0.2
Poria (StÃ¼cke)	1013	3.2	Testudinis plastrum (t)	15	0.0
Portulacae herba	1	0.0	Tetrapanacis medulla	2	0.0
Prunellae spica	105	0.3	Trachelospermi caulis	2	0.0
Pseudostellariae radix	23	0.1	Tribuli fructus	201	0.6

(continued)

Table 4.6 (continued)

TCM remedy (Latin)	*n*	%	TCM remedy (Latin)	*n*	%
Psoraleae fructus (semen)	20	0.1	Trichosanthis fructus	202	0.6
Puerariae radix	315	1.0	Trichosanthis pericarpium	48	0.2
Pyrrosiae folium	34	0.1	Trichosanthis radix	41	0.1
Raphani semen	1	0.0	Typhae pollen	1	0.0
Realgar (m)	1	0.0	Uncariae cum uncis ramulus	142	0.4
Rehmanniae praeparatae rhizoma	130	0.4	Vaccariae semen	2	0.0
Rehmanniae radix	220	0.7	Verbenae herba	10	0.0
Rhei radix et rhizoma	184	0.6	Viticis fructus	46	0.1
Rosae laevigatae fructus	7	0.0	Xanthii fructus	23	0.1
Salviae miltiorrhizae radix	247	0.8	Zedoariae rhizoma	4	0.0
Sanguisorbae radix	35	0.1	Zingiberis rhizoma	144	0.5
Sappan lignum	171	0.5	Ziziphi spinosae semen	111	0.3

Table 4.7 Frequency of TCM acupuncture points used in 2023 (n = 819); sorted alphabetically

Acupuncture point	*n*	%	Acupuncture point	*n*	%	Acupuncture point	*n*	%
3E1	51	0.1	Bl53	2	0.0	Dü4	344	0.4
3E11	2	0.0	Bl54	35	0.0	Dü5	288	0.3
3E14	47	0.1	Bl56	18	0.0	Dü6	20	0.0
3E17	186	0.2	Bl57	264	0.3	Dü8	57	0.1
3E21	110	0.1	Bl58	22	0.0	Dü9	273	0.3
3E23	30	0.0	Bl59	7	0.0	ExB2	894	1.1
3E3	358	0.4	Bl60	1184	1.4	ExB3	4	0.0
3E4	8	0.0	Bl61	1	0.0	ExB5	2	0.0
3E5	671	0.8	Bl62	26	0.0	ExB7	59	0.1
3E6	51	0.1	Bl63	6	0.0	ExB8	16	0.0
3E7	1	0.0	Bl65	299	0.4	ExCA1	37	0.0
Bl1	34	0.0	Bl66	733	0.9	ExHN1	284	0.3
Bl10	370	0.4	Bl67	48	0.1	ExHN14	2	0.0
Bl11	679	0.8	Bl7	24	0.0	ExHN15	609	0.7
Bl12	85	0.1	Bl8	3	0.0	ExHN2	12	0.0
Bl13	95	0.1	Bl9	29	0.0	ExHN3	1898	2.3
Bl14	63	0.1	Di1	683	0.8	ExHN4	6	0.0
Bl15	156	0.2	Di10	137	0.2	ExHN5	482	0.6
Bl16	52	0.1	Tue11	2032	2.4	ExHN7	1	0.0
Bl17	142	0.2	Di12	7	0.0	ExHN8	1	0.0
Bl18	284	0.3	Tue13	4	0.0	ExHNS1	1	0.0
Bl19	66	0.1	Tue14	189	0.2	ExHNS2	1104	1.3
Bl2	135	0.2	Tue15	521	0.6	ExHNS3	3	0.0
Bl20	89	0.1	Tue16	6	0.0	ExHNS5	2	0.0
Bl21	55	0.1	Tue19	5	0.0	ExLE10	9	0.0
Bl22	17	0.0	Di2	9	0.0	ExLE2	51	0.1
Bl23	1139	1.4	Tue20	197	0.2	ExLE3	34	0.0
Bl24	320	0.4	Di3	201	0.2	ExLE4	101	0.1
Bl25	1270	1.5	Di4	2730	3.3	ExLE5	75	0.1
Bl26	420	0.5	Di5	127	0.2	ExLE6	2	0.0
Bl27	143	0.2	Di6	1	0.0	ExLE7	1	0.0
Bl28	252	0.3	Di8	1	0.0	ExUE10	17	0.0
Bl3	4	0.0	Di9	2	0.0	ExUE4	3	0.0
Bl30	3	0.0	Dü1	81	0.1	ExUE7	77	0.1

(continued)

Table 4.7 (continued)

Acupuncture point	*n*	%	Acupuncture point	*n*	%	Acupuncture point	*n*	%
Bl31	18	0.0	Dü10	14	0.0	ExUE8	188	0.2
Bl32	53	0.1	Dü11	192	0.2	ExUE9	70	0.1
Bl33	13	0.0	Dü12	2	0.0	ExUES1	54	0.1
Bl34	5	0.0	Dü13	154	0.2	Gb1	34	0.0
Bl35	2	0.0	Dü14	28	0.0	Gb10	1	0.0
Bl36	34	0.0	Dü15	201	0.2	Gb11	5	0.0
Bl38	1	0.0	Dü18	16	0.0	Gb12	18	0.0
Bl39	1	0.0	Dü19	81	0.1	Gb13	21	0.0
Bl4	6	0.0	Dü2	346	0.4	Gb14	15	0.0
Bl40	1160	1.4	Dü3	983	1.2	Gb15	2	0.0
Gb17	2	0.0	KS8	9	0.0	Lg23	383	0.5
Gb18	2	0.0	KS9	1	0.0	Lg24	89	0.1
Gb19	16	0.0	Kg10	406	0.5	Lg26	6	0.0
Gb2	41	0.0	Kg11	128	0.2	Lg3	319	0.4
Gb20	2295	2.7	Kg12	1688	2.0	Lg4	220	0.3
Gb21	1204	1.4	Kg13	27	0.0	Lg5	20	0.0
Gb23	1	0.0	Kg14	3	0.0	Lg6	20	0.0
Gb25	2	0.0	Kg15	10	0.0	Lg7	4	0.0
Gb26	54	0.1	Kg17	277	0.3	Lg9	4	0.0
Gb28	9	0.0	Kg20	1	0.0	Lu10	22	0.0
Gb29	197	0.2	Kg22	101	0.1	Lu11	1727	2.1
Gb3	2	0.0	Kg23	12	0.0	Lu2	3	0.0
Gb30	821	1.0	Kg3	92	0.1	Lu3	6	0.0
Gb31	455	0.5	Kg4	1992	2.4	Lu4	14	0.0
Gb32	3	0.0	Kg5	53	0.1	Lu5	1076	1.3
Gb33	8	0.0	Kg6	943	1.1	Lu6	8	0.0
Gb34	1219	1.5	Kg7	1	0.0	Lu7	281	0.3
Gb35	1	0.0	Kg8	1	0.0	Lu8	1891	2.3
Gb36	146	0.2	Kg9	14	0.0	Lu9	765	0.9
Gb37	15	0.0	Le1	1798	2.1	MP1	10	0.0
Gb38	258	0.3	Le10	2	0.0	MP10	877	1.0
Gb39	29	0.0	Le11	15	0.0	MP12	2	0.0
Gb4	4	0.0	Le12	9	0.0	MP13	1	0.0
Gb40	164	0.2	Le13	16	0.0	MP14	2	0.0
Gb41	552	0.7	Le14	96	0.1	MP15	208	0.2
Gb43	363	0.4	Le2	916	1.1	MP19	1	0.0
Gb44	342	0.4	Le3	2267	2.7	MP2	83	0.1
Gb5	7	0.0	Le4	1772	2.1	MP20	1	0.0
Gb6	5	0.0	Le6	7	0.0	MP21	20	0.0
Gb7	102	0.1	Le7	10	0.0	MP3	1192	1.4
Gb8	678	0.8	Le8	867	1.0	MP4	268	0.3
Gb9	5	0.0	Lg10	4	0.0	MP5	251	0.3
Hz1	6	0.0	Lg11	3	0.0	MP6	1957	2.3
Hz2	1	0.0	Lg12	21	0.0	MP8	13	0.0
Hz3	234	0.3	Lg13	41	0.0	MP9	655	0.8
Hz4	170	0.2	Lg14	65	0.1	Ma10	1	0.0
Hz7	394	0.5	Lg16	5	0.0	Ma15	1	0.0
Hz8	973	1.2	Lg17	3	0.0	Ma18	1	0.0
Hz9	366	0.4	Lg18	4	0.0	Ma2	100	0.1

(continued)

Table 4.7 (continued)

Acupuncture point	*n*	%	Acupuncture point	*n*	%	Acupuncture point	*n*	%
KS3	118	0.1	Lg19	3	0.0	Ma20	4	0.0
KS4	2	0.0	Lg2	12	0.0	Ma21	9	0.0
KS5	7	0.0	Lg20	3068	3.7	Ma22	8	0.0
KS6	1243	1.5	Lg21	1	0.0	Ma23	5	0.0
KS7	126	0.2	Lg22	15	0.0	Ma24	222	0.3
Ma25	1346	1.6	Ma39	196	0.2	Ni11	1	0.0
Ma26	255	0.3	Ma4	77	0.1	Ni12	6	0.0
Ma27	12	0.0	Ma40	397	0.5	Ni13	15	0.0
Ma28	88	0.1	Ma41	53	0.1	Ni14	5	0.0
Ma29	34	0.0	Ma42	8	0.0	Ni16	75	0.1
Ma3	26	0.0	Ma43	5	0.0	Ni17	25	0.0
Ma30	5	0.0	Ma44	427	0.5	Ni18	1	0.0
Ma31	26	0.0	Ma45	348	0.4	Ni2	2	0.0
Ma32	17	0.0	Ma5	32	0.0	Ni3	2541	3.0
Ma33	6	0.0	Ma6	247	0.3	Ni4	78	0.1
Ma34	157	0.2	Ma7	120	0.1	Ni5	2	0.0
Ma35	381	0.5	Ma8	163	0.2	Ni6	1113	1.3
Ma36	2843	3.4	Ma9	18	0.0	Ni7	258	0.3
Ma37	197	0.2	Ni1	187	0.2	Ni9	1	0.0
Ma38	415	0.5	Ni10	1964	2.3	custom	102	0.1
Total							**83,955**	**100**

References

1. Geng J, Huang W, Ren T, Ma X. Materia medica der chinesischen Arzneimitteltherapie: Praxis der Chinesischen Arzneimitteltherapie [Materia Medica of Chinese Drug Therapy]. Band II. Bad Kötzting: Verlag für Systemische Medizin; 1993. ISBN: 978-3927344044.
2. Jingzhang Dai. Chinesisch-Deutsches Handbuch für häufig verwendete traditionelle chinesische Arzneimittel. Chinesisch-Deutsches Zentrum für Traditionelle Chinesische Medizin (Bad Kötzting). Die Buchreihe der TCM in der Ferne. China Press of Traditional Chinese Medicine. ISBN 978-7-5132-9212-2; 1. Auflage, Beijing, Volksrepublik China; 2024. p. 215–31.
3. Jingzhang Dai, Jing Wang. Theorien und Anwendungen von Yin und Yang, den fünf Elemente, den Funktionskreisen sowie den Haupt- und Netzleitbahnen. Chinesisch-Deutsches Zentrum für Traditionelle Chinesische Medizin (Bad Kötzting). Die Buchreihe der TCM in der Ferne. China Press of Traditional Chinese Medicine, 1. Auflage, Beijing; 2013. p. 234 ff.
4. Chen YJ, Shimizu Bassi G, Yang YQ. Classic Chinese acupuncture versus different types of control groups for the treatment of chronic pain: review of randomized controlled trials (2000–2018). Evid Based Complement Alternat Med. 2019;2019:6283912. https://doi.org/10.1155/2019/6283912.
5. Jingzhang Dai, Jinxi Zhao. Traditionelle chinesische Medizin—alte Gesundheitsweisheit. Chinesisch-Deutsches Zentrum für Traditionelle Chinesische Medizin (Bad Kötzting). Die Buchreihe der TCM in der Ferne. China Press of Traditional Chinese Medicine, 1. Auflage, Beijing; 2021. p. 118 ff.

Outcome Profile

5

Dieter Melchart, Jingzhang Dai, Likun Yang, Michael Frey, and Lara Isabel Jötten

5.1 General Evaluation of Patients on Admission, Discharge, and Follow-Up

As part of the Patient Care Evaluation Programme (PEP), quality assurance (QA) questionnaires have been used since the clinic was founded. These address key aspects of quality of outcomes and are available in three versions: one to be completed upon admission, one upon discharge, and one approximately 6 months after inpatient treatment as a post-inpatient follow-up survey. Outcome profile data are available for 821 of the 825 patients from the 2023 reporting period (99.5%) upon admission. Discharge data are available for 777 of these patients (94.6%). For the initial admission measurement, all data records were used that were documented within a maximum of 91 days before and 18 days after the admission date. Complete data on symptom severity at admission, discharge, and follow-up is available for 618 patients (74.9%). However, as not all patients complete all available

D. Melchart (✉) · M. Frey · L. I. Jötten
Faculty of Applied Healthcare Sciences, Deggendorf Institute of Technology (DIT), Competence Centre for Lifestyle Medicine and Naturopathy, Deggendorf, Germany
e-mail: dieter.melchart@th-deg.de

J. Dai · L. Yang
TCM-Klinik Bad Kötzting, Beijing University of Chinese Medicine (BUCM), Beijing, People's Republic of China

D. Melchart et al. (eds.), *TCM-Klinik Bad Kötzting*,
https://doi.org/10.1007/978-3-032-23307-3_5

questionnaires or items consistently, the actual number may vary slightly depending on the questionnaire and item. For descriptive evaluations of the follow-up data, all available data were considered (approximately 610–624 data points, depending on the item). The time at which the quality assurance (QA) questionnaires were completed could not be narrowed down to exactly 6 months after hospital discharge. Therefore, the follow-up survey includes all data collected between 154 days and 1 year after discharge. All results obtained should be considered in the context of an average inpatient care period of 4 weeks. The number of data points available from previous years also varies depending on the survey context. For comparisons between admission and discharge, and between admission and follow-up, only complete datasets available at the respective time points are considered.

5.1.1 Change in Subjective Health Status

5.1.1.1 At Hospital Discharge Compared to Admission (A-D)

At all survey points, patients are asked to describe their current subjective state of health. Upon admission to hospital in 2023, 38% rated their health as poor, 51.9% as fair, and 10% as good to excellent (in previous years, these figures were 33.8%, 53.0%, and 13.2%, respectively). Upon being discharged from hospital, patients gave a significantly better assessment: only 7.1% rated their health as poor, while 57.5% rated it as good to excellent (Table 5.1). In previous years, these figures were 6.5% and 60.5%, respectively.

Summarising the figures in the lower left triangle (each marked in green) of Table 5.1, it can be assumed that a total of 526 patients (68%) were in an improved condition compared to admission (previous years: 66.3%). For 28.7% of patients, their assessment of their state of health did not change (white fields; previous years: 29.2%), and for 3.4% of patients, a deterioration in their assessment was observed (previous years: 4.5%; upper right triangle, marked in red). Figure 5.1 provides an overview of the number of levels by which a change occurred.

5.1.1.2 At Follow-Up Compared to Admission (A-F)

A positive difference was also observed when comparing patients in 2023 between admission and follow-up (A-F), although this difference decreased slightly compared to discharge (Table 5.2).

Of the 625 patients, 89.3% reported poor or fair health on admission and 10.7% reported good or excellent health (in previous years, these figures were 86.1% and 13.9%, respectively). At the follow-up examination, patients' assessments were better: only 46.9% now classified their health as poor or less than good (compared to 51.3% in previous years), while 53.1% now classified it as good to excellent (compared to 48.7% in previous years).

Table 5.1 Changes in patients' self-reported health status at hospital discharge compared to admission, in 2023 ($n = 774$) and previous years ($n = 11{,}145$), including all patients with data available for both admission and discharge

2023		At discharge					
		excellent	very good	good	fair	poor	**Total**
On admission	excellent	0 0.0%	0 0.0%	1 0.1%	0 0.0%	0 0.0%	**1** **0.1%**
	very good	1 0.1%	0 0.0%	6 0.8%	1 0.1%	0 0.0%	**8** **1.0%**
	good	1 0.1%	13 1.7%	45 5.8%	10 1.3%	0 0.0%	**69** **8.9%**
	fair	1 0.1%	30 3.9%	233 30.1%	130 16.8%	8 1.0%	**402** **51.9%**
	poor	2 0.1%	6 0.8%	107 13.8%	132 17.1%	47 6.1%	**294** **38.0%**
	Total	**5** **0.6%**	**49** **6.3%**	**392** **50.6%**	**273** **35.3%**	**55** **7.1%**	**774** **100.0%**

Previous years		At discharge					
		excellent	very good	good	fair	poor	**Total**
On admission	excellent	6 0.1%	13 0.1%	3 0.0%	1 0.0%	0 0.0%	23 0.2%
	very good	9 0.1%	31 0.3%	36 0.3%	9 0.1%	3 0.0%	88 0.8%
	good	25 0.2%	216 1.9%	882 7.9%	219 2.0%	22 0.2%	1364 12.2%
	fair	37 0.3%	413 3.7%	3419 30.7%	1835 16.5%	199 1.8%	5903 53.0%
	poor	36 0.3%	125 1.1%	1491 13.4%	1615 14.5%	500 4.5%	3767 33.8%
	Total	113 1.0%	798 7.2%	5831 52.3%	3679 33.0%	724 6.5%	11145 100.0%

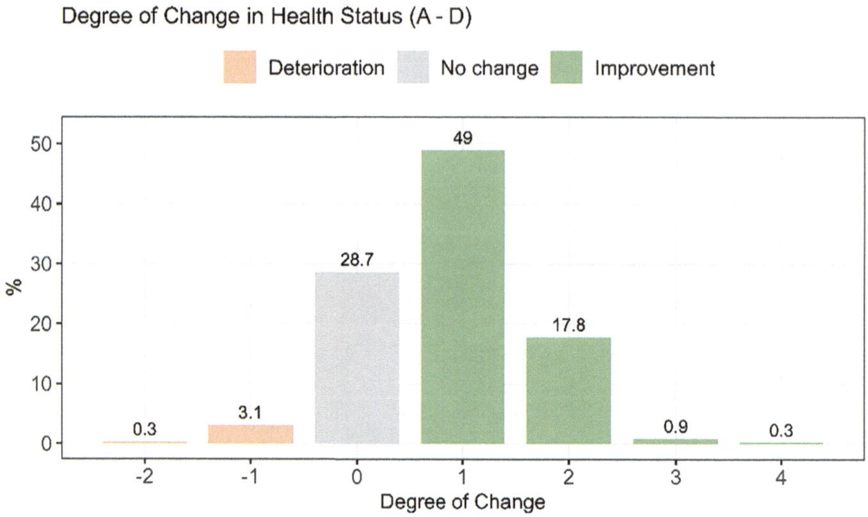

Fig. 5.1 Changes in patients' subjective health assessments at hospital discharge compared to admission in 2023 (n = 774), including all patients with data available for both admission and discharge. Larger positive values indicate greater improvement, while larger negative values indicate greater deterioration

Summarising the figures in the lower left triangle (each marked in green) of Table 5.2, 390 patients (62.4%) showed an improvement in their condition compared to admission (previous years: 55.1%). In 31.0% of cases, the health status assessment remained unchanged (previous years: 36.7%; white fields) and in 6.6% of cases, deterioration was observed (previous years: 8.2%; upper right triangle marked in red). Figure 5.2 provides an overview of the number of levels by which a change occurred.

5.1.2 Subjective Assessment of Symptom Change

5.1.2.1 At Discharge from Hospital

When asked about the perceived change in symptoms from admission to discharge, 36.8% of patients reported that their symptoms had either disappeared or become considerably weaker. 45% rated their symptoms as somewhat weaker. The remaining 18.2% rated their symptoms as unchanged (12%) or worse (6.2%) (Table 5.3). Figure 5.3 provides an overview of the levels at which a change occurred.

Table 5.2 Changes in patients' self-reported health status at hospital discharge compared to admission, in 2023 ($n = 774$) and previous years ($n = 11{,}145$), including all patients with data available for both admission and discharge

2023		At follow-up					
		excellent	very good	good	fair	poor	**Total**
On admission	excellent	0 0.0%	0 0.0%	1 0.2%	0 0.0%	0 0.0%	**1** **0.2%**
	very good	0 0.0%	2 0.3%	4 0.6%	1 0.2%	0 0.0%	**7** **1.1%**
	good	3 0.5%	7 1.1%	37 5.9%	12 1.9%	0 0.0%	**59** **9.4%**
	fair	2 0.3%	25 4.0%	170 27.2%	116 18.6%	23 3.7%	**336** **53.8%**
	bad	2 0.3%	3 0.5%	76 12.2%	102 16.3%	39 6.2%	**222** **35.5%**
	Total	**7** **1.1%**	**37** **5.9%**	**288** **46.1%**	**231** **37.0%**	**62** **9.9%**	**625** **100.0%**

Previous years		At follow-up					
		excellent	very good	good	fair	poor	**Total**
On admission	excellent	3 0.0%	2 0.0%	2 0.0%	5 0.1%	1 0.0%	13 0.2%
	very good	1 0.0%	18 0.2%	31 0.4%	14 0.2%	1 0.0%	65 0.8%
	good	18 0.2%	124 1.6%	559 7.1%	277 3.5%	38 0.5%	1016 12.9%
	fair	22 0.3%	210 2.7%	1998 25.3%	1744 22.1%	275 3.5%	4249 53.8%
	poor	9 0.1%	96 1.2%	751 9.5%	1123 14.2%	576 7.3%	2555 32.3%
	Total	53 0.7%	450 5.7%	3341 42.3%	3163 40.0%	891 11.3%	7898 100.0%

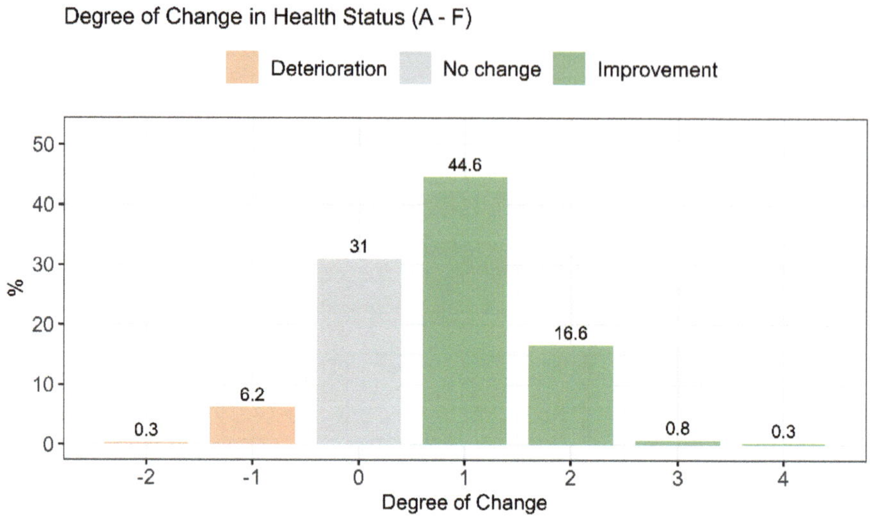

Fig. 5.2 Changes in patients' self-reported health status at follow-up compared to admission in 2023 ($n = 625$), including all patients with data available for both admission and follow-up. Larger positive values indicate greater improvement, while larger negative values indicate greater deterioration

Table 5.3 Subjective assessments of the extent of change in symptom complaints at hospital discharge in 2023 ($n = 777$) and in previous years ($n = 11{,}218$) were conducted, including all patients for whom data were available at both admission and discharge

	2023		Previous years	
Change in symptom complaints compared to admission (A-D)	*n*	%	*n*	%
No longer present	14	1.8	373	3.3
Considerably weaker	272	35.0	4220	37.6
Slightly weaker	350	45.0	4525	40.3
Unchanged	93	12.0	1501	13.4
Slightly stronger	39	5.0	416	3.7
Considerably stronger	9	1.2	183	1.6

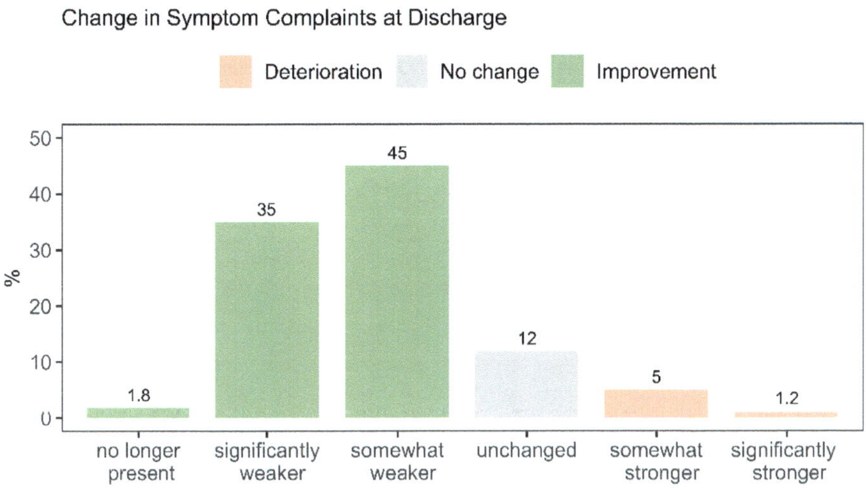

Fig. 5.3 Subjective assessments of the extent of the change in complaints at hospital discharge in 2023 ($n = 777$), including patients for whom data were available at both admission and discharge

Table 5.4 Subjective assessments of the extent of change in symptom complaints at follow-up in 2023 ($n = 625$) and in previous years ($n = 7961$), including all patients with available data for both admission and follow-up

	2023		Previous years	
Change in symptom complaints compared to admission (A-F)	*n*	%	*n*	%
No longer present	18	2.9	241	3.0
Considerably weaker	239	38.2	2754	34.6
Slightly weaker	208	33.3	2639	33.1
Unchanged	101	16.2	1523	19.1
Slightly stronger	40	6.4	543	6.8
Considerably stronger	19	3.0	262	3.3

5.1.2.2 At Follow-Up

When asked about perceived changes in symptoms at follow-up compared to admission, 41.1% of patients reported that their symptoms were either no longer present or significantly weaker. Meanwhile, 33.3% rated their symptoms as somewhat weaker. The remaining 25.6% rated their symptoms as unchanged (16.2%) or worse (9.4%) (Table 5.4). Figure 5.4 shows an overview of the levels at which changes occurred.

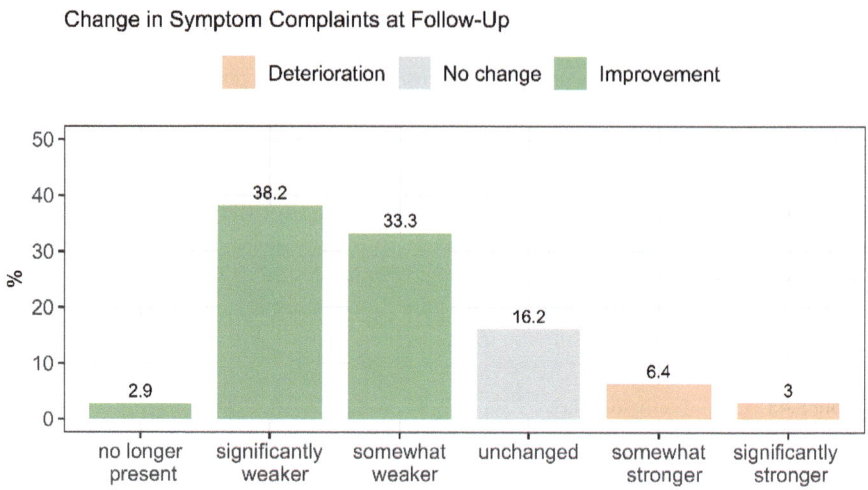

Fig. 5.4 Subjective assessments of the extent of change in complaints at the 2023 follow-up (n = 625), including patients for whom data was available at both admission and follow-up

5.1.3 Subjective Assessment of Treatment Success

5.1.3.1 At Discharge from Hospital

In addition, patients are asked upon discharge which therapies helped them the most. Due to the personalised therapy approach of the TCM clinic, not everyone receives all therapy elements. Therefore, Table 5.5 shows the number of patients who received each therapy element and the percentage who rated it as particularly helpful.

The different forms of therapy are listed in order of benefit, from the most beneficial to the least beneficial. The most common treatments were acupuncture, Chinese medicinal herbs, group Qigong, nutritional therapy, and psychological support. Conventional medicine was used by 51.6% of patients; individual Qigong, by 35.0%; matrix rhythm therapy, by 31.1%; physical therapy, by 37.3%; hydrotherapy, by 47.2%; and Tuina, by 34.7%. Many patients who received the respective therapy rated acupuncture (93.9%), Chinese herbal medicine (91.7%), physical therapy (90.7%), group Qigong (85.5%), individual Qigong (90.1%), Tuina (90.0%), and Matrix Rhythm Therapy (79.3%) as particularly helpful. A slightly lower proportion of patients found dietary changes (75.6%), psychological support (74.4%), nutritional therapy (66.9%), and hydrotherapy (70.0%) helpful. The lowest ratings were given to conventional drug treatment (62.3%) and the IHM lifestyle programme (62.0%). In this context, many patients perceived the distance from everyday life (87.1%) and the good atmosphere (87.0%) in the clinic as particularly helpful.

Table 5.5 The frequency of treatments received, and patients' subjective assessments of their effectiveness were surveyed at hospital discharge in 2023 (n = 777) and in previous years (n = 10,783). The data are sorted by descending perceived effectiveness in 2023

	2023 (n = 777)				Previous years (n = 10,783)			
	Received therapy		Of which: particularly helpful[a]		Received therapy		Of which: particularly helpful[a]	
Form of therapy	n	%	n	%	n	%	n	%
Acupuncture	774	99.6	727	93.9	10,758	99.8	9258	86.1
Chinese herbs/ medicinal teas	769	99.0	705	91.7	10,737	99.6	9647	89.8
Phys. Therapy/ physiotherapy	290	37.3	263	90.7	6262	58.1	3908	62.4
Individual qigong	272	35.0	245	90.1	5064	54.3	2872	56.7
Tuina	270	34.7	243	90.0	7368	68.3	4428	60.1
Group qigong	758	97.6	648	85.5	9220	98.9	7852	85.2
Matrix-rhythm-therapy	242	31.1	192	79.3	5604	52.0	2506	44.7
Change of diet	688	88.5	520	75.6	10,331	95.8	6982	67.6
Psychological support	759	97.7	565	74.4	10,636	98.7	6476	60.9
Hydrotherapy/foot baths/wraps	367	47.2	257	70.0	6551	60.8	2208	33.7
Nutritional therapy	717	92.3	480	66.9	10,364	96.1	7797	75.2
Drug therapy/ medication	401	51.6	250	62.3	6939	64.4	3808	54.9
Health training/IHM	681	87.6	422	62.0	10,256	95.2	7067	68.9
Other	583	75.0	234	40.1	9022	83.8	2838	31.5
Distance from everyday life	762	98.1	664	87.1	10,736	99.7	8667	80.7
Atmosphere	768	98.8	668	87.0	10,729	99.6	9295	86.6

[a]The percentages refer exclusively to patients who have received treatment

5.1.3.2 At Follow-Up

The results show that acupuncture (90.8%) and Qigong (84.6% for individuals and 88.5% for groups) are still considered very helpful. Physical therapy (87.0%) and Chinese herbal medicine (85.6%) follow closely behind (Table 5.6).

Table 5.6 The frequency of treatments received, and patients' subjective assessment of their effectiveness were surveyed at the 2023 follow-up ($n = 625$) and in previous years ($n = 7527$). The data are sorted by the descending frequency of perceived effectiveness in 2023

	2023 (n = 625)				Previous years (n = 7527)			
	Received therapy		Of which: particularly helpful[a]		Received therapy		Of which: particularly helpful[a]	
Form of therapy	n	%	n	%	n	%	n	%
Acupuncture	619	99.2	562	90.8	7491	99.6	6190	82.6
Chinese herbs/ medicinal teas	619	99.2	530	85.6	7479	99.4	6132	82.0
Phys. Therapy/ physiotherapy	316	50.6	275	87.0	5370	71.3	3699	68.9
Individual qigong	214	34.3	181	84.6	4666	62.0	2044	43.8
Tuina	231	37.0	194	84.0	5275	70.1	2996	56.8
Group qigong	617	98.9	546	88.5	7455	99.1	5763	77.3
Matrix-rhythm-therapy	188	30.1	136	72.3	4307	57.2	1884	43.7
Change of diet	568	91.0	454	79.9	7145	94.9	4795	67.1
Psychological support	618	99.0	456	73.8	7414	98.6	4548	61.3
Hydrotherapy/foot baths/wraps	234	37.5	155	66.2	4517	60.0	1190	26.3
Nutritional therapy	573	91.7	407	71.0	7113	94.5	4998	70.3
Drug therapy/ medication	322	51.6	172	53.4	5185	68.9	2582	49.8
Health training/IHM	575	92.0	368	64.0	7116	94.6	4609	64.8
Other	466	74.6	143	30.7	5842	89.3	1177	20.1
Distance from everyday life	623	99.8	550	88.3	6532	99.8	5258	80.5
Atmosphere	622	99.7	553	88.9	7503	99.8	5752	76.7

[a]The percentages refer exclusively to patients who have received treatment

5.1.4 Influence on the Progression of the Complaint

5.1.4.1 At Discharge from Hospital

Patients' assessments of their ability to influence the course of their symptoms change significantly upon discharge compared to hospital admission. Initially, only 34.9% of patients believed that they could influence the course of their illness to a moderate, quite strong, or strong extent, this proportion increased to 48.1% at discharge (compared to 32.5% and 49.4% in previous years, respectively). Summarising the figures in the green triangles at the bottom left of Table 5.7 shows an increase in estimated influenceability in 298 patients (38.5%) (compared to 43.4% in previous years). Conversely, a reduced ability to influence the course of the symptoms was observed in 17.1% of patients (previously 16.3%; red triangles), while no change was observed in this respect for 44.8% of patients (previously 40.3%; white fields). Figure 5.5 shows the degree to which the figures change when comparing admission and discharge.

Table 5.7 Patients' self-assessment of their ability to influence the course of symptoms upon discharge from hospital, compared to their assessment upon admission, in 2023 ($n = 774$) and in previous years ($n = 11,151$)

		At discharge					
2023		very strongly	quite strongly	moderately	slightly	not at all	**Total**
On admission	very strongly	27 3.5%	18 2.2%	6 0.8%	0 0.0%	0 0.0%	**51** **6.6%**
	quite strongly	37 4.8%	122 15.8%	52 6.7%	8 1.0%	0 0.0%	**219** **28.3%**
	moderately	10 1.3%	113 14.6%	145 18.7%	41 5.3%	1 0.1%	**310** **40.1%**
	slightly	4 0.5%	36 4.7%	67 8.7%	50 6.5%	3 0.4%	**160** **20.7%**
	not at all	1 0.1%	4 0.5%	16 2.1%	10 1.3%	3 0.4%	**34** **4.4%**
	Total	**79** **10.2%**	**293** **37.9%**	**286** **37.0%**	**109** **14.1%**	**7** **0.9%**	**774** **100%**

		At discharge					
Previous years		very strongly	quite strongly	moderately	slightly	not at all	**Total**
On admission	very strongly	371 3.3%	317 2.8%	94 0.8%	37 0.3%	5 0.1%	**824** **7.4%**
	quite strongly	559 5.0%	1506 13.5%	604 5.4%	112 1.0%	14 0.1%	**2795** **25.1%**
	moderately	262 2.4%	1593 14.3%	1805 16.2%	501 4.5%	51 0.5%	**4212** **37.8%**
	slightly	102 0.9%	611 5.5%	1021 9.2%	702 6.3%	84 0.8%	**2520** **22.6%**
	not at all	18 0.2%	162 1.5%	270 2.4%	239 2.1%	111 1.0%	**800** **7.2%**
	Total	**1312** **11.8%**	**4189** **37.6%**	**3794** **34.0%**	**1591** **14.3%**	**265** **2.4%**	**11151** **100%**

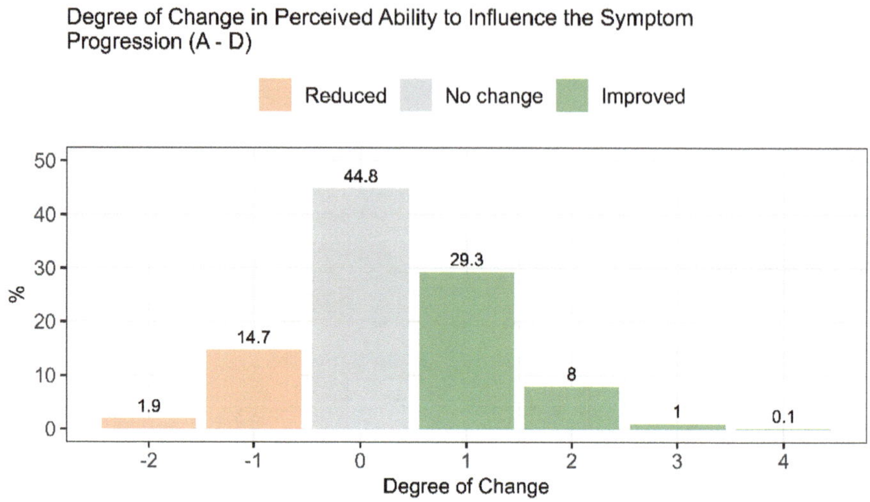

Fig. 5.5 Change in self-assessment of ability to influence symptoms at hospital discharge compared to admission in 2023 ($n = 774$)

5.1.4.2 At Follow-Up

Patients' assessments of their ability to influence the course of their symptoms change only slightly in the follow-up documentation compared to hospital admission. While initially, 35.8% of patients believed that they could influence the course of the disease moderately, quite strongly or very strongly, this proportion increased to 40.1% in the follow-up (compared to 32.6% and 35.9% in previous years, respectively). Summarising the figures in the green triangles at the bottom left of Table 5.8 shows an increase in estimated influenceability in 207 patients (33.2%) (previous years: 32.6%). Conversely, a reduced ability to influence the course of the symptoms was observed in 24.7% of patients (previously 27.5%; red triangles), while 42.1% of patients showed no change in this respect (previously 39.9%; white fields). Figure 5.6 shows the degree to which the figures change when comparing admission and follow-up.

Table 5.8 Patients' self-assessment of their ability to influence the course of their symptoms at follow-up, compared to their assessment upon admission, in 2023 ($n = 623$) and in previous years ($n = 7891$)

2023		**During the follow-up**					
		very strongly	quite strongly	moderately	slightly	not at all	**Total**
On admission	very strongly	15 2.4%	16 2.6%	8 1.3%	2 0.3%	0 0.0%	**41** **6.6%**
	quite strongly	26 4.2%	87 14.0%	54 8.7%	12 1.9%	3 0.5%	**182** **29.2%**
	moderately	13 2.1%	65 10.4%	118 18.9%	48 7.7%	4 0.6%	**248** **39.8%**
	slightly	2 0.3%	21 3.4%	62 10.0%	37 5.9%	7 1.1%	**129** **20.7%**
	not at all	2 0.2%	3 0.5%	6 1.0%	7 1.1%	5 0.8%	**23** **3.7%**
	Total	**58** **9.3%**	**192** **30.8%**	**248** **39.8%**	**106** **17.0%**	**19** **3.0%**	**623** **100%**

Previous years		**During the follow-up**					
		very strongly	quite strongly	moderately	slightly	not at all	**Total**
On admission	very strongly	177 2.2%	226 2.9%	133 1.7%	42 0.5%	13 0.2%	**591** **7.5%**
	quite strongly	250 3.2%	890 11.3%	612 7.8%	205 2.6%	24 0.3%	**1981** **25.1%**
	moderately	131 1.7%	768 9.7%	1363 17.3%	606 7.7%	123 1.6%	**2991** **37.9%**
	slightly	48 0.6%	281 3.6%	708 9.0%	590 7.5%	182 2.3%	**1809** **22.9%**
	not at all	16 0.2%	45 0.6%	171 2.2%	156 2.0%	131 1.7%	**519** **6.6%**
	Total	**622** **7.9%**	**2210** **28.0%**	**2987** **37.9%**	**1599** **20.3%**	**473** **6.0%**	**7891** **100%**

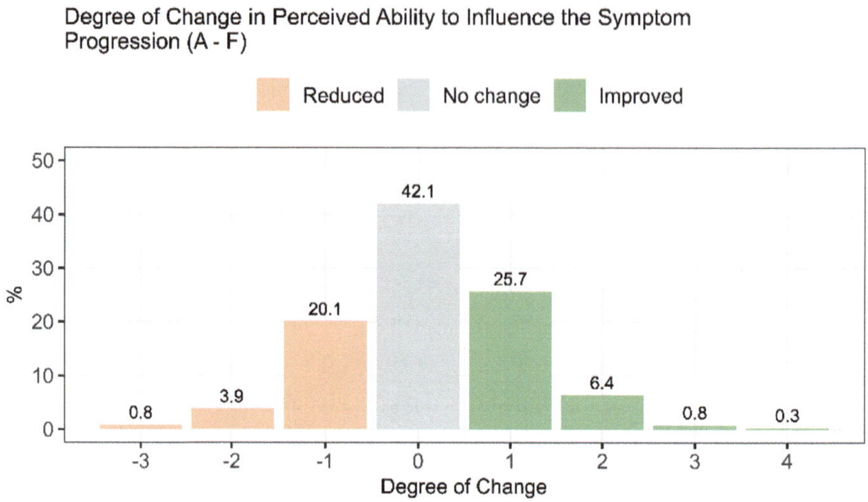

Fig. 5.6 Degree of change in the self-assessment of the ability to influence the course of symptoms at follow-up compared to admission in 2023 ($n = 623$)

5.1.5 Global Assessments of Treatment Success

5.1.5.1 At Discharge from Hospital

Finally, as part of the PEP survey at the end of their hospital stay, patients are asked to provide three global assessments of their previous treatment (Table 5.9). At the time of discharge from hospital, 64.9% of patients rated the overall success of the treatment as good or very good, 31.8% as moderate, and 3.3% were unable to determine any treatment success. Additionally, the vast majority of patients felt that the treatment had been worthwhile upon discharge (94.1%).

Regarding their own expectations, 55.4% of patients considered their expectations to be completely or largely fulfilled upon discharge. 35.0% considered their expectations to be only partially fulfilled, while 9.7% were disappointed and considered their expectations to be somewhat or entirely unfulfilled. Figure 5.7 shows the distribution of the overall assessment.

5.1.5.2 At Follow-Up

Approximately 6 months after discharge, 72.4% of patients rated the overall success of the treatments as good or very good, while 24.4% gave a moderate rating and 3.2% reported no noticeable success from the treatment (Table 5.10). Additionally, 93.9% of respondents said that they thought the treatment was worthwhile.

In terms of personal expectations, 57.5% felt that these were either fully or largely met, while 32.3% reported partial fulfilment. A further 10.2% expressed disappointment, indicating that their expectations were not met at all or only partially. Figure 5.8 illustrates how these overall assessments are distributed.

Table 5.9 Global assessments of treatment outcomes were surveyed at hospital discharge in 2023 ($n = 777$) and in previous years ($n = 11{,}211$)

		2023		Previous years	
Global judgment at discharge		*n*	%	*n*	%
Overall therapy success	Very good	118	15.2	1667	14.9
	Good	386	49.7	5574	49.7
	Moderate	247	31.8	3461	30.9
	No success	26	3.3	509	4.5
Treatment worthwhile	Very worthwhile	331	42.6	4857	43.3
	Worthwhile	400	51.5	5642	50.3
	Not worth it	42	5.4	647	5.8
	Rather harmed	4	0.5	65	0.6
Expectations fulfilled	Completely	135	17.4	1890	16.9
	Largely	295	38.0	4473	39.9
	Partially	272	35.0	3796	33.9
	Rather not	65	8.4	858	7.7
	Not at all	10	1.3	194	1.7

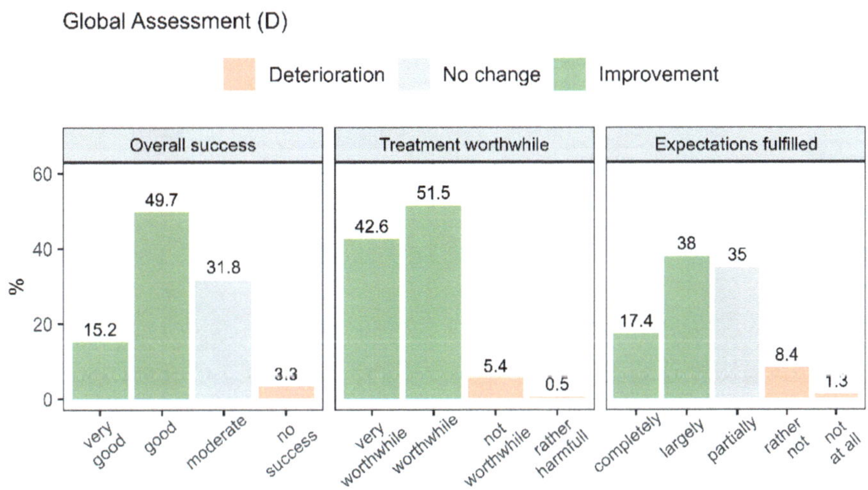

Fig. 5.7 Global assessments of overall success and whether the treatment was worthwhile as well as an evaluation whether expectations were met at the time of discharge ($n = 777$)

Table 5.10 Global assessments of the treatment outcome, surveyed at the follow-up in 2023 ($n = 623$) and previous years ($n = 7934$)

Global judgment at follow-up		2023		Previous years	
		n	%	*n*	%
Overall therapy success	Very good	169	27.1	1629	20.5
	Good	282	45.3	3443	43.4
	Moderate	152	24.4	2149	27.1
	No success	20	3.2	713	9.0
Treatment worthwhile	Very worthwhile	343	55.1	3536	44.6
	Worthwhile	242	38.8	3453	43.5
	Not worth it	37	5.9	869	11.0
	Rather harmed	1	0.2	76	1.0
Expectations fulfilled	Perfect	129	20.7	1177	14.8
	Largely	229	36.8	2662	33.6
	Partially	201	32.3	2688	33.9
	Rather not	57	9.1	972	12.3
	Not at all	7	1.1	435	5.5

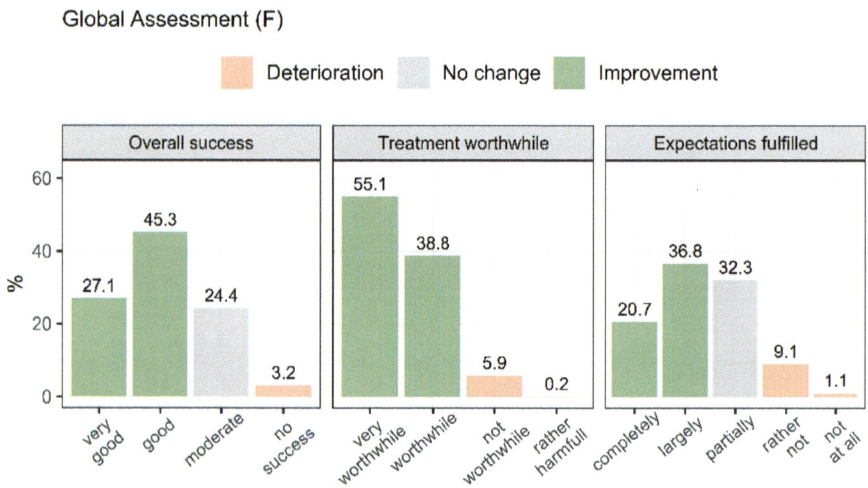

Fig. 5.8 Global assessments of the overall success and whether the treatment was worthwhile and an evaluation whether expectations were met at the time of the follow-up ($n = 623$)

5.1.5.3 Utilisation of Medical Services

Most patients (around 82%) saw a doctor for outpatient treatment between being discharged from hospital and completing the follow-up survey (Table 5.11). In this context, the majority of patients (61.4%) reported that their treatment was partially successful. Additionally, 14.4% of respondents indicated that they had been hospitalised during the discharge and follow-up period, while 44.7% were undergoing psychotherapeutic treatment.

Table 5.12 compares the data on incapacity for work and impairment of daily activities before hospital admission, as well as the period between hospital discharge and the follow-up survey.

Table 5.11 Information on the use of doctor and hospital visits, and psychotherapy, approximately 6 months after discharge from hospital in 2023 (n = 624), as well as in previous years (n = 6926)

		2023		Previous years	
		n	%	*n*	%
Doctor visits since discharge	None	103	16.5	1031	14.9
	1–3	198	31.7	1963	28.3
	4–10	223	35.7	2357	34.0
	11–25	72	11.5	1058	15.3
	>25	20	3.2	406	5.9
	Don't know	8	1.3	111	1.6
If yes,[a]	Without success	120	24.2	1588	26.8
	Partial success	304	61.4	3440	58.1
	Good success	71	14.3	896	15.1
Hospital visits since discharge	None	380	84.3	5887	85.0
	1–7 days	21	4.7	366	5.3
	8–14 days	11	2.4	209	3.0
	3–4 weeks	16	3.5	244	3.5
	>4 weeks	17	3.8	191	2.8
	Don't know	6	1.3	29	0.4
If yes,[a]	Without success	13	20.6	693	41.3
	Partial success	30	47.6	653	38.9
	Good success	20	31.7	333	19.8
Psychotherapy since discharge?	Yes	278	44.7	2265	32.7
	No	344	55.3	4661	67.3
If yes, how many **hours of psychotherapy**?	Up to 5	87	31.3	827	36.5
	6–25	169	60.8	1094	48.3
	26–160	22	7.9	294	13.0
	161–300	0	–	33	1.5
	>300 hrs	0	–	15	0.7

[a]Due to missing information, the figures do not match. However, since a correct answer was assumed for this response, no correction was made

At the time of the initial survey, 62.9% of patients reported being in employment. This figure declined slightly to 58.9% at the time of the follow-up survey. Of those who had been employed in the 6 months prior to hospital admission, 83.7% stated that they had been unable to work during that period. Following discharge, this proportion decreased to 52.9%, indicating partial recovery of work capacity.

The median number of sick leave days fell from 30 to 20. The average number of sick days decreased from 76.39 (SD = 74.17) to 72.11 (SD = 94.32). However, since a maximum sick leave of 6 months can be specified at admission, whereas values of up to 1 year are possible at follow-up, the actual reduction in sick days is likely to be even greater.

Table 5.12 Information on incapacity for work in a before-and-after comparison of 2023, 2022, and previous years

In the past 6 months (or since discharge) have you had to leave the hospital because of your sickness from time to time?												
	2023				**2022**				**Previous years**			
	In the past 6 months before admission $n = 821$		Since discharge at follow-up $n = 623$		In the past 6 months before admission $n = 725$		Since discharge at follow-up $n = 465$		In the past 6 months before admission $n = 11{,}915$		Since discharge at follow-up $n = 8011$	
	n	%	*n*	%	*n*	%	*n*	%	*n*	%	*n*	%
Not gainfully employed	305	37.1	256	41.1	218	30.1	175	33.9	4402	36.9	3233	40.4
Employed	516	62.9	367	58.9	507	69.9	341	66.1	7513	63.1	4778	59.6
Of which: Yes, with SL	432	83.7	194	52.9	400	78.9	175	51.3	5677	75.6	2249	47.1
≥ 1 month	196	50.8	101	61.2	185	50.8	76	55.5	3064	57.7	1372	67.3
≥ 2 months	27	7.0	8	4.8	28	7.7	11	8.0	626	11.8	153	7.5
≥ 3 months	20	5.2	3	1.8	20	5.5	8	5.8	334	6.3	74	3.6
≥ 4 months	22	5.7	12	7.3	29	8.0	5	3.6	339	6.4	68	3.3
≥ 5 months	5	1.3	5	3.0	14	3.8	9	6.6	170	3.2	72	3.5
≥ 6 months	116	30.1	36	21.9	88	24.2	38	20.4	779	14.7	301	14.7
Total	**386**	**100**	**165**	**100**	**364**	**100**	**137**	**100**	**5312**	**100**	**2040**	**100**
Missing data (SL)	46	10.7	29	15.0	36	9.0	38	21.7	364	6.4	209	9.3
SL days[a]: summary												
Median	30.0		20.0		30.0		24.0		26.0		15.0	
Mean (SD)	76.39 (74.17)		72.11 (94.32)		73.91 (69.63)		73.85 (89.95)		56.52 (62.09		53.48 (76.10)	
Total n: SL days[a]	**29,488**		**11,898**		**26,905**		**10,118**		**300,598**		**109,109**	

[a]*SL* sick leave. All data exceeding a duration of 6 months (183 days) at the time of admission or 1 year (365 days) at follow-up were changed to 183 or 365, respectively. As a period of up to 1 year is accepted at follow-up, these values cannot be compared directly

To obtain further information about possible impairments in everyday life, respondents were also asked about interruptions to their usual activities due to their illness. These figures also refer to the period before admission to the hospital (up to 6 months) and after discharge from the hospital (up to 1 year). The proportion of patients who reported interruptions to their activities due to their illness decreased from 84.9% before hospitalisation to 61.2% after discharge. The median number of days affected fell from 30 to 20 days (Table 5.13).

Table 5.13 Information on disability in everyday activities, presented as a comparison between 2023 and previous years

In the past 6 months (or since discharge) have you had to interrupt your usual activities because of your sickness?

	2023				2022				Previous years			
	In the past 6 months before admission *n* = 821		Since discharge at follow-up *n* = 623		In the past 6 months before admission *n* = 725		Since discharge at follow-up *n* = 465		In the past 6 months before admission *n* = 11,915		Since discharge at follow-up *n* = 8011	
	n	**%**	***n***	**%**	***n***	**%**	***n***	**%**	***n***	**%**	***n***	**%**
Yes, with interruption	697	84.9	381	61.2	590	81.4	295	57.2	9095	76.3	4288	53.5
≥ 1 month	280	50.5	173	64.3	240	53.1	141	71.2	4163	52.3	2444	69.6
≥ 2 months	83	15.0	32	11.9	75	16.6	20	10.1	1118	14.1	346	9.8
≥ 3 months	25	4.5	11	4.1	27	6.0	5	2.5	401	5.0	104	3.0
≥ 4 months	69	12.5	21	7.8	35	7.7	15	7.6	729	9.2	185	5.3
≥ 5 months	9	1.6	8	3.0	15	3.3	3	1.5	284	3.6	77	2.2
≥ 6 months	88	15.9	25	9.3	60	13.3	14	7.0	1258	15.8	358	10.2
Total	**554**	**100**	**270**	**100**	**452**	**100**	**198**	**100**	**7953**	**100**	**3514**	**100**
Missing data	143	20.5	111	29.1	138	23.4	97	32.8	1142	12.6	774	18.1
SL days: summary												
Median	30.0		20.0		30.0		16.0		30.0		20.0	
Mean (SD)	63.61 (59.46)		50.86 (68.55)		57.42 (58.44)		40.70 (58.00)		63.05 (62.10)		46.50 (67.83)	
Total n: SL days[a]	**35,241**		**13,733**		**25,955**		**8059**		**501,450**		**163,412**	

[a]All data exceeding a duration of 6 months (183 days) at the time of admission, or 1 year (365 days) at follow-up, were changed to 183 or 365, respectively. As a period of up to 1 year is accepted at follow-up, these values cannot be compared directly

As part of the follow-up, patients were asked about their medication use. While 59.0% stated that they were taking conventional medication, 67.4% reported taking herbal or homeopathic medication (Table 5.14). To compare medication use before and after hospital stays, patients were asked about any changes to their medication intake. Around 54.4% of patients stated that they took less conventional medication after their hospital stay (33.8% significantly less and 20.8% slightly less). For 39.2% of patients, their medication intake remained unchanged, while around 6.3% reported increased use. A similar pattern emerged when herbal medicines were considered (37.9% less, 44.8% unchanged, and 17.3% more). However, the effect of reducing intake is somewhat less pronounced here.

Table 5.14 Information on medication use, approximately 6 months after discharge in 2023 ($n = 625$) and in previous years ($n = 7243$)

		2023		Previous years	
		n	%	*n*	%
Currently taking **conventional medicine Medication**?	No, never taken	100	16.0	1214	16.8
	No more	156	25.0	1975	27.3
	Yes	369	59.0	4054	56.0
Compared to before hospital admission	Significantly less	211	33.8	2491	34.4
	Slightly less	130	20.8	1337	18.5
	About the same	245	39.2	3071	42.4
	A little more	28	4.5	239	3.3
	Significantly more	11	1.8	105	1.4
Currently taking **herbal/homeopathic medication**?	No, never taken	76	12.2	1145	15.8
	No more	127	20.4	1919	26.5
	Yes	420	67.4	4,179	57.7
Compared to before hospital admission	Significantly less	148	23.8	1831	25.3
	Slightly less	88	14.1	1134	15.7
	About the same	279	44.8	3529	48.7
	A little more	81	13.0	497	6.9
	Significantly more	27	4.3	252	3.5
New complaints occurred since discharge	Yes	158	25.4	2059	28.4
	No	465	74.6	5184	71.6

The follow-up survey revealed that 25.5% of patients had experienced new symptoms since being discharged from the clinic (Table 5.14). It is difficult to estimate the extent to which this circumstance affects people's state of mind regarding the original complaints.

5.1.6 Association Between Overall Assessment of Treatment Outcome and Side Effect Reports

Although there is a significant association ($p = 0.023$) between the reporting of adverse therapeutic effects (ATEs) and the assessment of treatment success, this has a negligible effect ($d = 0.16$). This suggests that 'side effects' or 'adverse events' occurring in connection with the treatment are only weakly associated with a poorer assessment of the therapy's overall success.

The largest difference is observed in the rating of therapy success as 'very good': 18.9% of patients without ATEs reported this level of satisfaction, compared to 11.8% of those with ATEs (Table 5.15). Although the proportion of patients who considered their treatment unsuccessful was slightly higher in those with ATE, it was still low in both groups (3.6% with ATE and 3.1% without). Of patients experiencing side effects, 33.6% rated their treatment success as moderate. In contrast, patients without side effects rated a moderate result in only 29.7% of cases. Analysis of larger datasets from previous years also revealed a statistically significant

Table 5.15 Association between overall assessment of treatment outcome and the reporting of side effects, surveyed at hospital discharge in 2023 ($n = 774$) and in previous years ($n = 11,215$); Cohen's d = effect measure ($d \geq 0.2$ = small, ≥ 0.5 = medium, ≥ 0.8 = strong effect)

	Side effects 2023						**Association: ATE and treatment outcome**	
Therapy success	**With side effects**		**No side effects**		**Total**			
	n	%	*n*	%	*n*	%	*p*	*d*
Very good	49	11.8	68	18.9	118	15.2		
Good	211	51.0	174	48.3	386	49.7		
Moderate	139	33.6	107	29.7	247	31.8		
No success	15	3.6	11	3.1	26	3.3		
Total	414	100	360	100	774	100	**0.023**	**0.16**
	Side effects previous years						**Association: ATE and treatment outcome**	
Therapy success	**With side effects**		**No side effects**		**Total**			
	n	%	*n*	%	*n*	%	*p*	*d*
Very good	626	12.3	1037	17.0	1667	14.9		
Good	2444	48.2	3114	51.0	5575	49.7		
Moderate	1745	34.4	1704	27.9	3463	30.9		
No success	260	5.1	248	4.1	510	4.5		
Total	5075	100	6103	100	11,215	100	**< 0.001**	**0.18**

correlation between satisfaction with treatment outcomes and reported side effects ($p < 0.001$), although the effect size remained small.

5.1.7 Adverse Therapeutic Side Effects (ATEs) Reported by Patients at Hospital Discharge

As part of the quality assurance process within the PEP, all patients being discharged are asked to describe any adverse therapeutic effects they experience in writing. This was completed in 414 cases and discussed with the attending physician at the end of the inpatient stay. These documents are reviewed by the CoCoNat scientific advisor when preparing the hospital report and are categorised primarily based on gastrointestinal complaints. Table 5.16 summarises the number and frequency of ATE, divided into corresponding categories. Overall, 50.2% ($n = 414$) of patients reported an adverse therapeutic effect (ATE). The following list of ATE highlights gastrointestinal complaints, which fall into the following categories: diarrhoea, constipation, nausea, vomiting, and flatulence. All entries containing these keywords were included and counted individually, including cases in which a single patient reported multiple symptoms.

The majority of ATE cases (62.3%) are related to patients' intolerance of Chinese medicines. From a toxicological point of view, vomiting is a particularly concerning symptom, but this was only reported by patients in four cases. Most ATE relate to other gastrointestinal intolerances, such as diarrhoea, flatulence, and nausea. Abdominal pain and stomach pain, as well as flatulence, are the most frequently documented ATE, with 58 and 43 hits, respectively. Once the ingredients of the

Table 5.16 Reported adverse therapeutic effects in the categories diarrhoea, constipation, nausea, vomiting, and flatulence (UTW) at hospital discharge in 2023 ($n = 414$)

Adverse therapeutic effects (ATE)	*n*
Diarrhoea	42
Constipation	19
Nausea	18
Vomiting	4
Blood in stool	1
Flatulence	43
Abdominal pain, cramps, Stomach ache	58
Toal	184

medicinal decoction have been individually tailored, most symptoms disappear again. All changes in liver values are documented by central transaminase monitoring. These are presented in the corresponding chapter on liver value screening.

Other important categories of side effects include ‘fatigue, exhaustion and tiredness’, ‘pain (general, headaches, etc.)’, ‘worsening of disease symptoms’, ‘dizziness and cardiovascular problems’, and ‘allergic symptoms’. The pain group is in the lead here with 74 mentions (general worsening of pain with 40 mentions and headaches with 34 mentions), followed by the fatigue and exhaustion symptom group with 67 individual entries. Allergic reactions are documented in 36 entries, and cardiovascular problems, including dizziness, are documented in 34 entries. Less common side effects reported by patients include restless legs (five reports), hair loss (three reports), and frequent urination (three reports). Patients may provide multiple answers.

5.1.8 Evaluation of Changes in Symptom Severity

A key measure of change in the patient’s predominant symptoms is the subjective assessment of the intensity of symptoms on admission and discharge (and again approximately 6 months later in the follow-up survey). Intensity is recorded on a numerical rating scale (from 0 = not present to 100 = extremely severe) and transformed into a visual analogue scale (VAS) according to the patient’s primary rating.

Table 5.17 summarises the descriptive statistics for all items related to the main complaint, including the severity ratings at admission, discharge, and follow-up, and the expected severity at discharge. Additionally, it presents the difference between the expected and actual values. For the reporting year, the descriptive analysis included all available data. However, only data from patients with complete data across all three time points were considered for the subsequent statistical evaluation of change over time.

The average severity of the primary complaint on admission was 71.16 points (SD = 18.95; $n = 821$). This decreased to 46.89 points at discharge (SD = 22.09; $n = 777$), before increasing slightly to 47.3 points at follow-up (SD = 24.2; $n = 629$). A similar pattern can be observed in data from previous years, although the severity

Table 5.17 This shows the cross-section of average complaint severity (scaled from 0 to 100) at all three survey points in 2023 and in previous years

	2023				Previous years			
Main complaint strength VAS 1	*n*	M	SD	Md	*n*	M	SD	Md
Admission (A)	821	71.16	18.95	70	11,862	66.56	19.26	70
Discharge (D)	777	46.89	22.09	50	11,216	42.46	21.74	40
Follow-up (F)	627	47.34	24.16	50	8934	45.78	23.42	50
Expected discharge value at admission	821	29.32	18.15	30	11,864	24.72	17.03	20
Difference A/D	777	−24.41	23.32	−20	11,155	−24.05	23.93	−20
Difference A/F	627	−23.29	26.97	−20	8815	−20.27	25.80	−20
Difference expected/actual	777	17.58	23.26	20	11,155	17.72	23.60	20
Second complaint strength VAS 2	*n*	M	SD	Md	*n*	M	SD	Md
Admission (A)	821	68.49	21.24	70	11,155	59.20	22.91	60
Discharge (D)	767	41.76	23.70	40	10,557	38.33	22.78	40
Follow-up (F)	610	43.00	25.86	40	7288	43.27	25.26	40
Expected discharge value at admission	821	27.69	19.16	20	11,383	22.67	17.47	20
Difference A/D	767	−26.68	26.88	−30	10,260	−21.16	27.85	−20
Difference A/F	610	−25.70	29.03	−30	7079	−15.89	30.25	−10
Difference expected/actual	767	14.25	25.95	10	10,259	15.54	24.87	10

of the complaint tended to be slightly lower. When asked to estimate the expected severity of their main complaint at discharge, patients anticipated an average value of 29.32 points (SD = 18.15, $n = 821$; 2023) and 24.7 points (SD = 17.0, $n = 11{,}864$; previous years), indicating a very low level of expected symptom burden. Considering the actual symptom severity at discharge (M = 46.89, SD = 22.09, $n = 777$ in 2023; M = 42.5, SD = 21.7, $n = 11{,}216$ in previous years), the expected outcome prior to hospital admission was clearly not achieved.

Like the main complaint, respondents have the option of providing information on an additional complaint. In the admission survey, all 821 patients in 2023 made use of this option, suggesting that all patients have at least one secondary complaint in addition to the main complaint. The average intensity decreased from 68.49 points (SD = 21.24; $n = 821$; 2023) and 59.20 points (SD = 22.91; $n = 11{,}155$; previous years) to 41.76 points (SD = 23.70; $n = 767$; 2023) and 38.33 points (SD = 22.78; $n = 10{,}557$; previous years) at discharge, followed by an increase to 43.00 points (SD = 25.86; $n = 610$) and 43.27 points (SD = 25.26; $n = 7288$; previous years) at follow-up.

As mentioned above, the figures for 2023 described in Table 5.17 are the result of cross-sectional analyses with different sample sizes. For this reason, the mean comparisons shown in Fig. 5.9 and Table 5.18 only include patients with complete follow-up data at all three time points. A *t*-test with a 95% confidence interval was used to compare the severity of symptoms between admission and discharge, and between admission and follow-up. A significance level of $p < 0.001$ was consistently observed, and the corresponding effect size (d) was calculated to quantify the magnitude of the observed differences. The effect sizes reported here are based on a formula previously established for dependent samples [1]. According to established conventions [2], values around 0.2 indicate a small effect, values around 0.5

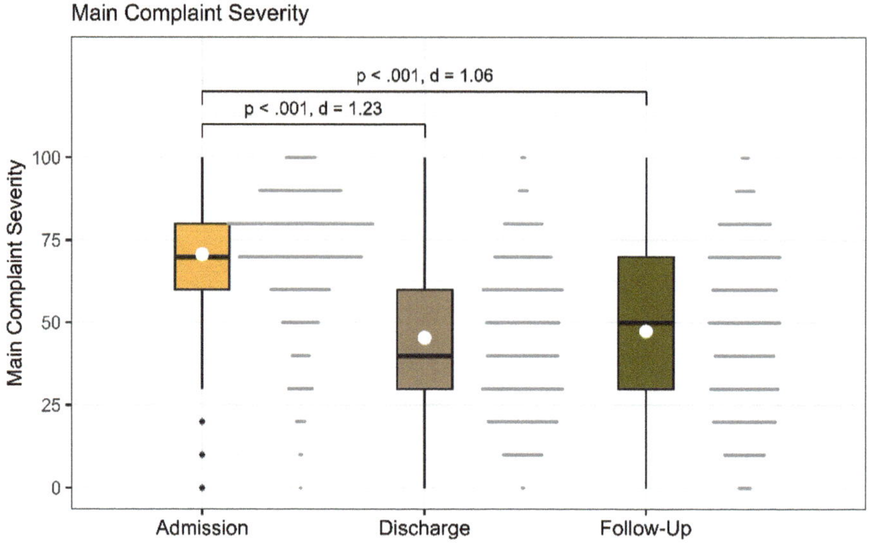

Fig. 5.9 Main complaint severity VAS 1 over the course of 2023 (complete follow-up samples A-E-F $n = 618$); white circles indicate the mean and the black lines the median

Table 5.18 Development of VAS scores for main (VAS 1) and secondary complaint (VAS 2) for complete follow-up data 2023 and previous years

		Course: A–D and A–F			Difference		
2023		***n***	**M**	**SD**	**M**	***p***	***d***
VAS 1	A	618	70.68	19.03	−25.32	<0.001	−1.23
	D		45.36	21.86			
	A	618	70.68	19.03	−23.24	<0.001	−1.06
	F		47.44	24.27			
VAS 2	A	595	68.47	20.82	−28.32	<0.001	−1.28
	D		40.15	23.39			
	A	595	68.47	20.82	−25.46	<0.001	−1.08
	F		43.01	25.93			
Previous years		***n***	**M**	**SD**	**M**	***p***	***d***
VAS 1	A	8571	66.08	19.13	−25.10	< 0.001	−1.24
	D		40.98	21.23			
	A	8571	66.08	19.13	−20.33	< 0.001	−0.95
	F		45.75	23.35			
VAS 2	A	6667	59.38	22.74	−21.93	< 0.001	−0.97
	D		37.44	22.44			
	A	6667	59.38	22.74	−16.15	< 0.001	−0.67
	F		43.22	25.27			

indicate a moderate effect, and values of 0.8 or higher indicate a large effect. Indicating the effect size underlines the significance of the results.

When considering only patients admitted in 2023 for whom admission, discharge, and follow-up values are available ($n = 618$), there was a reduction in symptom severity from an average of 70.68 (SD = 19.08) at baseline to an average of 45.31 (SD = 21.96) at discharge (an average reduction of 25.37 points). This corresponds to a strong effect size ($d = 1.23$, $p < 0.001$) according to Cohen (Table 5.18, Fig. 5.9). At follow-up, the score increased slightly to 47.30 (SD = 24.28). Nevertheless, this represents a substantial reduction of 23.39 points compared to admission, indicating a strong effect size ($d = 1.07$, $p < 0.001$). Based on the full 2023 dataset, the changes in symptom severity associated with the secondary complaint are comparable to those of the primary complaint, with large effect sizes at discharge ($d = 1.28$, $p < 0.001$) and at the follow-up ($d = 1.08$, $p < 0.001$).

In the complete reference dataset comprising 8571 patients, the average complaint severity decreased from 66.08 (SD = 19.13) points at baseline to 40.98 (SD = 21.23) points at discharge (an average reduction of 25.10 points). In the follow-up survey conducted approximately 6 months later, mean complaint severity increased slightly to 45.75 points (SD = 23.35), representing a mean decrease of 20.33 points compared to the level before hospitalisation. This corresponds to a significantly lower average severity of the main complaint at discharge, reflected in a large effect size ($d = 1.24$, $p < 0.001$). Although there was a slight increase in symptom severity between discharge and follow-up, a large, clinically relevant effect was still evident between the admission and follow-up values for the main complaint ($d = 0.95$, $p < 0.001$). Among the 8571 patients with complete data on the secondary complaint, the pattern mirrors that of the main complaint. However, the differences in complaint severity across the three measurement points are somewhat less pronounced. While discharge severity still reflects a strong effect ($d = 0.97$, $p < 0.001$), follow-up measurement shows a moderate effect ($d = 0.67$, $p < 0.001$).

In addition to the overall results presented in Table 5.17 and Table 5.18, the distribution of severity of the main complaint among patients with complete follow-up data is further broken down by sex and age category in Table 5.19 for 2023 and in Table 5.20 for previous years. The VAS changes reveal slight differences between gender and age. Younger patients benefit slightly more than older patients in terms of symptom reduction over time. Women benefit slightly more than men in this measurement.

To provide a more visual representation of the results, Fig. 5.10 illustrates the distribution of symptom severity upon hospital admission, discharge, and follow-up for those with complete follow-up data ($n = 618$), using the 2023 reporting year as an example. The bar charts demonstrate the skewed distribution of intensity values. Isolated values of 0 prior to treatment indicate medical conditions that are asymptomatic to the patient. At discharge and follow-up, there is a clear shift in the distribution towards lower intensity values.

Table 5.19 Main complaint severity VAS 1 (0–100) of patients with complete follow-up data; broken down by age and gender in 2023 ($n = 618$)

Main complaint strength VAS 1 in 2023									
		Number (%)		Admission		Discharge		Follow-up	
	Age in years	*n*	%	M	SD	M	SD	M	SD
Male	Up to 30	4	3.3	73.57	20.61	53.57	28.98	50.00	25.72
	31 to 40	8	6.5	71.67	17.10	50.24	21.24	44.29	25.58
	41 to 50	16	13.3	69.76	19.46	39.76	23.55	42.59	26.78
	51 to 60	56	45.5	72.17	18.28	46.99	21.93	48.55	23.56
	61 to 70	30	24.4	66.28	20.55	42.64	20.11	46.82	23.21
	Over 70	9	7.3	75.09	17.28	47.36	19.82	53.02	24.54
	Total	**123**	**100**	**70.41**	**18.39**	**44.88**	**20.97**	**48.62**	**24.00**
Female	Up to 30	10	2.0	87.50	18.93	67.50	34.03	45.00	28.87
	31 to 40	34	6.9	77.50	18.32	55.00	23.30	57.50	31.05
	41 to 50	69	13.9	63.75	19.96	40.62	17.69	42.50	27.20
	51 to 60	220	44.4	71.79	18.98	47.50	22.01	49.82	23.85
	61 to 70	118	23.8	69.33	15.52	39.33	16.60	48.67	20.47
	Over 70	44	8.9	63.33	16.58	35.56	15.09	45.56	25.06
	Total	**495**	**100**	**70.75**	**19.21**	**45.47**	**22.09**	**47.15**	**24.35**
Total	Up to 30	14	2.3	68.00	19.32	48.00	26.58	52.00	25.73
	31 to 40	42	6.8	70.29	16.78	49.12	20.94	41.18	23.58
	41 to 50	85	13.8	71.16	19.22	39.57	24.82	42.61	26.88
	51 to 60	276	44.7	72.27	18.14	46.86	21.95	48.23	23.53
	61 to 70	148	23.9	65.51	21.63	43.47	20.89	46.36	23.92
	Over 70	53	8.6	77.50	16.58	49.77	19.94	54.55	24.44
	Total	**618**	**100**	**70.68**	**19.03**	**45.36**	**21.86**	**47.44**	**24.27**

Table 5.20 Main complaint severity VAS 1 (0–100) of patients with complete follow-up data; broken down by age and gender in previous years ($n = 8571$)

Main complaint strength VAS 1 in previous years									
		Number (%)		Admission		Discharge		Follow-up	
	Age in years	*n*	%	M	SD	M	SD	M	SD
Male	Up to 30	80	3.7	60.50	22.44	36.62	21.28	35.00	23.38
	31 to 40	134	6.2	61.94	20.90	43.66	22.56	44.85	24.61
	41 to 50	401	18.6	63.79	18.96	39.85	22.25	46.36	23.52
	51 to 60	738	34.2	64.25	18.81	41.22	21.60	47.99	23.24
	61 to 70	489	22.7	64.40	20.18	40.63	22.10	48.63	23.61
	Over 70	313	14.5	64.66	18.91	42.59	20.13	51.09	22.82
	Total	**2155**	**100**	**63.98**	**19.44**	**41.01**	**21.69**	**47.61**	**23.57**
Female	Up to 30	237	3.7	61.18	20.86	40.21	23.50	37.30	24.28
	31 to 40	429	6.7	64.55	19.45	41.93	21.72	43.29	23.51
	41 to 50	1397	21.8	66.22	19.23	41.05	21.61	44.40	23.53
	51 to 60	2427	37.8	67.24	18.30	40.16	20.86	44.91	22.78
	61 to 70	1283	20.0	67.07	18.91	40.59	20.33	45.65	23.03
	Over 70	643	10.0	69.33	19.41	44.18	20.53	50.64	23.09
	Total	**6416**	**100**	**66.79**	**18.97**	**40.97**	**21.08**	**45.13**	**23.24**
Total	Up to 30	317	3.7	61.01	21.23	39.31	22.98	36.72	24.04
	31 to 40	563	6.6	63.93	19.81	42.34	21.91	43.66	23.76
	41 to 50	1798	21.0	65.68	19.19	40.78	21.76	44.83	23.54
	51 to 60	3165	36.9	66.54	18.46	40.41	21.04	45.63	22.92
	61 to 70	1772	20.7	66.33	19.30	40.60	20.83	46.47	23.22
	Over 70	956	11.2	67.80	19.36	43.66	20.40	50.78	22.99
	Total	**8571**	**100**	**66.08**	**19.13**	**40.98**	**21.23**	**45.75**	**23.35**

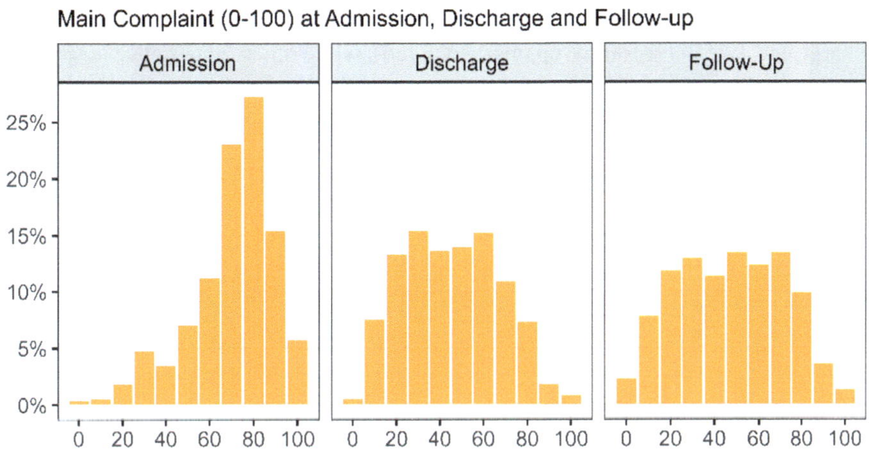

Fig. 5.10 Distribution of the VAS 1 assessments of main complaint severity (0 to 100) at hospital admission, discharge, and follow-up (complete follow-up data: $n = 618$) in 2023

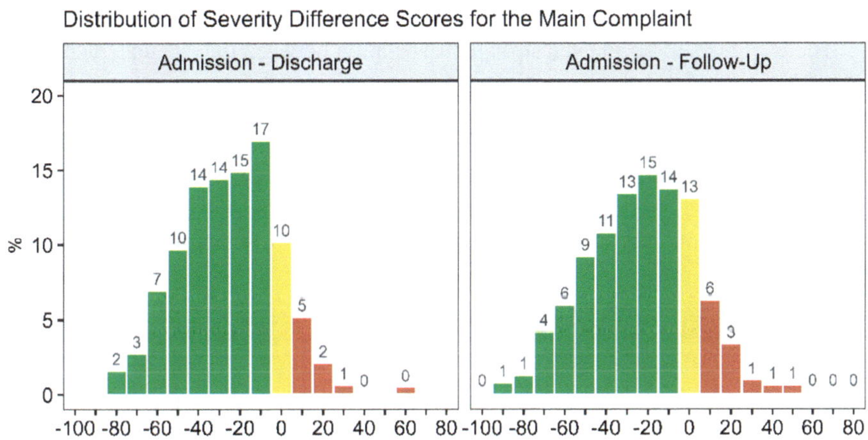

Fig. 5.11 Distribution of difference values for main complaint severity (VAS 1) between admission and discharge, and between admission and follow-up in 2023 ($n = 618$). Negative differences correspond to improvement

Additionally, Fig. 5.11 illustrates the extent of the change in terms of improvement, deterioration or unchanged symptom severity. The graphical representation of the calculated differences between discharge and admission (M = −25.32; $n = 618$), as well as admission and follow-up (M = −23.24; $n = 618$), reveals that reductions in complaints, reflected by negative differences ranging from −100 to −1 (highlighted in green), predominate. For most respondents (81.3% for discharge and 74.4% for follow-up), this indicates an improvement in symptoms compared to their condition at admission. However, it is also evident that some patients report an exacerbation of their symptoms upon hospital discharge (8.6% for discharge and 12.5% for follow-up, marked in red), while others experience no change in symptom severity (10.2% for discharge and 13.1% for follow-up, marked in yellow).

5.1.8.1 Association with the Average Treatment Success Rate (VAS 1)

The following analysis incorporates initial survey data on 'belief in help' to explore whether confidence in treatment success upon admission is associated with changes in the severity of the main complaint between admission and discharge. 'Belief in help' refers to patients' confidence that the treatment provided at the TCM-Klinik Bad Kötzting would be effective. The following analysis also incorporates initial survey data on 'belief in help' to explore whether confidence in treatment success at admission is associated with changes in main complaint severity between admission and discharge.

As shown in Fig. 5.12, data from 2023 indicate an association between patients' belief that they will receive effective help at the time of hospital admission and the observed change in the severity of their main complaint. On average, patients who expressed strong confidence in the success of their treatment experienced greater relief from their main complaint than those who were uncertain or sceptical.

There appears to be an even stronger association between the calculated changes in the severity of the main complaint and patients' global assessment of treatment success at hospital discharge (Fig. 5.13).

At the time of hospital discharge, each category of the Global Assessment of Treatment Success (GATS) is associated with a progressively greater reduction in symptom severity (Indirect Change Measurement). As expected, this indicates that the higher patients rate the success of their therapy at discharge, the greater the

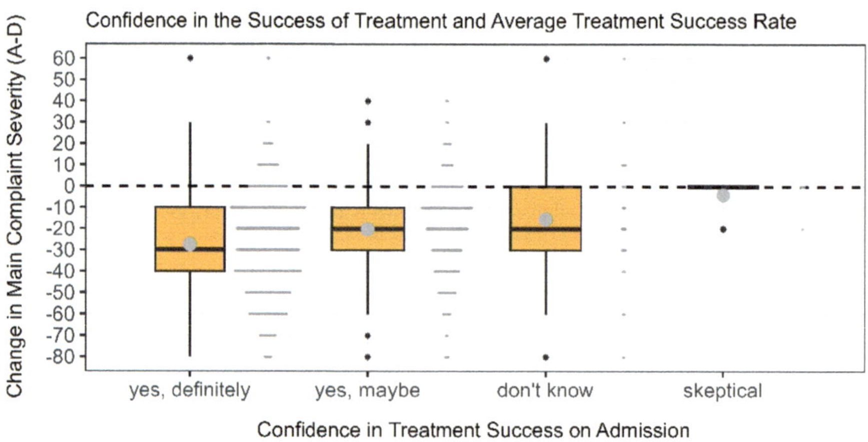

Fig. 5.12 Association between confidence in the success of treatment on admission and average treatment success, as measured by the change in VAS for the main complaint at hospital discharge in 2023. The dashed line indicates no change in the severity of the main complaint. Grey dots indicate the mean, black lines the median, and stars indicate outliers

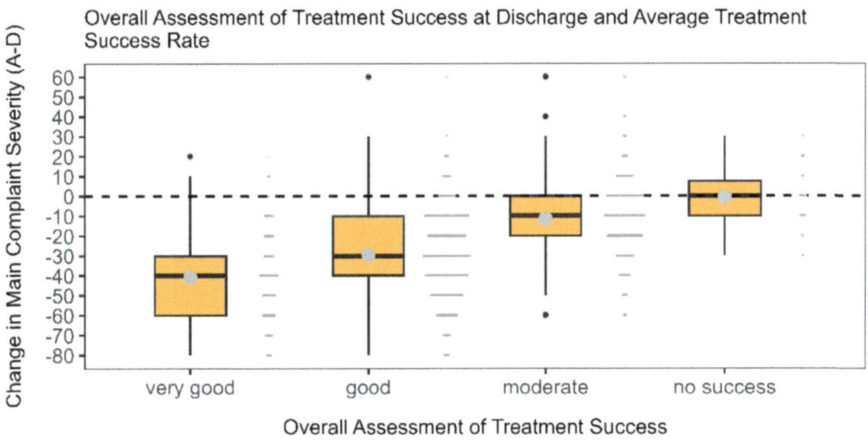

Fig. 5.13 Association between the overall assessment of treatment success at discharge and the average treatment success, as measured by the change in VAS for the main complaint at hospital discharge in 2023. The dashed line indicates no change in the severity of the main complaint. Grey dots indicate the mean, black lines the median, and stars indicate outliers

reduction in the severity of their main complaint. Conversely, patients who report no perceived treatment success at discharge show, on average, no change in symptom severity between admission and discharge.

5.1.9 Loss-of-Follow-Up Analyses as Part of the PEP Survey

As mentioned at the beginning of Sect. 5.1, follow-up data is available for approximately 75% of all patients. This means that approximately 25% of patients did not participate in the follow-up survey. The reasons for this were not determined. Since loss of follow-up can introduce bias and limit the interpretability of treatment outcomes, a separate analysis was conducted to compare patients with and without complete follow-up data. For this comparison, only patients with full documentation at both hospital admission and discharge ($n = 777$) were included. The aim was to examine adherence as a potential influencing factor and to counteract possible outcome distortions due to missing values by applying imputation methods (see Excursus). The key variables used in these analyses were the global assessment of treatment success and the severity of the main complaint. First, the two patient groups were examined for differences in gender and age distribution. As no significant differences were found in these characteristics, it can be assumed that the two subgroups are relatively homogeneous and therefore suitable for further comparison. Table 5.21 summarises the statistical results.

On admission, there was no significant difference in the severity or duration of the main complaint between patients with complete data sets ($n = 618$) and those without follow-up values ($n = 159$). However, the difference in severity was marginally non-significant ($p = 0.059$ and $p = 0.725$, respectively). At discharge, a

Table 5.21 A comparison of the patient groups with and without follow-up data in 2023 was conducted using the chi-square test for gender distribution and overall success (categorical), as well as the *t*-test for all other numerical comparisons

	No follow-up data			**With follow-up data**		**Comparison**		
	n	%	*n*		%	*p*	Cramer's *V*[a]	
Males	42	26.4%	123		19.9%	0.344	–	
Females	117	73.6%	495		80.1%			
Overall success on discharge						<0.001	0.18	
Very good success	15	9.4	103		16.7			
Good success	64	40.3	322		52.1			
Moderate success	69	43.4	178		28.8			
No success	11	6.9	15		2.4			
	n	**M**	**SD**	*n*	**M**	**SD**	**P**	*d*[b]
Age	159	54.24	13.83	618	56.46	10.98	0.061	–
Duration of the main complaint (days)	159	3878.3	4242.5	618	3747.5	3908.7	0.725	–
Main complaint severity on admission (0 to 100)	159	73.71	17.67	618	70.68	19.03	0.059	–
Main complaint severity at discharge (0 to 100)	159	52.83	22.05	618	45.36	21.86	<0.001	0.34
Complaint severity difference A/D	159	−20.88	21.71	618	−25.32	23.65	0.025	0.19

[a]Effect measure r and Cramer's *V* (< 0.3 = small, 0.3–0.5 = medium, ≥ 0.5 = strong effect)
[b]Effect measure Cohen's *d* (*d* ≥ 0.2 = small, ≥ 0.5 = medium, ≥ 0.8 = strong effect)

significant difference in the severity of the main complaint was observed between the groups, with a small effect size ($d = 0.34$, $p < 0.001$). Furthermore, assessment of treatment success at discharge also differed significantly between the groups, showing a small effect size ($V = 0.18$, $p < 0.001$). Overall, the results suggest that subsequent adherence to follow-up may be related to the benefit of treatment (in terms of both outcome scores and symptom severity at discharge).

To illustrate the differences in the results presented in Table 5.21 regarding the assessment of treatment success, Fig. 5.14. provides a graphical representation. The graph shows that patients with complete follow-up data rated their treatment as more successful at discharge than those without. While 31.2% of patients with complete follow-up data reported moderate or no success, this proportion was 50.3% among patients without follow-up data. Of the patients for whom follow-up data are available, half (52.8%) rate their treatment success at discharge as good. For patients without follow-up data, this figure is slightly lower at 40.3%. The difference between the two subgroups is particularly evident in the proportion of patients reporting very good treatment success, which falls from 16.7% to 9.4%. Conversely, the proportion of patients reporting no success increases almost threefold (2.4% vs. 6.9%).

5.1.9.1 Excursus: Analysis of Missing Values (Single Imputation)

To counteract any potential distortion of the outcomes caused by missing values, two imputation procedures were used to replace the missing values from the follow-up survey, thereby reducing the impact of non-response bias.

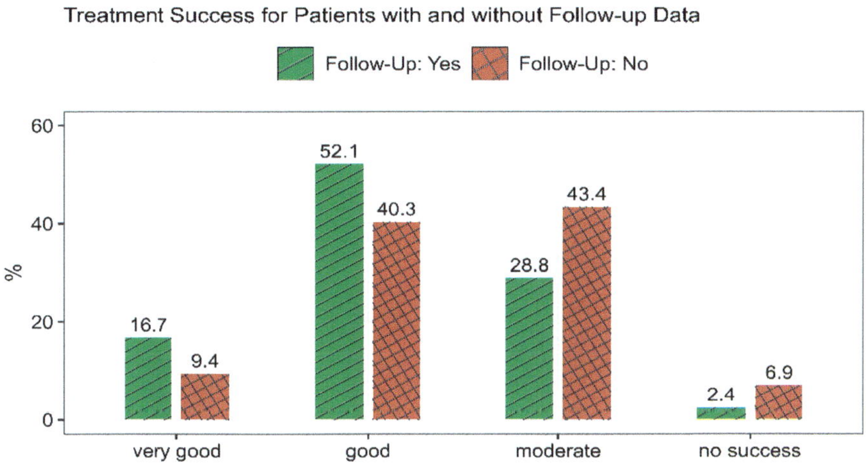

Fig. 5.14 Patients' overall assessment of treatment success at hospital discharge: comparison between patients with (n = 618) and without (n = 159) QA follow-up survey data on symptom severity

These were the Last Observation Carried Forward (LOCF) and Baseline Observation Carried Forward (BOCF) methods. In the LOCF method, each missing value for a patient is replaced by the last available value for that patient. In this case, missing follow-up survey values were replaced by the corresponding discharge survey values based on the assumption that the last observed value would remain unchanged over time. The BOCF method is a more conservative approach, replacing missing follow-up values with baseline values. This method assumes that patients still have the same symptoms at follow-up as they did before admission to hospital. Consequently, it does not consider any changes or improvements that may have occurred during their stay.

For the sensitivity analysis of overall treatment success, only the LOCF method was employed, since this outcome can only be evaluated at discharge. For severity of the main complaint, both the LOCF and BOCF methods were employed.

At discharge, treatment success was assessed in 777 patients. At follow-up, data was available for only 623 patients. For the remaining 154 cases with missing follow-up data, the LOCF method was used to impute values, assuming that the last observed condition remained unchanged.

Figure 5.15 shows the distribution of patient ratings of treatment success across all groups. Comparing discharge and follow-up ratings shows that the proportion of patients rating treatment success as 'good' or 'moderate' decreases, while the proportion rating it as 'very good' increases. Notably, a higher proportion of patients reported 'very good' treatment success at follow-up than at discharge, suggesting an overall positive shift in perceptions over time. Furthermore, comparing the available follow-up data with the imputed data using the LOCF method yields similar results, suggesting that bias due to patients lost to follow-up is minimal. The most noticeable differences appear in the 'very good' and 'moderate' ratings. While 27% of

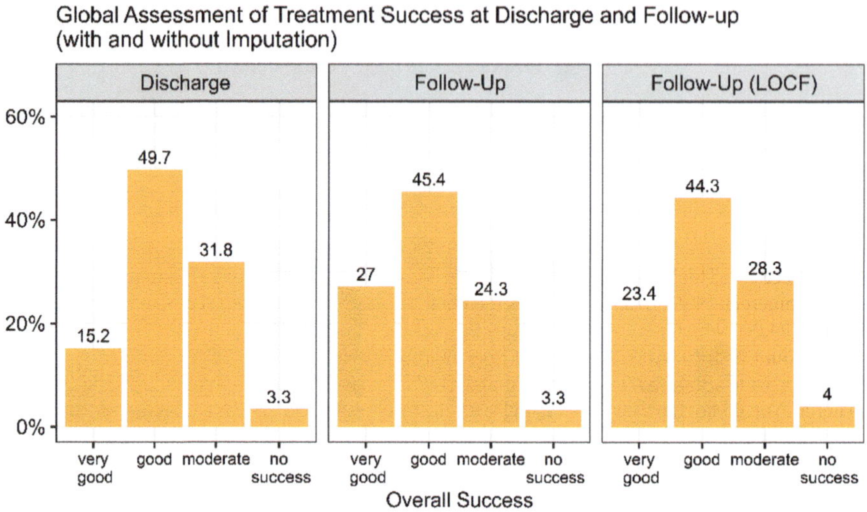

Fig. 5.15 Global assessment of treatment success at hospital discharge (left; $n = 777$), at follow-up (centre; $n = 614$), and at follow-up modified by the LOCF imputation where follow-up values were missing (right; $n = 777$) for 2023

patients rated treatment success as 'very good' and 24% as 'moderate' in the follow-up survey, the imputed data shows 23% and 28%, respectively.

In addition, the severity of the main complaints was compared between patients with and without follow-up data. The results also show that patients for whom follow-up data are available tend to report milder symptoms upon discharge from hospital (Fig. 5.16). While 64.1% of patients with complete data reported a main complaint severity score of 0–50 (low to moderate) upon discharge, this figure was just 50.3% for patients with no follow-up data.

In summary, the distribution of main complaint severity for the full dataset (without imputation; $n = 618$) is presented alongside the dataset with imputed follow-up data ($n = 777$). The corresponding descriptive statistics are presented in Table 5.22.

Comparing the severity of the main complaint at discharge with that at follow-up shows a slight increase in symptoms over time. After applying the LOCF imputation method, this increase becomes slightly more pronounced. Nevertheless, in both cases, symptom severity is clearly improved compared to the initial values at admission.

To allow for a more cautious interpretation of changes in symptoms, the BOCF method was applied as an alternative, more conservative approach to imputation. Compared to LOCF, this results in a more negative distribution of symptoms, emphasising its conservative nature by assuming no change at all.

To better interpret the results, a statistical test of the mean differences between admission and follow-up was conducted. A *t*-test with a 95% confidence interval was used to compare admission values with imputed follow-up values, and Cohen's d was calculated to assess the effect size. The results are summarised in Table 5.23.

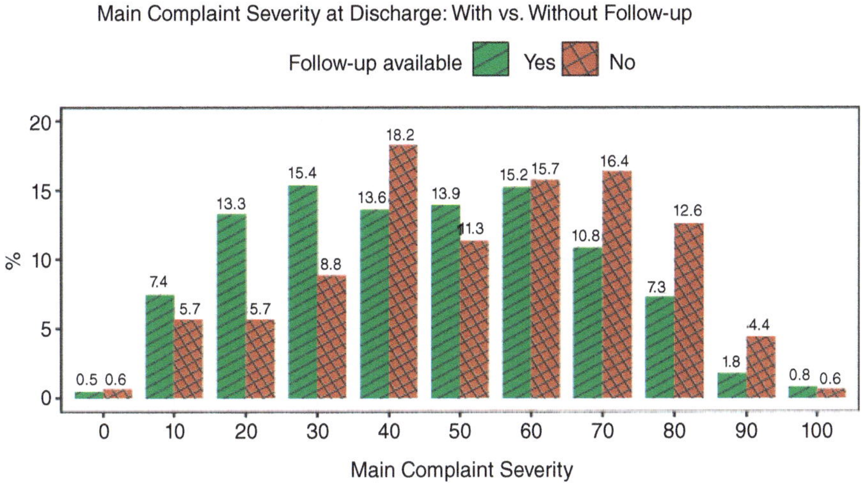

Fig. 5.16 Main complaint severity (0–100) at discharge in 2023; differentiated according to available QA follow-up survey data (with follow-up: $n = 618$/without follow-up: $n = 159$)

Table 5.22 Cross-sectional comparison of symptom severity (scaled from 0 to 100) with and without imputed follow-up data (2023)

Main complaint severity	*n*	M	SD	Median
Admission	777	71.30	18.79	70
Discharge	777	46.89	22.09	50
Follow-up LOCF	777	48.55	23.92	50
Follow-up BOCF	777	52.82	25.38	50
Admission (complete data)	618	70.68	19.03	70
Discharge (complete data)	618	45.36	21.86	40
Follow-up (complete data)	618	47.44	24.27	50

Table 5.23 A comparison of main complaint severity between hospital admission and the 2023 follow-up was conducted using the *t*-test for paired samples on complete and imputed data sets. According to Cohen's *d*, an effect size of ≥0.2 is considered small, ≥0.5 moderate, and ≥ 0.8 large

	Course: discharge/follow-up			Difference to admission		
Main complaint severity	*n*	M	SD	ΔM	*p*	*d*
	618	70.68	19.03	−23.24	< 0.001	1.06
Follow-up	618	47.44	24.27			
Admission	777	71.30	18.79	−22.75	< 0.001	1.05
Follow-up (LOCF)	777	48.55	23.92			
Admission	777	71.30	18.79	−18.48	< 0.001	0.82
Follow-up (BOCF)	777	52.82	25.38			

Both the LOCF method and the imputation based on baseline symptom severity show a highly significant reduction in main complaint severity at follow-up with a large effect size ($d = 1.05$, $p <. 001$; $d = 0.82$, $p <. 001$; respectively).

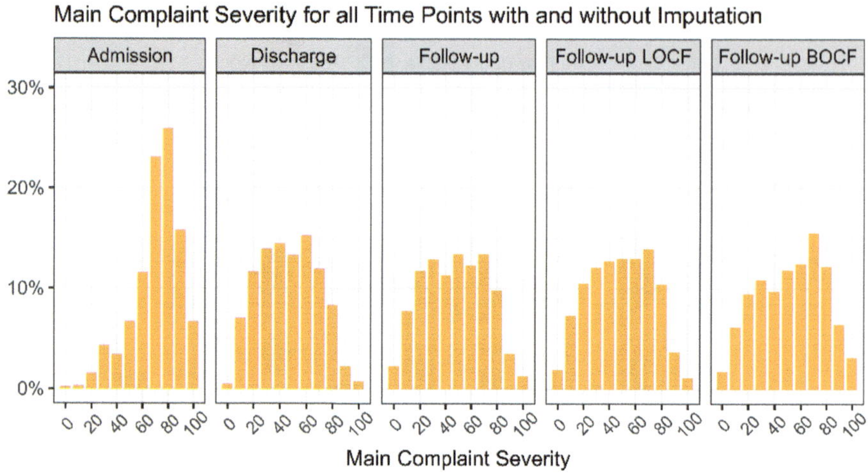

Fig. 5.17 Main complaint severity (0–100) on admission ($n = 777$), at discharge ($n = 777$), and at follow-up without imputation ($n = 618$), follow-up with LOCF method ($n = 777$), and follow-up with BOCF method ($n = 777$) in 2023

Since the baseline imputation method is more conservative than LOCF, the observed effect is slightly smaller, as expected. Nevertheless, the significant differences found with both methods confirm the positive impact of multimodal treatment at the TCM-Klinik Bad Kötzting on patients' main complaints. The actual change in symptom severity likely lies between the results of these two imputation approaches.

Figure 5.17 illustrates the distribution of each severity level for the complete dataset at admission and discharge ($n = 777$) and for all follow-up data, including both observed and imputed values (using LOCF and BOCF; $n = 777$). The substantial reduction in symptom severity from admission to follow-up is clearly visible regardless of the imputation method used and reflects the large effect size.

5.1.10 Pain-Disability Index (Self-Perceived Everyday Disability Due to the Complaints)

This questionnaire, which was developed specifically for patients with chronic pain, consists of seven items that cover the following areas of life: family and domestic responsibilities, recreation, social activities, occupation, sexual behaviour, self-care, and life-support activities [3, 4]. Each area is rated on an 11-point scale ranging from 0 (no disability) to 10 (complete disability), indicating the extent to which pain interferes with that particular aspect of life.

A total score is calculated by summing the responses to all seven items, resulting in a score ranging from 0 (no impairment) to 70 (maximum impairment). Although there are no standardised normative values for the PDI, extensive comparative data from various studies provide interpretive guidance [5]. A total score of ≥33 points is often considered to indicate conspicuous and significant impairment. However, the clinically relevant change in PDI scores depends on the patient's baseline level of disability.

Table 5.24 gives an overview of the target values for comparing the PDI total score at admission and discharge [5].

On admission in 2023, an average pain index of 28.95 points (SD = 15.67) was reported, which decreased to 25.01 points (SD = 15.10) at discharge (Table 5.25). Examining the individual items, the greatest impairment on admission was in the leisure category (5.36 points; 4.57 at discharge), followed by work (5.29 points;

Table 5.24 The minimal important change value (MIC) of the PDI is dependent on baseline values

PDI on admission	Target value of the reduced pain-related impairments at discharge
≤ 27	Min. 7 points
28–42	Min. 15 points
≥ 43	Min. 20 points

Table 5.25 Pain disability index in the before/after comparison 2023; t-test with paired samples; significance at $p < .05$; Cohen's d = effect size ($d \geq 0.2$= small, ≥0.5 = moderate, ≥0.8 = large effect)

		2023							
		Cross section A/D/F			Course A-D/A-F *n* = 589		Difference from admission A-D/A-F *n* = 589		
Pain disability index		*n*	M	SD	M	SD	ΔM	*p*	*d*
PDI total value	A	816	28.95	15.67	29.18	15.62	–4.62	<001	–.30
	D	776	25.01	15.10	24.56	15.03			
	F	600	23.84	16.38	23.91	16.38	–5.27	<.001	–.33
Family and domestic obligations	A	816	4.81	2.84	4.89	2.81	–0.80	<.001	–.29
	D	776	4.18	2.81	4.09	2.76			
	F	601	4.11	2.91	4.13	2.91	–0.76	<.001	–.27
Recreation	A	816	5.35	2.80	5.41	2.74	–0.96	<.001	–.34
	D	776	4.57	2.83	4.45	2.82			
	F	601	4.40	2.96	4.41	2.96	–1.00	<.001	–.35
Social activity	A	816	4.62	3.03	4.65	3.03	–0.65	<.001	–.22
	D	776	4.10	2.90	4.00	2.89			
	F	601	3.86	3.04	3.89	3.04	–0.76	<.001	–.25
Profession	A	816	5.28	3.27	5.29	3.24	–0.48	<.001	–.15
	D	776	4.90	3.19	4.81	3.18			
	F	600	4.11	3.31	4.11	3.31	–1.18	<.001	–.36
Sex life	A	816	4.56	3.69	4.57	3.68	–0.66	<.001	–.19
	D	776	3.88	3.42	3.91	3.42			
	F	600	3.98	3.61	3.99	3.61	–0.58	<.001	–.16
Self-sufficiency	A	816	2.27	2.60	2.28	2.57	–0.42	<.001	–.17
	D	776	1.93	2.46	1.86	2.43			
	F	600	1.88	2.54	1.88	2.54	-0.41	<.001	–.16
Essential activities	A	816	2.07	2.57	2.09	2.56	–0.65	<.001	–.27
	D	776	1.45	2.17	1.44	2.17			
	F	600	1.50	2.24	1.50	2.25	–0.59	<.001	–.25

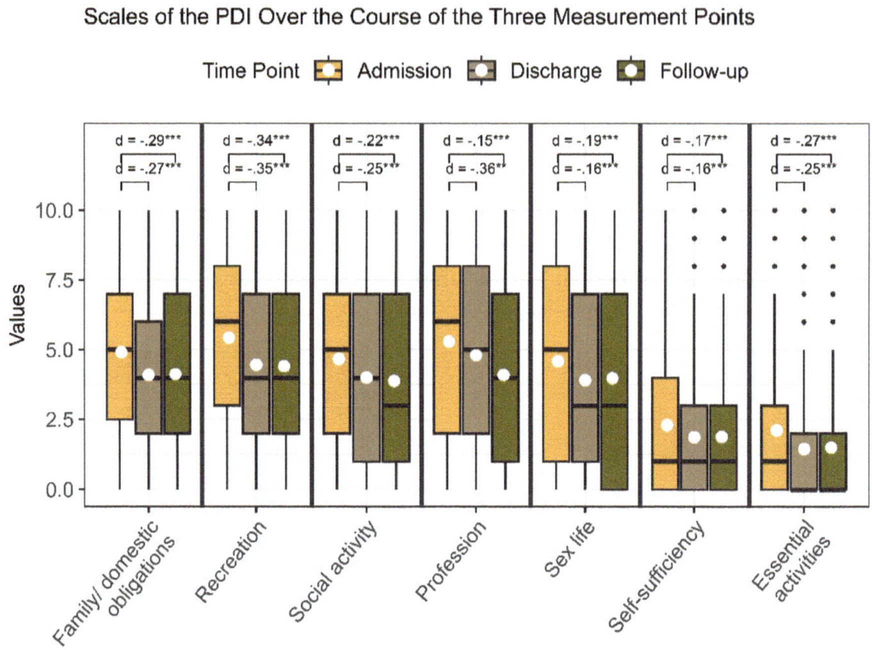

Fig. 5.18 Scales of the Pain Disability Index (PDI) over the course of the measurement points in 2023; *t*-test with paired samples; significance at $*p < 0.05$, $**p < 0.01$, $***p < 0.001$; significance at $p < 0.05$; Cohen's d = effect measure ($d \geq 0.2$ = small, ≥ 0.5 = moderate, ≥ 0.8 = large effect)

4.90 at discharge) and family and domestic responsibilities (4.81 points; 4.18 at discharge). Activities of daily living (2.07 points; 1.45 at discharge) and self-care (2.27 points; 1.93 at discharge) appear less frequently affected by pain. Figure 5.18 shows the distribution for all subcategories.

Statistical comparisons revealed significant improvements in all subcategories and in the total score from admission to discharge, as well as from admission to follow-up. However, the observed effect sizes ranged from minimal to small (Table 5.25). As Fig. 5.19 illustrates, the majority of patients did not exhibit a significant impairment in the total score at baseline. This explains why the average improvements appear only marginal.

5.1.11 Comparison of ICD-10 Symptom Rating (ISR) at Different Measurement Points

For the baseline measurement, all data sets documented within a few months before and up to 7 days after admission were included. For the second measurement, all questionnaires completed within 14 days before and 8 days after the discharge date were used. The follow-up survey includes data collected between 6 months and 1 year after discharge. A total of 824 ISR measurements were available at the start of

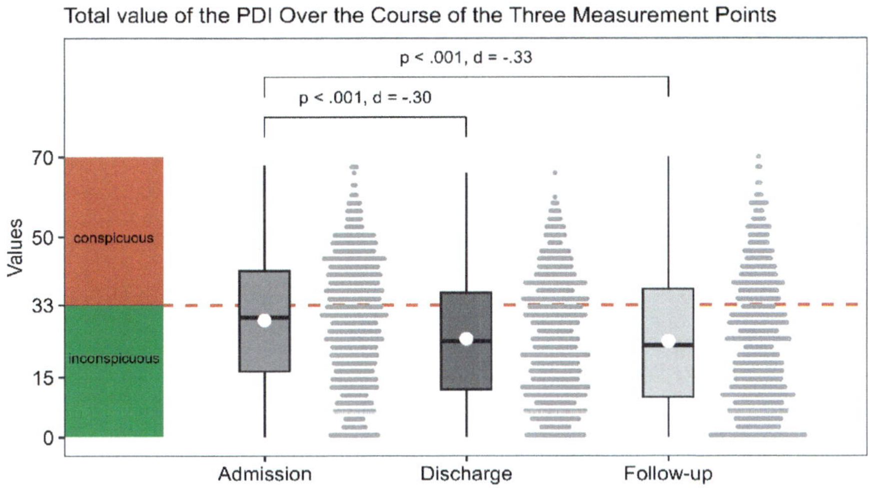

Fig. 5.19 Total value of the Pain Disability Index (PDI) over the course of the three measurement points in 2023 ($n = 587$); *t*-test with paired samples; significance at $p < 0.05$; Cohen's d = effect measure ($d \geq 0.2$ = small, ≥ 0.5 = moderate, ≥ 0.8 = large effect)

the hospital stay, 778 at discharge, and 608 at the 2023 follow-up. Data for all three survey dates are available for 603 patients. For the previous year's data, 11,032 measurements were available at hospital admission and 9250 at hospital discharge. A further 6180 patients from previous years also took part in the ISR follow-up survey approximately 6 months after hospital discharge. Complete data for all three survey dates are available for 5681 patients.

Tables 5.26, 5.27, 5.28, 5.29, 5.30, and 5.31 present data for all patients broken down by age category and gender, across all ISR subscales. Each table includes statistical dispersion measures (n, M, SD) for admission values, providing a descrip tive overview of the patient population upon arrival at the clinic.

When the values are distributed according to age and gender, both the 2023 data and the earlier annual reference data show significantly higher levels of depression and anxiety among younger patients of both genders. A comparison of the genders reveals that women experience a greater mental burden than men in these sub-scores. The same applies to the ICD-10 sub-score for somatoform disorder syndrome (DS), but not to the ISR sub-score for eating disorder syndrome, when considering men. This does not apply to the overall scores, where the values are the same for both women and men. Compared to the reference data from previous years, the ISR overall score values in 2023 are slightly higher (1.14 vs. 1.01, with an SD of 0.59 for both).

Table 5.32 provides an overview of the statistical results for comparing all measurement points. The first column shows the number, mean values, and standard deviations for the individual scales, as well as the total value, for the three survey points: admission, discharge, and the follow-up after approximately 6 months, using a cross-sectional approach. The middle column shows the same presentation for the

Table 5.26 ISR Depression Syndrome Disorder (SD) subscale for all patients on admission (2023: $n = 824$; previous years: $n = 11{,}032$); broken down by age and gender

Admission: ISR depression SD									
		2023				Previous years			
	Age group	*n*	%	M	SD	*n*	%	M	SD
Men	Up to 30	9	5.3	2.56	0.63	125	4.4	1.87	0.90
	31 to 40	13	7.6	2.38	0.94	191	6.8	2.07	0.96
	41 to 50	22	12.9	2.06	1.06	554	19.7	1.96	0.93
	51 to 60	64	37.6	2.22	0.94	942	33.5	1.89	0.96
	61 to 70	47	27.6	1.66	0.91	611	21.7	1.51	0.89
	Over 70	15	8.8	1.77	0.81	393	14.0	1.24	0.92
	Total	**170**	**100**	**2.04**	**0.95**	**2816**	**100**	**1.74**	**0.97**
Women	Up to 30	14	2.3	2.23	0.70	339	4.1	1.95	0.91
	31 to 40	50	7.6	2.10	0.72	584	7.1	2.09	0.96
	41 to 50	96	14.7	2.24	0.86	1822	22.2	2.09	0.91
	51 to 60	282	43.1	2.10	0.91	3108	37.8	2.02	0.90
	61 to 70	153	23.4	1.97	0.99	1541	18.8	1.74	0.92
	Over 70	59	9.0	1.89	0.95	822	10.0	1.50	0.90
	Total	**654**	**100**	**2.07**	**0.91**	**8216**	**100**	**1.93**	**0.93**
Total	Up to 30	23	2.9	2.36	0.68	464	4.2	1.93	0.91
	31 to 40	63	7.6	2.15	0.77	775	7.0	2.08	0.96
	41 to 50	118	14.3	2.20	0.90	2376	21.5	2.06	0.92
	51 to 60	346	41.9	2.12	0.91	4050	36.7	1.99	0.92
	61 to 70	200	24.2	1.90	0.97	2152	19.5	1.68	0.92
	Over 70	74	9.0	1.86	0.92	1215	11.0	1.42	0.91
	Total	**824**	**100**	**2.07**	**0.92**	**11,032**	**100**	**1.88**	**0.94**

Table 5.27 ISR Anxiety Disorder Syndrome (DS) subscale for all patients on admission (2023: $n = 824$; previous years: $n = 11{,}032$); broken down by age and gender

Admission: ISR anxiety DS									
		2023				Previous years			
	Age group	*n*	%	M	SD	*n*	%	M	SD
Men	Up to 30	9	5.3	1.89	0.63	125	4.4	1.11	1.07
	31 to 40	13	7.6	1.87	1.18	191	6.8	1.30	1.15
	41 to 50	22	12.9	1.25	1.14	554	19.7	1.19	1.05
	51 to 60	64	37.6	1.57	1.09	942	33.5	1.20	1.03
	61 to 70	47	27.6	0.98	1.00	611	21.7	0.85	0.96
	Over 70	15	8.8	0.98	1.02	393	14.0	0.73	0.88
	Total	**170**	**100**	**1.36**	**1.09**	**2816**	**100.0**	**1.06**	**1.03**
Women	Up to 30	14	2.3	1.57	1.12	339	4.1	1.25	1.08
	31 to 40	50	7.6	1.36	1.13	584	7.1	1.30	1.12
	41 to 50	96	14.7	1.60	1.12	1822	22.2	1.35	1.08
	51 to 60	282	43.1	1.44	1.05	3108	37.8	1.38	1.05
	61 to 70	153	23.4	1.40	1.05	1541	18.8	1.21	1.00
	Over 70	59	9.0	1.35	1.13	822	10.0	0.99	0.92
	Total	**654**	**100**	**1.44**	**1.07**	**8216**	**100.0**	**1.29**	**1.05**
Total	Up to 30	23	2.9	1.70	0.95	464	4.2	1.21	1.08
	31 to 40	63	7.6	1.47	1.15	775	7.0	1.30	1.12
	41 to 50	118	14.3	1.54	1.13	2376	21.5	1.32	1.07
	51 to 60	346	41.9	1.46	1.05	4050	36.7	1.34	1.05
	61 to 70	200	24.2	1.30	1.05	2152	19.5	1.11	1.00
	Over 70	74	9.0	1.28	1.11	1215	11.0	0.91	0.92
	Total	**824**	**100**	**1.43**	**1.08**	**11,032**	**100.0**	**1.23**	**1.05**

Table 5.28 ISR Compulsive-obsessive Disorder Syndrome (DS) subscale for all patients on admission (2023: $n = 824$; previous years: $n = 11{,}032$); broken down by age and gender

Admission: ISR compulsive-obsessive DS									
		2023				Previous years			
	Age group	*n*	%	M	SD	*n*	%	M	SD
Men	Up to 30	9	5.3	1.63	1.26	125	4.4	0.88	1.01
	31 to 40	13	7.6	1.08	1.02	191	6.8	1.12	1.14
	41 to 50	22	12.9	0.73	1.02	554	19.7	0.78	0.93
	51 to 60	64	37.6	1.28	1.05	942	33.5	0.84	0.95
	61 to 70	47	27.6	0.59	0.82	611	21.7	0.60	0.83
	Over 70	15	8.8	0.96	1.04	393	14.0	0.50	0.77
	Total	**170**	**100**	**0.99**	**1.03**	**2816**	**100**	**0.75**	**0.93**
Women	Up to 30	14	2.3	0.79	0.82	339	4.1	0.97	1.10
	31 to 40	50	7.6	1.11	1.11	584	7.1	0.91	1.05
	41 to 50	96	14.7	1.02	0.93	1822	22.2	0.92	1.00
	51 to 60	282	43.1	0.97	1.03	3108	37.8	0.92	0.96
	61 to 70	153	23.4	0.95	0.95	1541	18.8	0.81	0.93
	Over 70	59	9.0	0.82	0.92	822	10.0	0.59	0.80
	Total	**654**	**100**	**0.96**	**0.99**	**8216**	**100**	**0.86**	**0.97**
Total	Up to 30	23	2.9	1.12	1.08	464	4.2	0.94	1.08
	31 to 40	63	7.6	1.10	1.08	775	7.0	0.96	1.08
	41 to 50	118	14.3	0.96	0.95	2376	21.5	0.88	0.99
	51 to 60	346	41.9	1.03	1.04	4050	36.7	0.90	0.96
	61 to 70	200	24.2	0.86	0.93	2152	19.5	0.75	0.91
	Over 70	74	9.0	0.85	0.94	1215	11.0	0.56	0.79
	Total	**824**	**100**	**0.97**	**1.00**	**11,032**	**100**	**0.84**	**0.96**

Table 5.29 ISR Somatoform Disorder Syndrome (DS) subscale for all patients on admission (2023: $n = 824$; previous years: $n = 11{,}032$); broken down by age and gender

Admission: ISR somatoform DS									
		2023				Previous years			
	Age group	*n*	%	M	SD	*n*	%	M	SD
Men	Up to 30	9	5.3	1.96	0.56	125	4.4	0.96	1.01
	31 to 40	13	7.6	1.54	1.29	191	6.8	1.05	1.01
	41 to 50	22	12.9	0.83	1.09	554	19.7	0.80	0.86
	51 to 60	64	37.6	1.01	0.89	942	33.5	0.84	0.87
	61 to 70	47	27.6	0.84	0.95	611	21.7	0.73	0.84
	Over 70	15	8.8	1.18	1.15	393	14.0	0.64	0.81
	Total	**170**	**100**	**1.05**	**1.01**	**2816**	**100**	**0.80**	**0.88**
Women	Up to 30	14	2.3	1.05	0.75	339	4.1	0.83	0.93
	31 to 40	50	7.6	1.18	1.07	584	7.1	0.76	0.90
	41 to 50	96	14.7	0.93	0.95	1822	22.2	0.77	0.89
	51 to 60	282	43.1	0.76	0.81	3108	37.8	0.77	0.84
	61 to 70	153	23.4	0.79	0.86	1541	18.8	0.74	0.88
	Over 70	59	9.0	0.77	0.78	822	10.0	0.60	0.77
	Total	**654**	**100**	**0.83**	**0.87**	**8216**	**100**	**0.75**	**0.86**
Total	Up to 30	23	2.9	1.41	0.81	464	4.2	0.86	0.96
	31 to 40	63	7.6	1.25	1.12	775	7.0	0.84	0.94
	41 to 50	118	14.3	0.91	0.97	2376	21.5	0.78	0.88
	51 to 60	346	41.9	0.81	0.83	4050	36.7	0.78	0.85
	61 to 70	200	24.2	0.80	0.88	2152	19.5	0.74	0.87
	Over 70	74	9.0	0.86	0.88	1215	11.0	0.62	0.79
	Total	**824**	**100**	**0.88**	**0.90**	**11,032**	**100**	**0.76**	**0.87**

Table 5.30 ISR Eating Disorder Syndrome (DS) subscale for all patients on admission (2023: n = 824; previous years: n = 11,032); broken down by age and gender

Admission: ISR eating DS									
		2023				Previous years			
	Age group	*n*	%	M	SD	*n*	%	M	SD
Men	Up to 30	9	5.3	0.33	0.88	125	4.4	0.29	0.57
	31 to 40	13	7.6	0.44	0.70	191	6.8	0.48	0.75
	41 to 50	22	12.9	0.39	0.58	554	19.7	0.44	0.63
	51 to 60	64	37.6	0.58	0.79	942	33.5	0.50	0.69
	61 to 70	47	27.6	0.36	0.59	611	21.7	0.47	0.66
	Over 70	15	8.8	0.64	0.66	393	14.0	0.46	0.64
	Total	**170**	**100**	**0.48**	**0.70**	**2816**	**100**	**0.47**	**0.67**
Women	Up to 30	14	2.3	0.60	1.00	339	4.1	0.56	0.92
	31 to 40	50	7.6	0.49	0.77	584	7.1	0.64	0.93
	41 to 50	96	14.7	0.69	0.99	1822	22.2	0.64	0.88
	51 to 60	282	43.1	0.66	0.85	3108	37.8	0.66	0.84
	61 to 70	153	23.4	0.59	0.83	1541	18.8	0.58	0.82
	Over 70	59	9.0	0.53	0.80	822	10.0	0.38	0.66
	Total	**654**	**100**	**0.62**	**0.86**	**8216**	**100**	**0.61**	**0.84**
Total	Up to 30	23	2.9	0.49	0.94	464	4.2	0.49	0.84
	31 to 40	63	7.6	0.48	0.75	775	7.0	0.60	0.89
	41 to 50	118	14.3	0.63	0.93	2376	21.5	0.60	0.83
	51 to 60	346	41.9	0.65	0.83	4050	36.7	0.62	0.81
	61 to 70	200	24.2	0.54	0.78	2152	19.5	0.55	0.78
	Over 70	74	9.0	0.55	0.77	1215	11.0	0.41	0.65
	Total	**824**	**100**	**0.59**	**0.83**	**11,032**	**100**	**0.57**	**0.80**

Table 5.31 ISR total score for all patients on admission (2023: n = 824; previous years: n = 11,032); broken down by age and gender

Admission: ISR total score									
		2023				Previous years			
	Age group	*n*	%	M	SD	*n*	%	M	SD
Men	Up to 30	9	5.3	1.60	0.54	125	4.4	0.97	0.59
	31 to 40	13	7.6	1.41	0.76	191	6.8	1.14	0.64
	41 to 50	22	12.9	1.01	0.65	554	19.7	1.01	0.58
	51 to 60	64	37.6	1.28	0.61	942	33.5	1.03	0.62
	61 to 70	47	27.6	0.89	0.63	611	21.7	0.82	0.58
	Over 70	15	8.8	1.01	0.57	393	14.0	0.70	0.51
	Total	**170**	**100**	**1.14**	**0.65**	**2816**	**100**	**0.94**	**0.60**
Women	Up to 30	14	2.3	1.20	0.47	339	4.1	1.05	0.61
	31 to 40	50	7.6	1.23	0.61	584	7.1	1.09	0.60
	41 to 50	96	14.7	1.25	0.57	1822	22.2	1.11	0.60
	51 to 60	282	43.1	1.15	0.56	3108	37.8	1.10	0.58
	61 to 70	153	23.4	1.09	0.60	1541	18.8	0.96	0.57
	Over 70	59	9.0	1.02	0.57	822	10.0	0.76	0.49
	Total	**654**	**100**	**1.14**	**0.58**	**8216**	**100**	**1.04**	**0.59**
Total	Up to 30	23	2.9	1.36	0.53	464	4.2	1.03	0.60
	31 to 40	63	7.6	1.27	0.65	775	7.0	1.10	0.61
	41 to 50	118	14.3	1.21	0.59	2376	21.5	1.09	0.60
	51 to 60	346	41.9	1.17	0.57	4050	36.7	1.09	0.59
	61 to 70	200	24.2	1.04	0.61	2152	19.5	0.92	0.58
	Over 70	74	9.0	1.02	0.57	1215	11.0	0.74	0.50
	Total	**824**	**100**	**1.14**	**0.59**	**11,032**	**100**	**1.01**	**0.59**

Table 5.32 ISR scale values in the before/after comparison in 2023 and previous years; t-test for dependent samples; significance at $p < 0.05$; Cohen's d = effect measure ($d \geq 0.2$ = small, ≥ 0.5 = moderate, ≥ 0.8 = large effect)

		2023								Previous years			
		Cross-section: A/D/F			Course: A–D/A–F n = 603		Diff. From admission A–D/A–F n = 603			Course: A–D/A–F n = 5681		Diff. From admission A–D/A–F n = 5681	
		n	M	SD	M	SD	ΔM	p	d	M	p	ΔM	d
Depressive syndrome	**A**	824	2.07	0.92	2.07	0.91				1.88			
	D	778	1.22	0.89	1.19	0.88	−0.88	<0.001	**−0.98**	0.83	<0.001	−1.04	**−1.25**
	F	608	1.32	0.91	1.32	0.91	−0.75	<0.001	**−0.82**	1.20	<0.001	−0.68	−0.76
Anxiety syndrome	**A**	824	1.43	1.08	1.41	1.07				1.22			
	D	778	1.01	0.95	0.99	0.96	−0.41	<0.001	−0.40	0.75	<0.001	−0.47	−0.50
	F	608	0.93	0.91	0.93	0.91	−0.47	<0.001	−0.47	0.82	<0.001	−0.40	−0.42
Obsessive-compulsion syndrome	**A**	824	0.97	1.00	0.97	1.00				0.82			
	D	778	0.77	0.89	0.75	0.88	−0.23	<0.001	−0.24	0.61	<0.001	−0.21	−0.24
	F	608	0.66	0.82	0.67	0.82	−0.31	<0.001	−0.33	0.60	<0.001	−0.22	−0.26
Somatoform syndrome	**A**	824	0.88	0.90	0.84	0.88				0.73			
	D	778	0.63	0.78	0.59	0.76	−0.25	<0.001	−0.30	0.48	<0.001	−0.25	−0.32
	F	608	0.52	0.74	0.53	0.74	−0.32	<0.001	−0.38	0.49	<0.001	−0.23	−0.30
Eating disorder syndrome	**A**	824	0.59	0.83	0.61	0.82				0.58			
	D	778	0.52	0.77	0.53	0.78	−0.08	<0.001	−0.10	0.48	<0.001	−0.11	−0.14
	F	608	0.51	0.77	0.51	0.77	−0.10	<0.001	−0.13	0.51	<0.001	−0.08	−0.10
Total value	**A**	824	1.14	0.59	1.14	0.59				1.00			
	D	778	0.82	0.55	0.81	0.56	−0.33	<0.001	−0.58	0.64	<0.001	−0.37	−0.69
	F	608	0.78	0.55	0.78	0.55	−0.36	<0.001	−0.63	0.71	<0.001	−0.30	−0.54

valid data sets of the follow-up sample ($n = 604$). Additionally, the difference scores between the admission and discharge surveys, and between the admission and follow-up surveys, are shown in the right-hand column for the follow-up sample.

The highest scores on admission are observed for depressive syndrome, followed by anxiety syndrome. The mean scores for obsessive-compulsive syndrome, somatoform syndrome, and eating disorders are significantly lower. Possible improvements in these cases are therefore limited (floor effect).

A paired *t*-test was used to compare assessment times (admission–discharge and admission–follow-up). Significant improvements were observed for the total ISR score and all sub-scores at discharge and follow-up. The largest effect was seen in the depressive syndrome sub-score ($d = -0.98$ at discharge, $p < 0.001$; $d = -0.82$ at follow-up, $p < 0.001$). This is also reflected in the improvement of the total score ($d = -0.58$, $p < 0.001$ at discharge; $d = -0.63$, $p < 0.001$ at follow-up). Interestingly, anxiety, obsessions, somatisation, and eating disorders continued to improve during the follow-up period. Depression is the only factor that worsens slightly from discharge to follow-up. When comparing the 2023 data with that from previous years in Table 5.32, the statistically significant improvements at follow-up (difference between admission and follow-up) are usually less pronounced than those at discharge.

To illustrate the results, Figs. 5.20 and 5.21 present the frequency distributions for the ISR total score and its subscales at different measurement time points, based on data from 2023. The thresholds for each frequency distribution are indicated by a horizontal dashed line. The red lines show the thresholds for moderate and severe symptom burdens, indicating the need for action. The frequency distributions show a clear improvement in the overall ISR score over time. As shown in Fig. 5.20, there is a noticeable shift in values towards the less conspicuous range, indicating lower symptom severity. At both discharge and follow-up, a significantly higher proportion of patients fall below the threshold than at admission, reflecting a consistent trend towards low or inconspicuous symptom levels.

5.1.11.1 Excursus: Analysis of Missing Values

The following section compares symptom burden between patients with complete data sets and those without follow-up data, focusing on changes from admission to discharge. The analysis aims to explore whether the presence or absence of follow-up data is associated with differences in treatment outcomes. In this context, the results of 603 patients are compared with those of 175 patients (22.5%) without follow-up data from 2023. Comparing admission and discharge values between the two groups shows no significant difference in treatment success, except for depression, where a minor but statistically significant effect was observed (Table 5.33). These results suggest that adherence to follow-up may not systematically relate to improvement in symptoms. However, it is possible that patients whose depressive symptoms worsen during the follow-up period may be less inclined to participate in follow-up assessments.

Furthermore, as was done and described for the QA data (see Sect. 5.1.9), imputation methods were applied as a sensitivity analysis. The baseline observation

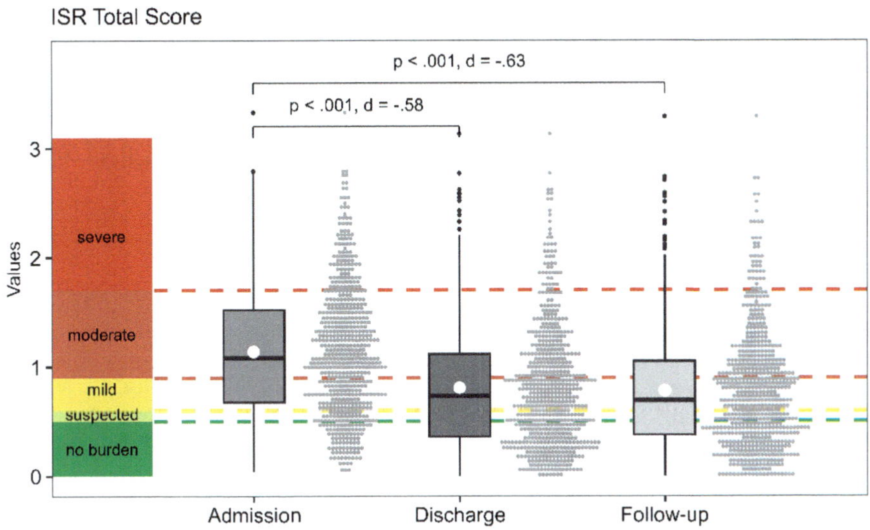

Fig. 5.20 The distribution of the ISR total score at admission (A), discharge (D), and follow-up (F) in 2023 is shown below ($n = 603$). The horizontal dashed lines mark the threshold values, the white circles indicate the mean, and the black lines indicate the median. Cohen's d is the effect measure ($d \geq 0.2$ = small effect, $d \geq 0.5$ = moderate effect, and $d \geq 0.8$ = large effect)

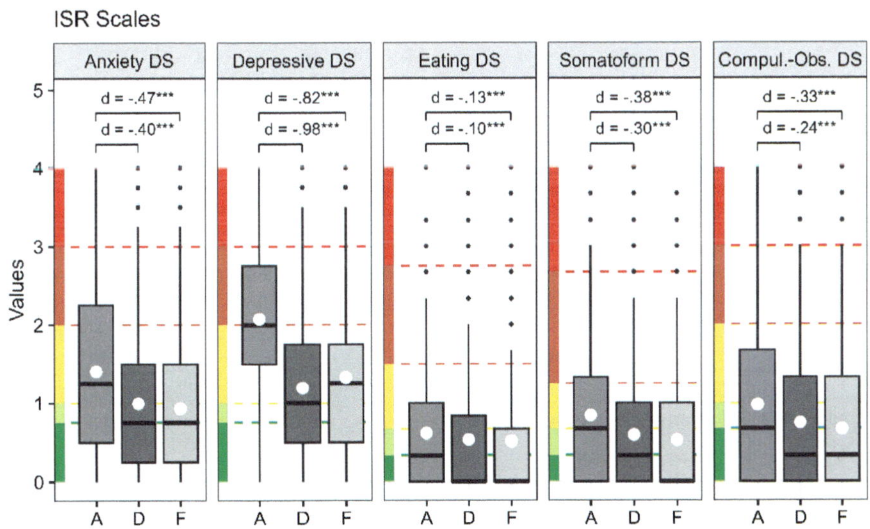

Fig. 5.21 Distribution of ISR scales at admission (A), discharge (D), and follow-up (F) in 2023 ($n = 603$); significance: $*p < 0.05$, $**p < 0.01$, $***p < 0.001$; Cohen's d = effect measure ($d \geq 0.2$ = small, ≥ 0.5 = moderate, ≥ 0.8 = large effect); DS = disorder syndrome

Table 5.33 ISR scale values in before/after comparison between patients with follow-up ($n = 603$) and without follow-up data ($n = 175$) in 2023; t-test for independent samples; significance: $p < 0.05$; Cohen's d = effect measure ($d \geq 0.2$ = small, ≥ 0.5 = moderate, ≥ 0.8 = large effect)

		Admission		Discharge		Comparison		
	Follow-up	M	SD	M	SD	ΔM	*p*	*d*
Depressive DS	Yes	2.07	0.91	1.19	0.88	−0.88	**0.042**	0.17
	No	2.06	0.91	1.33	0.91	−0.73		
Anxiety DS	Yes	1.41	1.07	0.99	0.96	−0.42	0.779	–
	No	1.48	1.08	1.05	0.90	−0.43		
Compulsive-Obs. DS	Yes	0.97	1.00	0.75	0.88	−0.22	0.260	–
	No	0.99	0.99	0.84	0.92	−0.15		
Somatoform DS	Yes	0.84	0.88	0.59	0.76	−0.25	0.605	–
	No	1.05	0.99	0.77	0.85	−0.28		
Eating DS	Yes	0.61	0.82	0.53	0.78	−0.08	0.655	–
	No	0.53	0.83	0.47	0.72	−0.06		
Total	Yes	1.14	0.59	0.81	0.56	−0.33	0.359	–
	No	1.18	0.58	0.88	0.53	−0.30		

DS disorder syndrome

Table 5.34 ISR scale values in a before/after comparison for complete datasets and datasets using the imputation methods BOCF and LOCF, t-test for independent samples; significance: $^{*}p < 0.05$, $^{**}p < 0.01$, $^{***}p < 0.001$; Cohen's d = effect measure ($d \geq 0.2$ = small, ≥ 0.5 = moderate, ≥ 0.8 = large effect)

		Complete data ($n = 603$)			BOCF ($n = 778$)			LOCF ($n = 778$)		
		M	SD	*d*	M	SD	*d*	M	SD	*d*
Depressive DS	A	2.07	0.91		2.07	0.91		2.07	0.91	
	F	1.32	0.91	**−0.82*****	1.49	0.96	−0.62***	1.33	0.91	**−0.82*****
Anxiety DS	A	1.41	1.07		1.42	1.07		1.42	1.07	
	F	0.93	0.91	−0.47***	1.06	0.98	−0.36***	0.96	0.91	−0.46***
Compulsive-Obs. DS	A	0.97	1.00		0.98	0.99		0.98	0.99	
	F	0.67	0.82	−0.33***	0.74	0.87	−0.25***	0.71	0.85	−0.29***
Somatoform DS	A	0.84	0.88		0.89	0.91		0.89	0.91	
	F	0.53	0.74	−0.38***	0.64	0.83	−0.28***	0.58	0.77	−0.36***
Eating DS	A	0.61	0.82		0.60	0.82		0.60	0.82	
	F	0.51	0.77	−0.13***	0.51	0.78	−0.10***	0.50	0.76	−0.12***
Total	A	1.14	0.59		1.15	0.59		1.15	0.59	
	F	0.78	0.55	−0.63***	0.87	0.58	−0.48***	0.80	0.55	−0.61***

A admission, *F* follow-up, *DS* disorder syndrome

carried forward (BOCF) and last observation carried forward (LOCF) methods were chosen to replace missing follow-up data with baseline or discharge values. Using the baseline value as the follow-up value for the 175 patients implies that no treatment took place, whereas using the discharge value implies the effect immediately after treatment. Despite loss of follow-up, the 778 patients (including the 175 patients for whom the conservative BOCF method was used) showed significant improvements on all ISR subscales and the total ISR score between baseline and follow-up. These results confirm the positive effect of multimodal treatment at the TCM-Klinik Bad Kötzting on ISR symptom burden (Table 5.34).

5.1.11.2 Load Levels for Each of the Individual ISR Dimensions

Due to the standardised evaluation of the ISR, it is possible to convert numerical scale values into stress levels, facilitating the interpretation of the measured values. It should be noted that the subscale and total ISR scores are partly based on different limit values, as outlined in Sect. 5.2.3.1.

Table 5.35 shows the frequencies of patients for stress levels for all ISR subscores and the total ISR score upon hospital admission ($n = 824$). Depression is the most prevalent syndrome. Here, 58.9% of patients reported moderate to severe symptom distress on admission (compared to 50.2% in previous years). For the total score, 62.8% of patients reported moderate to severe symptoms on admission (compared to 52.8% in previous years). It is possible to transform the numerical scale values into stress levels due to the standardised evaluation of the ISR, which facilitates the interpretation of the measured values. It should be noted here that both the subscale scores and the total value of the ISR score are partly based on different limit values (Sect. 5.2.3.1).

In addition to the baseline values ($n = 824$), which are collected on admission to hospital, the results for patients with complete data at all three survey times ($n = 603$) are also shown for all subscales in Table 5.36.

Using depressive syndrome as an example, the follow-up analysis ($n = 603$) shows that, at admission to hospital, 58.2% of patients reported moderate to severe symptoms. This proportion drops to 21.6% at discharge and decreases further to 24.9% at follow-up. Conversely, the proportion of patients with no overall burden increased more than fourfold, from 5.3% at admission to 29.7% at discharge, before decreasing slightly to 25.2% at follow-up.

Table 5.35 Distribution of ISR stress levels on hospital admission in 2023 (baseline; $n = 824$) and previous years ($n = 11{,}032$)

ISR 2023 admission	No indication		Possible burden		Mild burden		Moderate burden		Severe burden	
	n	%	*n*	%	*n*	%	*n*	%	*n*	%
Depressive DS	54	6.6	33	4.0	252	30.6	322	39.1	163	19.8
Anxiety DS	239	29.0	51	6.2	262	31.8	174	21.1	98	11.9
Compulsive-obsessive DS	356	43.2	68	8.3	224	27.2	124	15.0	52	6.3
Somatoform DS	256	31.1	218	26.5	84	10.2	218	26.5	48	5.8
Eating DS	411	49.9	87	10.6	209	25.4	95	11.5	22	2.7
Total score	123	14.9	46	5.6	138	16.7	360	43.7	157	19.1
ISR previous years admission	**No indication**		**Possible burden**		**Mild burden**		**Moderate burden**		**Severe burden**	
	n	%	*n*	%	*n*	%	*n*	%	*n*	%
Depressive DS	1126	10.2	617	5.6	3756	34.0	3726	33.8	1807	16.4
Anxiety DS	3958	35.9	864	7.8	3276	29.7	1941	17.6	993	9.0
Compulsive-obsessive DS	5450	49.4	946	8.6	2770	25.1	1339	12.1	527	4.8
Somatoform DS	3983	36.1	2970	26.9	1093	9.9	2400	21.8	586	5.3
Eating DS	5411	49.0	1400	12.7	2812	25.5	1148	10.4	261	2.4
Total score	2388	21.6	702	6.4	2169	19.7	4225	38.3	1548	14.0

Table 5.36 Distribution of ISR exposure levels over the course of time in 2023 (A–E–F: $n = 603$; previous years $n = 5681$)

ISR 2023 *n* = 603		**No indication**		**Possible burden**		**Mild burden**		**Moderate burden**		**Severe burden**	
		n	%	*n*	%	*n*	%	*n*	%	*n*	%
Depressive DS	A	32	5.3	29	4.8	191	31.7	234	38.8	117	19.4
	D	179	29.7	58	9.6	236	39.1	95	15.8	35	5.8
	F	152	25.2	55	9.1	246	40.8	103	17.1	47	7.8
Anxiety DS	A	180	29.9	40	6.6	182	30.2	136	22.5	65	10.8
	D	272	45.1	50	8.3	174	28.9	66	10.9	41	6.8
	F	272	45.1	65	10.8	169	28.0	73	12.1	24	4.0
Compulsive-obsessive DS	A	256	42.5	52	8.6	170	28.2	87	14.4	38	6.3
	D	309	51.2	56	9.3	168	27.9	50	8.3	20	3.3
	F	331	54.9	48	8.0	164	27.2	48	8.0	12	2.0
Somatoform DS	A	188	31.3	170	28.2	64	10.6	150	24.9	31	5.1
	D	268	44.4	152	25.2	65	10.8	103	17.1	15	2.5
	F	306	50.7	144	23.9	44	7.3	91	15.1	18	3.0
Eating DS	A	288	47.8	62	10.3	165	27.4	72	11.9	16	2.7
	D	313	51.9	72	11.9	147	24.4	55	9.1	16	2.7
	F	323	53.6	74	12.3	136	22.6	57	9.5	13	2.2
Total score	A	89	14.8	37	6.1	100	16.6	266	44.1	111	18.4
	D	208	34.5	43	7.1	129	21.4	175	29.0	48	8.0
	F	214	35.5	47	7.8	129	21.4	171	28.4	42	7.0
ISR previous years *n* = 5681		**No indication**		**Possible burden**		**Mild burden**		**Moderate burden**		**Severe burden**	
		n	%	*n*	%	*n*	%	*n*	%	*n*	%
Depressive DS	A	554	9.8	307	5.4	1975	34.8	1980	34.9	865	15.2
	D	2563	45.1	800	14.1	1821	32.1	416	7.3	81	1.4
	F	1616	28.4	680	12.0	2234	39.3	866	15.2	285	5.0
Anxiety DS	A	1999	35.2	467	8.2	1768	31.1	992	17.5	455	8.0
	D	3057	53.8	552	9.7	1525	26.8	450	7.9	97	1.7
	F	2911	51.2	546	9.6	1490	26.2	588	10.4	146	2.6
Compulsive-obsessive DS	A	2792	49.1	517	9.1	1470	25.9	651	11.5	251	4.4
	D	3175	55.9	526	9.3	1569	27.6	362	6.4	49	0.9
	F	3321	58.5	475	8.4	1412	24.9	393	6.9	80	1.4
Somatoform DS	A	2119	37.3	1562	27.5	553	9.7	1174	20.7	273	4.8
	D	2682	47.2	1609	28.3	602	10.6	725	12.8	63	1.1
	F	2788	49.1	1513	26.6	517	9.1	75	13.4	104	1.8
Eating DS	A	2721	47.9	718	12.6	1498	26.4	605	10.6	139	2.4
	D	2985	52.5	752	13.2	1403	24.7	473	8.3	68	1.2
	F	2981	52.5	683	12.0	1410	24.8	503	8.9	104	1.8
Total score	A	1193	21.0	386	6.8	1103	19.4	2271	40.0	728	12.8
	D	2617	46.1	503	8.9	1147	20.2	1241	21.8	173	3.0
	F	2372	41.8	431	7.6	1160	20.4	1421	25.0	297	5.2

DS disorder syndrome

Overall, the proportion of patients with moderate to severe symptom burden was 62.5% at hospital admission, 37.0% at discharge, and 35.4% at follow-up. This shows a clear trend towards improvement in symptom burden over time.

Comparative values are available for the clinical stress levels of the ISR, which allow patients at the TCM-Klinik Bad Kötzting to be compared with representative norm samples from the general population and from 10 specialist psychosomatic clinics [6, 7].

To illustrate this, the ISR total score and depressive syndrome are presented as examples. A comparison of ISR total scores reveals striking similarities between TCM patients prior to treatment in 2023 ($n = 603$) and the clinical reference sample ($n = 12,265$). In contrast, post-treatment scores among TCM patients show a clear shift towards the normative sample values ($n = 2512$), as depicted in Fig. 5.22. However, it should be noted that patients from the corresponding psychosomatic clinics still have slightly higher stress levels than those from the TCM-Klinik Bad Kötzting. Compared to the initial values, positive results can be observed at the time of the follow-up survey.

A similar picture emerges when we compare stress levels in people with depressive symptoms. In this case, the clinical sample comprises 8892 patients diagnosed with depression from ten psychosomatic specialist clinics. There is only a small difference between the TCM patients' admission scores and those of the clinical sample (Fig. 5.23). Changes in the frequency distribution of individual stress levels immediately after treatment at the TCM-Klinik Bad Kötzting are clearly visible. Figure 5.23 also shows that, about 6 months after discharge from the clinic, the proportion of critical stress levels increases again at the expense of the positive therapy results. However, the situation is still an improvement compared to admission to the clinic.

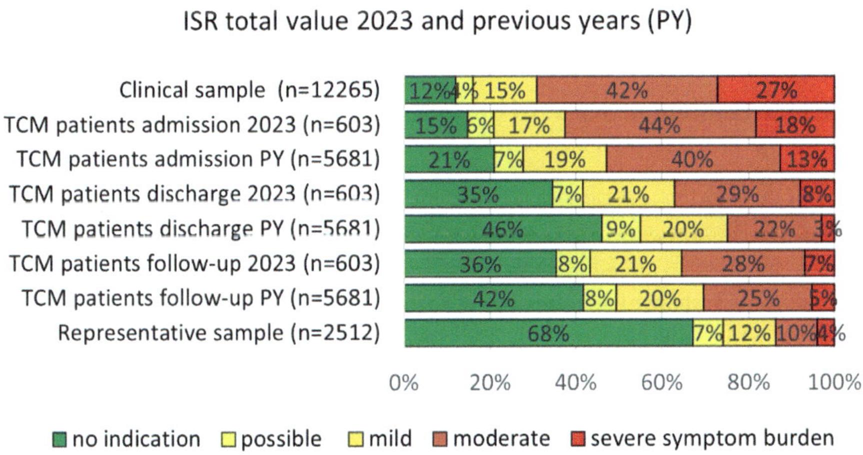

Fig. 5.22 Bar chart showing the frequency of individual clinical stress levels for the total ISR value in 2023 and previous years and comparing patients at the TCM-Klinik Bad Kötzting with clinical and normative samples

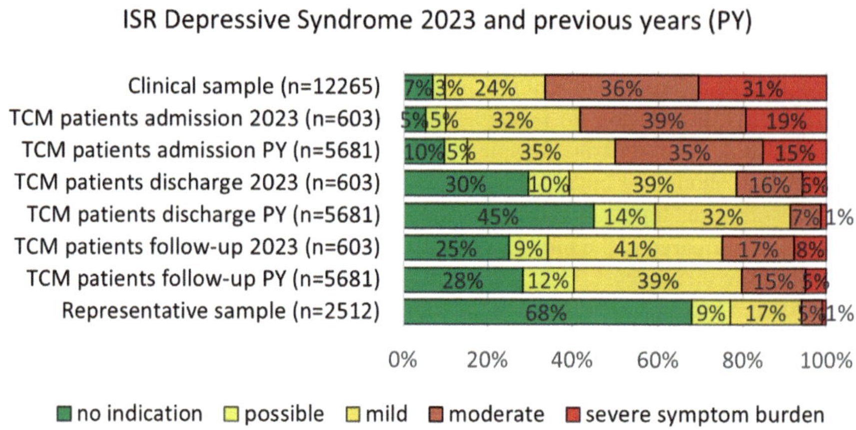

Fig. 5.23 Bar chart for the frequency of the individual clinical stress levels for depressive syndrome in 2023 and previous years; comparison of patients at the TCM-Klinik Bad Kötzting with a clinical sample and a norm sample

The subsequent section presents the ISR results for all patients with complete follow-up data, categorised by age group and gender. Descriptive statistics, including sample size (n), mean (M), and standard deviation (SD), are reported for admission, discharge, and follow-up scores. These values are displayed in separate tables for each ISR dimension (Tables 5.37, 5.38, 5.39, 5.40, 5.41, and 5.42).

5.1.11.3 Additional Scales of the ISR

As well as representing change in the total ISR score and its sub-dimensions, the additional scales are also very important. These scales screen for various psychological syndromes relevant to the findings, including the presence of suicidal thoughts. According to the literature, all item values of 1 ('hardly applies') and above should be explored in more detail.

Table 5.43 shows the frequency distribution of individual syndromes among patients with valid admission data. Notably, 3.1% of the 824 patients (n = 26) reported having suicidal thoughts. The most frequently reported issue was sleeping problems, affecting 73.7% of patients, which is consistent with previous screening procedures. In contrast, stress related to sexual preferences was reported very rarely, with 91.9% of patients indicating that this item did not apply to them.

Longitudinal comparisons indicate significant and sustained improvements, particularly in sleep problems ($d = -0.56$, $p < 0.001$), followed by psychological problems caused by everyday stress ($d = -0.41$, $p < 0.001$) and concentration difficulties ($d = -0.37$, $p < 0.001$). Table 5.44 presents all the statistical results, and Fig. 5.24 shows the distribution of mean responses for each scale (from 0 = does not apply to 4 = applies extremely).

Table 5.37 ISR Depression of patients with complete follow-up data (2023 $n = 603$; previous years n = 5681); broken down by age and gender

Depression		2023								Previous years							
				Admission		Discharge		Follow-up				Admission		Discharge		Follow-up	
	Age in years	*n*	%	M	SD	M	SD	M	SD	*n*	%	M	SD	M	SD	M	SD
Men	Up to 30	4	3.3	2.62	0.72	1.25	0.74	1.44	1.07	36	2.7	1.80	0.81	0.96	0.65	1.06	0.60
	31 to 40	7	5.7	2.57	0.97	1.86	1.40	1.75	1.31	67	5.0	2.06	0.92	1.11	0.91	1.29	0.93
	41 to 50	15	12.2	2.08	1.05	1.03	0.96	1.30	1.01	230	17.3	1.95	0.90	0.87	0.72	1.35	0.91
	51 to 60	56	45.5	2.27	0.94	1.42	1.02	1.54	1.01	492	37.0	1.89	0.93	0.92	0.76	1.31	0.88
	61 to 70	33	26.8	1.86	0.83	1.02	0.82	1.33	0.84	342	25.7	1.48	0.88	0.66	0.68	1.02	0.79
	Over 70	8	6.5	1.81	0.48	0.78	0.53	1.03	0.41	163	12.3	1.20	0.90	0.52	0.64	0.98	0.81
	Total	**123**	**100**	**2.14**	**0.91**	**1.24**	**0.97**	**1.43**	**0.96**	**1330**	**100**	**1.71**	**0.94**	**0.81**	**0.74**	**1.19**	**0.86**
Women	Up to 30	9	1.9	2.33	0.62	1.44	0.50	1.03	0.38	116	2.7	1.86	0.80	0.85	0.72	1.01	0.81
	31 to 40	31	6.5	2.03	0.77	1.20	0.81	1.14	0.99	238	5.5	2.12	0.93	0.98	0.71	1.20	0.88
	41 to 50	67	14.0	2.19	0.84	1.14	0.73	1.25	0.98	856	19.7	2.05	0.90	0.90	0.72	1.21	0.88
	51 to 60	212	44.2	2.09	0.89	1.28	0.93	1.38	0.92	1814	41.7	2.03	0.88	0.86	0.70	1.25	0.85
	61 to 70	118	24.6	1.97	1.01	1.08	0.82	1.27	0.81	907	20.8	1.74	0.91	0.75	0.65	1.10	0.84
	Over 70	43	9.0	1.84	0.92	0.97	0.83	1.23	0.89	420	9.7	1.53	0.89	0.75	0.68	1.22	0.86
	Total	**480**	**100**	**2.05**	**0.91**	**1.18**	**0.86**	**1.30**	**0.90**	**4351**	**100**	**1.92**	**0.91**	**0.84**	**0.70**	**1.20**	**0.86**
Total	Up to 30	13	2.2	2.42	0.64	1.38	0.56	1.15	0.65	152	2.7	1.84	0.80	0.87	0.70	1.02	0.76
	31 to 40	38	6.3	2.13	0.82	1.32	0.96	1.25	1.07	305	5.4	2.10	0.92	1.01	0.76	1.22	0.89
	41 to 50	82	13.6	2.17	0.88	1.12	0.77	1.26	0.98	1086	19.1	2.03	0.90	0.90	0.72	1.24	0.89
	51 to 60	268	44.4	2.13	0.90	1.31	0.95	1.41	0.94	2306	40.6	2.00	0.89	0.87	0.71	1.26	0.86
	61 to 70	151	25.0	1.95	0.97	1.07	0.82	1.28	0.82	1249	22.0	1.67	0.91	0.73	0.66	1.08	0.82
	Over 70	51	8.5	1.84	0.86	0.94	0.79	1.20	0.83	583	10.3	1.44	0.91	0.68	0.67	1.15	0.85
	Total	**603**	**100**	**2.07**	**0.91**	**1.19**	**0.88**	**1.32**	**0.91**	**5681**	**100**	**1.88**	**0.92**	**0.83**	**0.71**	**1.20**	**0.86**

Table 5.38 ISR Anxiety of patients with complete follow-up data (2023 $n = 603$; previous years $n = 5681$); broken down by age and gender

Anxiety		2023								Previous years							
				Admission		Discharge		Follow-up				Admission		Discharge		Follow-up	
	Age in years	*n*	%	M	SD	M	SD	M	SD	*n*	%	M	SD	M	SD	M	SD
Men	Up to 30	4	3.3	2.00	0.71	1.00	0.68	0.69	0.69	36	2.7	1.18	1.07	0.88	0.75	0.76	0.71
	31 to 40	7	5.7	1.71	1.27	1.32	1.19	1.14	0.83	67	5.0	1.25	1.06	0.79	0.74	0.80	0.81
	41 to 50	15	12.2	1.05	1.04	0.93	1.00	0.38	0.57	230	17.3	1.17	1.03	0.77	0.75	0.86	0.92
	51 to 60	56	45.5	1.62	1.11	1.24	1.15	1.17	1.09	492	37.0	1.21	0.99	0.81	0.82	0.87	0.88
	61 to 70	33	26.8	1.13	1.08	0.79	0.98	0.86	0.93	342	25.7	0.80	0.88	0.51	0.65	0.60	0.74
	Over 70	8	6.5	0.84	0.84	0.25	0.44	0.44	0.44	163	12.3	0.64	0.74	0.35	0.61	0.51	0.66
	Total	**123**	**100**	**1.39**	**1.10**	**1.01**	**1.06**	**0.93**	**0.97**	**1330**	**100**	**1.03**	**0.98**	**0.67**	**0.75**	**0.75**	**0.83**
Women	Up to 30	9	1.9	1.31	1.04	1.39	1.26	0.97	1.03	116	2.7	1.15	1.01	0.69	0.71	0.67	0.74
	31 to 40	31	6.5	1.24	1.09	0.98	0.90	0.86	1.02	238	5.5	1.28	1.12	0.81	0.80	0.81	0.88
	41 to 50	67	14.0	1.59	1.10	0.96	0.98	0.90	0.88	856	19.7	1.33	1.07	0.83	0.81	0.84	0.88
	51 to 60	212	44.2	1.40	1.06	1.04	0.97	0.98	0.89	1814	41.7	1.36	1.03	0.84	0.78	0.90	0.85
	61 to 70	118	24.6	1.44	1.06	0.96	0.87	0.90	0.90	907	20.8	1.21	0.99	0.69	0.74	0.82	0.81
	Over 70	43	9.0	1.22	0.97	0.78	0.80	0.89	0.79	420	9.7	1.00	0.88	0.63	0.69	0.74	0.76
	Total	**480**	**100**	**1.41**	**1.06**	**0.99**	**0.93**	**0.93**	**0.89**	**4351**	**100**	**1.28**	**1.02**	**0.78**	**0.77**	**0.85**	**0.84**
Total	Up to 30	13	2.2	1.52	0.98	1.27	1.10	0.88	0.92	152	2.7	1.16	1.02	0.74	0.73	0.69	0.73
	31 to 40	38	6.3	1.33	1.12	1.04	0.95	0.91	0.99	305	5.4	1.27	1.10	0.80	0.79	0.81	0.87
	41 to 50	82	13.6	1.49	1.10	0.95	0.98	0.80	0.86	1086	19.1	1.30	1.06	0.82	0.80	0.85	0.89
	51 to 60	268	44.4	1.45	1.07	1.08	1.01	1.02	0.93	2306	40.6	1.33	1.02	0.83	0.79	0.89	0.86
	61 to 70	151	25.0	1.37	1.07	0.93	0.90	0.89	0.90	1249	22.0	1.10	0.98	0.64	0.72	0.76	0.80
	Over 70	51	8.5	1.16	0.95	0.70	0.77	0.82	0.76	583	10.3	0.90	0.86	0.55	0.68	0.68	0.74
	Total	**603**	**100**	**1.40**	**1.07**	**0.99**	**0.96**	**0.93**	**0.91**	**5681**	**100**	**1.22**	**1.02**	**0.76**	**0.77**	**0.82**	**0.84**

Table 5.39 ISR Compulsion of patients with complete follow-up data (2023 n = 603; previous years n = 5681), broken down by age and gender

Compulsion		2023								Previous years							
				Admission		Discharge		Follow-up				Admission		Discharge		Follow-up	
	Age in years	*n*	%	M	SD	M	SD	M	SD	*n*	%	M	SD	M	SD	M	SD
Men	Up to 30	4	3.3	1.00	0.98	0.84	0.19	0.33	0.47	36	2.7	36	2.7	0.97	0.95	0.94	0.92
	31 to 40	7	5.7	1.19	1.15	1.19	1.21	1.33	1.07	67	5.0	67	5.0	1.02	1.11	0.85	0.94
	41 to 50	15	12.2	0.60	0.77	0.53	0.87	0.49	0.71	230	17.3	230	17.3	0.80	0.97	0.65	0.76
	51 to 60	56	45.5	1.31	1.08	1.05	1.03	0.91	0.95	492	37.0	492	37.0	0.82	0.89	0.69	0.76
	61 to 70	33	26.8	0.77	0.89	0.62	0.77	0.60	0.72	342	25.7	342	25.7	0.57	0.78	0.41	0.66
	Over 70	8	6.5	1.08	1.07	0.50	0.84	0.33	0.47	163	12.3	163	12.3	0.45	0.65	0.25	0.48
	Total	**123**	**100**	**1.05**	**1.02**	**0.84**	**0.94**	**0.74**	**0.86**	**1330**	**100**	**1330**	**100.0**	**0.72**	**0.88**	**0.57**	**0.74**
Women	Up to 30	9	1.9	1.04	0.79	0.85	0.77	0.37	0.59	116	2.7	116	2.7	0.85	1.08	0.70	0.76
	31 to 40	31	6.5	1.03	1.15	0.91	1.06	0.73	0.90	238	5.5	238	5.5	0.90	1.04	0.67	0.78
	41 to 50	67	14.0	1.07	0.94	0.75	0.87	0.72	0.84	856	19.7	856	19.7	0.86	0.98	0.66	0.78
	51 to 60	212	44.2	0.97	1.05	0.68	0.88	0.63	0.82	1814	41.7	1814	41.7	0.91	0.95	0.67	0.74
	61 to 70	118	24.6	0.91	0.92	0.74	0.74	0.66	0.81	907	20.8	907	20.8	0.82	0.92	0.54	0.67
	Over 70	43	9.0	0.71	0.90	0.69	0.89	0.58	0.72	420	9.7	420	9.7	0.62	0.80	0.51	0.64
	Total	**480**	**100**	**0.95**	**0.99**	**0.72**	**0.86**	**0.65**	**0.81**	**4351**	**100**	**4351**	**100.0**	**0.85**	**0.95**	**0.63**	**0.73**
Total	Up to 30	13	2.2	1.03	0.81	0.85	0.63	0.36	0.53	152	2.7	152	2.7	0.88	1.05	0.76	0.81
	31 to 40	38	6.3	1.06	1.13	0.96	1.08	0.84	0.94	305	5.4	305	5.4	0.93	1.05	0.71	0.82
	41 to 50	82	13.6	0.98	0.92	0.71	0.87	0.68	0.82	1086	19.1	1086	19.1	0.85	0.98	0.66	0.77
	51 to 60	268	44.4	1.04	1.06	0.75	0.92	0.69	0.86	2306	40.6	2306	40.6	0.89	0.93	0.67	0.74
	61 to 70	151	25.0	0.88	0.91	0.72	0.75	0.65	0.79	1249	22.0	1249	22.0	0.75	0.89	0.50	0.67
	Over 70	51	8.5	0.77	0.93	0.66	0.88	0.54	0.69	583	10.3	583	10.3	0.57	0.77	0.44	0.61
	Total	**603**	**100**	**0.97**	**1.00**	**0.75**	**0.88**	**0.67**	**0.82**	**5681**	**100**	**5681**	**100.0**	**0.82**	**0.93**	**0.61**	**0.73**

Table 5.40 ISR Somatisation of patients with complete follow-up data (2023 $n = 603$; previous years $n = 5681$); broken down by age and gender

Somatisation		2023								Previous years							
				Admission		Discharge		Follow-up				Admission		Discharge		Follow-up	
	Age in years	*n*	%	M	SD	M	SD	M	SD	*n*	%	M	SD	M	SD	M	SD
Men	Up to 30	4	3.3	1.92	0.69	1.50	0.58	0.42	0.63	36	2.7	0.94	1.00	0.75	0.72	0.60	0.78
	31 to 40	7	5.7	1.71	1.35	1.24	0.96	1.38	1.14	67	5.0	1.06	1.04	0.71	0.79	0.54	0.84
	41 to 50	15	12.2	0.51	0.71	0.42	0.46	0.33	0.62	230	17.3	0.77	0.86	0.56	0.66	0.55	0.71
	51 to 60	56	45.5	0.95	0.85	0.79	0.89	0.76	0.99	492	37.0	0.82	0.84	0.58	0.67	0.60	0.72
	61 to 70	33	26.8	0.91	0.97	0.84	0.79	0.67	0.81	342	25.7	0.67	0.76	0.53	0.63	0.54	0.71
	Over 70	8	6.5	0.75	0.64	0.29	0.42	0.21	0.35	163	12.3	0.63	0.83	0.43	0.65	0.50	0.71
	Total	**123**	**100**	**0.95**	**0.92**	**0.78**	**0.82**	**0.67**	**0.90**	**1330**	**100**	**0.77**	**0.84**	**0.56**	**0.67**	**0.56**	**0.72**
Women	Up to 30	9	1.9	1.07	0.66	0.44	0.41	0.37	0.42	116	2.7	0.76	0.93	0.47	0.59	0.34	0.59
	31 to 40	31	6.5	1.23	1.09	0.84	1.05	0.72	0.84	238	5.5	0.71	0.91	0.49	0.68	0.43	0.65
	41 to 50	67	14.0	0.98	1.05	0.54	0.87	0.51	0.79	856	19.7	0.75	0.87	0.47	0.65	0.47	0.67
	51 to 60	212	44.2	0.72	0.79	0.54	0.68	0.44	0.63	1814	41.7	0.74	0.83	0.47	0.61	0.48	0.67
	61 to 70	118	24.6	0.81	0.85	0.53	0.73	0.52	0.74	907	20.8	0.71	0.84	0.43	0.59	0.46	0.68
	Over 70	43	9.0	0.69	0.70	0.44	0.55	0.46	0.62	420	9.7	0.58	0.75	0.44	0.57	0.52	0.67
	Total	**480**	**100**	**0.81**	**0.87**	**0.55**	**0.74**	**0.49**	**0.69**	**4351**	**100**	**0.72**	**0.84**	**0.46**	**0.62**	**0.47**	**0.67**
Total	Up to 30	13	2.2	1.33	0.76	0.77	0.67	0.38	0.47	152	2.7	0.80	0.94	0.53	0.63	0.40	0.65
	31 to 40	38	6.3	1.32	1.14	0.91	1.03	0.84	0.93	305	5.4	0.79	0.95	0.54	0.71	0.45	0.69
	41 to 50	82	13.6	0.89	1.01	0.52	0.81	0.48	0.76	1086	19.1	0.75	0.87	0.49	0.66	0.49	0.68
	51 to 60	268	44.4	0.76	0.81	0.59	0.73	0.51	0.73	2306	40.6	0.75	0.83	0.49	0.62	0.51	0.68
	61 to 70	151	25.0	0.83	0.87	0.60	0.75	0.55	0.75	1249	22.0	0.70	0.82	0.46	0.60	0.48	0.69
	Over 70	51	8.5	0.70	0.69	0.42	0.53	0.42	0.59	583	10.3	0.60	0.77	0.44	0.59	0.51	0.68
	Total	**603**	**100**	**0.84**	**0.88**	**0.59**	**0.76**	**0.53**	**0.74**	**5681**	**100**	**0.73**	**0.84**	**0.48**	**0.63**	**0.49**	**0.68**

Table 5.41 ISR Eating Disorder of patients with complete follow-up data (2023 n = 603; previous years n = 5631); broken down by age and gender

Eating disorder		2023								Previous years							
				Admission		Discharge		Follow-up				Admission		Discharge		Follow-up	
	Age in years	*n*	%	M	SD	M	SD	M	SD	*n*	%	M	SD	M	SD	M	SD
Men	Up to 30	4	3.3	0.67	1.33	0.50	0.80	0.33	0.66	36	2.7	0.24	0.53	0.29	0.56	0.16	0.39
	31 to 40	7	5.7	0.33	0.51	0.28	0.49	0.38	1.01	67	5.0	0.42	0.66	0.33	0.52	0.36	0.54
	41 to 50	15	12.2	0.29	0.52	0.33	0.55	0.20	0.53	230	17.3	0.40	0.59	0.39	0.58	0.38	0.55
	51 to 60	56	45.5	0.54	0.76	0.55	0.86	0.54	0.82	492	37.0	0.52	0.71	0.49	0.65	0.51	0.67
	61 to 70	33	26.8	0.38	0.57	0.37	0.56	0.35	0.61	342	25.7	0.43	0.58	0.44	0.60	0.46	0.62
	Over 70	8	6.5	0.54	0.53	0.33	0.53	0.33	0.47	163	12.3	0.43	0.62	0.30	0.45	0.46	0.66
	Total	**123**	**100**	**0.46**	**0.68**	**0.44**	**0.71**	**0.42**	**0.72**	**1330**	**100**	**0.45**	**0.64**	**0.43**	**0.60**	**0.45**	**0.63**
Women	Up to 30	9	1.9	0.33	0.60	0.41	0.62	0.26	0.57	116	2.7	0.48	0.87	0.57	0.85	0.50	0.75
	31 to 40	31	6.5	0.62	0.84	0.53	0.74	0.49	0.74	238	5.5	0.69	0.96	0.50	0.76	0.52	0.85
	41 to 50	67	14.0	0.74	1.02	0.60	0.87	0.44	0.72	856	19.7	0.67	0.90	0.51	0.75	0.53	0.80
	51 to 60	212	44.2	0.69	0.82	0.54	0.76	0.60	0.82	1814	41.7	0.68	0.85	0.53	0.74	0.56	0.78
	61 to 70	118	24.6	0.62	0.84	0.60	0.89	0.57	0.86	907	20.8	0.59	0.81	0.45	0.67	0.49	0.74
	Over 70	43	9.0	0.57	0.81	0.48	0.71	0.33	0.49	420	9.7	0.40	0.64	0.36	0.59	0.39	0.66
	Total	**480**	**100**	**0.66**	**0.85**	**0.56**	**0.80**	**0.54**	**0.78**	**4351**	**100**	**0.63**	**0.85**	**0.49**	**0.72**	**0.52**	**0.77**
Total	Up to 30	13	2.2	0.44	0.84	0.44	0.64	0.28	0.58	152	2.7	0.42	0.81	0.50	0.80	0.42	0.69
	31 to 40	38	6.3	0.57	0.79	0.48	0.71	0.47	0.78	305	5.4	0.63	0.91	0.46	0.72	0.48	0.79
	41 to 50	82	13.6	0.66	0.96	0.55	0.83	0.40	0.69	1086	19.1	0.61	0.85	0.48	0.72	0.50	0.76
	51 to 60	268	44.4	0.65	0.81	0.54	0.78	0.59	0.82	2306	40.6	0.65	0.83	0.52	0.72	0.55	0.76
	61 to 70	151	25.0	0.57	0.79	0.55	0.83	0.52	0.81	1249	22.0	0.54	0.75	0.45	0.65	0.48	0.71
	Over 70	51	8.5	0.56	0.77	0.46	0.68	0.33	0.49	583	10.3	0.40	0.63	0.34	0.56	0.41	0.66
	Total	**603**	**100**	**0.62**	**0.82**	**0.53**	**0.78**	**0.51**	**0.77**	**5681**	**100**	**0.59**	**0.81**	**0.48**	**0.70**	**0.51**	**0.74**

Table 5.42 ISR total score of patients with complete follow-up data (2023 $n = 603$; previous years $n = 5681$); broken down by age and gender

ISR total score		2023								Previous years							
				Admission		Discharge		Follow-up				Admission		Discharge		Follow-up	
	Age in years	*n*	%	M	SD	M	SD	M	SD	*n*	%	M	SD	M	SD	M	SD
Men	Up to 30	4	3.3	1.58	0.73	0.93	0.24	0.60	0.34	36	2.7	0.97	0.57	0.73	0.45	0.63	0.41
	31 to 40	7	5.7	1.50	0.87	1.20	0.79	1.20	0.82	67	5.0	1.10	0.60	0.74	0.53	0.72	0.50
	41 to 50	15	12.2	0.91	0.50	0.70	0.60	0.56	0.44	230	17.3	0.99	0.56	0.65	0.47	0.76	0.56
	51 to 60	56	45.5	1.28	0.62	0.99	0.71	0.96	0.70	492	37.0	1.03	0.58	0.70	0.51	0.79	0.56
	61 to 70	33	26.8	1.00	0.66	0.71	0.54	0.77	0.57	342	25.7	0.79	0.52	0.52	0.44	0.61	0.47
	Over 70	8	6.5	0.93	0.46	0.43	0.39	0.50	0.33	163	12.3	0.67	0.48	0.40	0.39	0.56	0.46
	Total	**123**	**100**	**1.16**	**0.65**	**0.85**	**0.65**	**0.83**	**0.64**	**1330**	**100**	**0.92**	**0.57**	**0.61**	**0.49**	**0.70**	**0.53**
Women	Up to 30	9	1.9	1.18	0.38	0.82	0.38	0.59	0.26	116	2.7	0.95	0.54	0.65	0.46	0.59	0.46
	31 to 40	31	6.5	1.21	0.65	0.88	0.65	0.77	0.64	238	5.5	1.09	0.60	0.68	0.46	0.70	0.52
	41 to 50	67	14.0	1.26	0.59	0.79	0.55	0.74	0.57	856	19.7	1.08	0.58	0.68	0.47	0.72	0.54
	51 to 60	212	44.2	1.14	0.56	0.82	0.54	0.80	0.53	1814	41.7	1.10	0.56	0.69	0.47	0.76	0.53
	61 to 70	118	24.6	1.09	0.61	0.76	0.52	0.76	0.52	907	20.8	0.96	0.56	0.57	0.42	0.66	0.49
	Over 70	43	9.0	0.95	0.54	0.67	0.47	0.67	0.40	420	9.7	0.78	0.48	0.53	0.39	0.64	0.45
	Total	**480**	**100**	**1.13**	**0.58**	**0.79**	**0.54**	**0.77**	**0.52**	**4351**	**100**	**1.03**	**0.57**	**0.64**	**0.45**	**0.71**	**0.52**
Total	Up to 30	13	2.2	1.31	0.52	0.86	0.34	0.59	0.27	152	2.7	0.96	0.54	0.67	0.45	0.60	0.45
	31 to 40	38	6.3	1.26	0.69	0.94	0.68	0.85	0.68	305	5.4	1.09	0.60	0.69	0.48	0.70	0.51
	41 to 50	82	13.6	1.19	0.59	0.77	0.56	0.71	0.55	1086	19.1	1.06	0.57	0.67	0.47	0.73	0.55
	51 to 60	268	44.4	1.17	0.57	0.86	0.58	0.83	0.57	2306	40.6	1.08	0.57	0.69	0.48	0.76	0.53
	61 to 70	151	25.0	1.07	0.62	0.75	0.52	0.76	0.53	1249	22.0	0.91	0.55	0.56	0.42	0.64	0.49
	Over 70	51	8.5	0.94	0.52	0.63	0.46	0.65	0.40	583	10.3	0.75	0.48	0.49	0.40	0.61	0.46
	Total	**603**	**100**	**1.14**	**0.59**	**0.81**	**0.56**	**0.78**	**0.55**	**5681**	**100**	**1.00**	**0.57**	**0.64**	**0.46**	**0.71**	**0.52**

Table 5.43 Frequency distribution of the additional scales as part of the ISR on admission to hospital in 2023 ($n = 824$) and previous years ($n = 5681$)

	2023										Previous years									
	Does not apply		Hardly applies		Somewhat applies		Applies strongly		Applies extremely		Does not apply		Hardly applies		Somewhat applies		Applies strongly		Applies extremely	
ISR additional scales	*n*	%	*n*	%	*n*	%	*n*	%	*n*	%	*n*	%	*n*	%	*n*	%	*n*	%	*n*	%
Suicidal thoughts	679	81.6	119	14.4	20	2.4	5	0.6	1	0.1	4773	84.0	754	13.3	118	2.1	33	0.6	3	0.1
Sleep problems	56	6.8	161	19.5	190	23.1	191	23.2	226	27.4	721	12.7	1070	18.8	1360	23.9	1275	2.4	1255	22.1
Concentration difficulties	93	11.3	196	23.8	234	28.4	188	22.8	113	13.7	999	17.6	1705	30.0	1569	27.6	955	16.8	453	8.0
Poor appetite	489	59.3	237	28.8	67	8.1	19	2.3	12	1.5	3921	69.0	1268	22.3	324	5.7	122	2.1	46	0.8
Forgetfulness	83	10.1	283	34.3	229	27.8	144	17.5	85	10.3	769	13.5	2164	38.1	1581	27.8	801	14.1	366	6.4
Recurring dreams/ remembering memories of terrible experiences	366	44.4	251	30.5	109	13.2	68	8.3	30	3.6	2914	51.3	1654	29.1	620	10.9	353	6.2	140	2.5
Psy. problems due to everyday stress	260	31.6	181	22.0	180	21.8	112	13.6	91	11.0	2128	37.5	1201	21.1	1179	20.8	695	12.2	478	8.4
Alienation from own feelings and experiences	600	72.8	143	17.4	52	5.3	23	2.8	6	0.7	4428	77.9	862	15.2	247	4.3	113	2.0	31	0.5
People & surroundings appear unreal, distant, lifeless	616	74.8	141	17.1	50	5.1	13	1.6	4	0.5	4494	79.1	829	14.6	237	4.2	92	1.6	29	0.5
Feeling of impairment with exercise of sexuality	327	39.7	145	17.6	145	17.6	96	11.7	111	13.5	2312	40.7	1104	19.4	988	17.4	639	11.2	638	11.2
Permanent change through extreme load	589	71.5	82	10.0	83	10.1	41	5.0	29	3.5	4418	77.8	538	9.5	389	6.9	204	3.6	132	2.3
Sexual preferences are a load	757	91.9	49	5.9	12	1.5	4	0.5	2	0.2	5237	92.2	302	5.3	76	1.3	43	0.8	23	0.4

Table 5.44 Additional ISR scales in the pre/post comparison in 2023; significance at $p < 0.05$; t- test for paired samples; significance at $p < 0.05$; Cohen's d is the effect size measure ($d \geq 0.2$ = small, ≥ 0.5 = moderate, ≥ 0.8 = large effect); cross-section statistics are included for descriptive purposes and for full dataset comparisons (A–D–F $n = 600$)

		Cross-section: A/D/F			Course: A–D/A–F $n = 600$		Difference from admission: A–D/A–F $n = 600$		
ISR 2023 additional scales		n	M	SD	M	SD	ΔM	p	d
Suicidal thoughts	A	824	0.21	0.52	0.22	0.52			
	D	778	0.10	0.38	0.11	0.40	−0.11	<0.001	−0.22
	F	606	0.11	0.38	0.11	0.38	−0.11	<0.001	−0.23
Sleep problems	A	824	2.45	1.27	2.43	1.27			
	D	778	1.89	1.35	1.85	1.34	−0.58	<0.001	−0.45
	F	609	1.71	1.28	1.71	1.28	−0.72	<0.001	**−0.56**
Concentration difficulties	A	824	2.04	1.21	2.00	1.18			
	D	778	1.63	1.21	1.58	1.19	−0.43	<0.001	−0.36
	F	607	1.56	1.17	1.56	1.17	−0.44	<0.001	−0.37
Poor appetite	A	824	0.58	0.85	0.56	0.83			
	D	778	0.37	0.72	0.35	0.68	−0.22	<0.001	−0.28
	F	607	0.41	0.74	0.40	0.74	−0.17	<0.001	−0.21
Forgetfulness	A	824	1.84	1.14	1.83	1.12			
	D	778	1.61	1.12	1.56	1.10	−0.27	<0.001	−0.24
	F	607	1.51	1.09	1.52	1.09	−0.32	<0.001	−0.29
Recurring dreams/memory of terrible dream experiences	A	824	0.96	1.11	0.98	1.12			
	D	778	0.76	1.00	0.78	1.02	−0.20	<0.001	−0.19
	F	607	0.65	0.94	0.65	0.94	−0.32	<0.001	−0.31
Psychological problems due to everyday stress	A	824	1.50	1.35	1.50	1.36			
	D	778	1.19	1.25	1.15	1.26	−0.35	<0.001	−0.27
	F	607	0.98	1.19	0.98	1.20	−0.53	<0.001	−0.41
Alienation from own feelings and experiences	A	824	0.41	0.79	0.40	0.77			
	D	778	0.25	0.62	0.27	0.63	−0.14	<0.001	−0.19
	F	605	0.23	0.56	0.23	0.56	−0.17	<0.001	−0.25
People and surroundings appear unreal, distant, lifeless	A	824	0.36	0.71	0.36	0.71			
	D	778	0.21	0.53	0.21	0.53	−0.16	<0.001	−0.25
	F	605	0.21	0.54	0.22	0.54	−0.15	<0.001	−0.23
Feeling of impairment with exercise of sexuality	A	824	1.41	1.44	1.43	1.44			
	D	778	1.08	1.33	1.08	1.32	−0.35	<0.001	−0.25
	F	608	1.07	1.37	1.06	1.37	−0.37	<0.001	−0.26
Permanent change through extreme load	A	824	0.59	1.08	0.58	1.07			
	D	778	0.46	0.96	0.44	0.95	−0.14	<0.001	−0.14
	F	606	0.43	0.93	0.43	0.93	−0.16	<0.001	−0.16
Sexual preferences are a load	A	824	0.11	0.43	0.12	0.46			
	D	778	0.10	0.41	0.11	0.45	−0.01	0.564	–
	F	605	0.10	0.45	0.10	0.45	−0.02	0.266	–

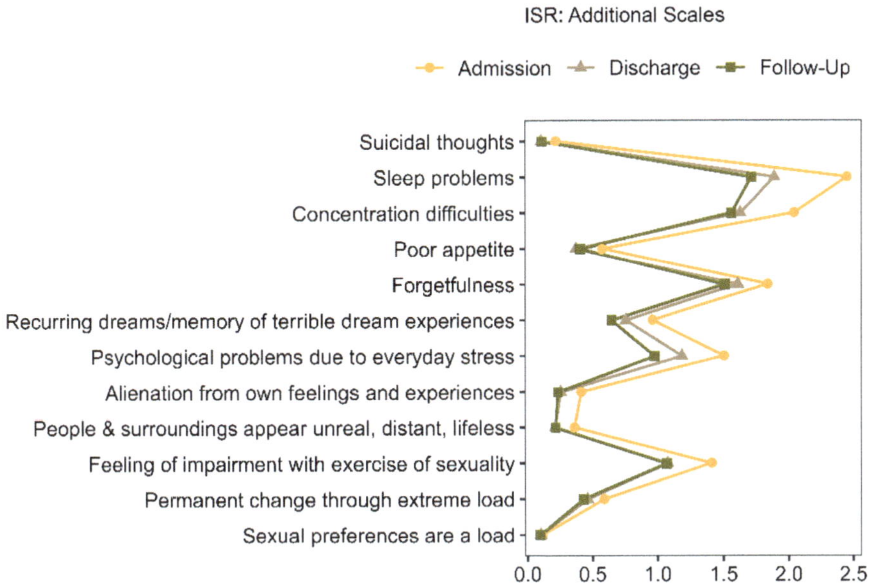

Fig. 5.24 Additional scales of the ICD-10 symptom rating (ISR) over the course of the 2023 measurement dates (A–D–F n = 600); the x-axis represents the mean values per scale, ranging from 0 = does not apply to 4 = applies extremely

5.2 Risk and Protective Factors in a Before-and-After Comparison

To evaluate potential inpatient effects, it is necessary to compare the risk-protective factor profile before and after the intervention in the form of an inpatient stay at the TCM-Klinik Bad Kötzting. Repeated questioning of patients on selected indicators via the VITERIO® health portal after discharge from the clinic became standard practice in September 2021. Until December 2021, only the Tedium Measure, Life Satisfaction, and Sense of Coherence (SOC) indicators were repeated at discharge. Subsequent follow-ups included the Tedium Measure, Life Satisfaction, and Pain Disability Index indicators. From January 2022 onwards, the following have been included at both discharge and follow-up: the Tedium Measure, the Perceived Stress Questionnaire (PSQ), Life Satisfaction (FLZ), Well-being (WHO-5), Vitality (SF-36), Sense of Coherence (SOC), Self-efficacy, Optimism, Pessimism (SWOP), Social Support Scale (SSS), Pittsburgh Sleep Quality Index (PSQI), Pain Disability Index (PDI), Generalised Anxiety Disorder Scale (GAD), and Functional Back Questionnaire (FFbH, if indicated). Since the 2022 revision, the Three-Level Stress Test, Stressors and Burdens, Movement Index, Nutrition Index and diabetes and high blood pressure risk are also collected at follow-up, in addition to the baseline assessment upon admission. These factors are not assessed at discharge, as changes in these domains typically require time to manifest. Comparisons of physical health risk factors requiring laboratory data are limited to admission and discharge, as these values cannot be collected during follow-up.

Prior to the implementation of the new indicator concept, repeated measurements via follow-up health checks were optional and only feasible for individuals with private internet access. Consequently, comparisons of the 2023 results with previous years are limited to data from 2022 for the risk and protective factors.

To examine changes in risk and protective factors between hospital admission, discharge, and follow-up, paired sample *t*-tests with 95% confidence intervals were conducted for comparisons between admission and discharge, and between admission and follow-up. To assess the practical relevance of statistically significant changes, effect sizes (Cohen's d) are reported, with thresholds of 0.2 indicating a small effect, 0.5 a moderate effect, and 0.8 a large effect. First, the pre-post results are presented for the psychological basic skills indicators (FLZ, SOC, WHO-5, Vitality, SWOP, and SSS), the IHM stress profile indicators (Tedium Measure, PSQ, Three-Level Stress Test, psycho-vegetative complaints, Stressors, and Burdens), and the mental stress indicator (WHO-5 Depression and GAD). These are followed by the results of the physiological resource profile (Movement Index, Nutrition Index, Psycho-Vegetative Stability, PSQI) and the risks to physical health (diabetes risk, hypertension risk, metabolic syndrome, fatty liver index).

Admission data were analysed in detail by age group and gender for all contexts, followed by a pre-post analysis for the entire patient sample.

5.2.1 Psychosocial Basic Skills (IHM Resource Profile) for the Mental Health

5.2.1.1 Life Satisfaction (FLZ)

Upon arrival at the TCM-Klinik Bad Kötzting, it is evident that older patients are slightly more satisfied with their lives than younger patients, although life satisfaction is below the desirable threshold for all age groups on average (Fig. 5.25). Overall, men (mean = 25.38, standard deviation = 37.56) report slightly higher life satisfaction than women (mean = 23.83, standard deviation = 34.22). Men are only less satisfied than women in the areas of 'friends', 'acquaintances', and 'general life situation'. However, these differences are only marginal. Table 5.45 provides an overview of all FLZ subscales, presenting the total score differentiated by gender. Table 5.46 shows the total FLZ score broken down by age group and gender. Figure 5.26 illustrates these results visually. Interestingly, despite all patients being diagnosed with primary psychological conditions, the lowest satisfaction ratings are found in the domain of general health domain—suggesting that physical aspects of life satisfaction are perceived as more problematic.

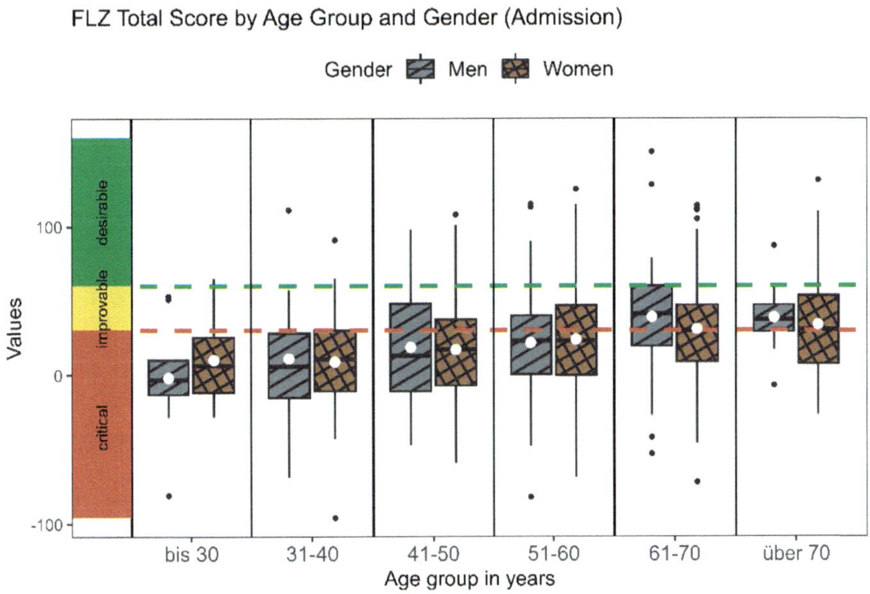

Fig. 5.25 Distribution of life satisfaction. Distribution of patients in the critical (red), improvable (yellow), and desirable (green) ranges, broken down by gender and age on admission in 2023 (n = 824, men: n = 170, women: n = 654). White circles indicate the mean and black lines the median

Table 5.45 Measures of dispersion for overall life satisfaction and its sub-dimensions; broken down by gender for 2023 (n = 824) and previous years (n = 12,570)

		2023				Previous years			
	Gender	*n*	M	SD	Md	*n*	M	SD	Md
FLZ total	Men	170	25.38	37.56	27.0	3260	33.00	35.71	32.0
	Women	654	23.83	34.22	24.0	9310	30.81	34.01	30.0
	Total	824	24.15	34.92	24.0	12,570	31.38	34.47	30.0
Friends/acquaintances	Men	170	3.59	7.01	2.0	3260	4.89	6.29	3.0
	Women	654	5.06	6.65	3.0	9310	6.01	6.66	6.0
	Total	824	4.76	6.75	3.0	12,570	5.72	6.59	6.0
Leisure time/hobbies	Men	170	1.63	6.31	1.0	3260	2.86	6.25	2.0
	Women	654	1.26	6.23	0.0	9310	2.57	5.94	2.0
	Total	824	1.33	6.24	0.0	12,570	2.65	6.02	2.0
Health	Men	170	−4.79	7.21	−4.0	3260	−4.37	7.17	−4.0
	Women	654	−5.25	5.85	−4.0	9310	−5.21	6.63	−4.0
	Total	824	−5.15	6.16	−4.0	12,570	−4.99	6.78	−4.0
Income	Men	170	3.88	7.10	3.0	3260	4.59	6.61	4.0
	Women	654	2.71	7.01	3.0	9310	4.12	6.84	3.0
	Total	824	2.95	7.04	3.0	12,570	4.24	6.79	3.0
Profession	Men	170	1.10	6.65	0.0	3260	2.97	7.03	2.0
	Women	654	0.91	6.87	0.0	9310	2.34	6.98	2.0
	Total	824	0.95	6.82	0.0	12,570	2.50	7.00	2.0

(continued)

Table 5.45 (continued)

		2023				Previous years			
	Gender	*n*	M	SD	Md	*n*	M	SD	Md
Living situation	Men	170	5.82	6.89	6.0	3260	8.19	6.92	9.0
	Women	654	6.84	7.71	9.0	9310	8.11	7.13	9.0
	Total	824	6.63	7.56	6.0	12,570	8.13	7.07	9.0
Family/children	Men	170	7.15	8.26	9.0	3260	8.08	8.17	9.0
	Women	654	7.06	8.41	6.0	9310	8.08	8.45	9.0
	Total	824	7.08	8.37	9.0	12,570	8.08	8.38	9.0
Partnership	Men	170	7.01	9.68	9.0	3260	5.79	8.99	4.0
	Women	653	5.26	9.39	3.0	9310	4.77	8.74	3.0
	Total	823	5.62	9.47	4.0	12,570	5.04	8.82	3.0

M mean, *SD* standard deviation, *Md* median

Table 5.46 Measures of distribution for life satisfaction (total score), broken down by gender and age in 2023 and previous years

FLZ total score									
		2023				Previous years			
	Age group	*n*	M	SD	Md	*n*	M	SD	Md
Men	Up to 30	9	−1.89	40.42	−3.00	154	18.11	39.64	154
	31 to 40	13	11.00	43.75	6.00	240	19.38	35.13	240
	41 to 50	22	18.59	38.56	13.00	666	25.42	33.50	666
	51 to 60	64	21.53	35.92	23.00	1069	29.82	35.38	1069
	61 to 70	47	38.85	36.52	41.00	686	40.61	32.43	686
	Over 70	15	38.40	20.93	37.00	445	52.78	32.72	445
	Total	170	25.38	37.56	27.00	3260	33.00	35.71	3260
Women	Up to 30	14	10.07	29.73	6.50	426	25.95	34.12	426
	31 to 40	50	8.82	33.77	10.50	702	18.81	33.92	702
	41 to 50	96	16.99	32.57	17.50	2110	26.21	34.01	2110
	51 to 60	282	23.77	34.80	23.00	3402	28.79	33.21	3402
	61 to 70	153	30.80	32.40	30.00	1750	38.77	33.04	1750
	Over 70	58	33.55	33.80	30.50	920	45.10	31.25	920
	Total	653	23.85	34.24	24.00	9310	30.81	34.01	9310
Total	Up to 30	23	5.39	33.94	0.00	580	23.87	35.80	580
	31 to 40	63	9.27	35.67	9.00	942	18.96	34.21	942
	41 to 50	118	17.29	33.60	16.50	2776	26.02	33.88	2776
	51 to 60	346	23.36	34.97	23.00	4471	29.04	33.74	4471
	61 to 70	200	32.69	33.49	31.50	2436	39.29	32.87	2436
	Over 70	73	34.55	31.52	32.00	1365	47.60	31.93	1365
	Total	823	24.17	34.94	24.00	12.570	31.38	34.47	12.570

M mean, *SD* standard deviation, *Md* median

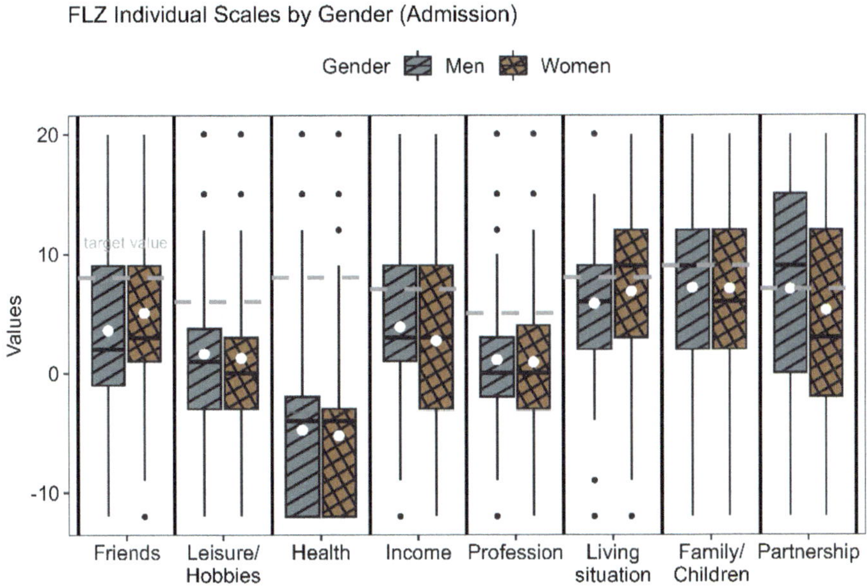

Fig. 5.26 Distribution of the individual scales for life satisfaction broken down by gender in 2023 on admission to hospital ($n = 824$, men: $n = 170$, women: $n = 654$); white circles indicate the mean, black lines the median

When comparing admission values with discharge and follow-up values, a significant difference was observed for the total score ($d = 0.53$, $p < 0.001$; $d = 0.47$, $p < 0.001$, respectively) and for all subcategories (Table 5.47).

The 'Health' subcategory shows the most pronounced change, with a moderate effect observed at both discharge ($d = 0.76$, $p < 0.001$) and follow-up ($d = 0.77$, $p < 0.001$). In contrast, all other subcategories exhibit changes of a small magnitude. As illustrated in Fig. 5.27, satisfaction with health has improved significantly, yet remains below the desired target level. Additionally, Fig. 5.28 demonstrates that, on average, overall 'life satisfaction' at hospital admission was within the critical range. By discharge, it had increased to the 'could be improved' range, where it remained through follow-up.

In addition to the statistical findings, Fig. 5.29 shows how the distribution of patients across the traffic light system levels for the overall FLZ score has changed over time. While 55% of patients had critical life satisfaction on admission, this proportion decreased to 35% at discharge and remained at 36% at follow-up. Conversely, the proportion of patients with sufficiently high life satisfaction increased from 15% at admission to 32% at discharge and 27% at follow-up.

5.2.1.2 Sense of Coherence (Health Literacy)

At the time of admission to the TCM-Klinik Bad Kötzting, patients had an average Sense of Coherence (SOC) score of 57.60 (SD = 12.42), which, according to the traffic light system described in the chapter 'Patient Profile' (Sect. 5.2.1.2), falls into the 'yellow' category ('could be improved'). Examining age and gender

Table 5.47 Life satisfaction in the before/after comparison in 2023; t-test with paired samples; significance at $p < 0.05$; Cohen's d = effect measure ($d \geq 0.2$ = small, ≥ 0.5 = moderate, ≥ 0.8 = large); cross-section statistics and full dataset comparisons (A–D–F $n = 611$); previous year's data since 2022

Life satisfaction		2023								Previous year 2022			
		Cross-section: A/D/F			Course: A–D/A–F $n = 611$		Difference from admission: A–D/A–F $n = 611$			Course: A–D/A–F $n = 508$	Difference from admission: A–D/A–F $n = 508$		
		n	M	SD	M	SD	ΔM	p	d	M	ΔM	p	d
Total score	**A**	823	24.17	34.94	25.31	33.61				28.78			
	D	777	41.95	37.61	44.09	36.77	18.78	<0.001	**0.53**	45.23	16.45	<0.001	0.46
	F	616	40.96	34.00	41.07	34.07	15.76	<0.001	0.47	41.91	13.13	<0.001	0.38
Friends/ acquaintances	**A**	823	4.75	6.76	4.92	6.67				5.07			
	D	777	6.59	6.70	6.70	6.56	1.79	<0.001	0.27	6.92	1.85	<0.001	0.28
	F	616	5.98	6.24	6.01	6.26	1.09	<0.001	0.17	6.09	1.02	<0.001	0.16
Leisure/hobbies	**A**	823	1.34	6.25	1.26	6.01				1.87			
	D	777	3.90	6.39	4.02	6.41	2.75	<0.001	0.44	4.06	2.19	<0.001	0.37
	F	616	3.73	5.57	3.73	5.56	2.47	<0.001	0.43	3.56	1.69	<0.001	0.29
Health	**A**	823	−5.15	6.16	−5.25	6.06				−4.62			
	D	777	−0.43	7.48	0.04	7.62	5.29	<0.001	**0.76**	−0.05	4.57	<0.001	**0.65**
	F	616	0.06	7.58	0.07	7.59	5.32	<0.001	**0.77**	−0.10	4.72	<0.001	**0.66**
Income	**A**	823	2.96	7.04	3.04	6.81				4.03			
	D	777	4.33	6.89	4.53	6.78	1.49	<0.001	0.22	5.24	1.21	<0.001	0.18
	F	616	4.20	6.29	4.22	6.30	1.84	<0.001	0.18	4.81	0.78	0.002	0.12
Profession	**A**	823	0.95	6.83	1.11	6.77				1.53			
	D	777	1.96	6.69	2.18	6.56	1.07	<0.001	0.16	2.20	0.67	0.017	0.09
	F	616	2.79	6.24	2.81	6.26	1.70	<0.001	0.26	2.77	1.24	<0.001	0.18
Housing situation	**A**	823	6.63	7.56	6.78	7.33				7.76			
	D	777	7.75	7.66	8.14	7.48	1.36	<0.001	0.18	8.91	1.15	<0.001	0.16
	F	616	7.68	6.82	7.67	6.83	0.89	<0.001	0.13	8.38	0.62	0.039	0.08
Family/children	**A**	823	7.08	8.38	7.53	8.32				7.82			
	D	777	9.62	8.03	9.87	7.94	2.34	<0.001	0.29	10.01	2.19	<0.001	0.26
	F	616	8.88	7.67	8.92	7.68	1.39	<0.001	0.17	9.00	1.18	<0.001	0.14
Partnership	**A**	823	5.62	9.47	5.92	9.37				5.20			
	D	777	8.23	9.41	8.63	9.18	2.71	<0.001	0.29	7.94	2.74	<0.001	0.29
	F	616	7.65	8.84	7.64	8.84	1.72	<0.001	0.19	7.20	2.00	<0.001	0.21

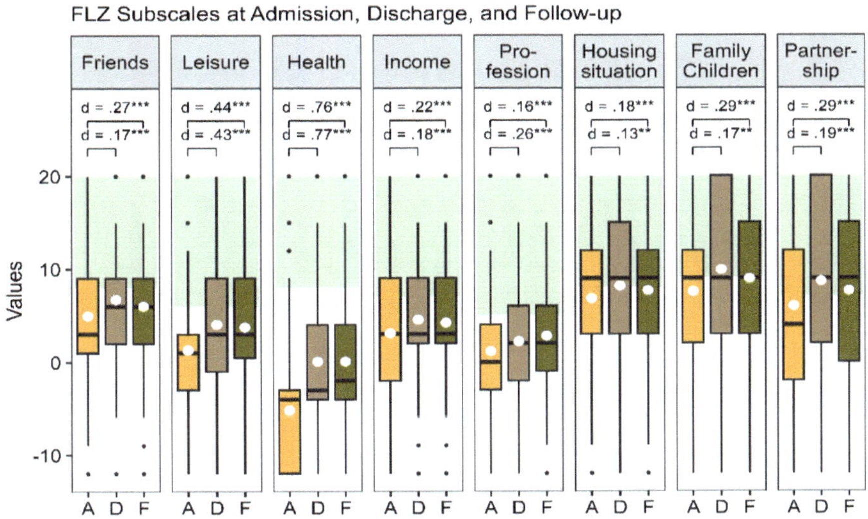

Fig. 5.27 Life satisfaction subscales over the course of 2023 (*A* admission, *D* discharge, *F* follow-up); *t*-test with paired samples; white circles indicate the mean, black lines the median; coloured background marks the desired area; significance at $*p < 0.05$, $**p < 0.01$, $***p < 0.001$; Cohen's d = effect measure ($d \geq 0.2$ = small, ≥ 0.5 = moderate, ≥ 0.8 = large)

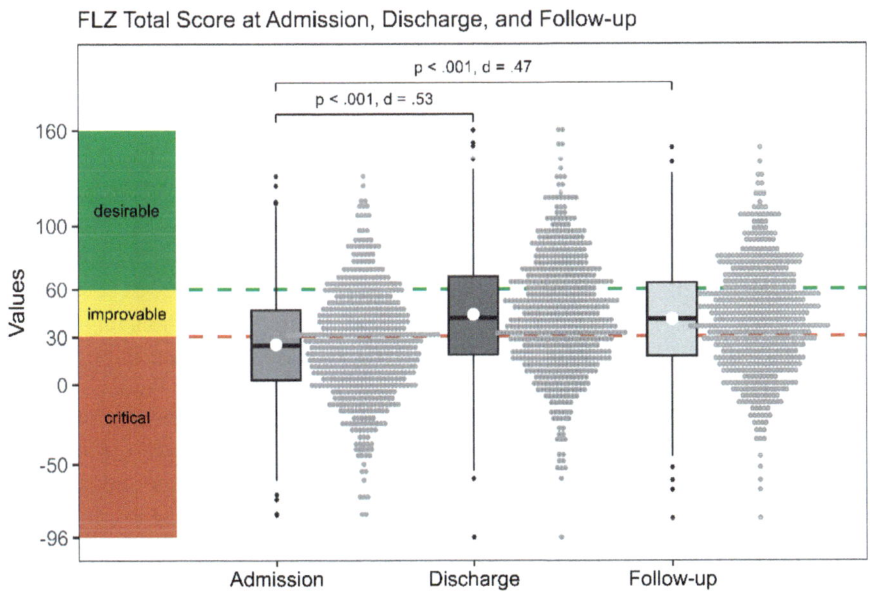

Fig. 5.28 Total FLZ score over the course of the measurement points in 2023. T-test with paired samples. Horizontal dashed lines mark the threshold values. White circles indicate the mean and black lines indicate the median. Cohen's d is the effect measure ($d \geq 0.2$ is small, $d \geq 0.5$ is moderate, and $d \geq 0.8$ is large)

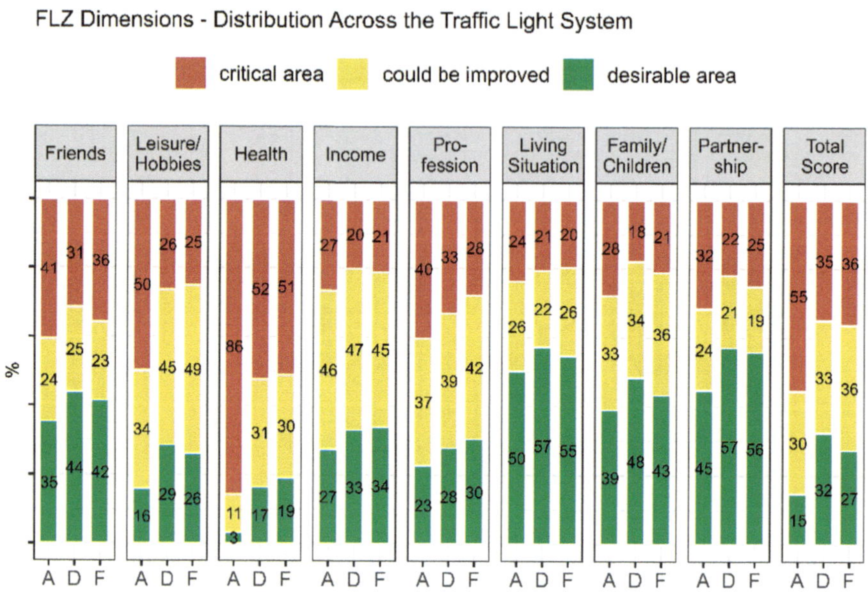

Fig. 5.29 Distribution of the FLZ scales across the levels of the traffic light system levels in 2023; *A* admission, *D* discharge, *F* follow-up

differences reveals that health literacy increases with age and is similar for men (M = 57.61, SD = 12.28) and women (M = 57.59, SD = 12.47). However, among younger patients (up to 40 years old), men demonstrate slightly higher health literacy (Fig. 5.30). Overall, both genders demonstrate deficiencies, particularly in terms of manageability, followed by meaningfulness (Fig. 5.31).

Compared to previous years, the level of sense of coherence is similar, albeit slightly lower than in previous years.

Tables 5.48 and 5.49 present the admission scores broken down by gender for all subscales and by age for the total SOC score. Figures 5.30 and 5.31 illustrate these results graphically.

The overall health literacy score, as well as those for the Meaningfulness, Comprehensibility and Manageability subscales, showed significant improvement between admission and discharge ($d = 0.37, p < 0.001$; $d = 0.30, p < 0.001$; $d = 0.35, p < 0.001$; $d = 0.31, p < 0.001$, respectively), and between admission and follow-up ($d = 0.38, p < 0.001$; $d = 0.26, p < 0.001$; $d = 0.39, p < 0.001$; $d = 0.31, p < 0.001$, respectively). The effect sizes for all scales fall within the small range and are similar to those observed in 2022 (Table 5.50). As shown in Fig. 5.32, the average overall health literacy score at admission was in the 'could be improved' range but had reached the 'desirable' range by discharge. This positive and significant development remained stable throughout the follow-up period. Figure 5.33 provides an overview of the subscales and their improvement at discharge and follow-up.

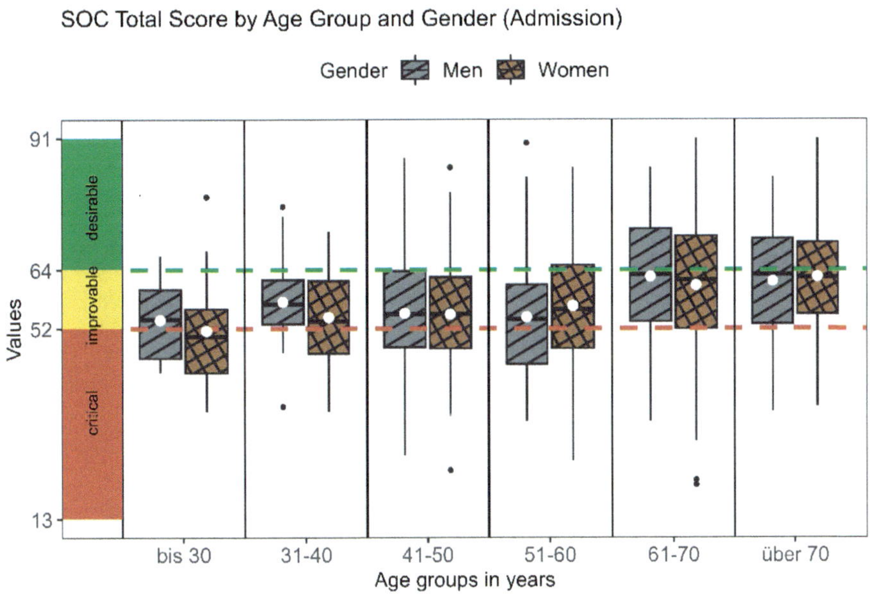

Fig. 5.30 Measures of distribution of the SOC total value in 2023 on admission, broken down by gender and age group ($n = 820$); white circles indicate the mean, the black line the median, and the coloured lines indicate the thresholds according to the traffic light system

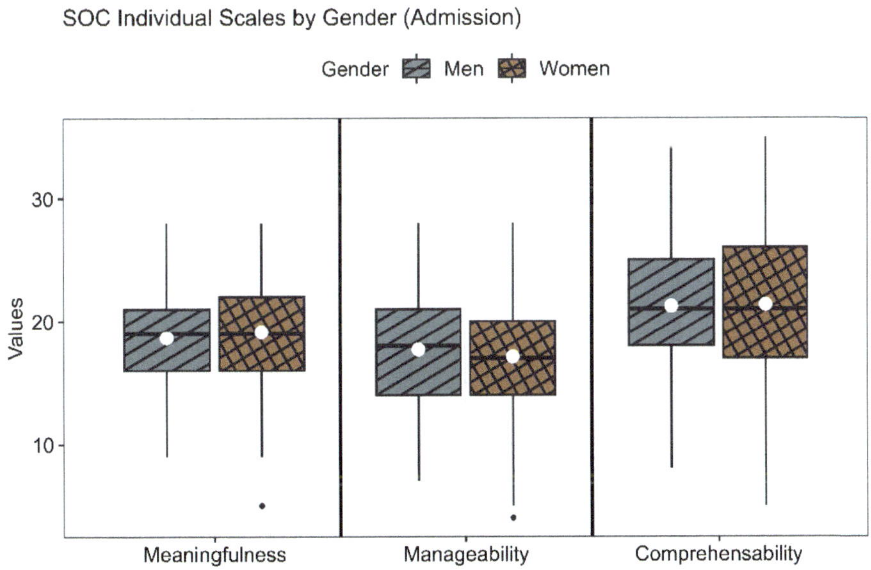

Fig. 5.31 Distribution values of the individual scales for health literacy by gender in 2023 ($n = 820$); white circles indicate the mean, the black line the median

Table 5.48 Measures of dispersion for the SOC, broken down by gender and age group for 2023 ($n = 820$) and previous years ($n = 12{,}482$)

SOC total score									
		2023				Previous years			
	Age group	*n*	M	SD	Md	*n*	M	SD	Md
Men	Up to 30	9	53.78	8.36	54.0	152	59.00	13.71	58.5
	31 to 40	13	57.46	10.84	57.0	238	56.61	13.48	56.0
	41 to 50	22	55.36	12.76	55.0	658	59.87	13.26	60.0
	51 to 60	64	54.34	11.69	54.0	1062	60.92	12.76	62.0
	61 to 70	47	62.57	11.99	63.0	677	64.71	12.65	66.0
	Over 70	15	61.67	13.43	63.0	437	67.98	11.28	69.0
	Total	**170**	**57.61**	**12.28**	**57.0**	**3224**	**62.05**	**13.14**	**63.0**
Women	Up to 30	14	51.57	11.94	50.5	423	57.35	13.96	57.0
	31 to 40	50	54.32	9.74	53.5	697	56.97	13.56	56.0
	41 to 50	95	54.95	11.66	55.0	2108	58.89	13.01	59.0
	51 to 60	280	56.57	12.23	56.0	3382	59.02	12.68	59.0
	61 to 70	153	60.85	13.24	62.0	1736	61.91	13.01	62.0
	Over 70	58	62.57	11.96	62.5	912	65.24	12.03	66.0
	Total	**650**	**57.59**	**12.47**	**57.0**	**9258**	**59.91**	**13.07**	**60.0**
Total	Up to 30	23	52.43	10.53	51.0	575	57.78	13.90	57.0
	31 to 40	63	54.97	9.97	55.0	935	56.88	13.54	56.0
	41 to 50	117	55.03	11.82	55.0	2766	59.13	13.08	59.0
	51 to 60	344	56.15	12.15	56.0	4444	59.47	12.72	59.0
	61 to 70	200	61.26	12.95	62.5	2413	62.70	12.97	63.0
	Over 70	73	62.38	12.18	63.0	1349	66.13	11.86	67.0
	Total	**820**	**57.60**	**12.42**	**57.0**	**12,482**	**60.47**	**13.12**	**61.0**

M mean, *SD* standard deviation, *Md* median

Table 5.49 Measures of dispersion for the overall value of health literacy and its sub-dimensions; separated by gender for 2023 ($n = 820$) and previous years ($n = 12{,}482$)

		2023				Previous years			
	Gender	*n*	M	SD	Md	*n*	M	SD	Md
SOC total	Males	170	57.61	12.28	57.0	3224	62.05	13.14	63.0
	Females	650	57.59	12.47	57.0	9258	59.91	13.07	60.0
	Total	820	57.60	12.42	57.0	12,482	60.47	13.12	61.0
Comprehensibility	Males	170	21.21	5.63	21.0	3224	23.38	5.85	24.0
	Females	650	21.35	5.68	21.0	9258	22.10	5.95	22.0
	Total	820	21.32	5.67	21.0	12,482	22.43	5.95	23.0
Manageability	Males	170	17.72	4.60	18.0	3224	18.74	4.84	19.0
	Females	650	17.11	4.76	17.0	9258	17.77	4.95	18.0
	Total	820	17.23	4.73	17.0	12,482	18.02	4.94	18.0
Meaningfulness	Males	170	18.68	3.99	19.0	3224	19.93	4.44	20.0
	Females	650	19.14	4.20	19.0	9258	20.04	4.29	20.0
	Total	820	19.04	4.16	19.0	12,482	20.01	4.33	20.0

M mean, *SD* standard deviation, *Md* median

Table 5.50 Sense of Coherence (SOC) in pre/post comparison in 2023; t-test for paired samples; significance at $p < 0.05$; Cohen's d = effect measure ($d \geq 0.2$ = small, ≥ 0.5 = moderate, ≥ 0.8 = large effect); previous year's data since 2022

		2023								Previous year 2022			
SOC		Cross-section: A/D/F			Course: A–D/A–F $n = 601$		Difference from admission: A–D/A–F $n = 601$			Course: A–D/A–F $n = 490$	Difference from admission: A–D/A–F $n = 490$		
		n	M	SD	M	SD	ΔM	p	d	M	ΔM	p	d
Total score	**A**	820	57.61	12.43	57.91	12.26				57.58			
	D	777	62.17	12.63	62.56	12.58	4.65	<0.001	0.37	62.49	4.91	<0.001	0.39
	F	608	62.73	12.93	62.71	12.89	4.80	<0.001	0.38	62.56	4.99	<0.001	0.39
Meaningfulness	**A**	820	19.04	4.15	19.14	4.03				19.44			
	D	777	20.27	4.10	20.35	4.07	1.21	<0.001	0.30	20.78	1.35	<0.001	0.33
	F	608	20.22	4.26	20.21	4.26	1.07	<0.001	0.26	20.33	0.89	<0.001	0.22
Comprehensibility	**A**	820	21.32	5.67	21.45	5.67				21.22			
	D	777	23.28	5.65	23.44	5.66	1.99	<0.001	0.35	23.25	2.02	<0.001	0.35
	F	608	23.72	5.84	23.72	5.82	2.47	<0.001	0.39	23.63	2.41	<0.001	0.41
Manageability	**A**	820	17.23	4.73	17.30	4.72				16.91			
	D	777	18.62	4.85	18.77	4.82	1.47	<0.001	0.31	18.46	1.55	<0.001	0.33
	F	608	18.79	4.79	18.78	4.78	1.48	<0.001	0.31	18.60	1.69	<0.001	0.36

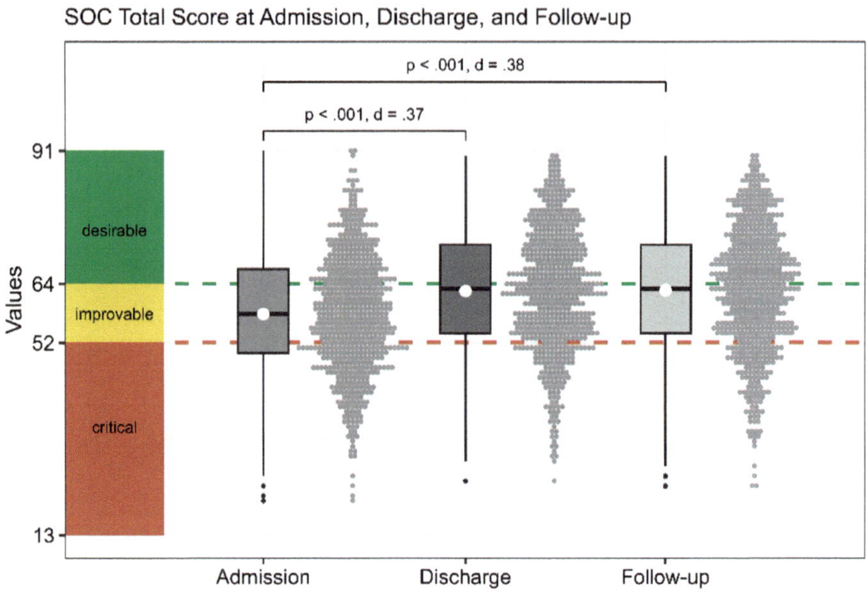

Fig. 5.32 Overall value for Sense of Coherence (SOC) over the course of the 2023 measurement points; *t*-test for paired samples; Cohen's d = effect measure ($d \geq 0.2$ = small, ≥ 0.5 = moderate, ≥ 0.8 = large effect); white circle indicates the mean, the black line the median

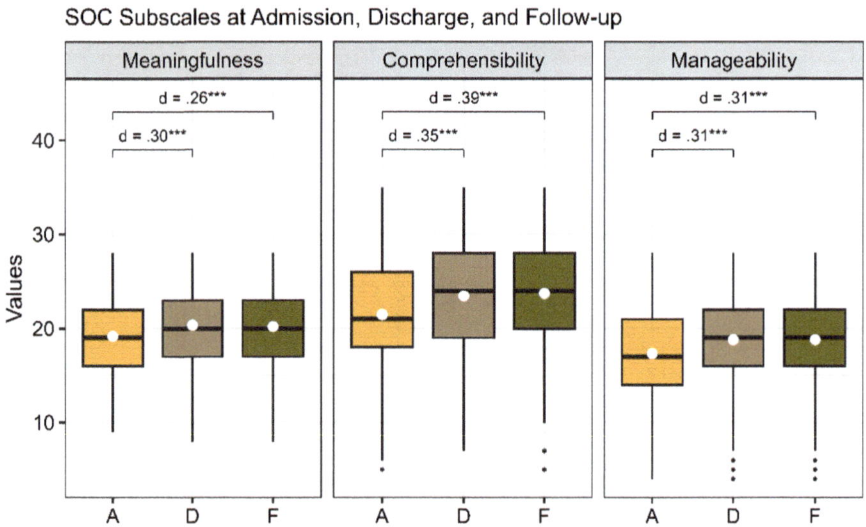

Fig. 5.33 Scales of the Sense of Coherence (SOC) over the course of the 2023 measurement points; *t*-test for paired samples; significance at $^{*}p < 0.05$, $^{**}p < 0.01$, $^{***}p < 0.001$; Cohen's d = effect measure ($d \geq 0.2$ = small, ≥ 0.5 = moderate, ≥ 0.8 = large effect); white circle indicates the mean, the black line the median; *A* admission, *D* discharge, *F* follow-up

Looking at the traffic light categories across the measurement points, we can see that, at admission, 30.9% of patients were in the desirable range. This proportion increased to 43.4% at discharge, rising further still to 46.8% at follow-up (Fig. 5.34).

5.2.1.3 Well-Being (WHO-5) and Vitality (SF-36)

Based on the traffic light system presented in the Patient Profile section of the previous chapter, both the average well-being and vitality scores fall within the critical area upon hospital admission (M = 28.78, SD = 19.35 and M = 27.78, SD = 17.78, respectively).

When broken down by gender and age group, however, noticeable differences emerge. Upon admission, men report higher levels of well-being and vitality across all age groups, except among those aged 31 to 40, where women score higher. On average, women reported a well-being score of 27.84 (SD = 18.83) and men a score of 32.40 (SD = 20.89). Women had an average vitality score of 26.84 (SD = 17.87) and men had an average vitality score of 31.38 (SD = 16.98).

For both indicators, average scores tend to increase with age. However, overall values remain below the desirable range, with vitality scores being particularly low; average values across all age groups fall within the critical range. Compared to previous years, patients in 2023 exhibit lower levels of vitality and well-being.

Table 5.51 summarises the results for the reporting year in comparing them with those from previous years. Figures 5.35 and 5.36 illustrate the figures graphically.

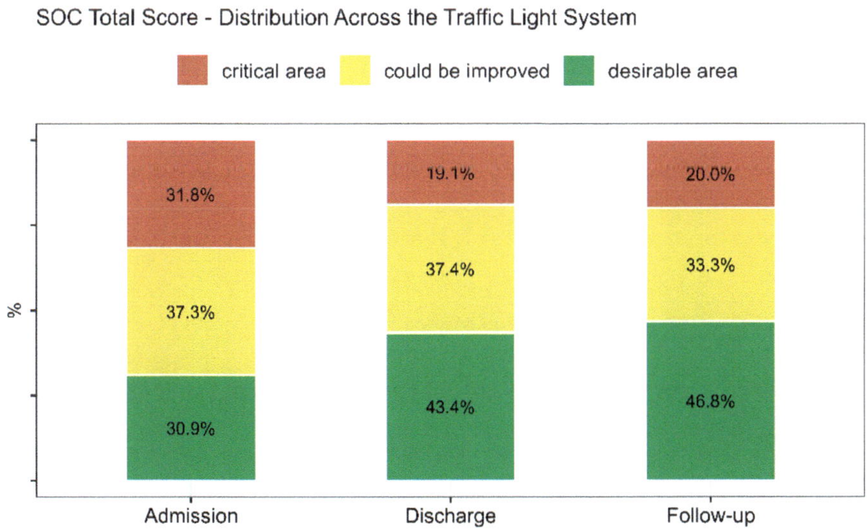

Fig. 5.34 Distribution of the SOC total score across the levels of the traffic light system levels in 2023

Table 5.51 Measures of dispersion for Well-being and Vitality, broken down by gender and age in 2023 and previous years

		Well-being								Vitality							
		2023				Previous years				2023				Previous years			
	Age group	*n*	M	SD	Md	*n*	M	SD	Md	*n*	M	SD	Md	*n*	M	SD	Md
Men	Up to 30	9	25.78	15.25	20.0	152	37.24	20.37	34.0	9	26.67	11.73	25.0	152	34.05	20.05	30.0
	31 to 40	13	21.54	15.54	16.0	232	32.66	20.89	28.0	13	21.54	15.99	20.0	232	32.28	19.18	30.0
	41 to 50	22	32.55	19.41	26.0	639	33.87	21.69	28.0	22	31.36	18.20	32.5	639	33.76	19.80	30.0
	51 to 60	64	26.62	17.43	24.0	1030	33.62	21.76	28.0	64	29.61	15.94	30.0	1030	34.01	19.50	30.0
	61 to 70	47	40.51	22.30	36.0	662	41.33	23.95	40.0	47	35.53	18.12	30.0	662	41.26	20.27	40.0
	Over 70	15	44.80	26.15	52.0	423	48.69	25.65	52.0	15	37.33	15.68	40.0	423	47.61	21.83	45.0
	Total	**170**	**32.40**	**20.89**	**28.0**	**3138**	**37.43**	**23.28**	**32.0**	**170**	**31.38**	**16.98**	**30.0**	**3138**	**37.20**	**20.68**	**35.0**
Women	Up to 30	14	22.00	13.47	18.0	414	33.80	20.18	32.0	14	19.64	8.87	20.0	414	32.04	19.39	30.0
	31 to 40	50	26.48	16.79	22.0	686	29.50	19.54	24.0	50	24.30	15.68	20.0	686	28.20	18.29	25.0
	41 to 50	96	24.96	17.22	20.0	2067	30.22	19.60	24.0	96	24.32	15.85	20.0	2067	28.70	18.14	25.0
	51 to 60	280	27.69	18.42	24.0	3343	29.88	19.39	24.0	280	26.38	17.69	25.0	3343	29.90	17.63	30.0
	61 to 70	153	30.20	20.87	24.0	1709	35.48	22.37	32.0	153	29.35	19.78	30.0	1708	36.24	19.19	35.0
	Over 70	59	29.69	19.99	28.0	892	37.96	23.38	32.0	59	30.51	18.91	30.0	892	38.02	20.25	40.0
	Total	**652**	**27.84**	**18.83**	**24.0**	**9111**	**31.95**	**20.69**	**28.0**	**652**	**26.84**	**17.87**	**25.0**	**9110**	**31.58**	**18.76**	**30.0**
Total	Up to 30	23	23.48	13.98	20	566	34.72	20.27	32.0	23	22.39	10.43	20.0	566	32.58	19.57	30.0
	31 to 40	63	25.46	16.54	20	918	30.30	19.92	24.0	63	23.73	15.66	20.0	918	29.23	18.60	25.0
	41 to 50	118	26.37	17.81	20	2706	31.08	20.17	28.0	118	25.64	16.47	20.0	2706	29.89	18.66	30.0
	51 to 60	344	27.49	18.22	24	4373	30.76	20.03	28.0	344	26.98	17.40	25.0	4373	30.87	18.17	30.0
	61 to 70	200	32.62	21.60	24	2371	37.11	22.97	32.0	200	30.80	19.54	30.0	2370	37.65	19.62	35.0
	Over 70	74	32.76	22.05	30	1315	41.41	24.64	40.0	74	31.89	18.41	35.0	1315	41.10	21.24	40.0
	Total	**822**	**28.78**	**19.35**	**24.0**	**12,249**	**33.35**	**21.52**	**28.0**	**822**	**27.78**	**17.78**	**25.0**	**12,248**	**33.02**	**19.43**	**30.0**

M mean, *SD* standard deviation, *Md* median

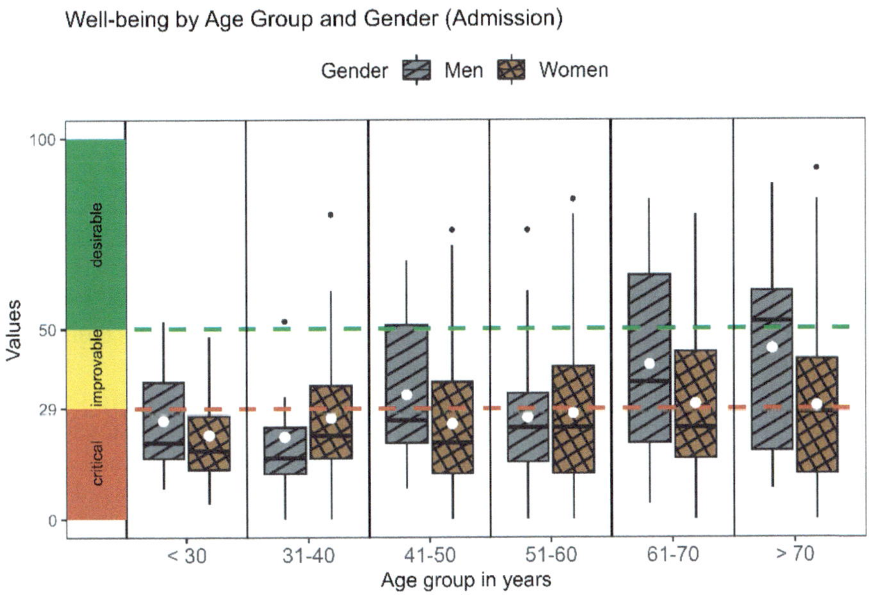

Fig. 5.35 Distribution of well-being (WHO-5) on admission in 2023, broken down by gender and age group. White circles indicate the mean and black lines indicate the median. Coloured lines indicate the thresholds according to the traffic light system

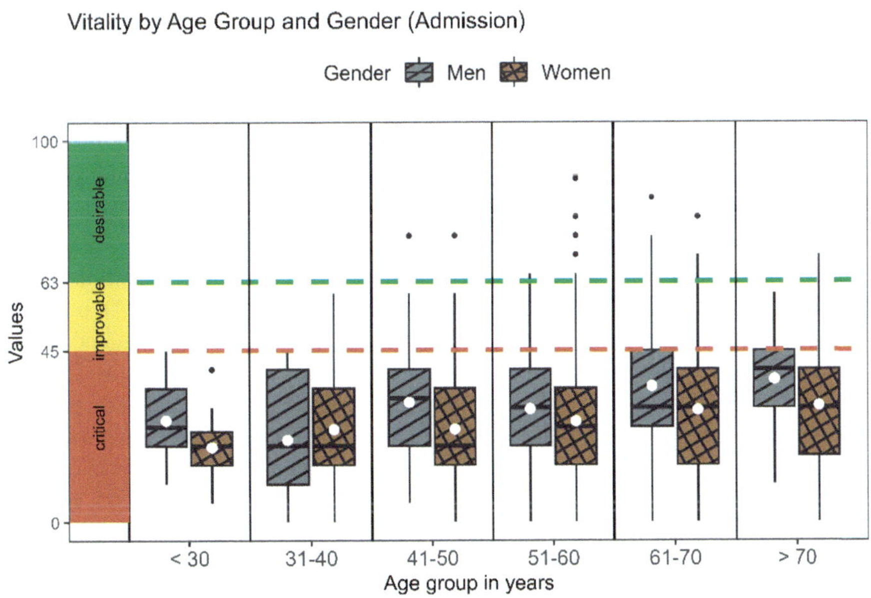

Fig. 5.36 Distribution of vitality (SF-36) on admission in 2023, broken down by gender and age group. White circles indicate the mean and black lines the median; the coloured lines indicate the thresholds according to the traffic light system

There was a significant improvement in both well-being and vitality, with a large effect size observed between hospital admission and discharge ($d = 1.22$, $p < 0.001$; $d = 0.97$, $p < 0.001$, respectively). By the time of the follow-up, the effect had diminished somewhat but was still moderate to large ($d = 0.76$, $p < 0.001$; $d = 0.74$, $p < 0.001$) (Table 5.52).

At the time of hospital admission, patients' well-being was, on average, at the threshold of the critical range. At hospital discharge, it was in the desirable range. At follow-up, it was just below this range (Fig. 5.37). A similar pattern was observed in vitality. At hospital admission, average vitality scores were clearly within the critical range. By discharge, they had improved to the 'could be improved' range. However, by the follow-up assessment, they had declined slightly again, falling just below that threshold (Fig. 5.38).

Taking a closer look at the distribution within the traffic light categories reveals that the proportion of patients in the desired range has increased significantly (Fig. 5.39). In terms of well-being, this proportion increased more than fourfold, rising from 14.1% to 59.6% by the time of discharge. Even at the follow-up stage, more than three times as many patients were in the desired range compared to before they were admitted to the clinic (42.7%).

Regarding vitality, only 3.7% of patients were in a desirable state upon admission. By the time of discharge, this proportion had increased to 26.2%—a rise of more than sevenfold. Although this figure declined slightly to 20.4% at follow-up, it still represented a more than fivefold improvement on the initial figure. Conversely, the proportion of patients in a critical state of vitality had almost halved by discharge, dropping from 82.1% to 42.2%. While 51.2% of patients remained in a critical state at the follow-up appointment, this still represented a significant improvement compared to their condition at admission.

5.2.1.4 Self-Efficacy, Optimism, Pessimism (SWOP)

Tables 5.53 and 5.54 present the dispersion measures for all SWOP scales for patients in the 2023 reporting year, differentiated by gender and age group. The average self-efficacy value in 2023 was 12.44 (SD = 3.01; in previous years, the average was 13.16, with an SD of 3.02). The respective averages for optimism and pessimism were 5.02 (SD = 1.46; previous years: M = 5.33, SD = 1.47) and 4.45 (SD = 1.41; previous years: M = 4.42, SD = 1.34). The mean optimism and pessimism scores fall within the 'could be improved' range for all age groups. The figures for self-efficacy show a similar pattern. However, on average, only women across all age groups fall into the 'could be improved' range, whereas this was only true for men in the 41–60 age group. Overall, men reported higher levels of self-efficacy than women (M = 13.01, SD = 2.76 and M = 12.29, SD = 3.05, respectively). Gender differences in optimism and pessimism are less pronounced and vary depending on the age group. Figures 5.40, 5.41, and 5.42 illustrate the self-efficacy, optimism, and pessimism values upon admission, broken down by gender and age group.

Table 5.52 Well-being and vitality in the before/after comparison in 2023; t-test for paired samples; significance at $p < 0.05$; *Cohen's d = effect measure ($d \geq 0.2$ = small, ≥ 0.5 = moderate, ≥ 0.8 = large effect); previous year's data since 2022

		2023								Previous year 2022			
		Cross-section: A/D/F			Course: A–D/A–F n = 602		Difference from admission: A–D/A–F n = 602			Course: A–D/A–F n = 493	Difference from admission: A–D/A–F n = 493		
		n	M	SD	M	SD	ΔM	p	d	M	ΔM	p	d
Well-being	**A**	822	28.78	19.35	28.62	18.54				27.93			
	D	777	53.29	23.45	54.55	23.12	25.93	<0.001	**1.22**	55.73	27.81	<0.001	**1.30**
	F	610	45.55	24.27	45.46	24.28	16.84	<0.001	**0.76**	45.99	18.06	<0.001	**0.82**
Vitality	**A**	822	27.78	17.78	27.96	17.29				27.56			
	D	777	46.09	22.11	47.42	21.77	19.46	<0.001	**0.97**	48.55	20.99	<0.001	**1.04**
	F	610	43.39	22.71	43.31	22.72	15.35	<0.001	**0.74**	42.70	15.14	<0.001	**0.75**

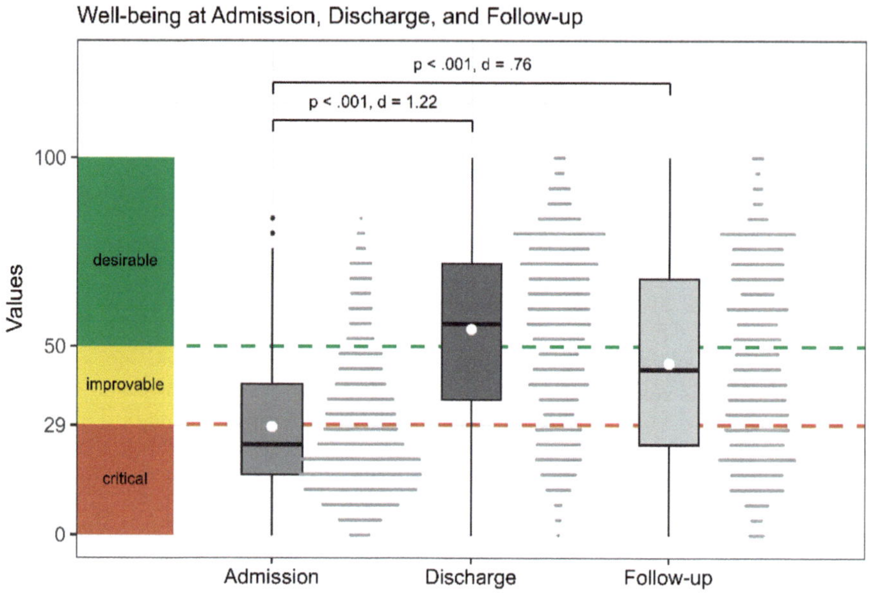

Fig. 5.37 Well-being over the course of the measurement points in 2023; t-test with paired samples; significance at $p < 0.05$; Cohen's d = effect measure ($d \geq 0.2$ = small, ≥ 0.5 = moderate, ≥ 0.8 = large effect); white circle indicates the mean, the black line the median; the coloured lines indicate the thresholds according to the traffic light system

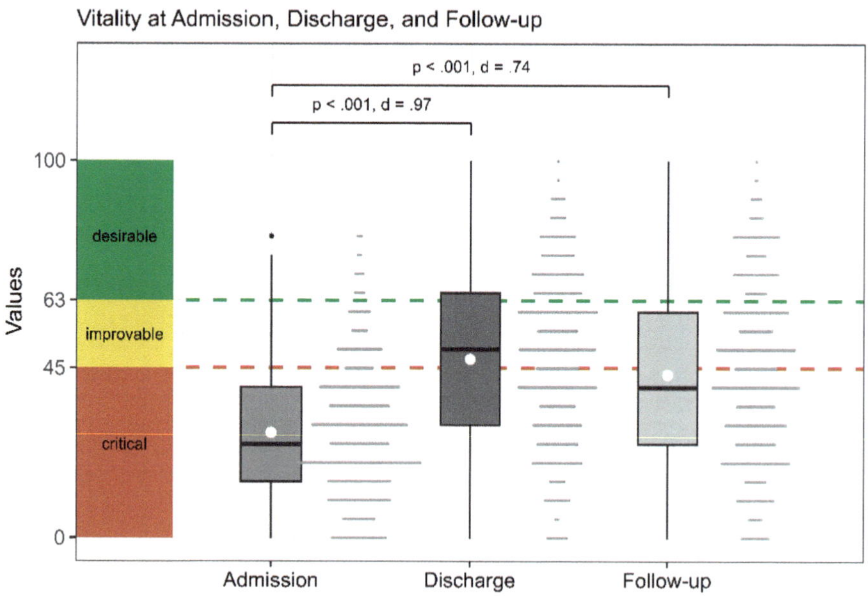

Fig. 5.38 Vitality over the course of the measurement points in 2023; t-test with paired samples; significance at $p < 0.05$; Cohen's d = effect measure ($d \geq 0.2$ = small, ≥ 0.5 = moderate, ≥ 0.8 = large effect); white circle indicates the mean, the black line the median; the coloured lines indicate the thresholds according to the traffic light system

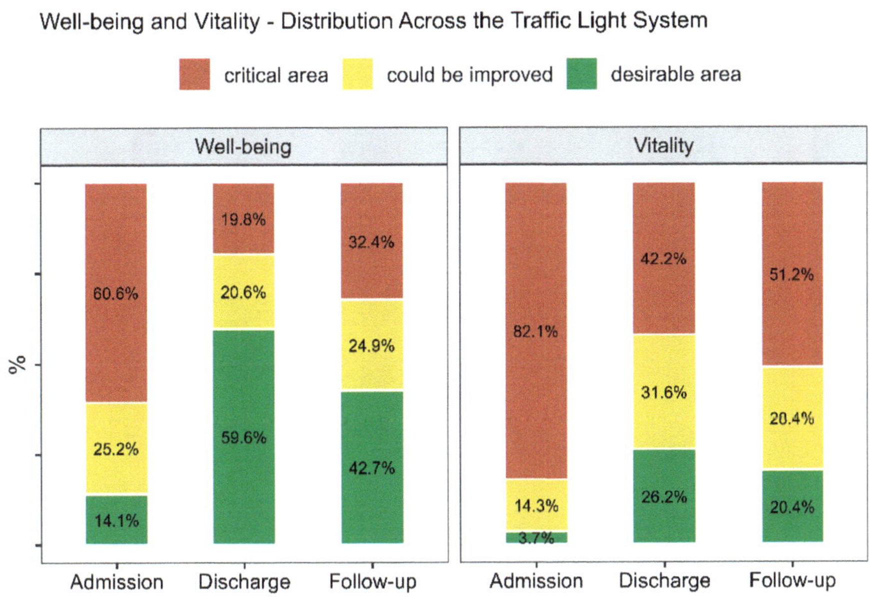

Fig. 5.39 Distribution of well-being and vitality across the levels of the traffic light system in 2023

Table 5.53 Measures of distribution for self-efficacy, broken down by gender and age in 2023 and previous years

Self-efficacy									
		2023				Previous years			
	Age group	*n*	M	SD	Md	*n*	M	SD	Md
Men	Up to 30	9	13.44	2.55	14.0	152	13.72	2.85	14.0
	31 to 40	13	13.23	2.42	14.0	232	13.50	2.97	14.0
	41 to 50	22	12.86	3.09	13.0	640	13.73	2.92	14.0
	51 to 60	64	12.17	2.26	12.0	1029	13.67	2.93	14.0
	61 to 70	47	13.70	3.09	14.0	662	14.49	2.81	15.0
	Over 70	15	14.20	2.86	15.0	424	15.38	2.72	15.0
	Total	**170**	**13.01**	**2.76**	**13.0**	**3139**	**14.08**	**2.94**	**15.0**
Women	Up to 30	14	11.50	3.16	11.0	414	12.77	2.93	13.0
	31 to 40	50	11.80	2.98	11.0	685	12.65	2.87	13.0
	41 to 50	96	12.25	3.09	12.0	2066	12.72	2.86	13.0
	51 to 60	279	12.25	3.12	13.0	3340	12.66	2.93	13.0
	61 to 70	153	12.57	2.81	13.0	1706	13.09	3.11	13.0
	Over 70	59	12.47	3.32	13.0	891	13.59	3.14	14.0
	Total	**651**	**12.29**	**3.05**	**13.0**	**9102**	**12.85**	**2.98**	**13.0**
Total	Up to 30	23	12.26	3.03	12.0	566	13.02	2.93	13.0
	31 to 40	63	12.10	2.92	12.0	917	12.86	2.92	13.0
	41 to 50	118	12.36	3.08	12.0	2706	12.96	2.91	13.0
	51 to 60	343	12.24	2.97	12.0	4369	12.89	2.96	13.0
	61 to 70	200	12.84	2.91	13.0	2368	13.48	3.09	14.0
	Over 70	74	12.82	3.29	13.0	1315	14.17	3.12	15.0
	Total	**821**	**12.44**	**3.01**	**13.0**	**12,241**	**13.16**	**3.02**	**13.0**

M mean, *SD* standard deviation, *Md* median

Table 5.54 Measures of distribution for optimism and pessimism, broken down by gender and age in 2023 and previous years

		Optimism								Pessimism							
		2023				Previous years				2023				Previous years			
	Age group	*n*	M	SD	Md	*n*	M	SD	Md	*n*	M	SD	Md	*n*	M	SD	Md
Men	Up to 30	9	5.33	1.22	5.0	152	5.22	1.56	5.0	9	4.67	1.50	5.0	152	4.47	1.21	4.0
	31 to 40	13	5.23	1.36	6.0	232	4.92	1.56	5.0	13	4.69	0.95	5.0	232	4.64	1.30	5.0
	41 to 50	22	4.86	1.83	4.0	640	5.21	1.48	5.0	22	4.50	1.74	4.0	640	4.42	1.30	4.0
	51 to 60	64	4.58	1.40	4.5	1029	5.30	1.43	6.0	64	4.62	1.60	4.0	1029	4.47	1.29	4.0
	61 to 70	47	5.11	1.55	5.0	662	5.51	1.46	6.0	47	4.13	1.47	4.0	662	4.46	1.29	4.0
	Over 70	15	4.80	1.97	4.0	424	6.03	1.46	6.0	15	4.13	1.60	4.0	424	4.50	1.46	4.0
	Total	**170**	**4.87**	**1.55**	**5.0**	**3139**	**5.39**	**1.50**	**6.0**	**170**	**4.44**	**1.53**	**4.0**	**3139**	**4.47**	**1.31**	**4.0**
Women	Up to 30	14	4.14	1.10	4.0	414	5.15	1.51	5.0	14	5.07	1.33	5.0	414	4.31	1.32	4.0
	31 to 40	50	4.84	1.36	5.0	685	5.15	1.54	5.0	50	4.34	1.47	4.0	685	4.45	1.38	4.0
	41 to 50	96	4.96	1.47	5.0	2066	5.29	1.38	6.0	96	4.46	1.28	4.0	2066	4.28	1.33	4.0
	51 to 60	279	5.07	1.42	5.0	3340	5.22	1.42	5.0	279	4.42	1.39	4.0	3340	4.42	1.32	4.0
	61 to 70	153	5.14	1.47	5.0	1706	5.41	1.49	6.0	153	4.48	1.35	4.0	1706	4.45	1.40	4.0
	Over 70	59	5.37	1.46	6.0	891	5.65	1.55	6.0	59	4.47	1.42	4.0	891	4.58	1.39	5.0
	Total	**651**	**5.06**	**1.44**	**5.0**	**9102**	**5.31**	**1.46**	**6.0**	**651**	**4.45**	**1.37**	**4.0**	**9102**	**4.41**	**1.35**	**4.0**
Total	Up to 30	23	4.61	1.27	4.0	566	5.17	1.52	5.0	23	4.91	1.38	5.0	566	4.35	1.29	4.0
	31 to 40	63	4.92	1.36	5.0	917	5.09	1.55	5.0	63	4.41	1.38	4.0	917	4.50	1.36	4.0
	41 to 50	118	4.94	1.54	5.0	2706	5.27	1.41	6.0	118	4.47	1.37	4.0	2706	4.32	1.32	4.0
	51 to 60	343	4.98	1.43	5.0	4369	5.24	1.43	6.0	343	4.45	1.43	4.0	4369	4.43	1.32	4.0
	61 to 70	200	5.13	1.49	5.0	2368	5.44	1.48	6.0	200	4.40	1.38	4.0	2368	4.45	1.37	4.0
	Over 70	74	5.26	1.58	6.0	1315	5.77	1.53	6.0	74	4.41	1.45	4.0	1315	4.56	1.41	5.0
	Total	**821**	**5.02**	**1.46**	**5.0**	**12,241**	**5.33**	**1.47**	**6.0**	**851**	**4.45**	**1.41**	**4.0**	**12,241**	**4.42**	**1.34**	**4.0**

M mean, *SD* standard deviation, *Md* median

Significant improvements were observed for all three SWOP subscales, with a small effect size (Table 5.55). The greatest improvement was observed in optimism at discharge ($d = 0.47$, $p < 0.001$), followed by self-efficacy ($d = 0.38$, $p < 0.001$). The change in pessimism was less pronounced ($d = -0.25$, $p < 0.001$). While the positive effect for optimism decreased slightly by follow-up ($d = 0.36$, $p < 0.001$), improvements in self-efficacy remained stable over time ($d = 0.38$, $p < 0.001$).

As can be seen in Fig. 5.43, the average self-efficacy value has risen from the 'could be improved' area to the 'desirable' area. For optimism and pessimism, the mean value remains in the 'improvable' range but is closer to the target value. Overall, the proportion of patients with 'critical' self-efficacy scores halved from 14.6% at admission to 7.7% at discharge, falling further to 7.2% at follow-up. Similarly, scores within the red area of the traffic light system halved for optimism, falling from 11.4% at admission to 5.0% at discharge and 6.4% at follow-up. Figure 5.44 provides an overview of the distribution across the traffic light system for all scales and measurement points.

5.2.1.5 Social Support (SSS)

The patients at the TCM-Klinik Bad Kötzting reported an average level of social support of 53.15 (SD = 17.08; in previous years, the average was 55.45 with an SD

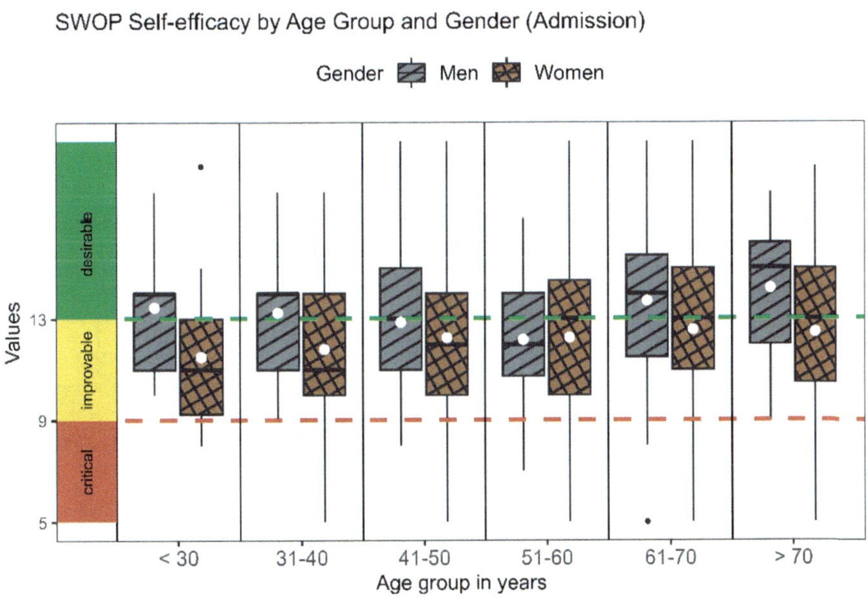

Fig. 5.40 Distribution of self-efficacy (SWOP9) at admission in 2023, broken down by gender and age group. White circles indicate the mean and black lines indicate the median. Coloured lines indicate the thresholds according to the traffic light system

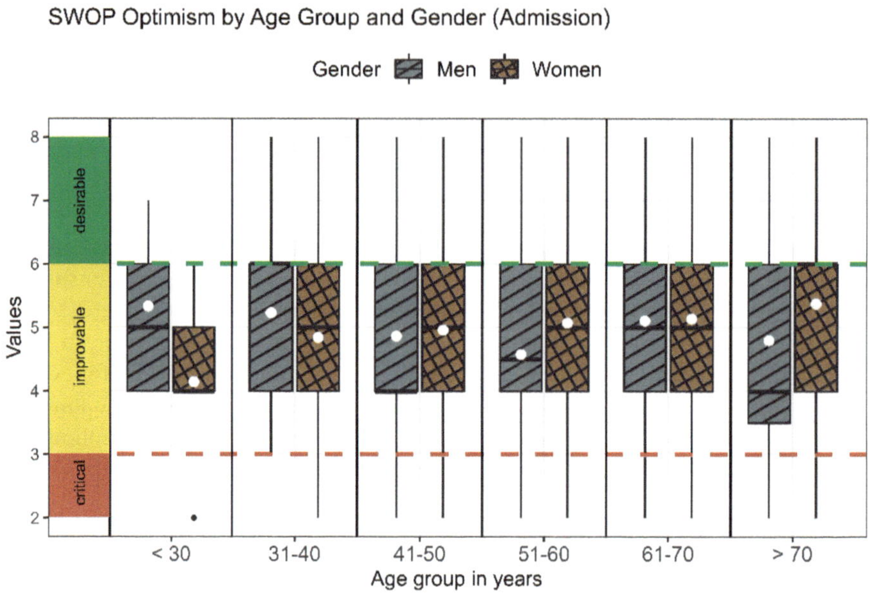

Fig. 5.41 Distribution of optimism (SWOP9) at admission in 2023, broken down by gender and age group. White circles indicate the mean, black lines the median; the coloured lines indicate the thresholds according to the traffic light system

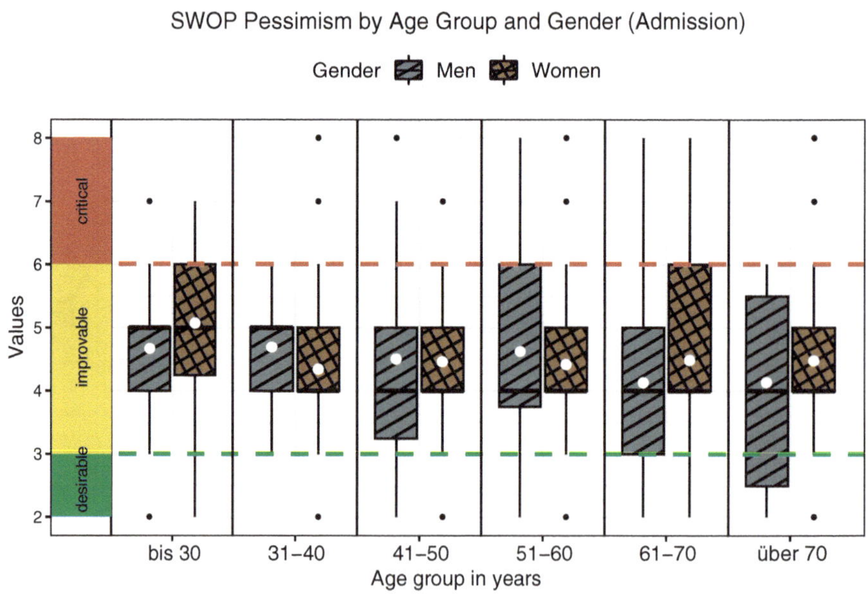

Fig. 5.42 Distribution of pessimism (SWOP9) at admission in 2023, broken down by gender and age group; white circles indicate the mean, black lines the median; the coloured lines indicate the thresholds according to the traffic light system

Table 5.55 SWOP scales in the before/after comparison in 2023; *t*-test for paired samples; significance at $p < 0.05$; Cohen's d = effect measure ($d \geq 0.2$ = small, ≥ 0.5 = moderate, ≥ 0.8 = large effect); previous year's data since 2022

SWOP		2023								Previous year 2022			
		Cross-section: A/D/F			Course: A–D/A–F $n = 597$		Difference from admission: A–D/A–F $n = 597$			Course: A–D/A–F $n = 490$	Difference from admission: A–D/A–F $n = 490$		
		n	M	SD	M	SD	ΔM	*p*	*d*	M	ΔM	*p*	*d*
Self-efficacy	**A**	821	12.44	3.01	12.48	2.34				12.52			
	D	777	13.44	2.79	13.54	2.74	1.06	<0.001	0.38	13.62	1.10	<0.001	0.39
	F	605	13.57	2.75	13.55	2.75	1.07	<0.001	0.38	13.72	1.20	<0.001	0.43
Optimism	**A**	821	5.02	1.46	5.04	1.44				5.15			
	D	777	5.68	1.40	5.70	1.39	0.66	<0.001	0.47	5.64	0.50	<0.001	0.35
	F	605	5.55	1.39	5.54	1.39	0.50	<0.001	0.36	5.64	0.49	<0.001	0.35
Pessimism	**A**	821	4.45	1.41	4.43	1.39				4.51			
	D	777	4.13	1.39	4.09	1.39	−0.35	<0.001	−0.25	4.17	−0.34	<0.001	−0.24
	F	605	4.20	1.42	4.22	1.41	−0.22	<0.001	−0.16	4.30	−0.21	<0.001	−0.15

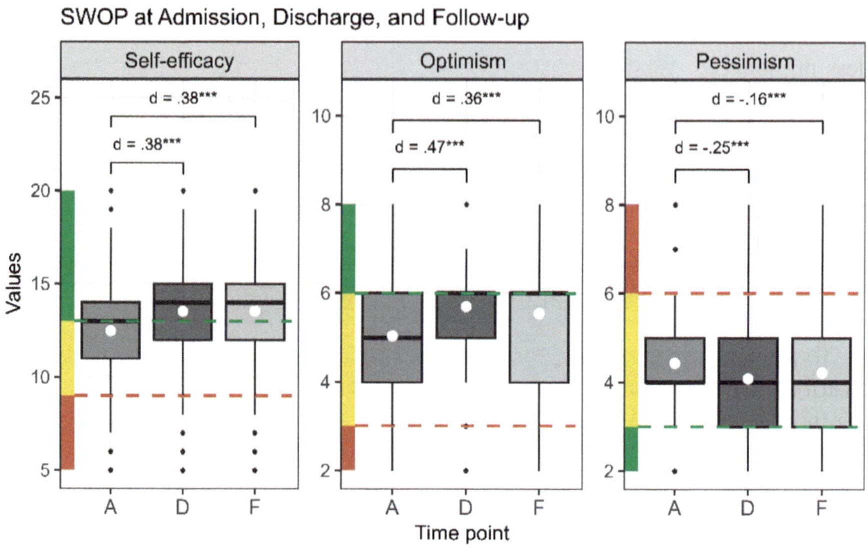

Fig. 5.43 SWOP scales over the course of the measurement points in 2023 (*A* admission, *D* discharge, *F* follow-up); *t*-test with paired samples; significance at $*p < 0.05$, $**p < 0.01$, $***p < 0.001$; Cohen's d = effect measure ($d \geq 0.2$ = small, ≥ 0.5 = moderate, ≥ 0.8 = large effect); red segment and line indicate the critical area, yellow the improvable area, and green the desirable area

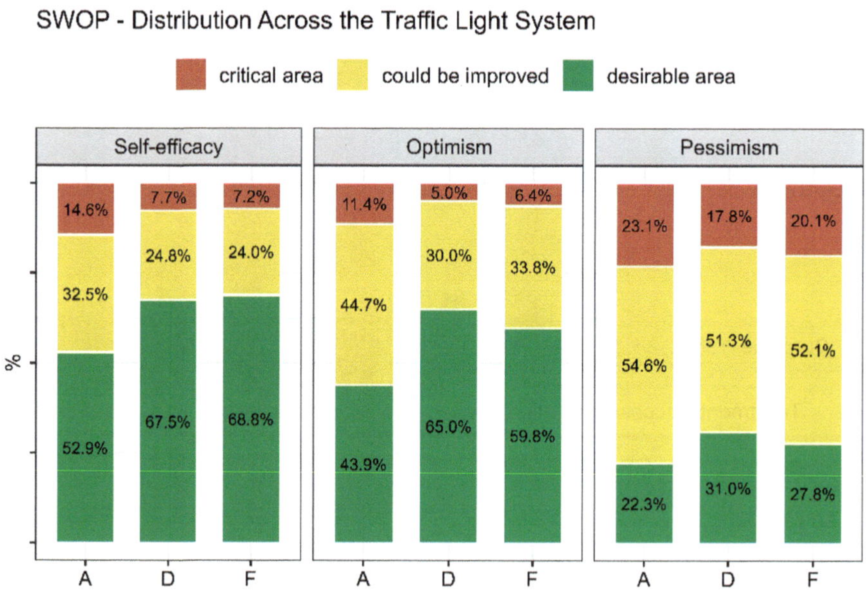

Fig. 5.44 Distribution of the SWOP scales across the levels of the traffic light system in 2023; *A* admission, *D* discharge, *F* follow-up

of 16.05). According to the traffic light system, this falls into the upper part of the 'could be improved' range. As illustrated in Fig. 5.45, there were no substantial differences across age groups, with all reporting levels of social support around the threshold between the 'improvable' and 'desirable' ranges. Although generally similar, men had slightly higher social support than women (M = 54.75, SD = 18.77; M = 52.73, SD = 16.60, respectively). The largest gender difference was observed among those aged over 70, with men indicating higher levels of social support (M = 57.07, SD = 17.49) than women (M = 49.03, SD = 17.12) (Table 5.56). Overall, the data show that social support among men needs improvement, particularly among those aged 31–40 and 51–60. For women, desirable levels of social support were only evident among those aged 30 or under.

Furthermore, men and women reported similar levels of social support across all subscales (Fig. 5.46 and Table 5.57), although men reported slightly higher levels of support in all areas except for the additional question about the number of people from whom one can expect support.

A comparison of the patients' assessment of their social support at admission and discharge shows a significant improvement ($d = 0.28$, $p < 0.001$), with an average improvement into the 'desirable' range. However, it drops back into the 'improvable' range by follow-up, indicating only a negligible, albeit significant, effect ($d = 0.13$, $p < 0.001$) (Fig. 5.47, Table 5.58). While there was no change in the emotional dimension of social support up to the follow-up assessment ($p = 0.084$), the

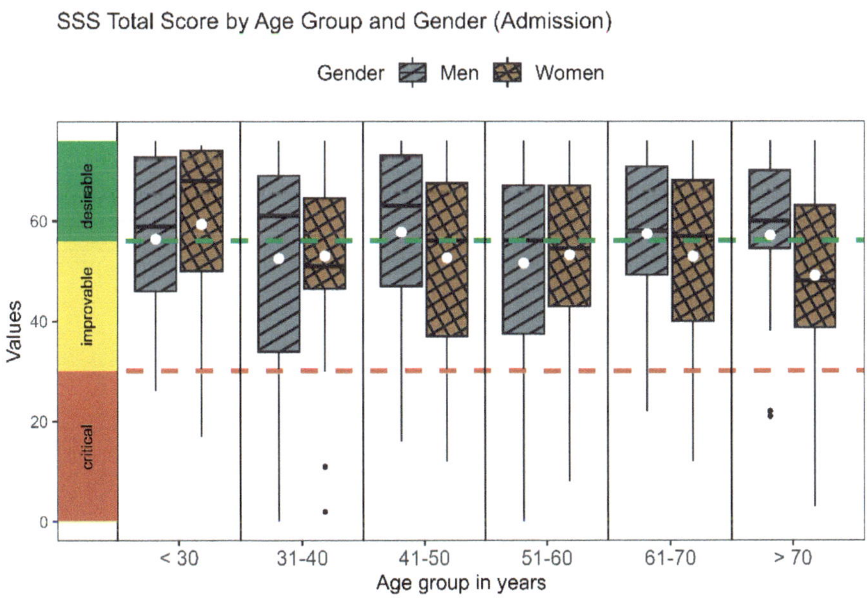

Fig. 5.45 Distribution of the social support protection factor (SSS) in the 2023 reporting year at admission, broken down by gender and age group; white circles indicate the mean, black lines the median; the coloured lines indicate the thresholds according to the traffic light system

Table 5.56 Measures of distribution for social support (total score), broken down by gender and age in 2023 and previous years

SSS total score									
		2023				Previous years			
	Age group	*n*	M	SD	Md	*n*	M	SD	Md
Men	Up to 30	8	56.38	18.84	59.0	152	56.5	15.8	59.0
	31 to 40	13	52.46	23.19	61.0	236	56.7	15.4	59.5
	41 to 50	21	57.76	16.96	63.0	657	55.1	15.7	57.0
	51 to 60	63	51.51	20.85	56.0	1056	56.1	16.2	59.0
	61 to 70	46	57.41	15.50	58.0	672	59.1	15.4	63.0
	Over 70	15	57.07	17.49	60.0	434	61.9	15.4	67.0
	Total	**166**	**54.75**	**18.77**	**58.0**	**3207**	**57.4**	**15.9**	**61.0**
Women	Up to 30	13	59.31	18.32	68.0	421	61.8	13.6	65.0
	31 to 40	48	52.92	15.81	51.0	696	56.3	14.6	58.0
	41 to 50	95	52.56	17.43	56.0	2099	54.5	15.7	56.0
	51 to 60	270	53.18	15.92	54.5	3358	53.2	16.1	55.0
	61 to 70	149	52.85	17.16	57.0	1733	55.6	16.4	58.0
	Over 70	58	49.03	17.12	48.0	910	55.2	17.2	59.0
	Total	**633**	**52.73**	**16.60**	**55.0**	**9217**	**54.8**	**16.1**	**57.0**
Total	Up to 30	21	58.19	18.11	63.0	573	60.4	14.4	64.0
	31 to 40	61	52.82	17.42	52.0	932	56.4	14.8	58.0
	41 to 50	116	53.50	17.39	56.0	2756	54.7	15.7	56.0
	51 to 60	333	52.86	16.94	55.0	4414	53.9	16.1	56.0
	61 to 70	195	53.92	16.86	58.0	2405	56.6	16.2	60.0
	Over 70	73	50.68	17.39	53.0	1344	57.3	16.9	62.0
	Total	**799**	**53.15**	**17.08**	**56.0**	**12,424**	**55.5**	**16.1**	**58.0**

M mean, *SD* standard deviation, *Md* median

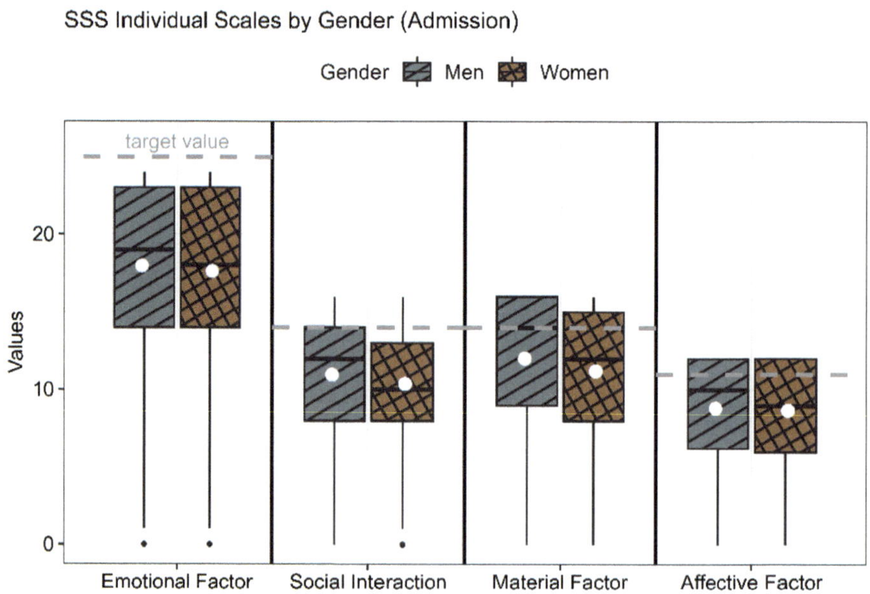

Fig. 5.46 Distribution values of the individual scales for social support, broken down by gender in 2023; white circles indicate the mean, black lines the median; the grey lines indicate the threshold value for the desirable area according to the traffic light system

Table 5.57 Measures of distribution for social support including all subscales, broken down by gender in 2023 and previous years

		2023				Previous years			
SSS	Gender	*n*	M	SD	Md	*n*	M	SD	Md
Total score	Men	166	54.75	18.77	58	3207	57.38	15.89	61.0
	Women	633	52.73	16.60	55	9217	54.78	16.05	57.0
	Total	799	53.15	17.08	56	12,424	55.45	16.05	58.0
Emotional	Men	166	17.96	5.90	19	3207	21.22	6.23	22.0
	Women	633	17.62	5.49	18	9217	20.73	6.18	21.0
	Total	799	17.69	5.58	18	12,424	20.86	6.19	22.0
Social interaction	Men	166	10.95	4.09	12	3207	11.60	3.72	12.0
	Women	633	10.37	3.70	10	9218	10.86	3.68	11.0
	Total	799	10.49	3.79	11	12,425	11.05	3.70	12.0
Material	Men	166	12.02	4.75	14	3207	13.10	3.91	15.0
	Women	633	11.20	4.47	12	9218	11.98	4.20	13.0
	Total	799	11.37	4.54	12	12,425	12.27	4.16	13.0
Affective	Men	166	8.83	3.36	10	3207	9.29	3.03	10.0
	Women	633	8.68	3.12	9	9218	8.94	3.04	10.0
	Total	799	8.71	3.17	9	12,425	9.03	3.04	10.0
Additional question	Men	170	3.39	2.57	3	3216	3.86	3.57	3.0
	Women	652	3.78	2.41	3	9246	4.23	3.62	3.0
	Total	822	3.70	2.45	3	12,462	4.13	3.61	3.0

M mean, *SD* standard deviation, *Md* median

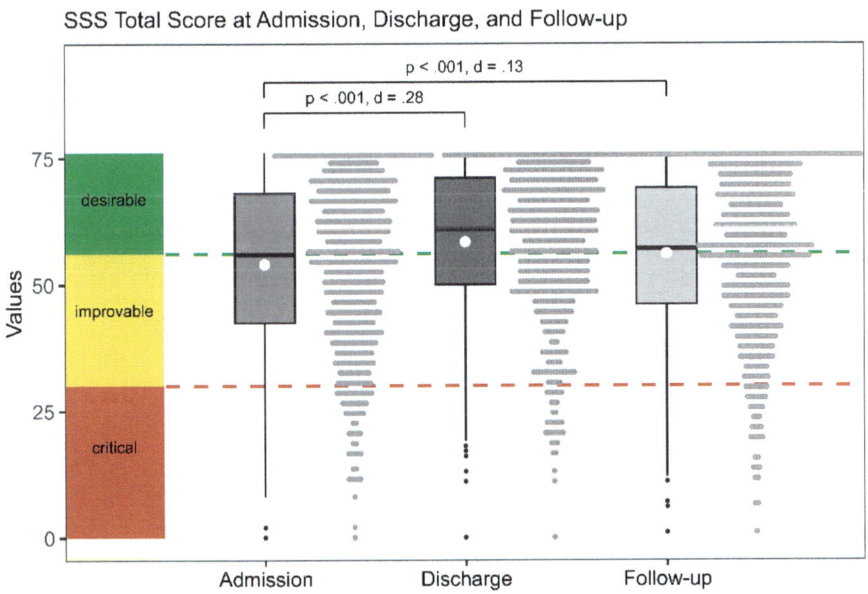

Fig. 5.47 Total social support score (SSS) over the course of the measurement time points in 2023; *t*-test with paired samples; Cohen's *d* = effect measure ($d \geq 0.2$ = small, ≥ 0.5 = moderate, ≥ 0.8 = large effect); white circle indicates the mean, the black line the median

Table 5.58 Social support scale before/after comparison in 2023; t-test for paired samples; significance at $p < 0.05$; Cohen's d = effect measure ($d \geq 0.2$ = small, ≥ 0.5 = moderate, ≥ 0.8 = large effect); previous year's data since 2022

SSS		2023								Previous year 2022			
		Cross-section: A/D/F			Course: A–D/A–F $n = 602$		Difference from admission: A–D/A–F $n = 602$			Course: A–D/A–F $n = 460$	Difference from admission: A–D/A–F $n = 460$		
		n	M	SD	M	SD	ΔM	p	d	M	ΔM	p	d
Total score	**A**	799	53.15	17.08	54.02	16.43				53.15			
	D	777	57.95	15.35	58.41	14.92	4.38	<0.001	0.28	57.95	4.60	<0.001	0.28
	F	602	56.10	15.62	56.07	15.63	2.04	<0.001	0.13	57.33	2.90	<0.001	0.18
Emotional	**A**	799	17.69	5.58	17.97	5.42				17.69			
	D	777	18.80	5.11	18.94	5.00	0.97	<0.001	0.19	18.80	1.29	<0.001	0.24
	F	602	18.27	5.10	18.25	5.12	0.28	0.084	–	18.66	0.62	<0.001	0.11
Social interaction	**A**	799	10.49	3.79	10.65	3.67				10.49			
	D	777	11.61	3.40	11.66	3.35	1.01	<0.001	0.29	11.61	0.85	<0.001	0.24
	F	602	11.24	3.50	11.24	3.48	0.60	<0.001	0.17	11.38	0.55	<0.001	0.15
Material	**A**	799	11.37	4.54	11.65	4.33				11.37			
	D	777	12.68	3.81	12.79	3.75	1.14	<0.001	0.28	12.68	1.19	<0.001	0.29
	F	602	12.33	4.00	12.31	4.03	0.66	<0.001	0.16	12.78	1.01	<0.001	0.24
Affective	**A**	799	8.71	3.17	8.87	3.10				8.71			
	D	777	9.42	2.83	9.54	2.75	0.67	<0.001	0.23	9.42	0.69	<0.001	0.22
	F	602	9.07	2.92	9.08	2.91	0.22	0.010	0.07	9.26	0.29	0.003	0.09

social interaction and material support domains demonstrated the most notable improvements, albeit with effect sizes ranging from minimal to small (Fig. 5.48, Table 5.58).

Closer examination of the severity levels based on the traffic light system reveals a particular need for improvement in the emotional aspect of social support. Notably, none of the patients reported receiving support within the 'desirable' range for this factor. However, only a small proportion of patients were categorised as 'critical', and this proportion decreased slightly by the follow-up examination for all subscales (Fig. 5.49).

5.2.2 IHM Stress Profile

5.2.2.1 Tedium Scale (Burnout)

Upon admission to the clinic in 2023, the average total burnout score was around 4.24 points (SD = 0.94), slightly higher than in previous years (M = 4.03, SD = 0.98). Men exhibited a slightly lower level of stress (M = 4.12, SD = 1.02), whereas women demonstrated a higher level (M = 4.27, SD = 0.92). Women indicated a higher risk of burnout, particularly in the 41–50, 61–70, and over 70 age groups. As can be seen in Fig. 5.50 and Table 5.59, the severity of burnout syndromes tends to decrease with age. Additionally, the majority of patients experience pre-burnout syndromes or are in an acute crisis upon admission to the clinic.

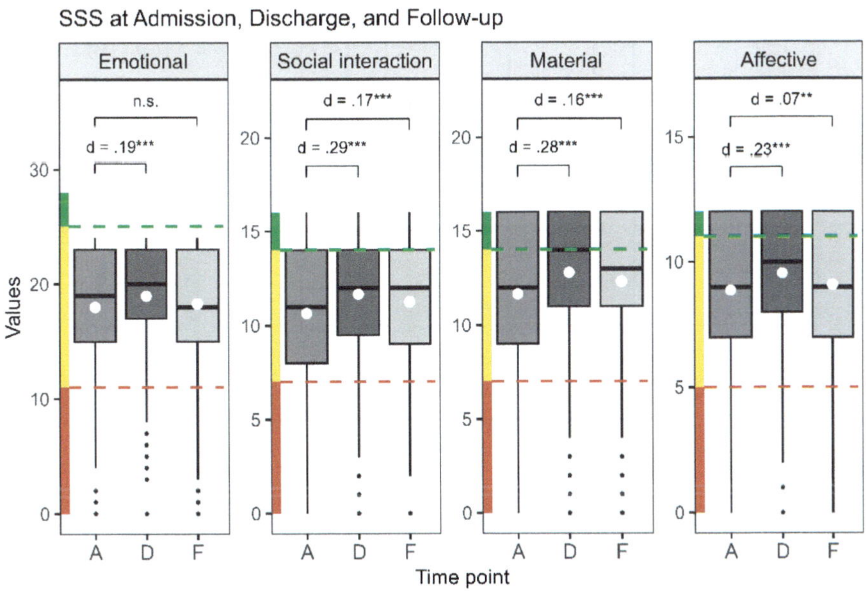

Fig. 5.48 Scales of social support (SSS) over the course of the 2023 measurement time points (*A* admission, *D* discharge, *F* follow-up); *t*-test with paired samples; significance at $^{*}p < 0.05$, $^{**}p < 0.01$, $^{***}p < 0.001$; Cohen's d = effect measure ($d \geq 0.2$ = small, ≥ 0.5 = moderate, ≥ 0.8 = large); the red line shows the critical, yellow the improvable, and green the desirable area

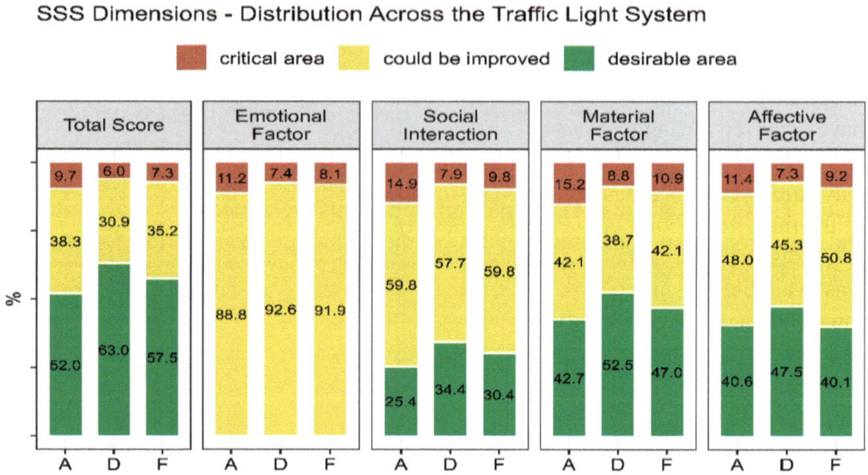

Fig. 5.49 Distribution of the SSS scales across the levels of the traffic light system in 2023; *A* admission, *D* discharge, *F* follow-up

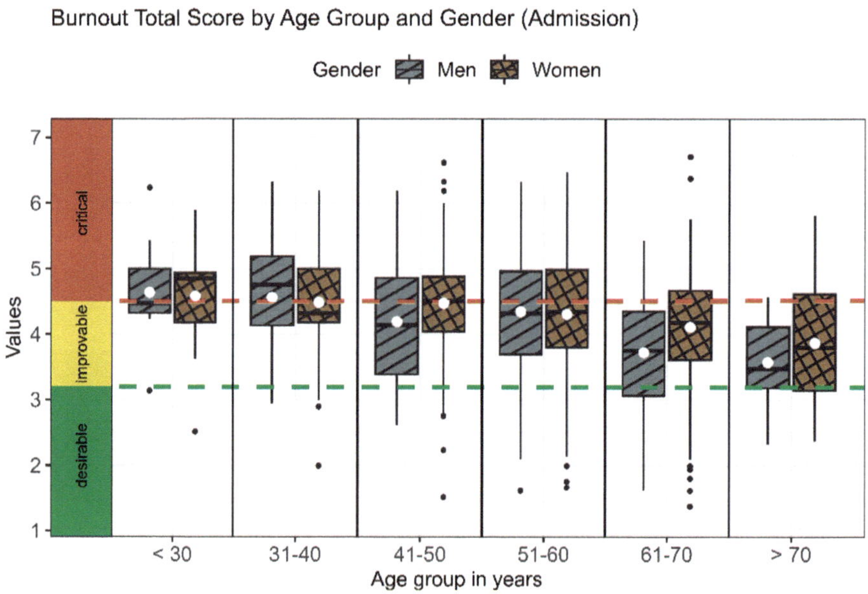

Fig. 5.50 Distribution measures of the burnout score in the 2023 reporting year at admission, broken down by gender and age group; white circles indicate the mean, black lines the median; the coloured lines indicate the thresholds according to the traffic light system

Table 5.59 Measures of distribution for the overall burnout score, broken down by gender and age in 2023 and previous years

Burnout total score									
		2023				Previous years			
	Age group	*n*	M	SD	Md	*n*	M	SD	Md
Men	Up to 30	9	4.64	0.86	4.48	133	3.86	1.04	3.86
	31 to 40	13	4.56	1.00	4.76	203	4.08	1.02	4.19
	41 to 50	22	4.20	1.03	4.14	595	4.06	0.99	4.10
	51 to 60	64	4.35	1.02	4.33	990	4.04	1.03	4.10
	61 to 70	47	3.73	0.97	3.76	623	3.57	0.99	3.57
	Over 70	15	3.58	0.65	3.48	398	3.13	0.98	3.12
	Total	**170**	**4.12**	**1.02**	**4.19**	**2942**	**3.82**	**1.06**	**3.90**
Women	Up to 30	14	4.58	0.87	4.86	371	4.03	1.01	4.10
	31 to 40	50	4.49	0.85	4.33	625	4.27	0.97	4.29
	41 to 50	96	4.48	0.82	4.52	1926	4.24	0.92	4.29
	51 to 60	282	4.31	0.90	4.36	3217	4.22	0.89	4.29
	61 to 70	153	4.12	0.98	4.19	1602	3.89	0.94	3.95
	Over 70	58	3.87	0.89	3.81	836	3.59	0.94	3.62
	Total	**653**	**4.27**	**0.92**	**4.33**	**8577**	**4.10**	**0.95**	**4.14**
Total	Up to 30	23	4.60	0.85	4.52	504	3.98	1.02	4.05
	31 to 40	63	4.50	0.88	4.38	828	4.22	0.98	4.29
	41 to 50	118	4.42	0.86	4.48	2521	4.20	0.94	4.24
	51 to 60	346	4.32	0.92	4.33	4207	4.18	0.92	4.24
	61 to 70	200	4.03	0.99	4.14	2225	3.80	0.97	3.86
	Over 70	73	3.81	0.85	3.67	1234	3.44	0.97	3.48
	Total	**823**	**4.24**	**0.94**	**4.29**	**11,519**	**4.03**	**0.98**	**4.10**

M mean, *SD* standard deviation, *Md* median

Table 5.60 displays the distribution values for the total Tedium score and its three subscales: Discouragement, Exhaustion, and Loss of Motivation. Of all the burnout dimensions, Exhaustion was found to be the most affected. Notably, women reported higher levels of exhaustion than men, indicating a greater burden in this domain. The discouragement factor is less pronounced for both women and men and is a typical effect of a later stage in the development of burnout syndrome. Figure 5.51 illustrates the results, showing the distribution of the three subscales and the total score separately by gender.

Following treatment at the clinic, patients showed significant improvement in all burnout dimensions, with moderate effect sizes. The total burnout score decreased by 0.67 points until discharge ($d = -0.67$, $p < 0.001$) and remained relatively stable until the follow-up assessment ($d = -0.62$, $p < 0.001$). Table 5.61 summarises the statistical results for all burnout dimensions and the total score. The largest improvement was observed for the Exhaustion subscale at discharge ($d = -0.77$, $p < 0.001$), which also showed the strongest effect size until follow-up ($d = -0.67$, $p < 0.001$). Figures 5.52 and 5.53 illustrate the results graphically.

Table 5.60 Measures of distribution for the total burnout value including all subscales, broken down by gender in 2023 and previous years

		2023				Previous years			
Burnout	Gender	*n*	M	SD	Md	*n*	M	SD	Md
Total score	Men	170	4.12	1.02	4.19	2942	3.82	1.06	3.90
	Women	653	4.27	0.92	4.33	8577	4.10	0.95	4.14
	Total	823	4.24	0.94	4.29	11,519	4.03	0.98	4.10
Discouragement	Men	170	3.68	1.22	3.75	2943	3.40	1.20	3.40
	Women	653	3.80	1.09	3.90	8577	3.66	1.12	3.70
	Total	823	3.77	1.12	3.90	11,520	3.59	1.14	3.70
Exhaustion	Men	170	4.75	1.13	4.83	2942	4.39	1.21	4.50
	Women	653	5.06	1.04	5.00	8579	4.80	1.09	4.83
	Total	823	5.00	1.06	5.00	11,521	4.70	1.13	4.83
Loss of motivation	Men	170	4.24	0.91	4.20	2942	3.96	1.02	4.00
	Women	653	4.27	0.89	4.40	8578	4.12	0.90	4.20
	Total	823	4.26	0.89	4.40	11,520	4.08	0.93	4.20

M mean, *SD* standard deviation, *Md* median

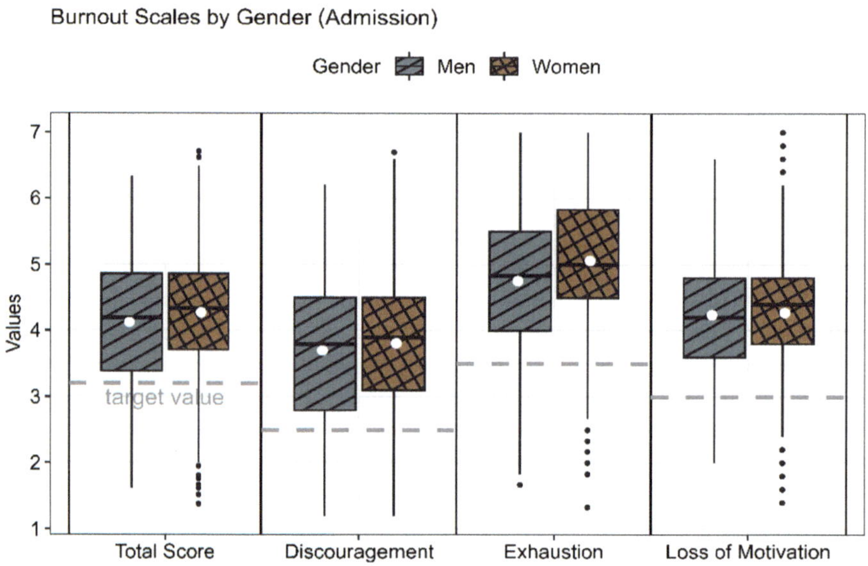

Fig. 5.51 Distribution of the burnout subscales, broken down by gender in 2023; white circles indicate the mean, black lines the median; the grey lines indicate the threshold value for the desirable area according to the traffic light system

Additionally, the data shows that nearly 40% of patients exhibited clear signs of burnout upon hospital admission, whereas only 15% showed no signs of burnout syndromes. At discharge, the proportion of patients with an acute burnout crisis halved to 19.8%, while the proportion without signs of burnout syndromes more than doubled to 37.7%. This positive change was maintained until follow-up. Similar improvements were observed in the subscales. For example, 'Loss of Motivation' was present in only 9.8% of patients upon admission, but by discharge,

Table 5.61 Burnout before/after comparison in 2023; *t*-test for paired samples; significance at $p < 0.05$; Cohen's d = effect measure ($d \geq 0.2$ = small, ≥ 0.5 = moderate, ≥ 0.8 = large effect); previous year's data since 2022

Burnout		2023								Previous year 2022			
		Cross-section: A/D/F			Course: A–D/A–F $n = 612$		Difference from admission: A–D/A–F $n = 612$			Course: A–D/A–F $n = 508$	Difference from admission: A–D/A–F $n = 508$		
		n	M	SD	M	SD	ΔM	*p*	*d*	M	ΔM	*p*	*d*
Total score	**A**	823	4.24	0.94	4.21	0.93				4.25			
	D	777	3.59	1.05	3.54	1.04	−0.67	<0.001	**−0.67**	3.53	−0.72	<0.001	**−0.74**
	F	617	3.60	1.04	3.60	1.04	−0.60	<0.001	**−0.62**	3.60	−0.65	<0.001	**−0.68**
Loss of motivation	**A**	823	4.26	0.89	4.23	0.87				4.24			
	D	777	3.71	0.99	3.67	0.98	−0.56	<0.001	**−0.60**	3.65	−0.59	<0.001	**−0.65**
	F	617	3.71	0.98	3.71	0.98	−0.57	<0.001	**−0.50**	3.70	−0.54	<0.001	**−0.60**
Exhaustion	**A**	823	5.00	1.06	4.98	1.05				4.99			
	D	777	4.16	1.22	4.10	1.20	−0.88	<0.001	**−0.77**	4.07	−0.92	<0.001	**−0.79**
	F	617	4.21	1.22	4.21	1.22	−0.77	<0.001	**−0.67**	4.26	−0.74	<0.001	**−0.64**
Discouragement	**A**	823	3.77	1.12	3.74	1.11				3.81			
	D	777	3.19	1.15	3.14	1.15	−0.60	<0.001	**−0.53**	3.14	−0.67	<0.001	**−0.61**
	F	617	3.17	1.16	3.18	1.16	−0.52	<0.001	**−0.56**	3.15	−0.66	<0.001	**−0.60**

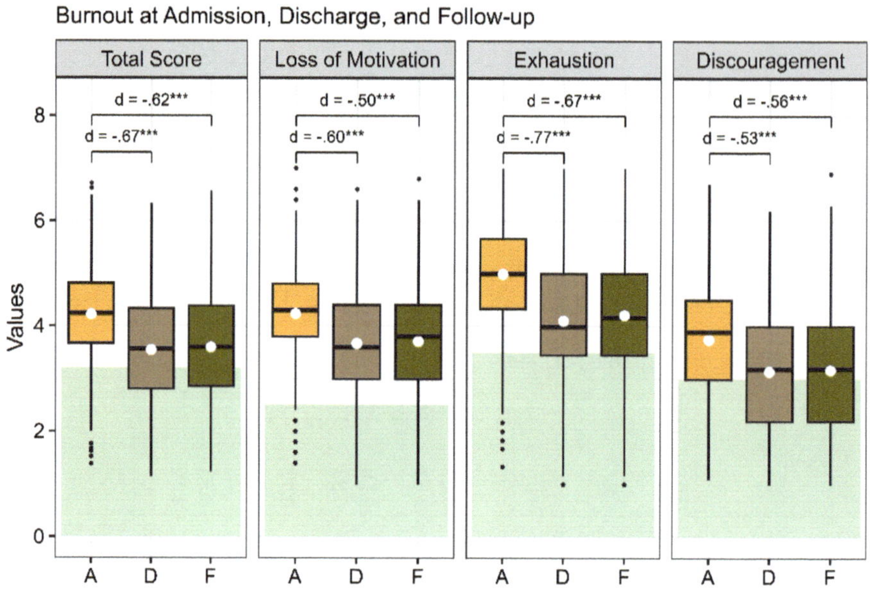

Fig. 5.52 Burnout scales over the course of the 2023 measurement time points (*A* admission, *D* discharge, *F* follow-up); *t*-test with paired samples; significance at $*p < 0.05$, $**p < 0.01$, $***p < 0.001$; Cohen's d = effect measure ($d \geq 0.2$ = small, ≥ 0.5 = moderate, ≥ 0.8 = large); the coloured background marks the desired area

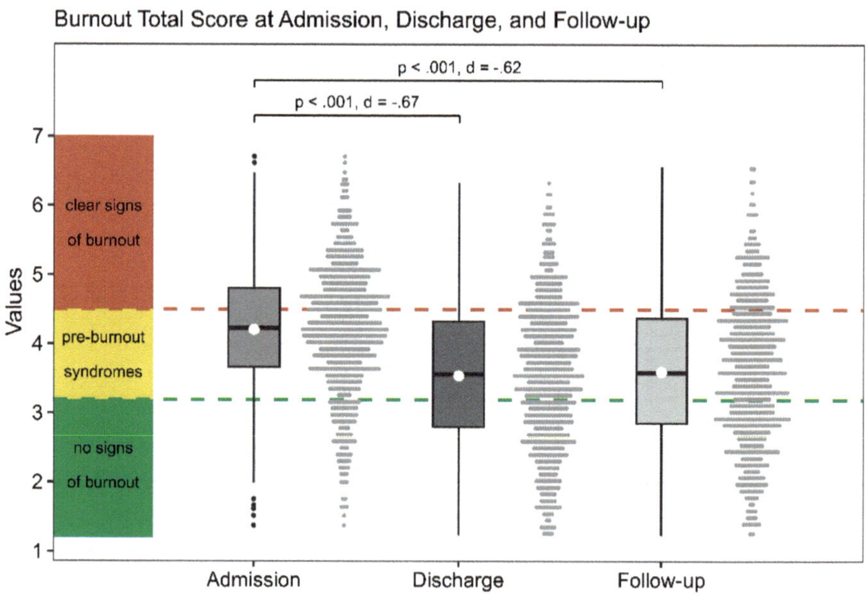

Fig. 5.53 Burnout total score over the course of the measurement time points in 2023; *t*-test with paired samples; Cohen's d = effect measure ($d \geq 0.2$ = small, ≥ 0.5 = moderate, ≥ 0.8 = large effect); white circle indicates the mean, the black line the median

this figure had almost tripled to 28.1%. This positive change was also maintained until the follow-up stage (27.8%). Figure 5.54 provides an overview of the distribution across the traffic light system for all burnout scales and measurement points.

5.2.2.2 Perceived Stress Questionnaire (PSQ)

On average, patients reported a perceived stress level of 57.63 (SD = 18.07) upon admission, close to the critical range threshold of 58.5, indicating significantly increased stress levels. Men reported lower levels of perceived stress in all age groups except the 51–60 age group, where men and women reported similar levels. Overall, men reported a perceived stress level of 54.63 (SD = 18.62), while women reported a level of 58.42 (SD = 17.86). Stress levels were particularly high among younger patients and decreased with increasing age. Figure 5.55 and Table 5.62 present the data broken down by age group and gender for the total score. A closer look at the subscales reveals that tension was the most affected area (mean = 67.14, standard deviation = 21.43), followed by worries (mean = 50.30, standard deviation = 23.71) and demands (mean = 46.78, standard deviation = 25.16). Figure 5.56 and Table 5.63 show the figures for all PSQ subscales categorised by gender.

Following treatment at the clinic, the overall perceived stress load decreased significantly, with a large effect size ($d = 1.05$, $p < 0.001$). The improvements were most pronounced regarding Demands ($d = 0.97$, $p < 0.001$) and Tension ($d = 0.99$, $p < 0.001$) but Worries and Joy also improved significantly with moderate effects

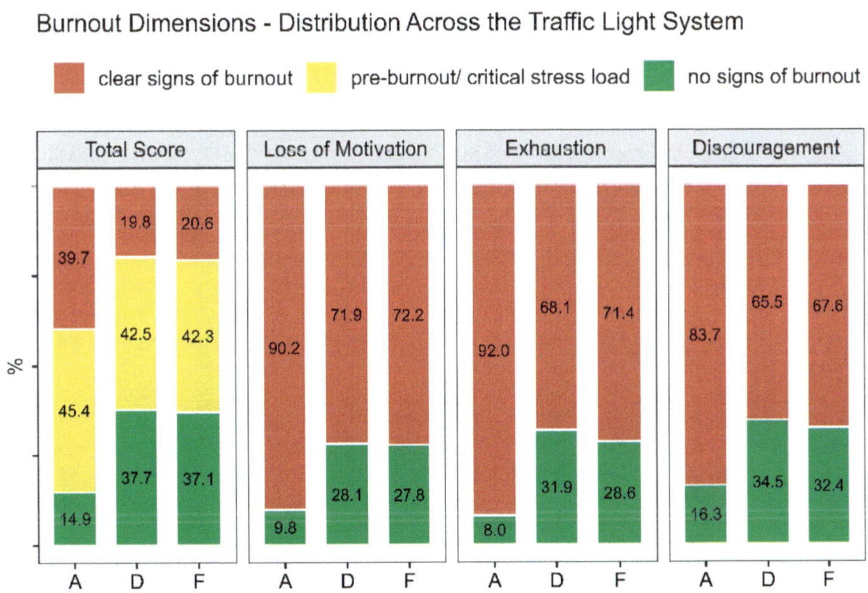

Fig. 5.54 Distribution of all burnout dimensions across the levels of the traffic light system in 2023; *A* admission, *D* discharge, *F* follow-up; in the burnout subscales, categorisation according to the traffic light system is limited to 'desirable' and 'action required'; the red area should therefore be interpreted as part of the yellow category

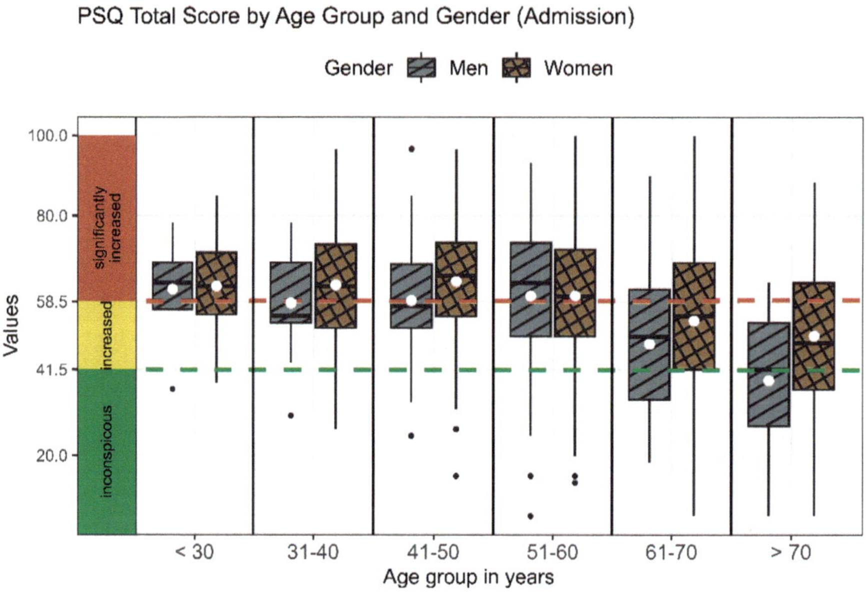

Fig. 5.55 Distribution measures of the PSQ score in the 2023 reporting year at admission, broken down by gender and age group; white circles indicate the mean, black lines the median; the coloured lines indicate the thresholds according to the traffic light system

Table 5.62 Measures of distribution for the overall PSQ score, broken down by gender and age in 2023 and previous years

PSQ total score									
		2023				Previous years			
	Age group	*n*	M	SD	Md	*n*	M	SD	Md
Men	Up to 30	9	61.67	11.63	63.33	56	58.81	11.92	58.33
	31 to 40	13	58.20	14.18	55.00	95	62.77	13.26	63.33
	41 to 50	22	58.86	17.14	57.50	292	60.39	14.90	60.00
	51 to 60	64	59.97	18.33	63.34	511	61.14	15.31	60.00
	61 to 70	47	48.05	17.71	50.00	251	54.22	15.66	53.33
	Over 70	15	38.89	18.39	41.67	108	46.71	15.38	45.84
	Total	**170**	**54.63**	**18.62**	**55.00**	**1313**	**58.48**	**15.65**	**58.33**
Women	Up to 30	14	62.38	13.82	62.50	155	60.29	14.73	60.00
	31 to 40	50	62.67	15.91	62.50	331	64.26	14.94	65.00
	41 to 50	96	63.59	14.78	65.00	1037	63.20	14.63	63.33
	51 to 60	280	59.97	16.75	60.00	2064	62.87	14.23	63.33
	61 to 70	153	53.80	19.61	55.00	865	58.30	15.11	58.33
	Over 70	59	50.03	20.14	48.33	385	52.27	14.89	51.67
	Total	**652**	**58.42**	**17.86**	**60.00**	**4837**	**61.29**	**14.95**	**61.67**
Total	Up to 30	23	62.10	12.73	63.33	211	59.90	14.03	60.00
	31 to 40	63	61.75	15.57	60.00	426	63.92	14.58	64.16
	41 to 50	118	62.71	15.28	62.50	1329	62.59	14.73	63.33
	51 to 60	344	59.97	17.03	61.67	2575	62.53	14.47	61.67
	61 to 70	200	52.45	19.29	53.33	1116	57.38	15.32	57.50
	Over 70	74	47.77	20.19	47.50	493	51.05	15.16	50.00
	Total	**822**	**57.63**	**18.07**	**58.33**	**6150**	**60.69**	**15.14**	**60.00**

M mean, *SD* standard deviation, *Md* median

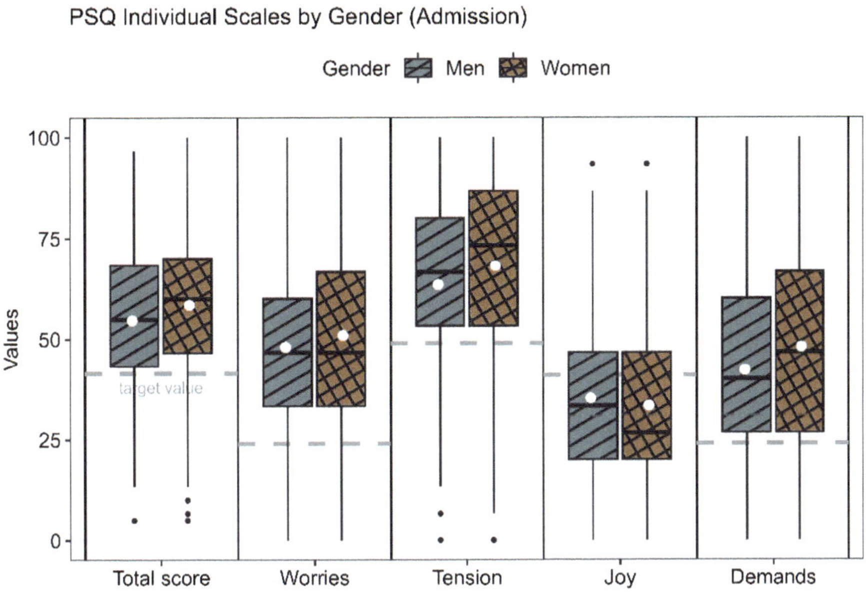

Fig. 5.56 The distribution values of the PSQ scales are shown below, divided by gender in 2023. White circles indicate the mean and black lines represent the median. Grey lines show the threshold value for the desirable area according to the traffic light system

Table 5.63 Measures of distribution for the total PSQ value including all subscales, broken down by gender in 2023 and previous years

		2023				Previous years			
PSQ	Gender	*n*	M	SD	Md	*n*	M	SD	Md
Total score	Men	170	54.63	18.62	55.00	1313	58.48	15.65	58.33
	Women	652	58.42	17.86	60.00	4837	61.29	14.95	61.67
	Total	822	57.63	18.07	58.33	6150	60.69	15.14	60.00
Worries	Men	170	48.00	24.54	46.67	1313	51.64	20.63	53.33
	Women	652	50.90	23.47	46.67	4837	53.16	20.15	53.33
	Total	822	50.30	23.71	46.67	6150	52.83	20.26	53.33
Tension	Men	170	63.49	23.24	66.67	1313	66.93	19.46	66.67
	Women	652	68.09	20.85	73.33	4837	70.58	17.84	73.33
	Total	822	67.14	21.43	66.67	6150	69.80	18.26	73.33
Joy	Men	170	35.18	19.00	33.33	1313	31.27	16.68	33.33
	Women	652	33.30	19.74	26.67	4837	30.70	16.19	26.67
	Total	822	33.69	19.59	33.33	6150	30.82	16.29	30.00
Demands	Men	170	42.20	23.84	40.00	1313	46.64	24.29	46.67
	Women	652	47.98	25.37	46.67	4837	52.14	24.16	53.33
	Total	822	46.78	25.16	46.67	6150	50.97	24.29	53.33

M mean, *SD* standard deviation, *Md* median

($d = 0.69$, $p < 0.001$; $d = 0.79$, $p < 0.001$, respectively). Despite a slight reduction in effect during the follow-up phase, the overall improvement remained statistically significant, with a moderate effect size ($d = 0.64$, $p < 0.001$). Table 5.64 summarises all statistical results.

A positive trend can also be seen in the traffic light categories for the overall score. While patients were, on average, at the threshold of the critical range upon admission, they had reached the desirable range by discharge time and remained relatively close to the desirable range threshold until the follow-up (Fig. 5.57). The average scores for the Tension and Joy subcategories also reached desirable levels at discharge and follow-up. Figure 5.58 illustrates the results for all PSQ subscales.

Figures showing the distribution across the traffic light system indicate that, upon admission, nearly half of patients (49.3%) reported significantly increased stress levels, while only 16.7% had inconspicuous stress levels. At discharge, over half of the patients indicated inconspicuous stress levels (57.0%), while only 15.4% still had significantly increased stress levels. Although the effect was less pronounced after follow-up, 40.2% still had an inconspicuous stress level. Notable positive improvements in desirable values were seen in the areas of tension and joy. Figure 5.59 illustrates the results for all subscales in more detail.

5.2.2.3 Three-Level Stress Test (3-LST)

Table 5.65 and Fig. 5.60 show that, in 2023, both men and women are most susceptible to stress at the motor level (M = 27.76, SD = 8.79). At the vegetative and motor levels, women tend to be more affected than men: M = 20.10, SD = 7.59 and M = 28.41, SD = 8.62, respectively, versus M = 16.84, SD = 8.03 and M = 25.27, SD = 9.00, respectively. At the cognitive-emotional level, women (M = 23.12, SD = 9.90) and men (M = 22.11, SD = 10.95) experience similar levels of distress. These figures are consistent with the PSQ sub-dimension ‘Tension’.

Taking a closer look at the different levels differentiated by age group reveals an age difference, particularly at the cognitive-emotional level, where stress decreases with age—more so in men than in women. At the motor and vegetative level, older men tend to exhibit fewer symptoms. By contrast, this age effect is less pronounced in women, who exhibit a relatively consistent level of symptoms across all age groups (Figs. 5.61, 5.62, 5.63, Tables 5.66, 5.67).

Table 5.64 PSQ before/after comparison in 2023; t-test for paired samples; significance at $p < 0.05$; Cohen's d = effect measure ($d \geq 0.2$ = small, ≥ 0.5 = moderate, ≥ 0.8 = large effect); previous year's data since 2022

		2023								Previous year 2022			
PSQ		Cross-section: A/D/F			Course: A–D/A–F $n = 609$		Difference from admission: A–D/A–F $n = 609$			Course: A–D/A–F $n = 495$	Difference from admission: A–D/A–F $n = 495$		
		n	M	SD	M	SD	ΔM	p	d	M	ΔM	p	d
Total score	**A**	822	57.63	18.07	57.55	17.92				58.52			
	D	777	39.47	19.37	38.12	19.12	−19.43	<0.001	**−1.05**	38.22	−20.30	<0.001	**−0.1.07**
	F	616	45.65	19.06	45.71	19.03	−11.84	<0.001	**−0.64**	45.70	−12.82	<0.001	**−0.70**
Worries	**A**	822	50.30	23.71	49.98	23.09				50.96			
	D	777	35.65	23.45	34.13	23.13	−15.85	<0.001	**−0.69**	34.52	−16.44	<0.001	**−0.72**
	F	617	37.19	23.40	37.12	23.35	−12.86	<0.001	**−0.55**	36.59	−14.37	<0.001	**−0.65**
Demands	**A**	822	46.78	25.16	46.98	25.05				48.51			
	D	777	25.25	21.76	24.31	21.48	−22.67	<0.001	**−0.97**	24.69	−23.61	<0.001	**−1.03**
	F	617	37.95	23.12	37.95	23.23	−9.03	<0.001	−0.37	37.60	−16.20	<0.001	**−0.75**
Joy	**A**	822	33.69	19.59	33.91	19.49				33.25			
	D	777	49.38	22.49	50.66	22.61	16.75	<0.001	**0.79**	50.59	17.33	<0.001	**0.81**
	F	617	44.99	23.03	44.85	22.96	10.54	<0.001	**0.51**	43.06	9.81	<0.001	0.47
Tension	**A**	822	67.14	21.43	67.15	21.32				67.87			
	D	777	46.34	24.26	44.71	23.66	−22.44	<0.001	**−0.99**	44.26	−23.83	<0.001	**−0.97**
	F	617	52.53	22.72	52.61	22.75	−14.54	<0.001	**−0.66**	51.66	−10.91	<0.001	−0.45

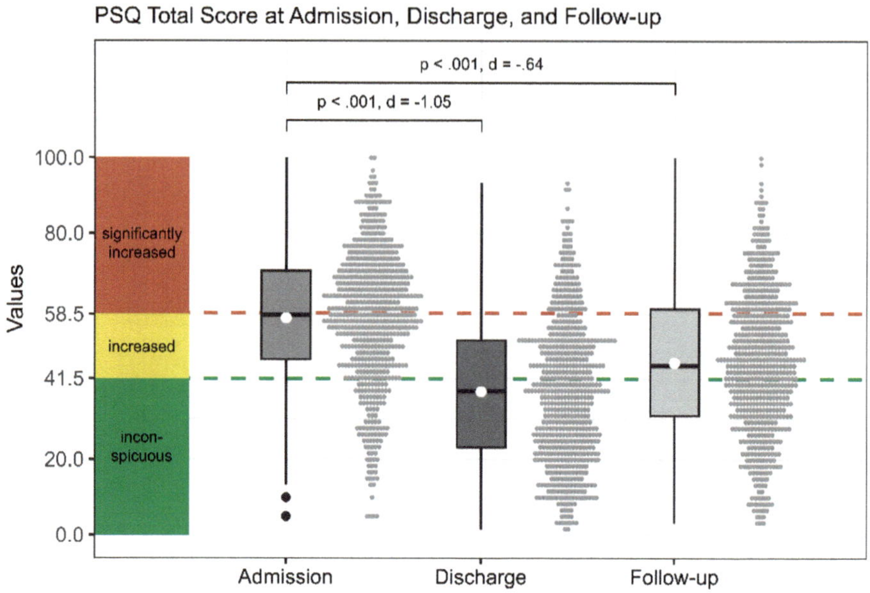

Fig. 5.57 PSQ total score over the course of the measurement time points in 2023; *t*-test with paired samples; Cohen's *d* = effect measure ($d \geq 0.2$ = small, ≥ 0.5 = moderate, ≥ 0.8 = large effect); white circle indicates the mean, the black line the median

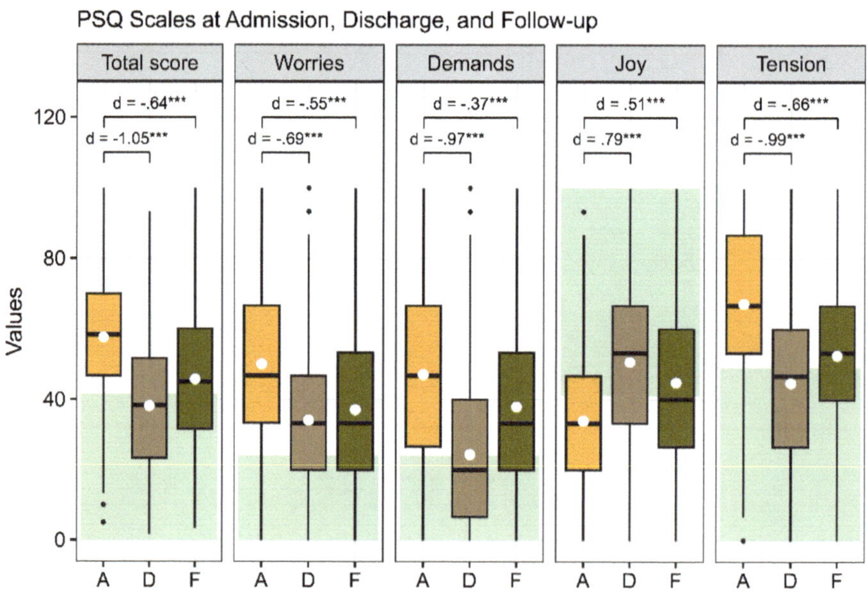

Fig. 5.58 PSQ scales over the course of the 2023 measurement time points (*A* admission, *D* discharge, *F* follow-up); *t*-test with paired samples; significance at $^{*}p < 0.05$, $^{**}p$, $^{***}p < 0.001$; Cohen's *d* = effect measure ($d \geq 0.2$ = small, ≥ 0.5 = moderate, ≥ 0.8 = large); the coloured background marks the desired area

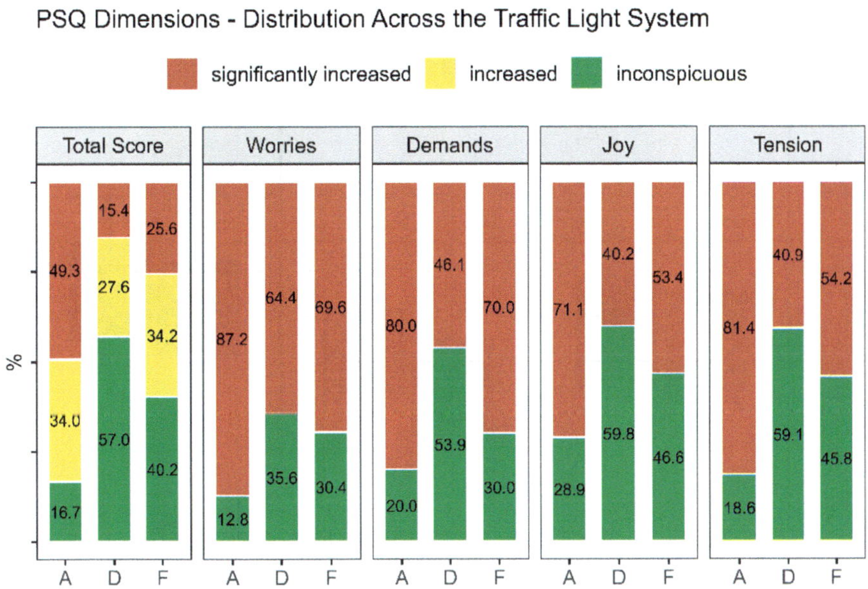

Fig. 5.59 Distribution of all PSQ dimensions across the levels of the traffic light system in 2023; *A* admission, *D* discharge, *F* follow-up; in the burnout subscales, categorisation according to the traffic light system is limited to 'desirable' and 'action required'; the red area should therefore be interpreted as part of the yellow category

Table 5.65 Measures of distribution for the Three-level Stress Test, broken down by gender in 2023 and previous years

		2023				Previous years			
3-LST	Gender	*n*	M	SD	Md	*n*	M	SD	Md
Cognitive	Men	170	22.11	10.95	22	3141	18.58	10.30	18.0
	Women	651	23.12	9.90	22	9048	20.82	9.97	20.0
	Total	**821**	**22.91**	**10.13**	**22**	**12,189**	**20.24**	**10.11**	**20.0**
Vegetative	Men	170	16.84	8.03	16	3141	15.65	8.02	14.0
	Women	651	20.10	7.59	20	9048	18.98	7.70	18.0
	Total	**821**	**19.43**	**7.79**	**18**	**12,189**	**18.12**	**7.92**	**18.0**
Motor	Men	170	25.27	9.00	24	3141	23.13	9.83	24.0
	Women	651	28.41	8.62	28	9048	26.93	9.17	28.0
	Total	**821**	**27.76**	**8.79**	**28**	**12,189**	**25.95**	**9.49**	**26.0**

M mean, *SD* standard deviation, *Md* median

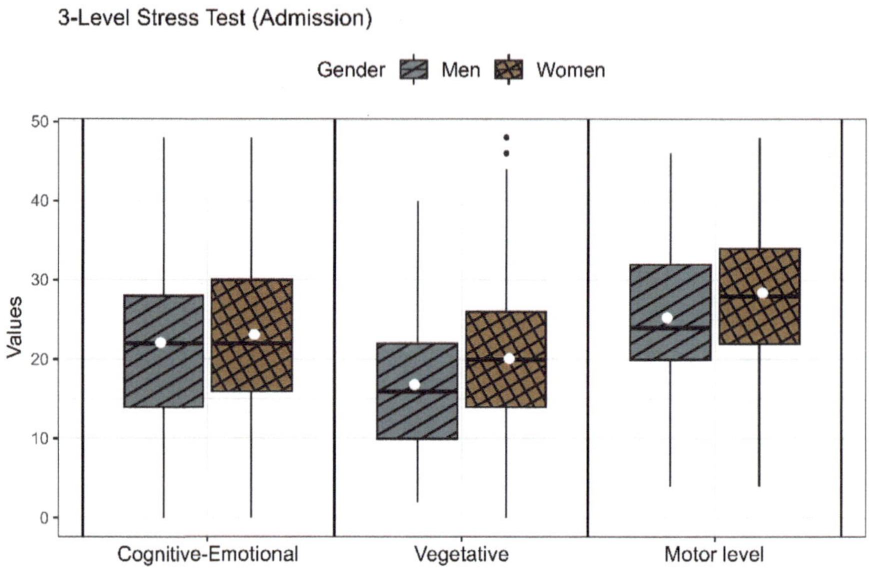

Fig. 5.60 Distribution values of the 3-LST scales, broken down by gender in 2023; white circles indicate the mean, black lines the median

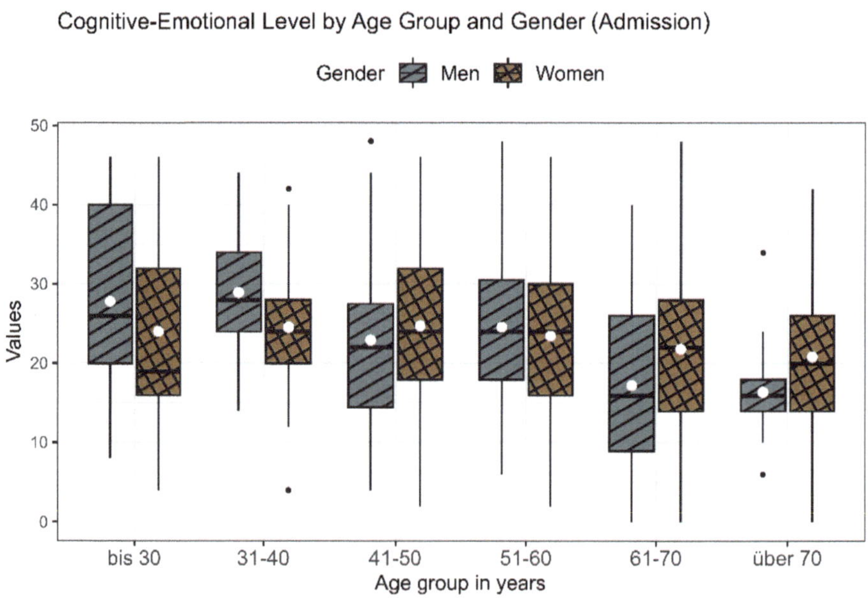

Fig. 5.61 Distribution measures of the Cognitive-Emotional Level in the 2023 reporting year at admission, broken down by gender and age group; white circles indicate the mean, black lines the median

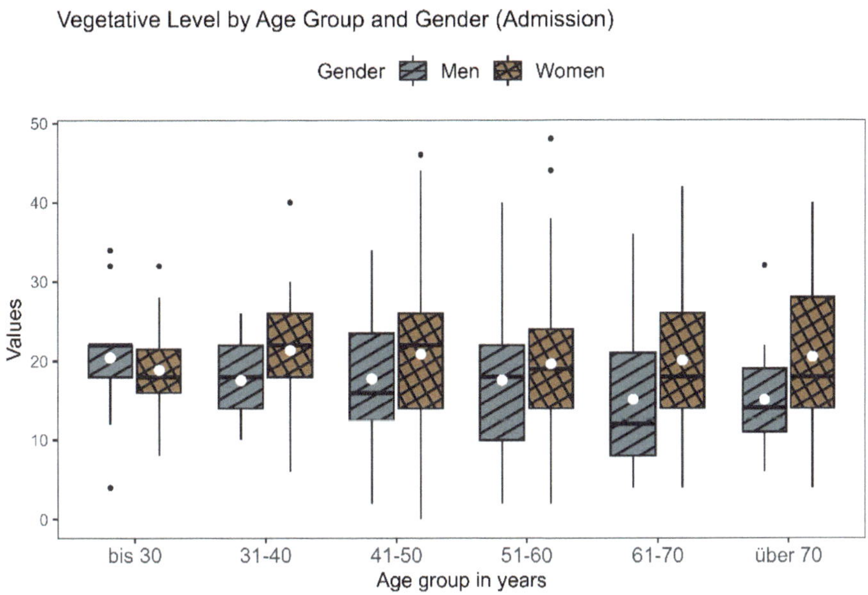

Fig. 5.62 Distribution measures of the Vegetative Level in the 2023 reporting year at admission, broken down by gender and age group; white circles indicate the mean, black lines the median

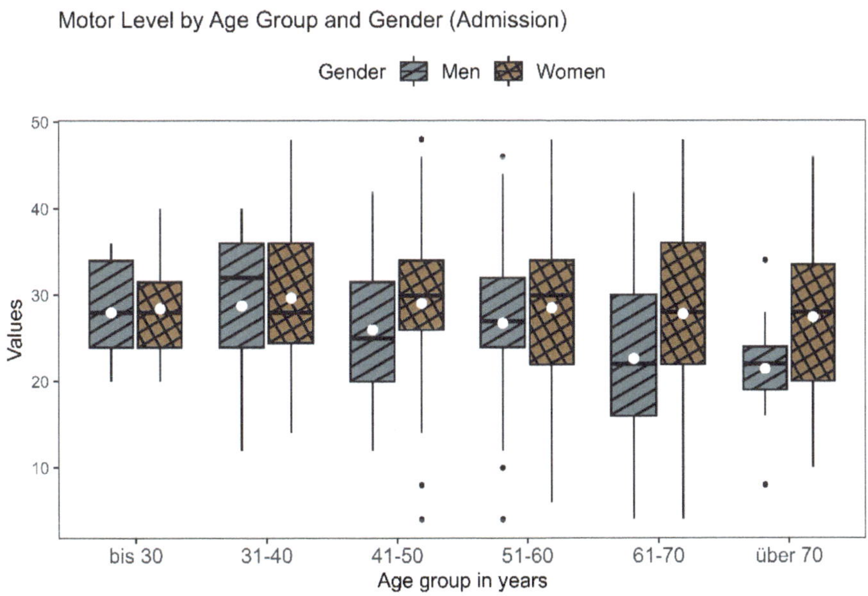

Fig. 5.63 Distribution measures of the Motor Level in the 2023 reporting year at admission, broken down by gender and age group; white circles indicate the mean, black lines the median

Table 5.66 Measures of distribution for the Cognitive-Emotional Level, broken down by gender and age in 2023 and previous years

Cognitive-emotional level									
		2023				Previous years			
	Age group	*n*	M	SD	Md	*n*	M	SD	Md
Men	Up to 30	9	27.78	13.02	26	145	20.31	11.19	145
	31 to 40	13	28.92	9.30	28	236	20.18	10.46	236
	41 to 50	22	22.91	11.80	22	636	19.91	10.21	636
	51 to 60	64	24.56	10.21	24	1038	20.19	10.43	1038
	61 to 70	47	17.23	10.30	16	655	16.33	9.38	655
	Over 70	15	16.40	6.51	16	431	14.70	9.44	431
	Total	170	22.11	10.95	22	3141	18.58	10.30	3141
Women	Up to 30	14	24.00	12.00	19	412	19.10	10.91	412
	31 to 40	50	24.52	7.73	24	678	21.36	10.40	678
	41 to 50	96	24.69	10.30	24	2030	22.20	9.99	2030
	51 to 60	280	23.44	10.01	24	3336	22.04	9.63	3336
	61 to 70	153	21.79	9.96	22	1703	19.14	9.76	1703
	Over 70	58	20.83	9.37	20	889	16.70	9.12	889
	Total	651	23.10	9.91	22	9048	20.82	9.97	9048
Total	Up to 30	23	25.48	12.26	20	557	19.42	10.99	557
	31 to 40	63	25.43	8.19	26	914	21.06	10.43	914
	41 to 50	118	24.36	10.56	24	2666	21.65	10.09	2666
	51 to 60	344	23.65	10.04	24	4374	21.60	9.85	4374
	61 to 70	200	20.72	10.20	20	2358	18.36	9.74	2358
	Over 70	73	19.92	9.00	18	1320	16.04	9.27	1320
	Total	821	22.89	10.14	22	12.189	20.24	10.11	12.189

M mean, *SD* standard deviation, *Md* median

Comparing the different symptom levels between admission and follow-up shows significant changes at each level. After approximately 6 months, susceptibility to stress was reduced at all reaction levels, with moderate effect sizes for the cognitive-emotional ($d = -0.51$, $p < 0.001$) and motor levels ($d = -0.54$, $p < 0.001$) and a small-to-moderate effect size for the vegetative level ($d = -0.44$, $p < 0.001$). An overview of the results is given in Table 5.68 and Fig. 5.64.

Table 5.67 Measures of distribution for the Vegetative and Motor Level, broken down by gender and age in 2023 and previous years

		Vegetative level								Motor level							
		2023				Previous years				2023				Previous years			
	Age group	*n*	M	SD	Md	*n*	M	SD	Md	*n*	M	SD	Md	*n*	M	SD	Md
Men	Up to 30	9	20.44	9.21	22	145	15.74	8.42	145	9	28.00	6.24	28	145	21.31	9.98	145
	31 to 40	13	17.54	5.55	18	236	16.42	8.27	236	13	28.77	10.08	32	236	23.91	9.93	236
	41 to 50	22	17.73	8.05	16	636	16.47	8.17	636	22	26.00	8.68	25	636	25.08	9.37	636
	51 to 60	64	17.56	8.42	18	1038	16.76	7.93	1038	64	26.75	9.01	27	1038	24.87	9.50	1038
	61 to 70	47	15.11	8.03	12	655	14.43	7.71	655	47	22.64	9.39	22	655	21.57	9.64	655
	Over 70	15	15.07	7.00	14	431	13.18	7.46	431	15	21.47	5.83	22	431	18.59	9.51	431
	Total	170	16.84	8.03	16	3141	15.65	8.02	3141	170	25.27	9.00	24	3141	23.13	9.83	3141
Women	Up to 30	14	18.86	6.36	18	412	17.21	7.63	412	14	28.43	6.89	28	412	23.62	9.75	412
	31 to 40	50	21.36	7.08	22	678	18.88	7.79	678	50	29.64	8.03	28	678	27.06	9.17	678
	41 to 50	96	20.85	7.88	22	2030	19.03	7.67	2030	96	29.04	8.52	30	2030	28.04	8.99	2030
	51 to 60	280	19.62	7.27	19	3336	19.74	7.45	3336	280	28.51	8.35	30	3336	28.20	8.55	3336
	61 to 70	153	20.07	7.90	18	1703	18.71	7.86	1703	153	27.79	9.35	28	1703	25.47	9.44	1703
	Over 70	58	20.52	8.51	18	889	17.36	7.95	889	58	27.41	9.02	28	889	23.90	9.59	889
	Total	651	20.10	7.59	20	9048	18.98	7.70	9048	651	28.41	8.62	28	9048	26.93	9.17	9048
Total	Up to 30	23	19.48	7.44	18	557	16.83	7.86	557	23	28.26	6.50	28	557	23.02	9.85	557
	31 to 40	63	20.57	6.93	20	914	18.25	7.99	914	63	29.46	8.41	30	914	26.25	9.46	914
	41 to 50	118	20.27	7.97	20	2666	18.42	7.87	2666	118	28.47	8.60	28	2666	27.33	9.16	2666
	51 to 60	344	19.24	7.53	18	4374	19.04	7.67	4374	344	28.18	8.49	28	4374	27.41	8.89	4374
	61 to 70	200	18.90	8.18	18	2358	17.52	8.05	2358	200	26.58	9.59	26	2358	24.38	9.66	2358
	Over 70	73	19.40	8.47	18	1320	16.00	8.04	1320	73	26.19	8.77	26	1320	22.17	9.88	1320
	Total	821	19.43	7.79	18	12.189	18.12	7.92	12.189	821	27.76	8.79	28	12.189	25.95	9.49	12.189

M mean, *SD* standard deviation, *Md* median

Table 5.68 Three-Level Stress Test before/after comparison in 2023; t-test for paired samples; significance at $p < 0.05$; Cohen's d = effect measure ($d \geq 0.2$ = small, ≥ 0.5 = moderate, ≥ 0.8 = large effect); previous year's data since 2022

		2023								Previous year 2022			
Level		Cross-section: A/D/F			Course: A–D/A–F $n = 612$		Difference from admission: A–D/A–F $n = 612$			Course: A–D/A–F $n = 514$	Difference from admission: A–D/A–F $n = 514$		
		n	M	SD	M	SD	ΔM	p	d	M	ΔM	p	d
Cognitive-emotional	**A**	821	22.89	10.14	22.68	9.89				22.54			
	F	612	17.69	9.69	17.71	9.69	−4.97	<0.001	**−0.51**	17.62	−4.92	<0.001	**−0.50**
Motor	**A**	821	27.76	8.79	19.34	7.87				27.51			
	F	612	22.53	10.33	15.79	8.16	−5.26	<0.001	**−0.54**	22.34	−5.17	<0.001	**−0.56**
Vegetative	**A**	821	19.43	7.79	27.82	8.70				19.23			
	F	612	15.78	8.16	22.56	10.31	−3.55	<0.001	−0.44	15.56	−3.67	<0.001	−0.48

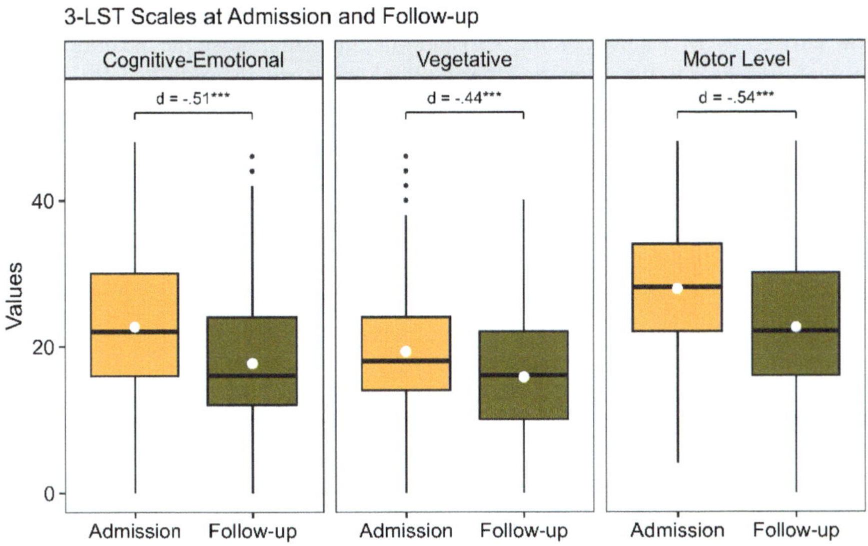

Fig. 5.64 3-LST over the course of the measurement time points in 2023; *t*-test with paired samples; Cohen's *d* = effect measure ($d \geq 0.2$ = small, ≥ 0.5 = moderate, ≥ 0.8 = large effect); white circle indicates the mean, the black line the median

Table 5.69 Measures of distribution for the Psycho-Vegetative Stability, broken down by gender in 2023 and previous years

		2023				Previous years			
	Gender	*n*	M	SD	Md	*n*	M	SD	Md
Total score	Men	170	55.62	17.36	55.0	3269	49.00	19.25	48.0
	Women	653	62.73	16.74	63.0	9344	58.38	18.03	59.0
	Total	**823**	**61.26**	**17.11**	**62.0**	**12,615**	**55.95**	**18.81**	**56.0**
Complaint index	Men	170	0.46	0.64	0.0	3269	0.62	0.65	1.0
	Women	653	0.27	0.49	0.0	9339	0.35	0.54	0.0
	Total	**823**	**0.31**	**0.53**	**0.0**	**12,610**	**0.42**	**0.59**	**0.0**

M mean, *SD* standard deviation, *Md* median

5.2.2.4 Psycho-Vegetative Complaints (Somatic Stress Disorders)

As explained in the previous chapter Patient Profile, the psycho-vegetative complaints questionnaire was developed to describe the main ICD-10 mental health diagnosis, Functional Somatic Disorder (FSD). Based on the 42 symptoms, a total value is calculated that can reach a maximum of 126 points. In addition, a total complaint index is created and divided into traffic light categories. On admission, patients had an average complaint score of 61.26 (SD = 17.11), with men reporting less severe symptoms (M = 55.62, SD = 17.36) than women (M = 62.73, SD = 17.11). On a scale from 0 to 2, where 0 indicates a high level of somatic functional stress disorder, the TCM patients had an average index value of 0.31 (SD = 0.53) at admission (men: M = 0.46, SD = 0.64; women: M = 0.27, SD = 0.49). Table 5.69 summarises the results categorised by gender. Compared to previous years, a greater proportion of patients reported severe symptoms of somatic stress disorder (M = 61.26 vs. M = 55.95). Table 5.70 and Fig. 5.65 summarise the mean frequencies of responses in the categories 'fairly often' and 'strong/very frequently' for all measurement points across individual functional and organ systems. Since the number of items varies between organ systems, the mean values should be interpreted in relation to the number of symptoms assessed within each system. A value of 0 indicates that the respective response was not selected on average; depending on the organ system, values can range from 0 to 8. The percentages reflect the relative distribution of responses per category and highlight the most frequently affected systems.

All cases in Table 5.70 and Fig. 5.65 were counted if they indicated at least one symptom as fairly/often (2) or strongly/very often (3). If several symptoms within a category were indicated at the two degrees of severity, the cases were counted accordingly.

Taking a closer look at the assessment of individual categories of the psycho-vegetative profile, according to the severity and frequency of stress experienced by patients, reveals that musculoskeletal symptoms are the most prevalent. These are followed by gastrointestinal complaints and emotional disorders, with disorders affecting heat regulation ranking fourth.

Responses in the 'fairly/often' and 'strongly/very often' categories were less common in all organ systems at hospital discharge and follow-up than at hospital admission. The total number of complaints of symptoms present 'fairly/often' decreased from 30.1% to 20% by discharge, increasing slightly again to 22.9% by follow-up. Symptoms experienced 'strongly/very frequently' decreased from 17% at admission to 7.9% at discharge, increasing slightly to 8.9% at follow-up.

Figure 5.66 illustrates the distribution of answers for the individual items per category across all measurement points for patients with a complete dataset at admission, discharge, and follow-up.

Statistical comparison of response frequencies shows highly significant differences between admission and discharge, as well as between admission and follow-up, which can be classified as having a moderate effect (fairly/often: $d = -0.79$, $p < 0.001$; $d = -0.55$, $p < 0.001$; respectively; strong/very frequently: $d = -0.75$, $p < 0.001$; $d = -0.66$, $p < 0.001$; respectively). Table 5.71 and Fig. 5.67 show the results in more detail.

Furthermore, as previously mentioned, an overall symptom index is formed across all complaints, ranging from 0 (= high somatic functional stress disorder) to 1 (= moderate somatic functional stress disorder) to 2 (= no relevant somatic functional stress disorder). The total score and total index of the Psycho-Vegetative Stability test show significant improvement between hospital admission and discharge, with large effect sizes ($d = -1.02$, $p < 0.001$; $d = -0.93$, $p < 0.001$, respectively). At follow-up, the effect size is somewhat weaker but remains in the moderate to large range for both the total score and the index ($d = -0.75$, $p < 0.001$; $d = -0.84$, $p < 0.001$, respectively) (Table 5.71). Figure 5.68 illustrates the difference for the complaint index graphically.

Table 5.70 Summary of symptom frequencies for the functional symptom disorder (FSD) profile by organ system in 2023, sorted by descending frequency of the response 'very/very frequent' (A–D–F: $n = 611$)

	Admission				Discharge				Follow-up			
Functional symptom disorder profile	Quite/often		Strong/very frequently		Quite/often		Strong/very frequently		Quite/often		Strong/very frequently	
	M (SD)	%	M (SD)	%	M (SD)	%	M (SD)	%	M (SD)	%	M (SD)	%
Musculoskeletal system (3)	0.88 (0.86)	29.2	1.00 (0.96)	33.2	0.83 (0.88)	27.7	0.37 (0.69)	12.3	0.90 (0.91)	29.9	0.58 (0.87)	19.3
Gastrointestinal system (1)	0.34 (0.47)	34.0	0.28 (0.45)	28.2	0.30 (0.46)	30.0	0.16 (0.36)	15.5	0.32 (0.47)	32.2	0.13 (0.34)	13.1
Fatigue and sleep-related symptoms (6)	2.35 (1.39)	39.1	1.65 (1.51)	27.5	1.72 (1.43)	28.7	0.77 (1.26)	12.9	1.84 (1.49)	30.6	0.84 (1.35)	14.0
(thermal) regulation-related symptoms (7)	2.04 (1.57)	29.1	1.28 (1.59)	18.3	1.47 (1.54)	21.0	0.64 (1.24)	9.1	1.85 (1.67)	26.5	0.72 (1.27)	10.2
Affective symptoms (8)	3.05 (1.81)	38.1	1.31 (1.63)	16.4	1.66 (1.79)	20.8	0.55 (1.12)	6.9	1.92 (1.89)	24.0	0.61 (1.19)	7.7
Urogenital system (1)	0.31 (0.46)	30.8	0.16 (0.36)	15.5	0.33 (0.47)	33.1	0.11 (0.31)	11.0	0.27 (0.45)	27.3	0.10 (0.30)	9.8
Brain-related symptoms (4)	1.33 (1.07)	33.2	0.55 (0.86)	13.7	0.77 (1.00)	19.3	0.28 (0.68)	6.9	0.91 (1.02)	22.8	0.29 (0.67)	7.3
Immune system (1)	0.22 (0.42)	22.4	0.09 (0.29)	9.2	0.10 (0.30)	9.8	0.04 (0.19)	3.8	0.16 (0.36)	15.7	0.05 (0.22)	4.9
Allergy-related symptoms (5)	0.89 (1.03)	17.9	0.38 (0.78)	7.6	0.56 (0.9)	11.2	0.17 (0.50)	3.4	0.61 (0.97)	12.1	0.17 (0.51)	3.5
Cardiovascular system (6)	1.25 (1.31)	20.9	0.45 (0.88)	7.5	0.67 (1.04)	11.2	0.22 (0.66)	3.7	0.82 (1.11)	13.6	0.23 (0.68)	3.9
Total (42)	**12.66 (5.06)**	**30.1**	**7.15 (5.59)**	**17.0**	**8.42 (5.62)**	**20.0**	**3.30 (4.37)**	**7.9**	**9.60 (5.98)**	**22.9**	**3.72 (4.75)**	**8.9**

Note: The number corresponds to the total amount of information from all patients, while the percentages correspond to the proportion within each category. It is possible for bias to be introduced by individual items in systems with many different symptom options

A value of 0 means that, on average, the respective answer was not given (values between 0 and 8 are possible, depending on the organ system). % figures correspond to the mean relative proportion of answers per category. Sorted by descending frequency of answers 'strongly/very frequently' on admission

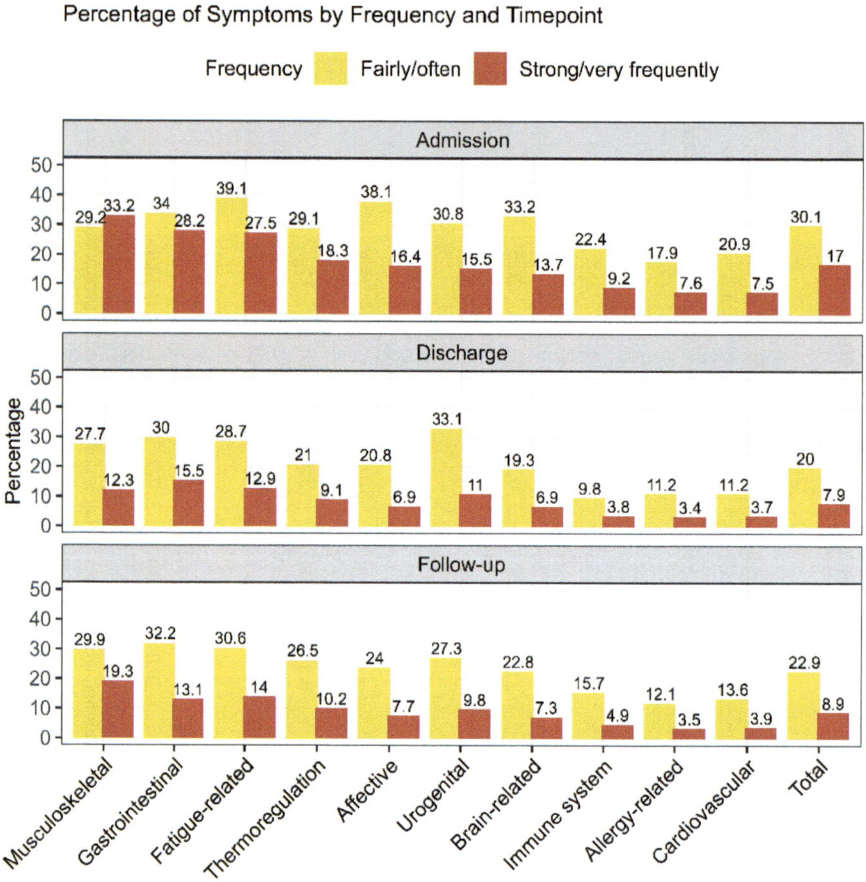

Fig. 5.65 Distribution of symptom frequencies for the FSD disorder profile by functional and organ system in 2023 (complete dataset A–D–F: n = 611); sorted in descending frequency of answers 'strongly/very frequently' on admission

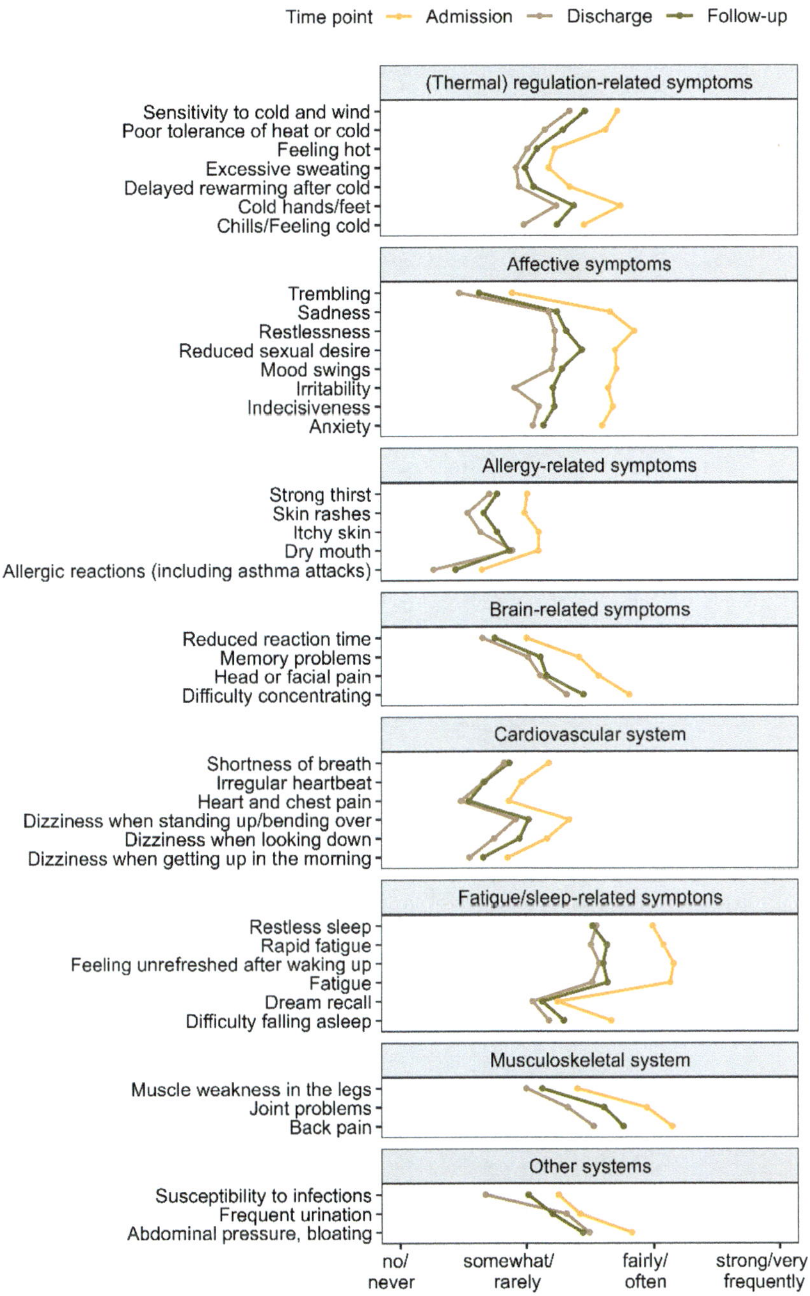

Fig. 5.66 Distribution of symptom frequencies for the FSD profile in 2023 (A-E-F: $n = 613$)

Table 5.71 FSD disturbance profile in pre/post comparison in 2023 for complete data sets and psycho-vegetative complaints in pre/post comparison in 2023 for complete data sets t-test for paired samples; significance at $p < 0.05$; Cohen's d = effect measure ($d \geq 0.2$ = small, ≥ 0.5 = moderate, ≥ 0.8 = large effect); previous year's data since 2022

		2023								Previous year 2022			
FSD		Cross-section: A/D/F			Course: A–D/A–F $n = 611$		Difference from admission: A–D/A–F $n = 611$			Course: A–D/A–F $n = 504$	Difference from admission: A–D/A–F $n = 504$		
		n	M	SD	M	SD	ΔM	p	d	M	ΔM	p	d
Answer: Fairly/often	**A**	823	12.54	5.06	12.66	5.06				12.48			
	D	777	8.66	5.63	8.42	5.62	−4.24	<0.001	**−0.79**	8.14	−4.34	<0.001	**−0.84**
	F	618	9.59	5.98	9.60	5.98	−3.06	<0.001	**−0.55**	9.55	−2.93	<0.001	**−0.56**
Answer: Strong/very frequently	**A**	823	7.22	5.68	7.15	5.59				7.19			
	D	777	3.46	4.44	3.30	4.37	−3.84	<0.001	**−0.75**	3.29	−3.90	<0.001	**−0.78**
	F	618	3.72	4.74	3.72	4.75	−3.43	<0.001	**−0.66**	3.74	−3.45	<0.001	**−0.67**
Complaint index	**A**	823	0.31	0.53	0.31	0.52				0.29			
	D	777	0.89	0.78	0.94	0.79	0.64	<0.001	**−0.93**	0.93	0.64	<0.001	**−0.94**
	F	618	0.86	0.75	0.86	0.76	0.55	<0.001	**−0.84**	0.85	0.56	<0.001	**−0.85**
Total score	**A**	823	61.26	17.11	61.45	16.72				60.89			
	D	777	43.78	18.79	43.11	18.86	−18.34	<0.001	**−1.02**	42.17	−18.72	<0.001	**−1.04**
	F	618	47.74	19.21	47.74	19.27	−13.71	<0.001	**−0.75**	46.96	−14.93	<0.001	**−0.78**

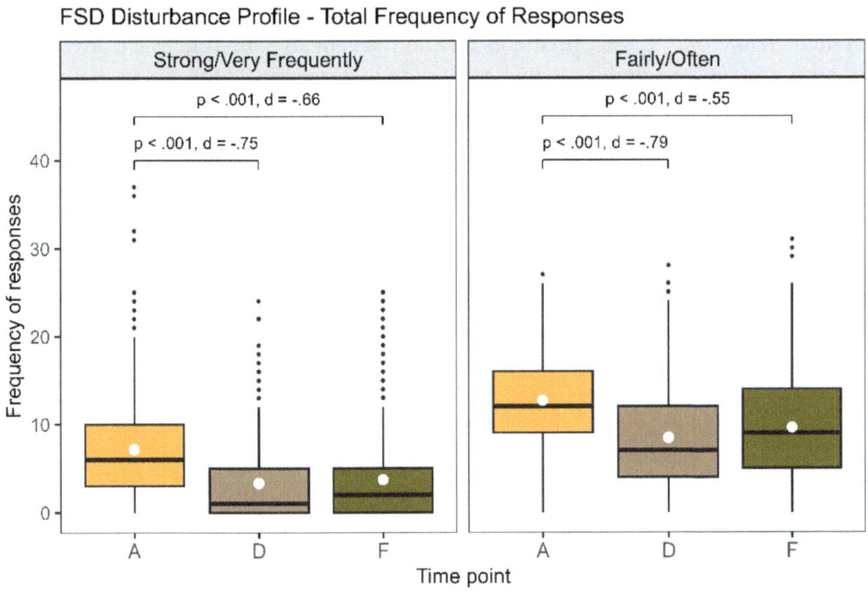

Fig. 5.67 FSD disturbance profile: total frequency of 'fairly/often' and 'strong/very frequently' responses over the course of the 2023 measurement points (*A* admission, *D* discharge, *F* follow-up); *t*-test for paired samples; Cohen's *d* = effect measure ($d \geq 0.2$ = small, 0.5 = moderate, $\geq$ 0.8 = large effect)

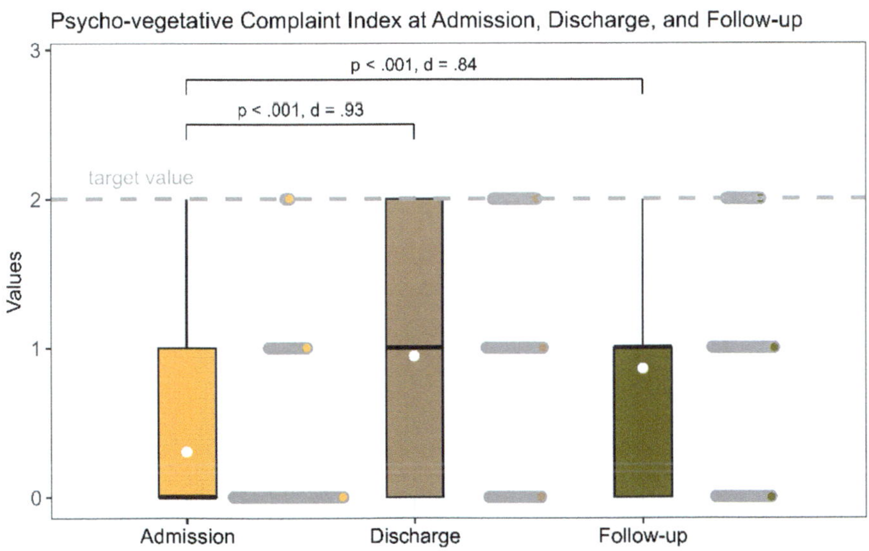

Fig. 5.68 FSD disturbance profile: complaint index over the course of the 2023 measurement points; *t*-test for paired samples; Cohen's d = effect size measure ($d \geq 0.2$ = small effect, $\geq$ 0.5 = moderate effect, 0.8 = large effect); the grey dashed line indicates the target value

Figure 5.69 shows the distribution of the complaint index across the traffic light system. While only 2.8% of patients had no relevant somatic functional stress disorder symptoms on admission, this proportion increased to 28.6% by discharge and remained relatively high at 22.6% at follow-up. Conversely, the proportion of patients experiencing high somatic functional stress disorder symptoms halved from 72.2% at admission to 34.2% at discharge, remaining at 36.5% at follow-up.

5.2.2.5 Stressors and Burdens

The stressors and burdens questionnaire is completed on admission and at follow-up. The value distributions of patients on the individual scales can be seen in Table 5.72 and Fig. 5.70. When it comes to stress factors, domestic/everyday life and work-related stress are the main contributors. The greatest gender difference is observed in domestic/everyday life stressors, where women tend to report higher levels of stress. Figure 5.71 shows the percentage distribution of responses within each age group, separated by gender. The total for each subgroup (e.g. women aged 31–40) adds up to 100%. Apart from patients aged 61–70, women report higher stressors and burdens in all age categories. Table 5.73 presents the numerical results for each subgroup.

Between admission and the follow-up examination, the total value of the stressors decreased significantly with a small effect size ($d = -0.22$, $p < 0.001$). This decrease was primarily due to the subcategories of occupational stress, domestic/everyday life, and major life events, which had all decreased significantly by the time of the follow-up examination approximately 6 months later ($d = -0.17$, $p < 0.001$; $d = -0.21$, $p < 0.001$; $d = -0.21$, $p < 0.001$, respectively). The financial burden subscale showed no significant change. Table 5.74 and Fig. 5.72 illustrate the results in more detail.

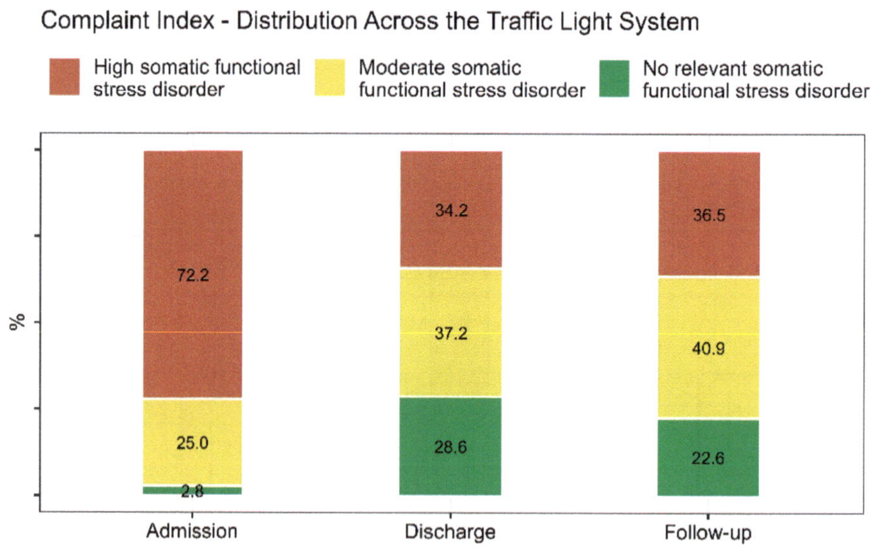

Fig. 5.69 Distribution of the complaint index across the levels of the traffic light system in 2023

Table 5.72 Measures of distribution for the total Stressors and Burdens value including all subscales, broken down by gender in 2023 and previous years

		2023				Previous years			
Stressors and burdens	Gender	*n*	M	SD	Md	*n*	M	SD	Md
Total score	Men	170	1.84	0.39	2	3210	1.81	0.43	2
	Women	652	1.89	0.37	2	9166	1.87	0.38	2
	Total	822	1.88	0.37	2	12,376	1.85	0.40	2
Occupational stress	Men	170	1.26	0.91	2	3210	1.30	0.88	2
	Women	652	1.30	0.90	2	9166	1.32	0.89	2
	Total	822	1.29	0.9	2	12,376	1.31	0.89	2
Domestic/everyday life	Men	170	1.61	0.60	2	3210	1.59	0.58	2
	Women	652	1.71	0.53	2	9166	1.69	0.55	2
	Total	822	1.69	0.54	2	12,376	1.66	0.56	2
Financial burdens	Men	170	0.45	0.71	0	3210	0.44	0.67	0
	Women	652	0.47	0.68	0	9166	0.44	0.67	0
	Total	822	0.47	0.69	0	12,376	0.44	0.67	0
Major life events	Men	170	1.06	0.75	1	3210	0.95	0.83	1
	Women	652	1.09	0.79	1	9166	1.11	0.82	1
	Total	822	1.09	0.78	1	12,376	1.07	0.82	1

M mean, *SD* standard deviation, *Md* median

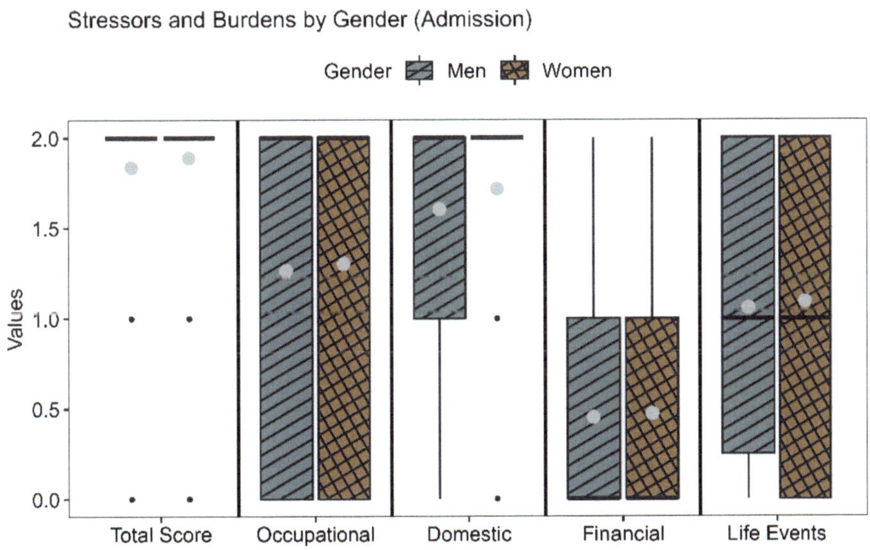

Fig. 5.70 Distribution of the Stressors and Burdens subscales, divided by gender in 2023. Grey circles indicate the mean and black lines represent the median. Due to the highly skewed response distribution on the limited three-point scale (0–2), some items show no visible bar in the chart. This occurs when almost all patients select the same response category. Consequently, only the median and mean indicators are displayed, accurately reflecting the lack of dispersion

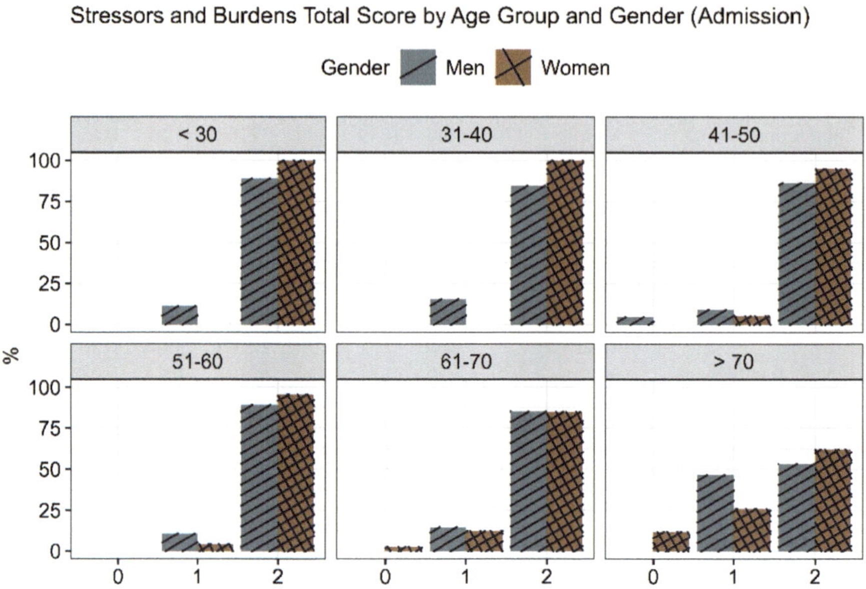

Fig. 5.71 Percentage distribution of the overall Stressors and Burdens score within each age group, separated by gender; for each subgroup (e.g. women <30), the total adds up to 100%

Table 5.73 Measures of distribution for the overall Stressors and Burdens score, broken down by gender and age in 2023 and previous years

Stressors and burdens total score									
		2023				Previous years			
	Age group	*n*	M	SD	Md	*n*	M	SD	Md
Men	Up to 30	9	1.89	0.33	2	150	1.83	0.41	2
	31 to 40	13	1.85	0.38	2	244	1.95	0.22	2
	41 to 50	22	1.82	0.50	2	651	1.94	0.24	2
	51 to 60	64	1.89	0.31	2	1059	1.91	0.30	2
	61 to 70	47	1.85	0.36	2	669	1.69	0.51	2
	Over 70	15	1.53	0.52	2	437	1.47	0.62	2
	Total	170	1.84	0.39	2	3210	1.81	0.43	2
Women	Up to 30	14	2.00	0.00	2	421	1.91	0.30	2
	31 to 40	50	2.00	0.00	2	690	1.97	0.18	2
	41 to 50	96	1.95	0.22	2	2073	1.95	0.24	2
	51 to 60	280	1.96	0.20	2	3358	1.93	0.27	2
	61 to 70	153	1.82	0.45	2	1724	1.77	0.48	2
	Over 70	58	1.50	0.71	2	900	1.54	0.65	2
	Total	651	1.89	0.37	2	9166	1.87	0.38	2
Total	Up to 30	23	1.96	0.21	2	571	1.89	0.34	2
	31 to 40	63	1.97	0.18	2	934	1.96	0.19	2
	41 to 50	118	1.92	0.30	2	2724	1.94	0.24	2
	51 to 60	344	1.94	0.23	2	4417	1.93	0.28	2
	61 to 70	200	1.83	0.43	2	2393	1.75	0.49	2
	Over 70	73	1.51	0.67	2	1337	1.52	0.64	2
	Total	821	1.88	0.37	2	12.376	1.85	0.40	2

M mean, *SD* standard deviation, *Md* median

Table 5.74 Stressors and Burdens before/after comparison in 2023; t-test for paired samples; significance at $p < 0.05$; Cohen's d = effect measure ($d \geq 0.2$ = small, ≥ 0.5 = moderate, ≥ 0.8 = large effect); previous year's data since 2022

		2023								Previous year 2022			
Stressors and burdens		Cross-section: A/D/F			Course: A–D/A–F $n = 614$		Difference from admission: A–D/A–F $n = 614$			Course: A–D/A–F $n = 513$	Difference from admission: A–D/A–F $n = 513$		
		n	M	SD	M	SD	ΔM	p	d	M	ΔM	p	d
Total value	**A**	821	1.88	0.37	1.88	0.36				1.91			
	F	614	1.79	0.45	1.79	0.45	−0.09	<0.001	−0.22	1.84	−0.07	<0.001	−0.18
Occupational stress	**A**	821	1.29	0.90	1.30	0.89				1.43			
	F	614	1.15	0.92	0.15	0.92	−0.15	<0.001	−0.17	1.27	−0.16	<0.001	−0.19
Domestic/everyday life	**A**	821	1.69	0.54	1.70	0.53				1.74			
	F	614	1.58	0.56	1.58	0.56	−0.12	<0.001	−0.21	1.65	−0.09	<0.001	−0.19
Financial burdens	**A**	821	0.47	0.69	0.45	0.68				0.43			
	F	614	0.42	0.67	0.42	0.67	−0.03	0.185	–	0.42	−0.02	0.466	–
Major life events	**A**	821	1.09	0.78	1.08	0.78				1.10			
	F	614	0.92	0.79	0.92	0.79	−0.17	<0.001	−0.21	1.04	−0.07	0.060	–

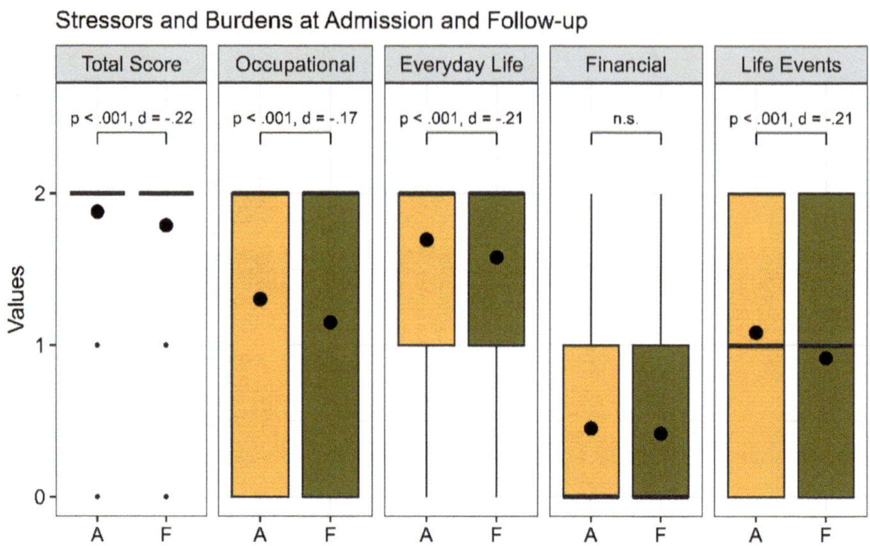

Fig. 5.72 Stressors and Burdens scales over the course of the 2023 measurement time points (*A* admission, *F* follow-up); *t*-test with paired samples; significance at $p < 0.05$; Cohen's d = effect measure ($d \geq 0.2$ = small, ≥ 0.5 = moderate, ≥ 0.8 = large); black circles indicate the mean, black lines the median

As can be seen in Fig. 5.73, the percentage distribution across the traffic light system improved slightly, reflecting the statistical results.

5.2.3 Mental Stress

5.2.3.1 WHO-5 Depression

The WHO-5 well-being figures were presented in Sect. 5.2.1.3. As the depression score corresponds to the well-being score but uses different thresholds to categorise the severity of depression symptoms, only the visual results relating to the traffic light colour categories are shown here. Refer to the Sect. 5.2.1.3 for the results tables.

As can be seen in Fig. 5.74, the average value for women across all age groups indicates minor depression. Older age groups tend towards the 'could be improved' threshold, while younger age groups tend towards 'major depression'.

For men, the picture is somewhat different: the age groups under 30, 31–40, and 51–60 can be classified as 'minor depression', while the age groups 41–50, 61–70, and over 70 falls into the 'could be improved' category.

Comparing the measurement points shows that, while most patients indicate minor or major depression at admission, this proportion decreases significantly by discharge, with moderate to large improvement still evident at follow-up (Fig. 5.75).

The positive effect of the treatment is evident in the percentage distribution: while 34.7% of patients showed signs of severe depression upon admission, this

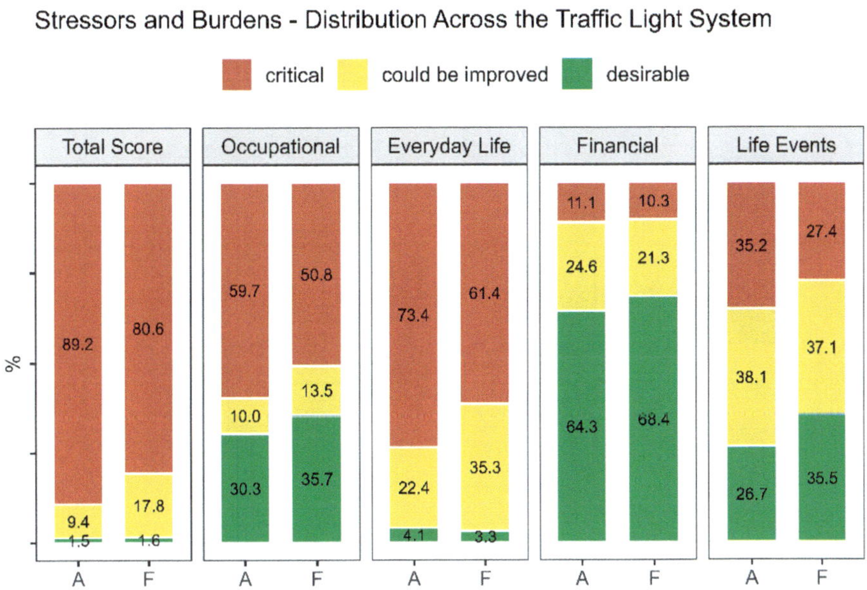

Fig. 5.73 Percentage distribution of all Stressors and Burdens dimensions across the levels of the traffic light system in 2023; *A* admission, *F* follow-up

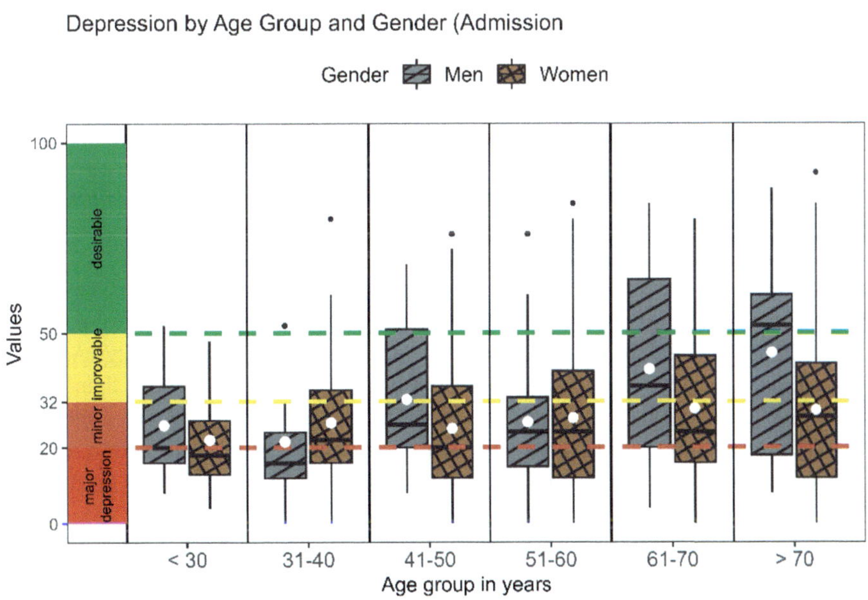

Fig. 5.74 Distribution measures of the WHO-5 Depression (well-being) score in the 2023 reporting year at admission, broken down by gender and age group; white circles indicate the mean, black lines the median; the coloured lines indicate the thresholds according to the traffic light system

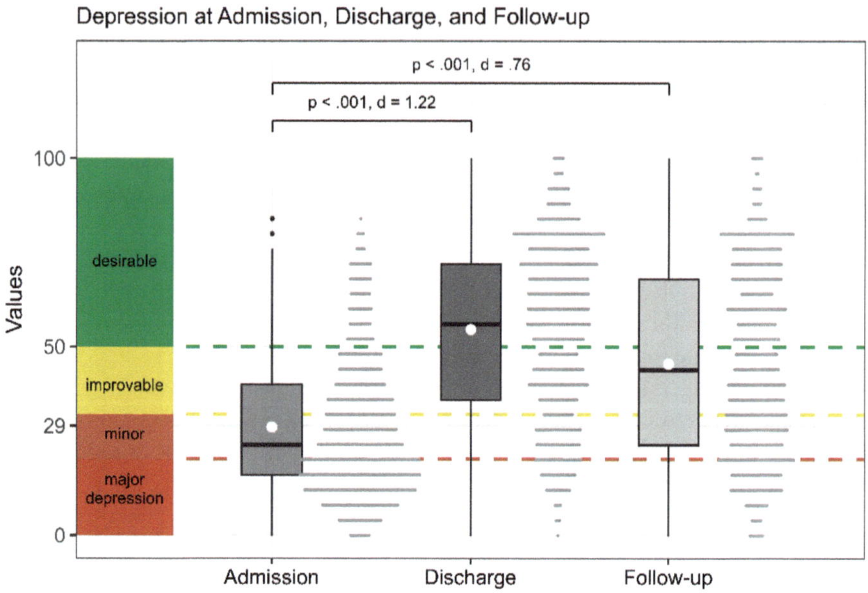

Fig. 5.75 Depression score (WHO-5) over the course of the measurement time points 2023; *t*-test with paired samples; Cohen's d = effect measure ($d \geq 0.2$ = small, ≥ 0.5 = moderate, ≥ 0.8 = large effect); white circle indicates the mean, the black line the median

figure fell to 7.0% at discharge and to less than half of that number (14.3%) at the follow-up examination. Conversely, the proportion of patients achieving desirable scores on the depression scale increased from 14.1% at admission to 59.6% at discharge. Although the proportion fell between discharge and the follow-up examination, it remained three times higher than at admission (14.15% vs. 42.7%) Fig. 5.76 illustrates the results for all categories.

5.2.3.2 Generalised Anxiety Disorder (GAD)

Upon admission to the clinic, most patients presented with moderate anxiety symptoms (mean = 10.36, standard deviation = 4.81). Men had slightly less severe symptoms than women, with mean scores of 9.56 and 10.56 respectively. Anxiety symptoms are somewhat more pronounced in the younger age groups than in the older age groups, but there are some fluctuations between the years, especially among men. Women show relatively consistent symptom severity across all age groups. Table 5.75 presents the figures broken down by gender and age group, and Fig. 5.77 illustrates the results graphically.

There was a significant improvement in anxiety disorder symptoms between admission and discharge, as well as between admission and follow-up, with large ($d = -0.98$, $p < 0.001$) and moderate-to-large ($d = -0.75$, $p < 0.001$) effects, respectively. Table 5.76 and Fig. 5.78 present the results in more detail.

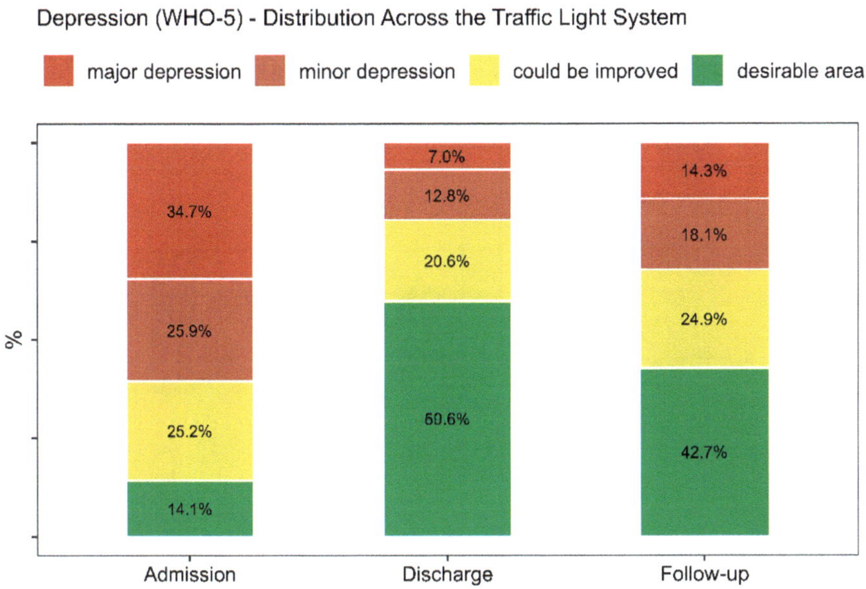

Fig. 5.76 Distribution of the depression score (WHO-5 Well-being) across the levels of the traffic light system in 2023; *A* admission, *D* discharge, *F* follow-up

Table 5.75 Measures of distribution for the GAD, broken down by gender and age in 2023 and previous years

GAD									
		2023				Previous year[a]			
	Age group	*n*	M	SD	Md	*n*	M	SD	Md
Men	Up to 30	9	11.44	4.93	10	1	9	–	9.0
	31 to 40	13	10.69	4.55	12	7	13.70	3.40	16.0
	41 to 50	22	8.91	4.05	8	14	8.86	6.10	7.0
	51 to 60	63	10.95	4.85	10	32	9.59	4.58	9.0
	61 to 70	45	7.76	5.00	8	19	8.79	4.02	10.0
	Over 70	14	7.86	4.05	8	10	7.60	5.44	8.5
	Total	**166**	**9.56**	**4.88**	**9**	**83**	**9.39**	**4.86**	**9.0**
Women	Up to 30	14	11.86	5.39	12	5	13.40	5.90	12.0
	31 to 40	50	10.64	4.95	11	21	9.19	4.17	9.0
	41 to 50	96	10.27	4.70	10	45	11.80	4.39	12.0
	51 to 60	278	10.64	4.34	10	140	10.20	4.88	10.0
	61 to 70	153	10.52	5.09	10	76	9.95	4.56	11.0
	Over 70	58	10.40	5.72	10	36	9.19	5.01	10.0
	Total	**649**	**10.56**	**4.77**	**10**	**323**	**10.30**	**4.79**	**10.0**
Total	Up to 30	23	11.7	5.10	11	6	12.70	5.57	10.5
	31 to 40	63	10.65	4.84	11	28	10.30	4.41	10.5
	41 to 50	118	10.02	4.6	10	59	11.10	4.96	11.0
	51 to 60	341	10.7	4.43	10	172	10.10	4.82	10.0
	61 to 70	198	9.89	5.19	9	95	9.72	4.46	10.0
	Over 70	72	9.90	5.50	9	46	8.85	5.09	9.0
	Total	**815**	**10.36**	**4.81**	**10**	**406**	**10.10**	**4.79**	**10.0**

M mean, *SD* standard deviation, *Md* median

[a]Since the GAD7 questionnaire was introduced in May 2022, only data from the previous year, 2022, is available

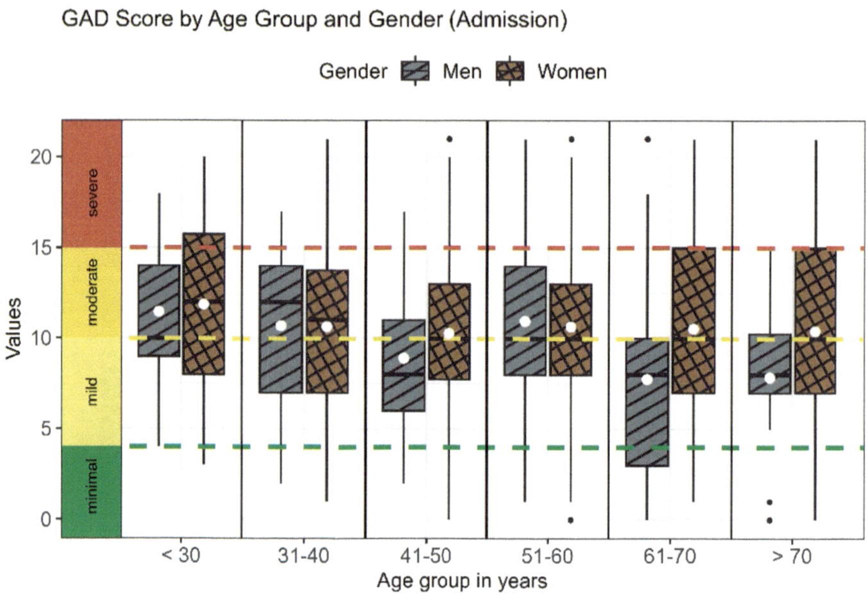

Fig. 5.77 Distribution of GAD in 2023 at admission, broken down by gender and age group; white circles indicate the mean, black lines the median; the coloured lines indicate the thresholds according to the traffic light system

The shift towards mild or minimal anxiety symptoms after treatment is clearly visible in both Figs. 5.78 and 5.79. While only 10.8% of patients had minimal anxiety symptoms upon admission, this proportion increased more than fourfold (44.6%) by discharge and showed a further threefold increase (37.2%) at follow-up. Conversely, the proportion of patients with severe anxiety symptoms fell dramatically, from 20.9% at admission to 5.0% at discharge and 7.7% at follow-up.

5.2.4 Physiological Resource Profile

5.2.4.1 IHM Movement Index

Upon admission, the average IHM Movement Index score for all patients is around 3.90 points (SD = 2.74). The overall result for men (M = 4.12, SD = 2.63) differs slightly from that for women (M = 3.84, SD = 2.77), with the latter having a lower average physical activity index. Further analysis of the individual age categories by gender indicates only minimal age differences (Table 5.77). Regardless of gender, all patients in every age group are, on average, classified as 'could be improved' upon admission, except women over 70, who are, on a mean basis, classified as 'critical' (Fig. 5.80).

There was a significant improvement in the Movement Index, which can be described as a small effect size ($d = 0.26$, $p < 0.001$). The average Movement Index improved by 0.71 points at the time of follow-up. Figure 5.81 illustrates the results

Table 5.76 GAD before/after comparison in 2023; *t*-test for paired samples; significance at $p < 0.05$; Cohen's d = effect measure ($d \geq 0.2$ = small, ≥ 0.5 = moderate, ≥ 0.8 = large effect); previous year's data since 2022

		2023								Previous year 2022			
		Cross-section: A/D/F			Course: A–D/A–F $n = 583$		Difference from admission: A–D/A–F $n = 583$			Course: A–D/A–F $n = 258$	Difference from admission: A–D/A–F $n = 258$		
		n	M	SD	M	SD	ΔM	*p*	*d*	M	ΔM	*p*	*d*
GAD	**A**	815	10.36	4.81	10.30	4.78				10.29			
	D	776	5.95	4.41	5.78	4.37	−4.52	<0.001	**−0.98**	5.67	−4.62	<0.001	**−1.01**
	F	593	6.72	4.65	6.67	4.66	−3.54	<0.001	**−0.75**	6.46	−3.63	<0.001	**−0.83**

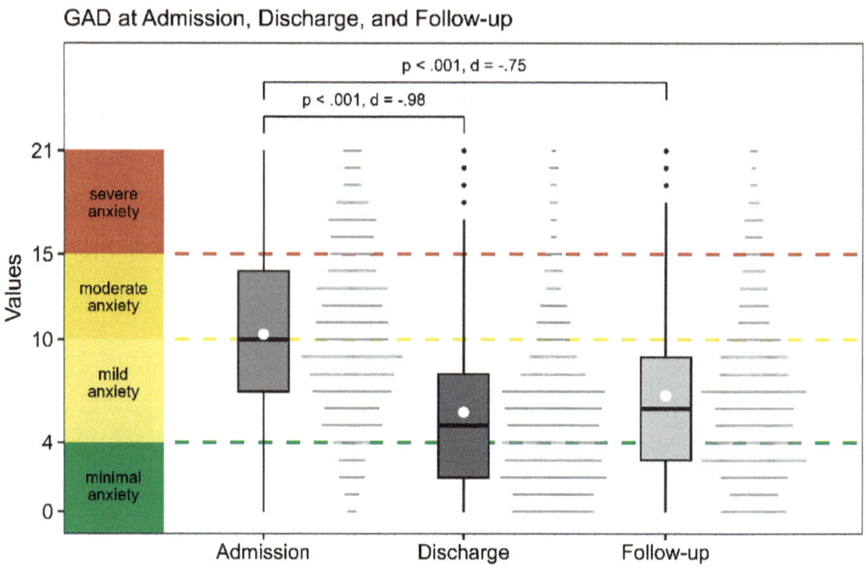

Fig. 5.78 GAD score over the course of the measurement time points in 2023; *t*-test with paired samples; Cohen's *d* = effect measure ($d \geq 0.2$ = small, ≥ 0.5 = moderate, ≥ 0.8 = large effect); white circle indicates the mean, the black line the median

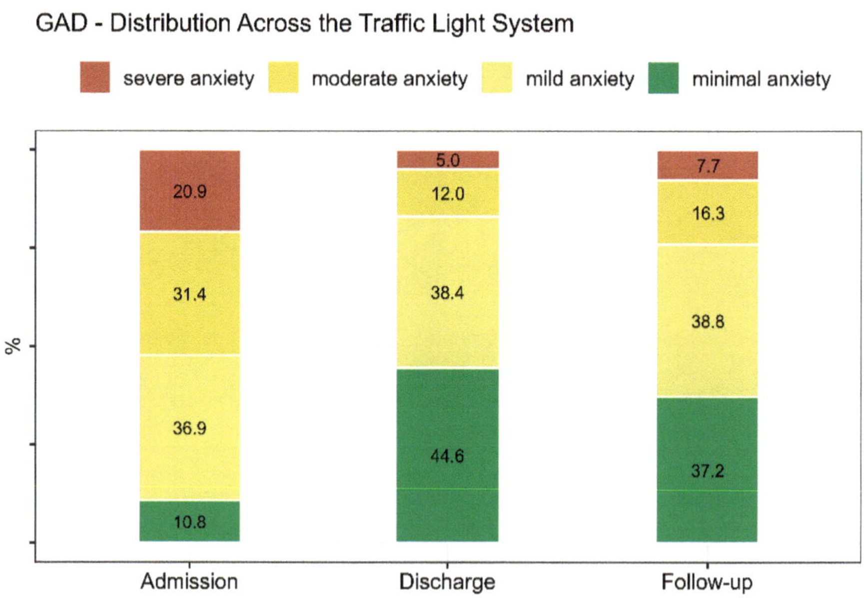

Fig. 5.79 Distribution of the GAD index across the levels of the traffic light system in 2023

Table 5.77 Measures of distribution for the movement index, broken down by gender and age in 2023

Movement index									
		2023				Previous years[a]			
	Age group	*n*	M	SD	Md	*n*	M	SD	Md
Men	Up to 30	9	3.67	2.12	4.0	–	–	–	–
	31 to 40	13	4.62	2.63	6.0	–	–	–	–
	41 to 50	21	4.24	2.55	4.0	–	–	–	–
	51 to 60	63	4.03	2.8	4.0	–	–	–	–
	61 to 70	47	4.15	2.46	4.0	–	–	–	–
	Over 70	15	4.13	3.16	4.0	–	–	–	–
	Total	**168**	**4.12**	**2.63**	**4.0**	–	–	–	–
Women	Up to 30	14	3.36	2.92	2.5	–	–	–	–
	31 to 40	50	3.56	2.39	4.0	–	–	–	–
	41 to 50	95	4.01	2.77	4.0	–	–	–	–
	51 to 60	279	3.82	2.68	4.0	–	–	–	–
	61 to 70	150	4.19	3.02	4.0	–	–	–	–
	Over 70	58	3.09	2.69	2.5	–	–	–	–
	Total	**646**	**3.84**	**2.77**	**4.0**	–	–	–	–
Total	Up to 30	23	3.48	2.59	4.0	–	–	–	–
	31 to 40	63	3.78	2.46	4.0	–	–	–	–
	41 to 50	116	4.05	2.72	4.0	–	–	–	–
	51 to 60	342	3.86	2.7	4.0	–	–	–	–
	61 to 70	197	4.18	2.89	4.0	–	–	–	–
	Over 70	73	3.3	2.8	3.0	–	–	–	–
	Total	**814**	**3.90**	**2.74**	**4.0**	–	–	–	–

M mean, *SD* standard deviation, *Md* median

[a]A revised version of the Movement Index has been in use since the beginning of 2023, so no comparative data is available yet

in graph form, and Table 5.78 presents the numerical data. Figure 5.82 presents the distribution across the levels of the traffic light system, showing a clear shift from the critical area towards the desirable area at follow-up.

5.2.4.2 IHM Nutrition Index

On admission, the average physical activity index value for all patients was around 9.45 (SD = 2.13). The overall result for women (M = 9.53, SD = 2.09) differs slightly from that for men (M = 9.15, SD = 2.26), with the latter having a lower average Nutrition Index. The distribution in the individual age categories by gender indicates only minimal age differences (Table 5.79 and Fig. 5.83). Across genders, most patients are in the 'could be improved' range on admission.

Approximately 6 months after discharge from hospital, the average Nutrition Index had improved by an average of 0.40 points, corresponding to a small effect size ($d = 0.20$, $p < 0.001$). Table 5.80 and Fig. 5.84 illustrate the results.

Upon admission, 19.5% of patients had a critical Nutrition Index; at follow-up, this figure was 11.4%. This suggests that more than 40% of patients initially categorised as critical improved to reach the 'could be improved' or 'desirable' categories. Figure 5.85 shows the percentage distribution of admissions and follow-ups across the traffic light system in detail.

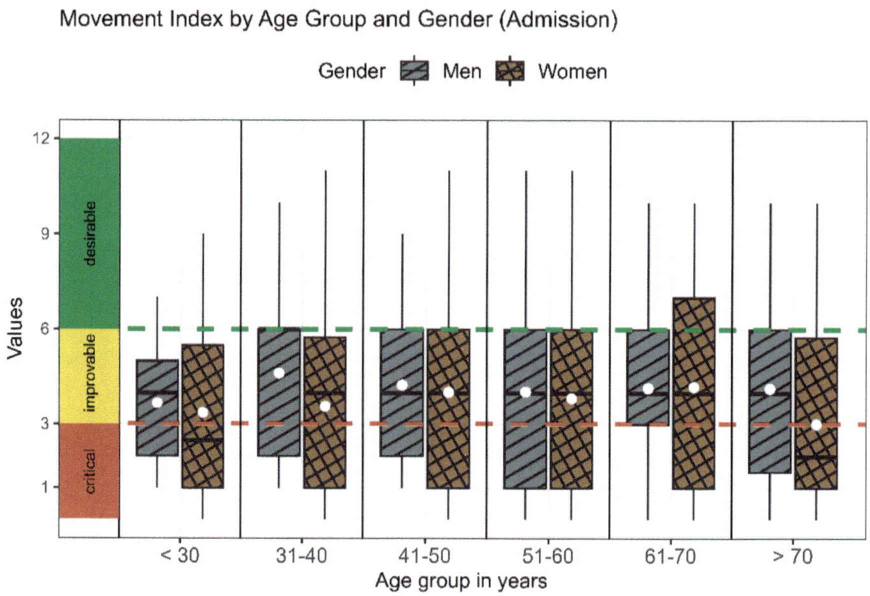

Fig. 5.80 Distribution measures of the Movement Index in the 2023 reporting year at admission, broken down by gender and age group; white circles indicate the mean, black lines the median; the coloured lines indicate the thresholds according to the traffic light system

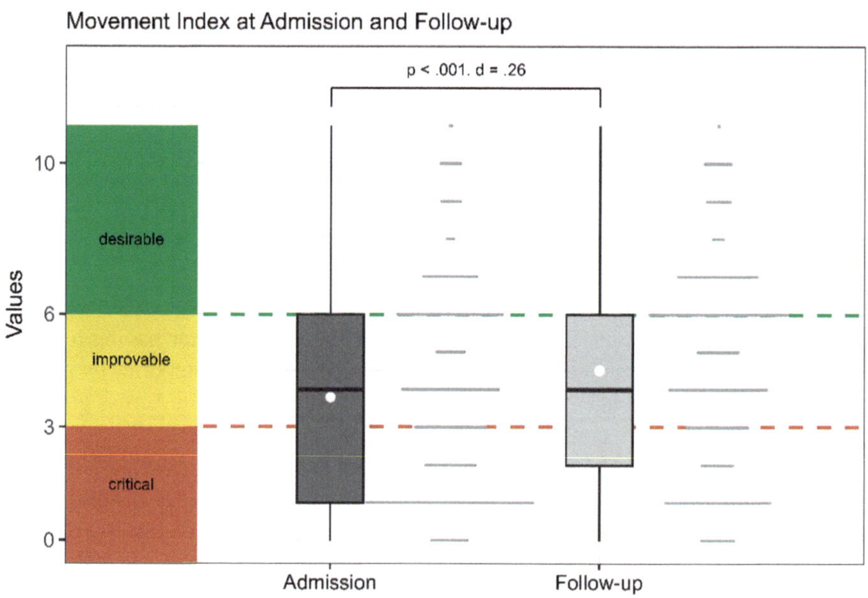

Fig. 5.81 Movement Index over the course of the measurement time points in 2023; *t*-test with paired samples; Cohen's *d* = effect measure ($d \geq 0.2$ = small, ≥ 0.5 = moderate, ≥ 0.8 = large effect); white circle indicates the mean, the black line the median

Table 5.78 Movement Index before/after comparison in 2023; *t*-test for paired samples; significance at $p < 0.05$; Cohen's d = effect measure ($d \geq 0.2$ = small, ≥ 0.5 = moderate, ≥ 0.8 = large effect); previous year's data is not available yet

Movement index		2023							
		Cross-section: A/D/F			Course: A–D/A–F $n = 598$		Difference from admission: A–D/A–F $n = 598$		
		n	M	SD	M	SD	ΔM	p	d
Index	**A**	814	3.89	2.74	3.80	2.70			
	F	607	4.50	2.67	4.50	2.68	0.71	<0.001	0.26

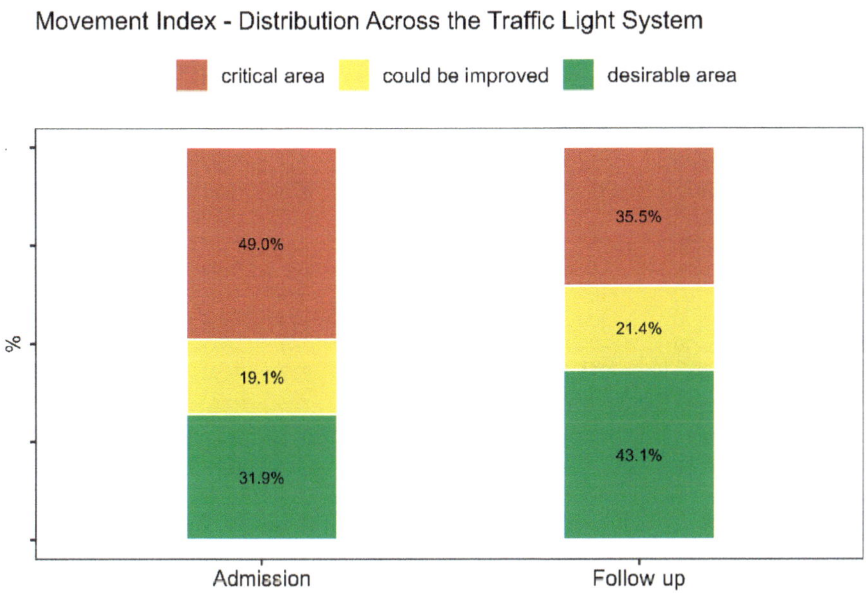

Fig. 5.82 Distribution of the Movement Index across the levels of the traffic light system in 2023

5.2.4.3 Psycho-Vegetative Stability (Sleep, Dizziness, and Heat Balance)

Sleep, heat balance, and dizziness (here primarily of orthostatic origin) are interpreted as indicators of neuro-vegetative stability in relation to thermoregulation, cardiovascular regulation, and emotional regulation, and are therefore considered protective factors for physical health.

On admission, the average scores for all patients were 7.06 (SD = 2.21) for sleep, 3.36 (SD = 2.23) for dizziness, and 5.61 (SD = 2.79) for heat balance. Overall, women reported more problems with sleep, dizziness, and heat balance than men (Tables 5.81 and 5.82). For both men and women, sleep is most affected, with more than 76% reporting a critical state. While dizziness is more prevalent in older age groups, sleep problems decrease slightly with age.

Table 5.79 Measures of distribution for the nutrition index, broken down by gender and age in 2023 and the previous year 2022

Nutrition index									
		2023				Previous year[a]			
	Age group	*n*	M	SD	Md	*n*	M	SD	Md
Men	Up to 30	9	8.33	2.45	9	4	8.75	2.22	8.0
	31 to 40	13	8.77	3.14	10	10	8.70	2.21	8.5
	41 to 50	22	8.55	2.2	8.5	21	8.05	2.52	9.0
	51 to 60	64	8.92	2.18	9	58	9.10	2.47	9.0
	61 to 70	47	9.74	1.92	10	36	9.17	2.14	9.0
	Over 70	15	9.93	2.4	11	15	10.30	2.15	11.0
	Total	**170**	**9.15**	**2.26**	**9**	**144**	**9.05**	**2.37**	**9.0**
Women	Up to 30	14	9.36	2.73	9.5	10	8.40	2.07	8.5
	31 to 40	50	9.04	2.28	9	43	9.33	2.08	9.0
	41 to 50	96	9.33	2.14	9.5	81	9.32	1.89	9.0
	51 to 60	280	9.49	2.14	10	251	9.79	2.18	10.0
	61 to 70	153	9.81	1.95	10	137	9.77	2.08	10.0
	Over 70	58	9.72	1.75	10	52	9.88	1.74	10.0
	Total	**651**	**9.53**	**2.09**	**10**	**574**	**9.67**	**2.08**	**10.0**
Total	Up to 30	23	8.96	2.62	9	14	8.50	2.03	8.0
	31 to 40	63	8.98	2.45	9	53	9.21	2.10	9.0
	41 to 50	118	9.19	2.16	9	102	9.06	2.09	9.0
	51 to 60	344	9.39	2.15	10	309	9.66	2.25	10.0
	61 to 70	200	9.8	1.94	10	173	9.64	2.10	10.0
	Over 70	73	9.77	1.88	10	67	9.97	1.83	10.0
	Total	**821**	**9.45**	**2.13**	**10**	**718**	**9.54**	**2.15**	**10.0**

M mean, *SD* standard deviation, *Md* median

[a]Since the Movement Index questionnaire was revised in 2022, only data from the previous year, 2022, is available

Figures 5.86, 5.87, and 5.88 illustrates the data on sleep, dizziness and heat balance in graphical form.

Between admission and discharge, all categories (sleep, dizziness, and heat balance) improved significantly, with moderate effect sizes ($d = -0.72$, $p < 0.001$; $d = -0.54$, $p < 0.001$; $d = -0.68$, $p < 0.001$, respectively) (Table 5.83). After approximately 6 months, the effect size was smaller but still significant, ranging from moderate to small ($d = -0.64$, $p < 0.001$; $d = -0.35$, $p < 0.001$; $d = -0.45$, $p < 0.001$). While the average values for dizziness and heat balance were in the critical range upon admission, the majority fell into the 'could be improved' range at hospital discharge and follow-up (Fig. 5.89). The mean sleep value also shows significant improvement, though it does not exceed the threshold for the 'could be improved' range. Nevertheless, while 76.6% of patients reported critical sleep values upon admission, this proportion decreased to 45.7% at follow-up. This indicates that approximately 40% of patients who were initially in the critical range improved to the 'could be improved' or 'desirable' categories 6 months after treatment. Similarly, while 2.8% of patients reported desirable sleep values at admission, this proportion increased to 11.9% at discharge and remained at 8.5% at follow-up. Similar improvements were observed for heat balance and dizziness (see Fig. 5.90 for more details).

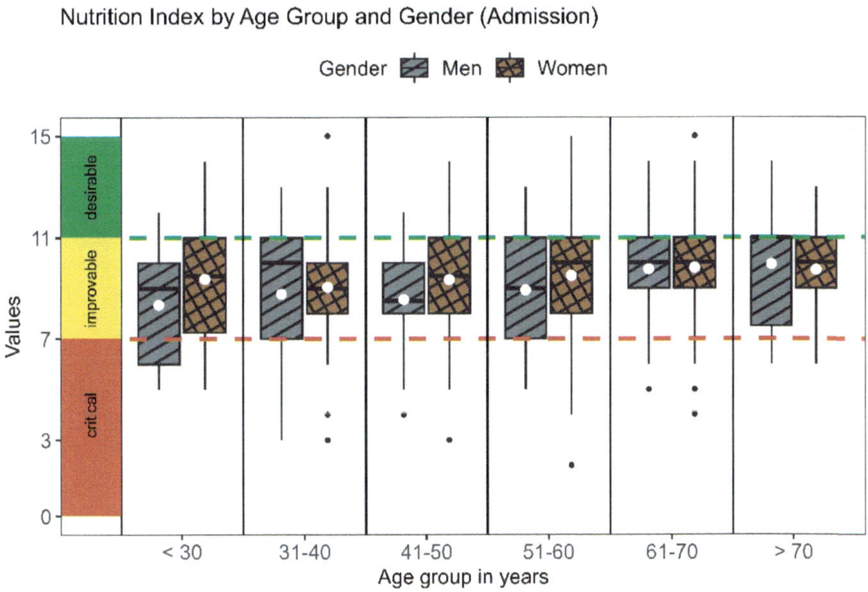

Fig. 5.83 Distribution measures of the Nutrition Index in the 2023 reporting year at admission, broken down by gender and age group; white circles indicate the mean, black lines the median; the coloured lines indicate the thresholds according to the traffic light system

Table 5.80 Nutrition index before/after comparison in 2023; *t*-test for paired samples; significance at $p < 0.05$; Cohen's d = effect measure ($d \geq 0.2$ = small, ≥ 0.5 = moderate, ≥ 0.8 = large effect); previous year's data since 2022

		2023								Previous year 2022			
		Cross-section: A/D/F			Course: A–D/A–F $n = 605$		Difference from admission: A–D/A–F $n = 605$			Course: A–D/ A–F $n = 508$	Difference from admission: A–D/A–F $n = 508$		
		n	M	SD	M	SD	ΔM	*p*	*d*	M	ΔM	*p*	*d*
Nutrition index	**A**	821	9.45	2.13	9.43	2.05				9.46			
	F	607	9.83	1.95	9.83	1.95	0.40	<0.001	0.20	9.74	0.29	0.002	0.14

5.2.4.4 Pittsburgh Sleep Quality Index (PSQI)

PSQI for All Patients Upon Admission

On admission, the average PSQI total score for all patients is around 10.45 (SD = 3.99). Consistent with the results of the Psycho-Vegetative Stability Questionnaire, the PSQI indicates that women report lower overall sleep quality than men. Specifically, women's mean score is 10.66 (SD = 4.03), while men's is 9.67 (SD = 3.75).

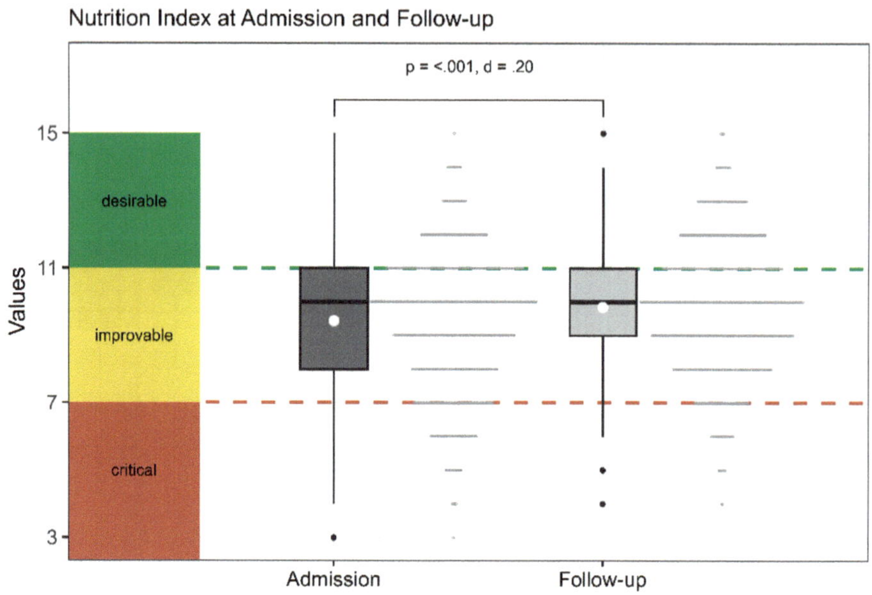

Fig. 5.84 Nutrition index over the course of the measurement time points in 2023; *t*-test with paired samples; Cohen's d = effect measure ($d \geq 0.2$ = small, ≥ 0.5 = moderate, ≥ 0.8 = large effect); white circle indicates the mean, the black line the median

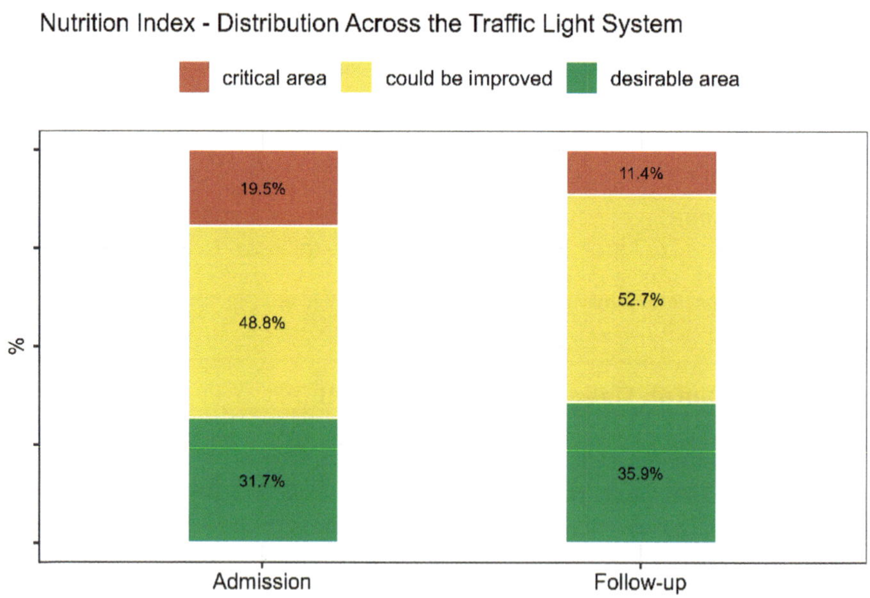

Fig. 5.85 Distribution of the nutrition index across the levels of the traffic light system in 2023

Further analysis of the data broken down by age and gender indicates only minimal age differences (Table 5.84, Fig. 5.91). Sleep disturbances are most prevalent among men aged 51–60, while the greatest impact is felt by women aged 61–70.

Although women and men report similar sleep durations and latencies, women consistently report slightly more difficulties in all other areas, including sleep efficiency, sleep pill usage, sleep quality, sleep disturbances, and daytime sleepiness. Of all the categories, sleep efficiency appears to be the least affected for both genders, with sleep pill usage reported at the lowest levels overall. Table 5.85 and Fig. 5.92 show the figures for each subscale.

PSQI for Patients with Diagnosed Sleep Disorder Upon Admission

A total of 255 patients were diagnosed with a sleep disorder in 2023. PSQI values on admission are available for 250 of these patients. The average sleep quality score for all these patients on admission is around 11.64 (SD = 3.55), which is slightly above the critical range threshold (>11 points).

While the overall trends in this subgroup are similar to those observed in the full sample, the highest levels of impairment are seen in women under 30 and over 70, and in men aged 31–40 and over 70 (Table 5.86, Fig. 5.93).

The biggest difference between men and women regarding the subscales can be seen in sleep efficiency. On this subscale, women reported an average value of 1.72 (SD = 1.11), whereas men reported an average value of 1.16 (SD = 1.03). Table 5.87 and Fig. 5.94 present the figures in more detail.

The results of the pre/post comparison for all patients are presented in the section below. Please refer to the relevant Sect. 5.4.2 for the pre/post comparisons for the patients with a diagnosed sleep disorder.

PSQI Pre/Post-treatment Comparison for All Patients

All Pittsburgh Sleep Quality Index subscales, except sleep duration, showed significant changes at discharge (Table 5.89). Sleep quality ($d = -0.55$, $p < 0.001$), sleep latency ($d = -0.25$, $p < 0.001$) and sleep efficiency ($d = -0.16$, $p < 0.001$) increased, while sleep dysfunction ($d = -0.33$, $p < 0.001$) and daytime sleepiness ($d = -0.89$, $p < 0.001$) decreased. Although sleeping pill consumption also increased significantly during the patients' stay in hospital, showing a moderate effect size ($d = 0.53$, $p < 0.001$), by the follow-up, medication intake had returned to pre-admission levels ($p = 0.448$). In contrast, however, improvements in sleep problems were still significant, especially with regard to sleep efficiency ($d = -0.35$, $p < 0.001$).

Overall sleep quality improved with a small effect size until discharge ($d = -0.26$, $p < 0.001$) and a small to moderate effect size until the follow-up ($d = -0.47$, $p < 0.001$). Table 5.88, Figs. 5.95, and 5.96 present the results in more detail.

Furthermore, Fig. 5.97 shows the percentage distribution across the traffic light system. It illustrates that the proportion of patients with clear signs of a sleep disorder decreased from 49.3% at admission to 29.0% at follow-up. Conversely, the proportion of patients reporting good sleep quality rose from 12.3% on admission to 29.5% at follow-up. Conversely, while only 12.3% reported a good sleep quality on admission, this proportion rose to 29.5% until follow-up.

Table 5.81 Measures of distribution for sleep, broken down by gender and age in 2023 and previous years

Sleep									
		2023				Previous years			
	Age group	*n*	M	SD	Md	*n*	M	SD	Md
Men	Up to 30	9	7.56	0.73	7	155	5.63	2.62	5
	31 to 40	13	6.62	2.40	7	240	6.42	2.71	6
	41 to 50	22	6.45	2.30	7	667	6.39	2.64	6
	51 to 60	64	6.73	2.46	7	1072	6.36	2.52	6
	61 to 70	47	5.94	2.14	6	687	5.70	2.52	6
	Over 70	15	6.00	2.07	6	448	5.02	2.67	5
	Total	**170**	**6.45**	**2.27**	**7**	**3269**	**6.02**	**2.63**	**6**
Women	Up to 30	14	7.50	2.10	7	428	6.51	2.64	6
	31 to 40	50	7.26	2.14	8	702	6.92	2.57	7
	41 to 50	96	7.18	2.40	7	2117	7.03	2.44	7
	51 to 60	281	7.31	2.10	7	3410	7.18	2.32	7
	61 to 70	153	7.24	2.22	8	1757	6.48	2.51	7
	Over 70	59	6.75	1.94	7	927	6.03	2.71	6
	Total	**653**	**7.22**	**2.16**	**7**	**9341**	**6.85**	**2.49**	**7**
Total	Up to 30	23	7.52	1.68	7	583	6.28	2.66	6
	31 to 40	63	7.13	2.19	7	942	6.79	2.61	7
	41 to 50	118	7.04	2.39	7	2784	6.88	2.50	7
	51 to 60	345	7.21	2.18	7	4482	6.99	2.39	7
	61 to 70	200	6.93	2.27	7	2444	6.26	2.54	6
	Over 70	74	6.59	1.98	7	1375	5.71	2.74	6
	Total	**823**	**7.06**	**2.21**	**7**	**12,610**	**6.64**	**2.55**	**7**

M mean, *SD* standard deviation, *Md* median

5.2.5 Risks to Physical Health

5.2.5.1 10-Year Risk of Developing a Cardiovascular Disease (SCORE2 ESC)

Upon admission, the average probability of patients developing cardiovascular disease within the next 10 years is around 6.58% (SD = 5.84). The overall result for men (M = 9.43, SD = 6.90) differs from that for women (M = 5.85, SD = 5.31), with women having a lower probability of developing cardiovascular disease than men across all age groups. As can be seen in Table 5.89 and Fig. 5.98, the risk generally increases with age, and the gender differences are even more pronounced. With an average value of 25.40% (SD = 6.86), men over 70 have a very high probability of developing cardiovascular disease within the next 10 years.

There was no significant difference in the risk of developing cardiovascular disease within the next 10 years between admission and discharge ($p = 0.446$). It is highly plausible that changes in vital signs and laboratory parameters require more time to become apparent. It is likely that a period of three to 4 weeks is insufficient to observe clinically meaningful alterations. Table 5.90 and Fig. 5.99 present the statistical results, while Fig. 5.100 illustrates the distribution across the traffic light system. At discharge, 44.3% of patients had a desirable low value, while 15% had a critical value.

Table 5.82 Measures of distribution for dizziness and heat balance, broken down by gender and age in 2023 and previous years

		Dizziness								Heat balance							
		2023				Previous years				2023				Previous years			
	Age group	*n*	M	SD	Md	*n*	M	SD	Md	*n*	M	SD	Md	*n*	M	SD	Md
Men	Up to 30	9	2.11	1.62	2	155	2.06	2.09	1	9	5.44	3.32	5	155	3.70	2.83	3
	31 to 40	13	3.38	2.14	3	240	2.59	2.11	2	13	4.23	3.32	3	240	4.04	2.97	4
	41 to 50	22	3.68	1.89	4	667	2.91	2.31	3	22	5.09	2.56	4.5	667	4.25	2.95	4
	51 to 60	64	2.98	2.01	3	1072	2.89	2.15	3	64	4.86	2.61	5	1072	4.35	2.81	4
	61 to 70	47	3.04	2.36	3	687	2.69	2.05	3	47	4.83	2.92	5	687	4.08	2.67	4
	Over 70	15	3.93	2.89	4	448	2.84	2.27	3	15	4.00	2.85	3	448	3.86	2.98	3.5
	Total	**170**	**3.16**	**2.18**	**3**	**3269**	**2.78**	**2.18**	**3**	**170**	**4.79**	**2.79**	**5**	**3269**	**4.15**	**2.85**	**4**
Women	Up to 30	14	2.57	2.31	1.5	428	2.85	2.30	3	14	6.14	2.14	6	428	6.07	2.98	6
	31 to 40	50	2.98	1.99	3	702	3.06	2.17	3	50	6.46	2.56	7	702	6.51	2.84	7
	41 to 50	96	3.33	2.46	3	2117	3.33	2.18	3	96	6.70	2.71	7	2117	6.24	2.93	6
	51 to 60	281	3.26	2.09	3	3410	3.34	2.19	3	281	5.77	2.60	6	3410	5.51	2.78	5
	61 to 70	153	3.74	2.34	3	1757	3.11	2.21	3	153	5.34	3.01	5	1757	5.13	2.76	5
	Over 70	59	4.05	2.27	4	927	3.09	2.33	3	59	5.29	2.78	5	927	4.98	2.94	5
	Total	**653**	**3.42**	**2.24**	**3**	**9341**	**3.23**	**2.21**	**3**	**653**	**5.82**	**2.76**	**6**	**9341**	**5.65**	**2.89**	**6**
Total	Up to 30	23	2.39	2.04	2	583	2.64	2.27	2	23	5.87	2.62	6	583	5.44	3.12	5
	31 to 40	63	3.06	2.02	3	942	2.94	2.16	3	63	6.00	2.85	6	942	5.88	3.07	6
	41 to 50	118	3.40	2.36	3	2784	3.23	2.22	3	118	6.40	2.74	7	2784	5.76	3.05	6
	51 to 60	345	3.21	2.07	3	4482	3.23	2.19	3	345	5.60	2.63	6	4482	5.23	2.83	5
	61 to 70	200	3.58	2.36	3	2444	2.99	2.17	3	200	5.22	2.99	5	2444	4.83	2.78	5
	Over 70	74	4.03	2.39	4	1375	3.01	2.31	3	74	5.03	2.82	5	1375	4.62	3.00	4
	Total	**823**	**3.36**	**2.23**	**3**	**12,610**	**3.11**	**2.21**	**3**	**823**	**5.61**	**2.79**	**6**	**12,610**	**5.26**	**2.95**	**5**

M mean, *SD* standard deviation, *Md* median

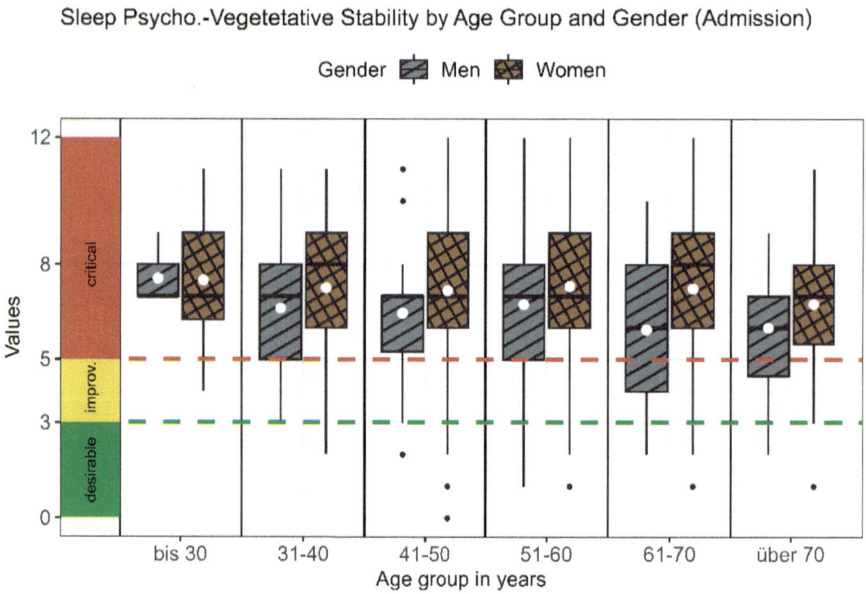

Fig. 5.86 Distribution of Sleep (Psycho-Vegetative Stability) at admission in 2023, broken down by gender and age group; white circles indicate the mean, black lines the median; the coloured lines indicate the thresholds according to the traffic light system

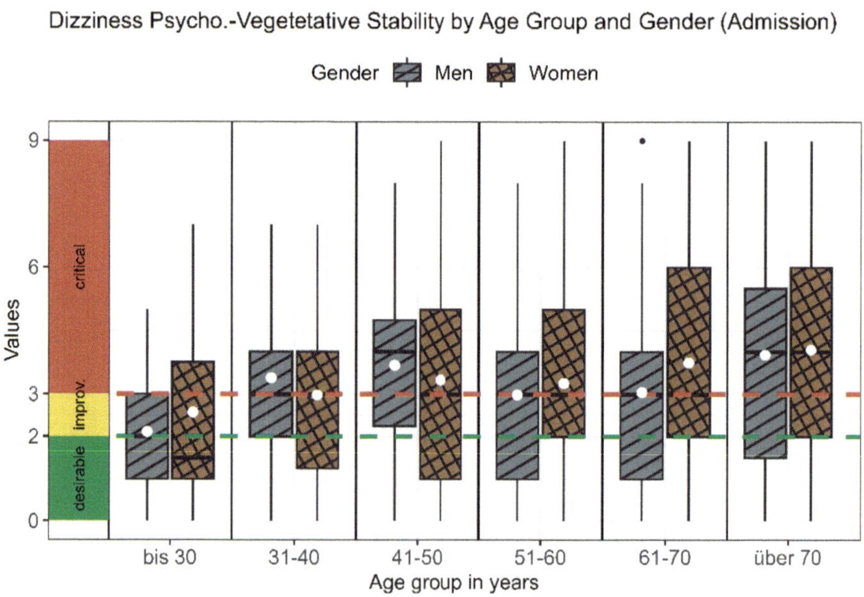

Fig. 5.87 Distribution of dizziness (Psycho-Vegetative Stability) at admission in 2023, broken down by gender and age group. White circles indicate the mean and black lines the median. Coloured lines indicate the thresholds according to the traffic light system

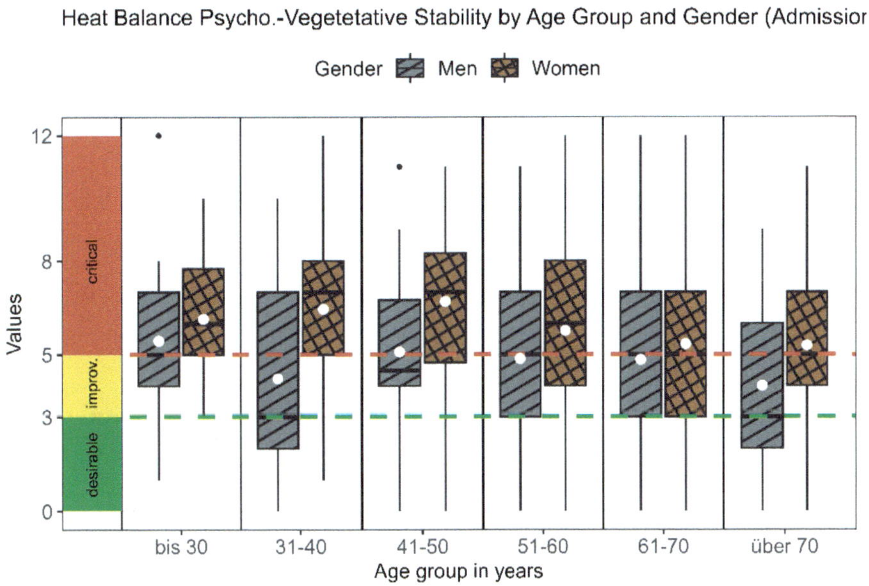

Fig. 5.88 Distribution of Heat Balance (Psycho-Vegetative Stability) 2023 at admission, broken down by gender and age group; white circles indicate the mean, black lines the median; the coloured lines indicate the thresholds according to the traffic light system

5.2.5.2 Risk of Developing Diabetes (FINDRISK)

Upon admission in 2023, the average risk of developing diabetes mellitus within the next 10 years was 10.62 points (SD = 5.00), i.e. approx. 4%. The probability of developing the disease differs slightly between men (mean = 9.54, SD = 5.14) and women (mean = 10.89, SD = 4.93), with women having a higher probability (Table 5.91, Fig. 5.101). The average risk for women is slightly higher than for men across all age groups except for 31–40. The gender difference is particularly pronounced in the under-30 s and over-60 s age groups. Generally, the risk increases with age for both men and women.

Although women are at a higher risk of developing diabetes mellitus, the disease has already developed in more men (8.3%) than women (4.2%). Patients between the ages of 51 and 70 are the most likely to have developed diabetes.

To provide a more detailed picture of these figures, Table 5.92 presents the frequency distributions within the individual risk groups, broken down by gender and age. The data reveal that, upon admission, 22.8% of patients were classified as having a low risk, 34.6% as having a slightly increased risk, and 42.6% as having an increased to very high risk of developing diabetes within the next 10 years.

Examining the full dataset for admission and follow-up revealed that patients had an average risk score of 10.63 (SD = 2.00) at admission, with only a slight reduction during follow-up (M = 10.53; SD = 5.18).

Table 5.93 shows the results for the point value. Figure 5.102 illustrates these results graphically.

Table 5.83 Psycho-Vegetative Stability in pre/post comparison in 2023; *t*-test for paired samples; significance at $p < 0.05$; Cohen's d = effect measure ($d \geq 0.2$ = small, ≥ 0.5 = moderate, ≥ 0.8 = large effect); previous year's data since 2022

		2023								Previous year 2022			
Psycho-vegetative stability		Cross-section: A/D/F			Course: A–D/A–F $n = 611$		Difference from admission: A–D/A–F $n = 611$			Course: A–D/A–F $n = 504$	Difference from admission: A–D/A–F $n = 504$		
		n	M	SD	M	SD	ΔM	*p*	*d*	M	ΔM	*p*	*d*
Sleep	**A**	823	7.06	2.21	7.06	2.21				7.14			
	D	777	5.44	2.57	5.35	2.53	−1.71	<0.001	**−0.72**	5.33	−1.81	<0.001	**−0.74**
	F	618	5.54	2.46	5.55	2.48	−1.52	<0.001	**−0.64**	5.63	−1.51	<0.001	**−0.64**
Dizziness	**A**	823	3.36	2.23	3.36	2.17				3.41			
	D	777	2.26	2.18	2.21	2.13	−1.15	<0.001	**−0.54**	2.17	−1.24	<0.001	**−0.57**
	F	618	2.62	2.10	2.62	2.10	−0.74	<0.001	−0.35	2.61	−0.80	<0.001	−0.37
Heat balance	**A**	823	5.61	2.79	5.67	2.81				5.63			
	D	777	3.84	2.61	3.82	2.64	−1.85	<0.001	**−0.68**	3.86	−1.77	<0.001	**−0.65**
	F	618	4.48	2.59	4.46	2.59	−1.21	<0.001	−0.45	4.48	−1.15	<0.001	−0.43

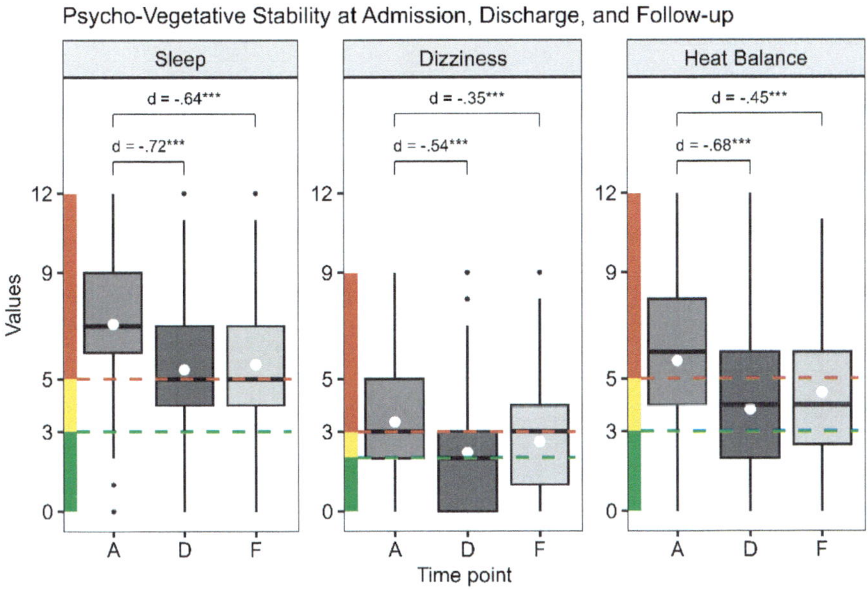

Fig. 5.89 Psycho-Vegetative Stability scales over the course of the measurement points in 2023 (*A* admission, *D* discharge, *F* follow-up); *t*-test with paired samples; significance at $*p < 0.05$, $**p < 0.01$, $***p < 0.001$; Cohen's d = effect measure ($d \geq 0.2$ = small, ≥ 0.5 = moderate, ≥ 0.8 = large effect)

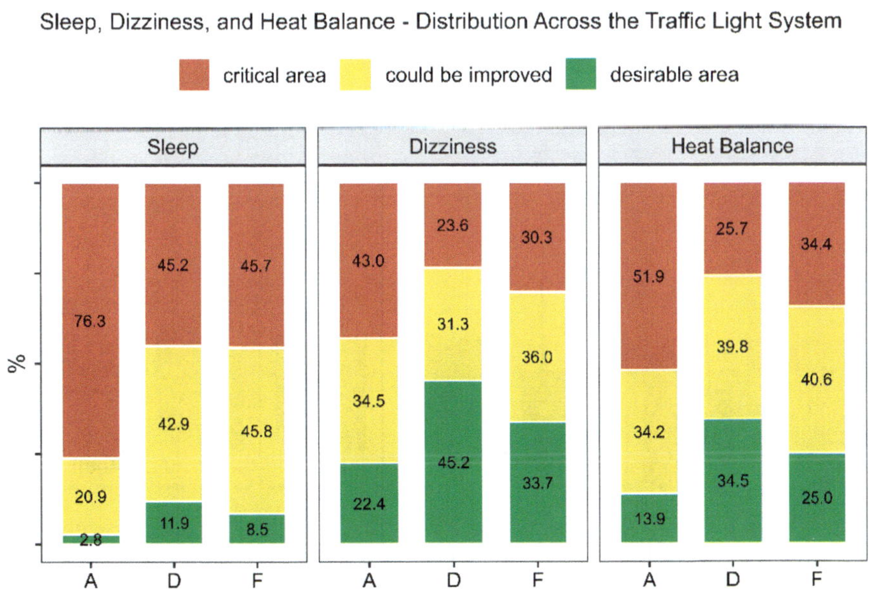

Fig. 5.90 Distribution of the Psycho-Vegetative Stability scales across the levels of the traffic light system in 2023; *A* admission, *D* discharge, *F* = follow-up

Table 5.84 Measures of distribution for the PSQI total score, broken down by gender and age in 2023 and previous years

PSQI total score									
		2023				Previous year[a]			
	Age group	*n*	M	SD	Md	*n*	M	SD	Md
Men	Up to 30	9	9.33	3.08	10.0	4	9.25	1.71	9.5
	31 to 40	13	8.77	4.00	9.0	10	9.60	3.20	9.5
	41 to 50	22	9.91	3.60	9.0	22	9.95	4.46	9.5
	51 to 60	63	10.11	3.93	10.0	58	9.60	4.28	10.0
	61 to 70	46	9.33	3.71	8.5	35	8.89	3.44	9.0
	Over 70	15	9.53	3.78	10.0	15	9.07	3.59	8.0
	Total	**168**	**9.67**	**3.75**	**9.0**	**144**	**9.42**	**3.89**	**9.0**
Women	Up to 30	14	8.79	3.96	7.0	9	10.33	5.20	11.0
	31 to 40	48	9.10	3.51	9.5	44	9.84	4.06	9.0
	41 to 50	94	10.04	4.19	9.0	80	11.16	3.48	12.0
	51 to 60	281	10.95	3.90	11.0	254	11.13	3.80	11.0
	61 to 70	150	11.13	4.03	12.0	137	10.53	4.12	10.0
	Over 70	59	10.73	4.40	10.0	54	10.50	4.42	11.0
	Total	**646**	**10.66**	**4.03**	**11.0**	**578**	**10.80**	**3.94**	**11.0**
Total	Up to 30	23	9.00	3.58	9.0	13	10.00	4.36	10.0
	31 to 40	61	9.03	3.59	9.0	54	9.80	3.89	9.0
	41 to 50	116	10.02	4.07	9.0	102	10.90	3.72	11.0
	51 to 60	344	10.80	3.91	11.0	312	10.80	3.93	11.0
	61 to 70	196	10.70	4.02	11.0	172	10.20	4.27	11.0
	Over 70	74	10.49	4.28	10.0	69	10.20	4.27	11.0
	Total	**814**	**10.45**	**3.99**	**10.0**	**722**	**10.50**	**3.97**	**11.0**

M mean, *SD* standard deviation, *Md* median

[a]As the PSQI was introduced in the course of 2021, only comparative data from 2022 is available

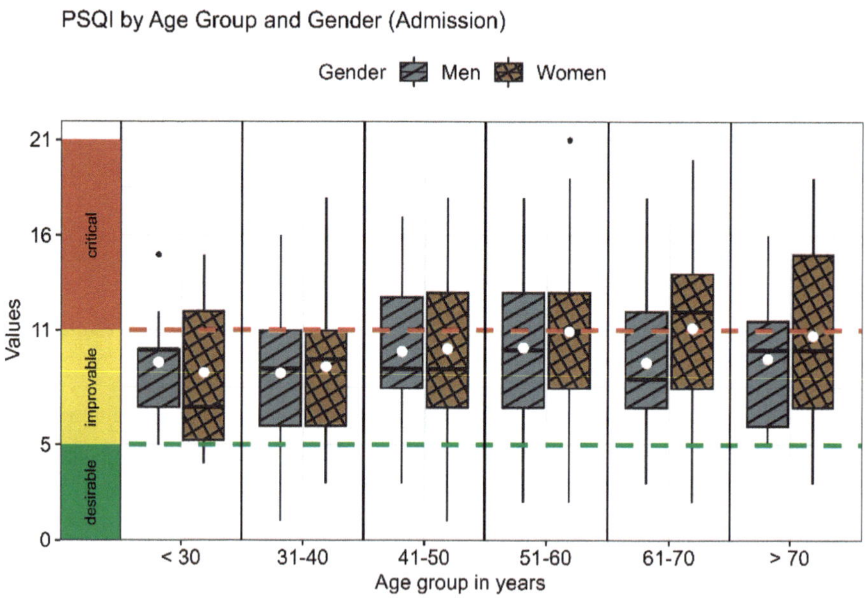

Fig. 5.91 Distribution of the PSQI total score on admission in 2023 ($n = 814$), broken down by gender and age group; white circles indicate the mean, black lines the median; the coloured lines indicate the thresholds according to the traffic light system

Table 5.85 Measures of distribution for the total PSQI value including all subscales, broken down by gender in 2023 and previous years

		2023				Previous year[a]			
PSQI	Gender	*n*	M	SD	Md	*n*	M	SD	Md
Total score	Men	168	9.67	3.75	9	144	9.42	3.89	9
	Women	646	10.66	4.03	11	578	10.8	3.94	11
	Total	814	10.45	3.99	10	722	10.5	3.97	11
Sleep quality	Men	168	1.69	0.73	2	144	1.73	0.69	2
	Women	646	1.82	0.66	2	578	1.82	0.68	2
	Total	814	1.79	0.67	2	722	1.80	0.68	2
Sleep latency	Men	168	1.67	1.02	2	144	1.44	1.07	1
	Women	646	1.75	1.06	2	578	1.81	1.04	2
	Total	814	1.74	1.05	2	722	1.73	1.06	2
Sleep duration	Men	168	1.52	0.88	2	144	1.50	0.91	2
	Women	646	1.53	0.94	2	578	1.63	0.91	2
	Total	814	1.53	0.93	2	722	1.60	0.91	2
Sleep efficiency	Men	168	1.12	1.13	1	144	1.11	1.18	1
	Women	646	1.33	1.18	1	578	1.36	1.18	1
	Total	814	1.29	1.17	1	722	1.31	1.18	1
Sleep malfunction	Men	168	1.59	0.64	2	144	1.56	0.63	2
	Women	646	1.76	0.64	2	578	1.79	0.64	2
	Total	814	1.73	0.64	2	722	1.74	0.64	2
Sleeping pill consumption	Men	168	0.46	0.94	0	144	0.43	0.96	0
	Women	646	0.65	1.14	0	578	0.62	1.12	0
	Total	814	0.61	1.1	0	722	0.58	1.09	0
Daytime sleepiness	Men	168	1.61	0.80	2	144	1.65	0.70	2
	Women	646	1.81	0.74	2	578	1.79	0.75	2
	Total	814	1.77	0.76	2	722	1.76	0.75	2
Sleep efficiency in %	Men	168	78.53	16.25	77.78	144	80.1	17.6	80.0
	Women	646	75.42	17.02	76.56	578	74.9	16.6	75.0
	Total	814	76.06	16.9	77.35	722	75.9	16.9	76.9

M mean, *SD* standard deviation, *Md* median

[a]As the PSQI was introduced in the course of 2021, only comparative data from 2022 is available

Figure 5.103 provides a graphical overview of the percentage distribution across the traffic light system for the entire dataset.

5.2.5.3 Risk of Developing High Blood Pressure (Framingham Hypertension Risk Score)

On average, patients in 2023 have a 5.6% risk of developing hypertension within the following year (Table 5.94, Fig. 5.104). This increases to an average of 10.5% over a two-year period (Table 5.95, Fig. 5.105), and to 18.9% after 4 years (Table 5.96, Fig. 5.106). There is a clear age-related trend: the risk of developing hypertension increases steadily with advancing age. Among younger age groups, men exhibit a higher average risk than women. However, in older age groups (61–70 and over 70), women are at a higher risk. Notably, individuals of both sexes aged 61–70 are most frequently classified as having hypertension.

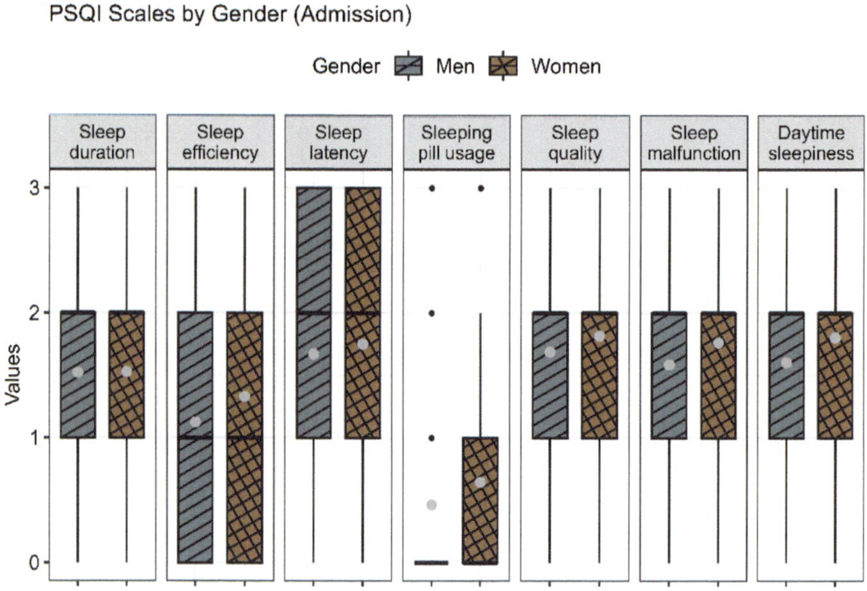

Fig. 5.92 Distribution of the individual scales for the PSQI; broken down by gender, for patients admitted to hospital in 2023 (n = 814, men: n = 168, women: n = 646); grey circles indicate the mean, black lines the median; the target value for all subscales is 0

When comparing pre- and post-treatment risks, patients show an initial hypertension risk of 19.47% (SD = 17.28) at admission, which drops only imperceptibly to 18.20% (SD = 15.96) at follow-up (p = 0.052) (Table 5.97, Fig. 5.107).

5.2.5.4 Metabolic Syndrome Index

Upon admission, the average Metabolic Syndrome Index was 1.88 (SD = 1.28). Women tended to have a slightly lower index (M = 1.84, SD = 1.27) than men (M = 2.07, SD = 1.33). The index generally increases with age. Compared to previous years, the index in 2023 is marginally lower (M = 1.88 vs. M = 1.91) Table 5.98 and Fig. 5.108 present the figures in more detail.

For the complete dataset (admission and discharge), the metabolic syndrome index was, on average, 1.87 (SD = 1.29) at admission and 1.82 (SD = 1.29) at discharge. This difference is not statistically significant (p = 0.110; Table 5.99, Fig. 5.109). However, it should be noted that changes in vital signs and laboratory parameters often take longer to become evident.

5.2.5.5 Fatty Liver Index (FLI)

The distribution of the Fatty Liver Index for patients in 2023 is shown in Table 5.100. On average, the Fatty Liver Index was 37.62 (SD = 30.12) upon admission. Men were more likely to have fatty liver disease than women, with mean scores of 50.10 (SD = 29.21) and 34.29 (SD = 29.50), respectively. According to Fig. 5.110, the risk

Table 5.86 Measures of distribution for the PSQI total score for patients with a diagnosed sleep disorder, broken down by gender and age in 2023 and previous years

PSQI total score									
		2023				Previous year[a]			
	Age group	*n*	M	SD	Md	*n*	M	SD	Md
Men	Up to 30	3	8.33	2.08	9.0	3	9.00	2.00	9.0
	31 to 40	2	12.00	1.41	12.0	2	9.00	2.83	9.0
	41 to 50	6	10.33	2.16	10.5	12	10.42	3.65	11.0
	51 to 60	26	9.88	3.94	10.0	25	12.12	3.33	12.0
	61 to 70	21	11.14	3.51	11.0	18	10.50	3.45	11.0
	Over 70	5	11.80	3.11	11.0	7	9.29	3.5.0	8.0
	Total	**63**	**10.49**	**3.49**	**10.0**	**67**	**10.85**	**3.45**	**11.0**
Women	Up to 30	4	13.50	1.29	13.5	6	13.17	3.76	12.5
	31 to 40	13	10.54	3.84	10.0	23	12.04	3.87	13.0
	41 to 50	28	12.11	3.73	12.0	48	12.69	2.59	13.0
	51 to 60	89	12.09	3.53	12.0	136	12.39	3.39	12.0
	61 to 70	41	11.80	3.13	12.0	76	11.89	3.97	12.0
	Over 70	12	13.25	3.96	14.5	21	12.33	4.23	12.0
	Total	**187**	**12.03**	**3.50**	**12.0**	**310**	**12.30**	**3.52**	**12.0**
Total	Up to 30	7	11.29	3.15	12.0	9	11.78	3.77	11.0
	31 to 40	15	10.73	3.61	10.0	25	11.80	3.84	13.0
	41 to 50	34	11.79	3.54	12.0	60	12.23	2.94	12.5
	51 to 60	115	11.59	3.73	12.0	161	12.35	3.37	12.0
	61 to 70	62	11.58	3.25	12.0	94	11.63	3.90	11.0
	Over 70	17	12.82	3.70	14.0	28	11.57	4.22	11.5
	Total	**250**	**11.64**	**3.55**	**12.0**	**377**	**12.04**	**3.55**	**12.0**

M mean, *SD* standard deviation, *Md* median

[a]As the PSQI was introduced in the course of 2021, only comparative data from 2022 is available

of developing a fatty liver increase with age. However, men aged 41–50 are almost as likely to have fatty liver disease as those aged over 70.

There was a statistically significant improvement regarding fatty liver, although the effect size can be considered minimal ($d = -0.05$, $p < 0.001$) (Table 5.101). At the time of admission, the mean value was 37.62 (SD = 30.17), decreasing slightly to 36.94 (SD = 29.94) at discharge. Figure 5.111 illustrates the results in a graph.

Figure 5.112 presents the distribution across the traffic light system upon admission and discharge. Similarly to other laboratories and vital measures, it is likely that a longer observation period is required to see meaningful changes.

5.2.5.6 High Blood Pressure

High blood pressure (hypertension) is a widespread disease. In Germany, 20–30 million people suffer from it [8]. In the long term, high blood pressure damages the blood vessels and thus contributes to the development of secondary diseases such as heart attacks and strokes.

Antihypertensive drugs (antihypertensives) are for drug treatment:

- ACE inhibitors: e.g. enalapril, perindopril, lisinopril.
- Sartans: e.g. valsartan, irbesartan, candesartan.

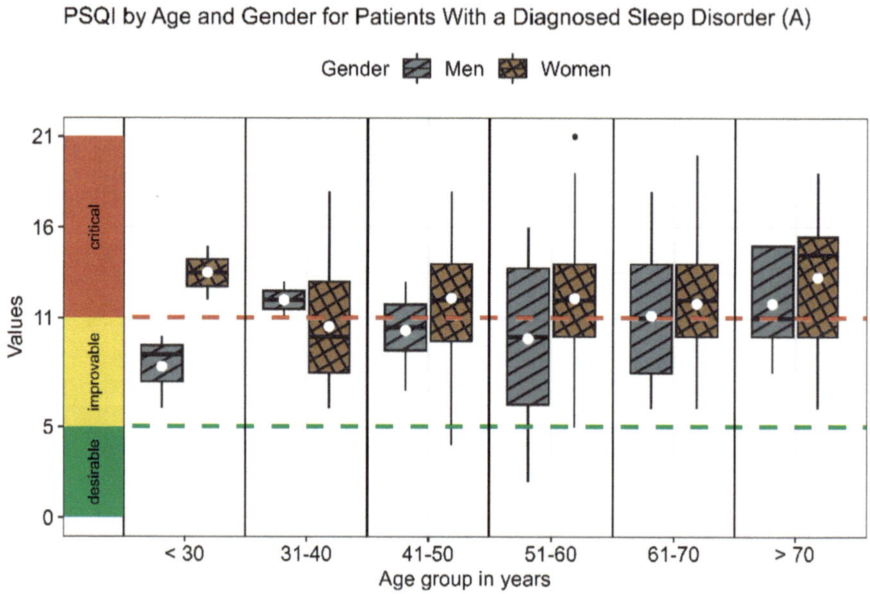

Fig. 5.93 This shows the distribution of the PSQI total score in 2023 for patients with a diagnosed sleep disorder at admission (n = 250), broken down by gender and age group. The white circles indicate the mean, and the black lines indicate the median. The coloured lines indicate the thresholds according to the traffic light system

- Renin inhibitors: aliskiren.
- Calcium channel blockers: e.g. amlodipine.
- Beta-blockers: e.g. metoprolol, bisoprolol, nebivolol.

In the clinic, 200 patients were coded as having essential hypertension. In the systemic anamnesis, 228 people identified themselves as having hypertension. Of these, 194 were taking medication and 85 stated that their everyday life was restricted by high blood pressure (Chap. 3, Table 3.9). The people who received a diagnosis of hypertension (ICD- I10) are described in more detail below (Table 5.102). Of the 200 patients, between 183 and 192 had data available on admission and discharge, depending on the measured value.

Table 5.87 Measures of distribution for the total PSQI value including all subscales for patients with a diagnosed sleep disorder, broken down by gender in 2023 and previous years

		2023				Previous year[a]			
PSQI	Gender	*n*	M	SD	Md	*n*	M	SD	Md
Total score	Men	63	10.49	3.49	10	67	10.85	3.45	11.0
	Women	187	12.03	3.50	12	310	12.30	3.52	12.0
	Total	250	11.64	3.55	12	377	12.04	3.55	12.0
Sleep quality	Men	63	1.90	0.67	2	67	1.91	0.60	2.0
	Women	187	2.02	0.58	2	310	2.06	0.57	2.0
	Total	250	1.99	0.60	2	377	2.03	0.58	2.0
Sleep latency	Men	63	1.89	1.09	2	67	1.63	1.13	2.0
	Women	187	1.96	1.06	2	310	2.09	0.97	2.0
	Total	250	1.94	1.07	2	377	2.00	1.01	2.0
Sleep duration	Men	63	1.59	0.84	2	67	1.76	0.85	2.0
	Women	187	1.80	0.83	2	310	1.85	0.82	2.0
	Total	250	1.74	0.84	2	377	1.83	0.83	2
Sleep efficiency	Men	63	1.16	1.03	1	67	1.54	1.20	1.0
	Women	187	1.72	1.11	2	310	1.70	1.14	2.0
	Total	250	1.58	1.12	2	377	1.67	1.15	2.0
Sleep malfunction	Men	63	1.70	0.66	2	67	1.66	0.59	2.0
	Women	187	1.91	0.57	2	310	1.94	0.60	2.0
	Total	250	1.86	0.60	2	377	1.89	0.61	2.0
Sleeping pill consumption	Men	63	0.52	1.05	0	67	0.60	1.10	0.0
	Women	187	0.75	1.19	0	310	0.84	1.23	0.0
	Total	250	0.69	1.16	0	377	0.79	1.21	0.0
Daytime sleepiness	Men	63	1.73	0.72	2	67	1.76	0.65	2.0
	Women	187	1.87	0.71	2	310	1.83	0.76	2.0
	Total	250	1.84	0.72	2	377	7.81	0.75	2.0
Sleep efficiency in %	Men	63	78.61	15.89	76.92	67	73.5	12.9	75.0
	Women	187	69.54	16.08	70.59	310	70.3	16.2	71.4
	Total	250	71.82	16.48	71.43	377	70.85	15.7	71.4

M mean, *SD* standard deviation, *Md* median

[a]As the PSQI was introduced in the course of 2021, only comparative data from 2022 is available

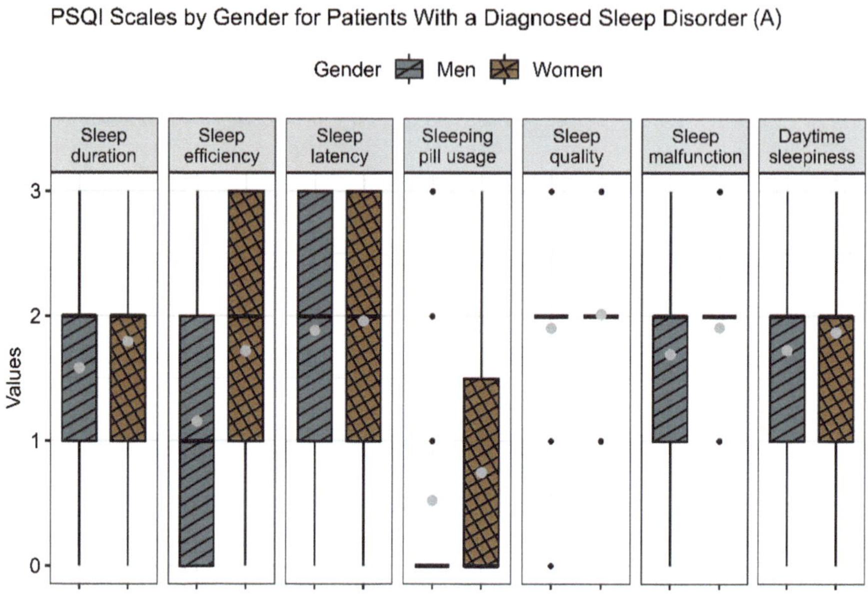

Fig. 5.94 Distribution of the individual scales for the PSQI; broken down by gender in 2023 for patients with a diagnosed sleep disorder on admission to hospital (n = 250, men: n = 63, women: n = 187); grey circles indicate the mean, black lines the median; the target value for all subscales is 0

Table 5.88 PSQI in the before/after comparison in 2023; *t*-test with paired samples; significance at $p < 0.05$; Cohen's d = effect measure ($d \geq 0.2$ = small, ≥ 0.5 = moderate, ≥ 0.8 = large); cross-section statistics and full dataset comparisons (A–D–F $n = 611$); previous year's data since 2022

PSQI		2023 Cross-section: A/D/F			Course: A–D/A–F $n = 599$		Difference from admission: A–D/A–F $n = 599$			Previous year 2022 Course: A–D/A–F $n = 500$	Difference from admission: A–D/A–F $n = 500$		
		n	M	SD	M	SD	ΔM	*p*	*d*	M	ΔM	*p*	*d*
Total score	**A**	814	10.45	3.99	10.43	4.02				10.62			
	D	777	9.55	4.44	9.36	4.39	−1.08	<0.001	−0.26	9.11	−1.50	<0.001	−0.36
	F	615	8.52	4.14	8.52	4.14	−1.92	<0.001	−0.47	8.67	−1.95	<0.001	−0.49
Sleep quality	**A**	814	1.79	0.67	1.79	0.68				1.80			
	D	777	1.43	0.70	1.41	0.69	−0.38	<0.001	**−0.55**	1.35	−0.45	<0.001	**−0.63**
	F	615	1.44	0.71	1.44	0.71	−0.35	<0.001	**−0.50**	1.47	−0.33	<0.001	−0.49
Sleep latency	**A**	813	1.74	1.05	1.69	1.04				1.74			
	D	777	1.48	1.03	1.44	1.02	−0.26	<0.001	−0.25	1.44	−0.30	<0.001	−0.29
	F	615	1.43	1.01	1.43	1.01	−0.26	<0.001	−0.25	1.43	−0.31	<0.001	−0.30
Sleep duration	**A**	814	1.53	0.93	1.51	0.93				1.62			
	D	777	1.47	0.91	1.46	0.91	−0.05	0.167	–	1.55	−0.07	0.074	–
	F	615	1.27	0.90	1.27	0.90	−0.24	<0.001	−0.26	1.42	−0.20	<0.001	**−0.**23
Sleep efficiency	**A**	814	1.29	1.17	1.29	1.17				1.34			
	D	777	1.15	1.18	1.10	1.16	−0.19	<0.001	−0.16	1.13	−0.21	<0.001	−0.18
	F	615	0.89	1.09	0.38	1.09	−0.40	<0.001	−0.35	0.95	−0.40	<0.001	−0.35
Sleep malfunction	**A**	814	1.73	0.64	1.75	0.65				1.77			
	D	777	1.55	0.61	1.54	0.60	−0.21	<0.001	−0.33	1.50	−0.26	0.017	−0.44
	F	615	1.51	0.65	1.50	0.64	−0.24	<0.001	−0.37	1.50	−0.27	<0.001	−0.42

(continued)

Table 5.88 (continued)

PSQI		2023 Cross-section: A/D/F			Course: A–D/A–F $n = 611$		Difference from admission: A–D/A–F $n = 611$			Previous year 2022 Course: A–D/A–F $n = 500$	Difference from admission: A–D/A–F $n = 500$		
		n	M	SD	M	SD	ΔM	p	d	M	ΔM	p	d
Sleeping pill consumption	**A**	814	0.61	1.10	0.62	1.12				0.57			
	D	777	1.33	1.41	1.30	1.41	0.68	<0.001	**0.53**	1.07	0.50	<0.001	0.41
	F	615	0.59	1.08	0.59	1.08	−0.03	0.448	–	0.52	−0.05	0.276	–
Daytime sleepiness	**A**	814	1.77	0.76	1.79	0.75				1.78			
	D	777	1.14	0.81	1.11	0.79	−0.68	<0.001	**−0.89**	1.07	−0.72	<0.001	**−0.92**
	F	615	1.39	0.82	1.39	0.82	−0.40	<0.001	**−0.50**	1.39	−0.40	<0.001	**−0.51**
Sleep efficiency in %	**A**	814	76.06	16.90	76.43	16.80				75.20			
	D	777	78.10	16.78	78.58	15.90	2.15	0.003	0.13	77.99	2.79	<0.001	0.17
	F	615	81.19	14.74	81.23	14.82	4.80	<0.001	0.30	79.79	4.58	<0.001	0.29

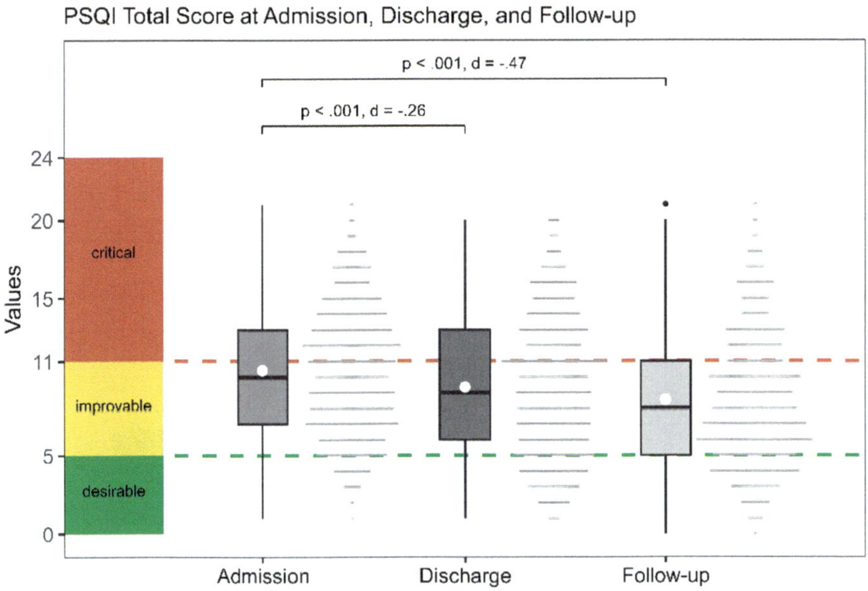

Fig. 5.95 PSQI total score over the course of the measurement time points in 2023; *t*-test with paired samples; Cohen's *d* = effect measure ($d \geq 0.2$ = small, ≥ 0.5 = moderate, ≥ 0.8 = large effect); white circle indicates the mean, the black line the median

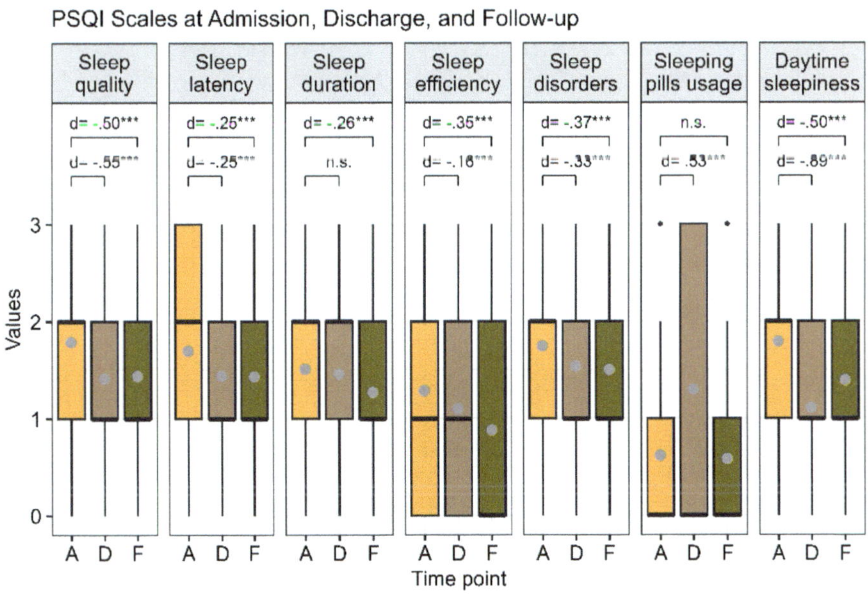

Fig. 5.96 PSQI scales over the course of the 2023 measurement time points (*A* admission, *D* discharge, *F* follow-up); *t*-test with paired samples; significance at $^{*}p < 0.05$, $^{**}p < 0.01$, $^{***}p < 0.001$; Cohen's *d* = effect measure ($d \geq 0.2$ = small, ≥ 0.5 = moderate, ≥ 0.8 = large)

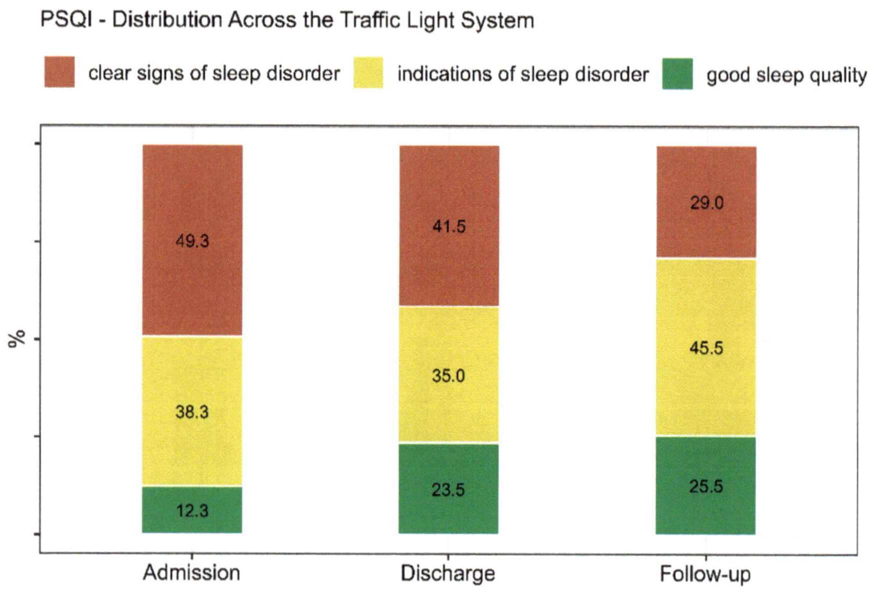

Fig. 5.97 Distribution of the PSQI total score across the levels of the traffic light system in 2023

Table 5.89 Measures of distribution for the cardiovascular risk score (SCORE2), broken down by gender and age in 2023 and previous years

SCORE2 in %									
		2023				Previous year[a]			
	Age group	*n*	M	SD	Md	*n*	M	SD	Md
Men	Up to 30	0	–	–	–	2	2	0	2.0
	31 to 40	1	3.00	–	3.0	4	2.50	1.29	2.5
	41 to 50	22	3.73	1.39	4.0	17	3.71	1.72	4.0
	51 to 60	60	7.05	2.88	6.0	32	5.94	3.69	5.5
	61 to 70	47	10.19	2.60	10.0	28	6.50	4.99	7.5
	Over 70	15	25.40	8.68	24.0	12	21.83	13.08	24.0
	Total	**145**	**9.43**	**6.90**	**7.0**	**95**	**7.48**	**7.99**	**5.0**
Women	Up to 30	0	–	–	–	3	2.33	1.15	3.0
	31 to 40	2	1.50	0.71	1.5	22	2.14	0.99	3.0
	41 to 50	93	1.98	1.78	2.0	49	2.47	1.71	2.0
	51 to 60	274	3.91	2.21	3.0	170	3.53	2.02	3.0
	61 to 70	148	7.47	3.12	7.0	94	5.34	3.46	5.0
	Over 70	57	17.49	6.72	16.0	38	12.24	7.96	11.0
	Total	**574**	**5.85**	**5.31**	**4.0**	**376**	**4.63**	**4.37**	**3**
Total	Up to 30	0	–	–	–	5	2.20	0.84	2.0
	31 to 40	3	2.00	1.00	2.0	26	2.19	1.02	3.0
	41 to 50	115	2.31	1.84	2.0	66	2.79	1.78	3.0
	51 to 60	334	4.47	2.64	3.0	202	3.91	2.51	3.0
	61 to 70	195	8.13	3.22	7.0	122	5.61	3.87	5.0
	Over 70	72	19.14	7.81	17.5	50	14.54	10.17	13.0
	Total	**719**	**6.58**	**5.84**	**5.0**	**471**	**5.21**	**5.41**	**3.0**

M mean, *SD* standard deviation, *Md* median

[a]Since the SCORE2 was introduced in the course of 2022, only partial data from the previous year, 2022, is available

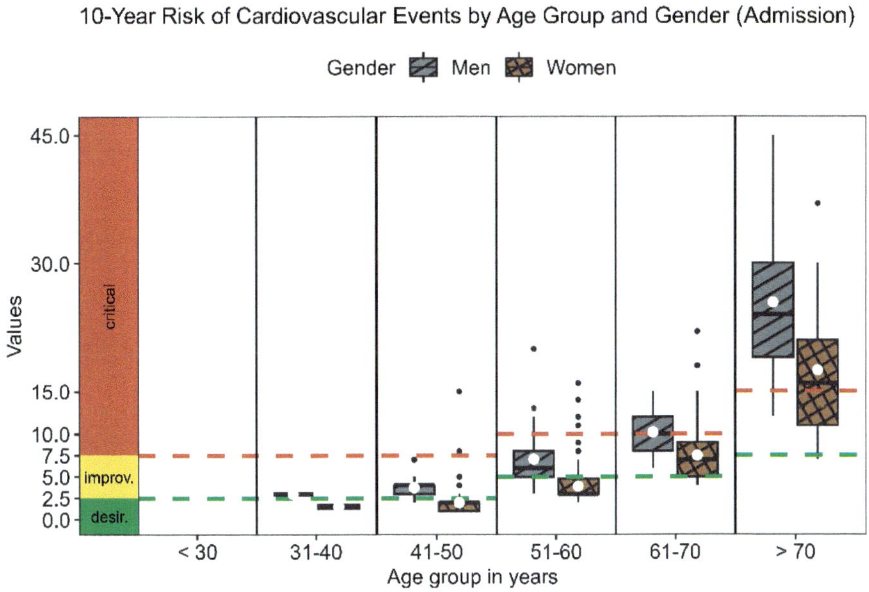

Fig. 5.98 Distribution measures of the 10-year cardiovascular risk in the 2023 reporting year on admission ($n = 719$), broken down by gender and age group; white circles indicate the mean, black lines the median; the coloured lines indicate the thresholds according to the traffic light system (the category thresholds vary depending on the age group)

Table 5.90 Cardiovascular risk score before/after comparison in 2023; t-test for paired samples; significance at $p < 0.05$; Cohen's d = effect measure ($d \geq 0.2$ = small, ≥ 0.5 = moderate, ≥ 0.8 = large effect); previous year's data since 2022

		2023								Previous year 2022			
SCORE2		Cross-section: A/D			Course: A–D $n = 705$		Difference from admission: A–D $n = 705$			Course: A–D $n = 743$	Difference from admission: A–D $n = 743$		
		n	M	SD	M	SD	ΔM	p	d	M	ΔM	p	d
Risk score	**A**	719	6.58	5.84	6.54	5.85				5.18			
	D	726	6.49	5.78	6.48	5.80	−0.06	0.446	–	5.26	0.08	0.414	–

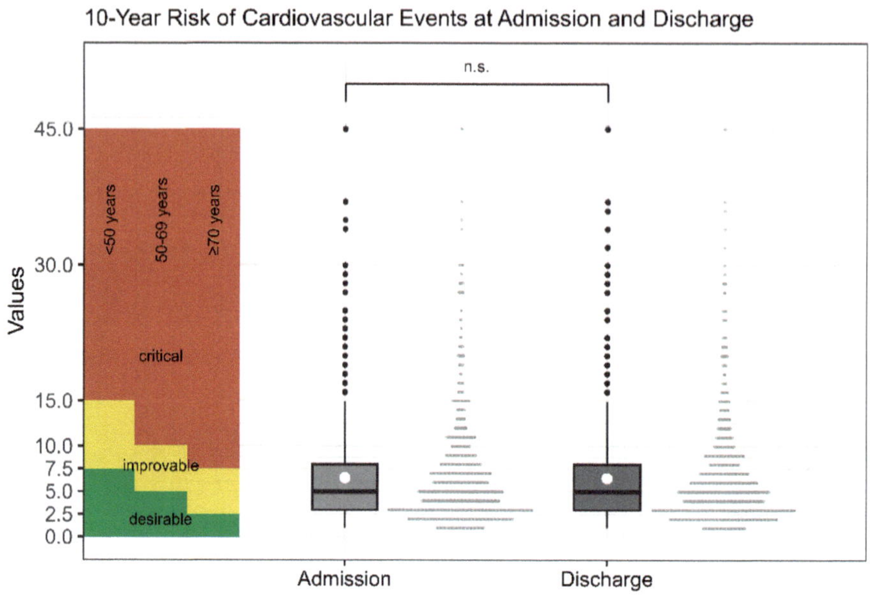

Fig. 5.99 Cardiovascular risk score (SCORE2) over the course of the measurement time points in 2023; *t*-test with paired samples; Cohen's d = effect measure ($d \geq 0.2$ = small, ≥ 0.5 = moderate, ≥ 0.8 = large effect); white circle indicates the mean, the black line the median

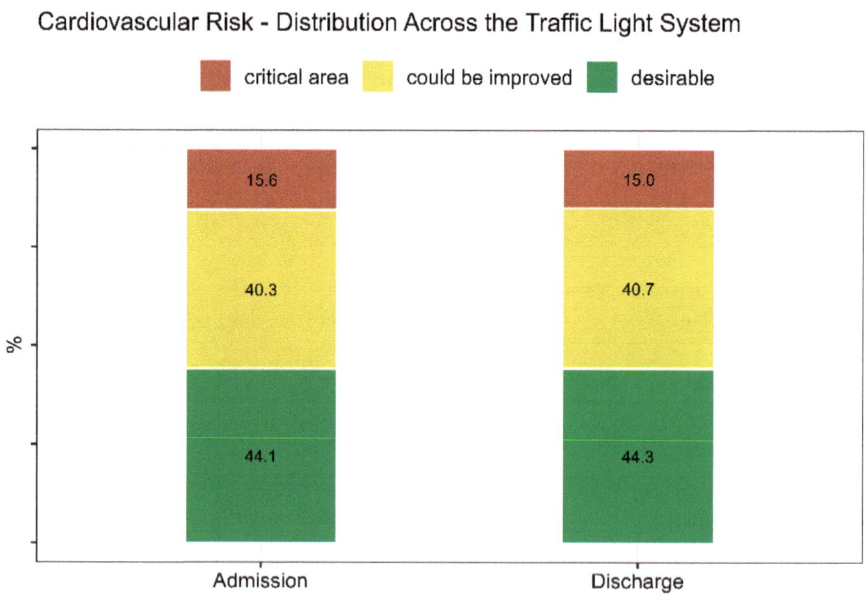

Fig. 5.100 Distribution of the cardiovascular risk score across the levels of the traffic light system in 2023

Table 5.91 Measures of distribution for the FINDRISK score, broken down by gender and age in 2023 and previous years; *M* mean, *SD* standard deviation, *Md* median; the distribution of patients who already have diabetes are presented in separated columns (already ill)

FINDRISK													
		2023						Previous years					
						Already ill						Already ill	
	Age group	*n*	M	SD	Md	*n*	%	*n*	M	SD	Md	*n*	%
Men	Up to 30	9	3.67	2.45	2.0	0	0.0	92	4.15	3.22	3.0	1	0.1
	31 to 40	13	6.08	3.25	6.0	0	0.0	148	6.91	4.46	6.0	0	0.0
	41 to 50	19	8.53	5.34	8.0	2	1.2	414	9.46	4.50	9.0	11	0.5
	51 to 60	60	10.72	5.28	11.0	4	2.4	701	10.83	4.61	10.0	49	2.3
	61 to 70	43	9.81	4.47	9.0	4	2.4	433	11.96	4.41	12.0	62	2.8
	Over 70	11	12.64	4.65	13.0	4	2.4	231	11.88	4.17	11.0	39	1.8
	Total	**155**	**9.54**	**5.14**	**9.0**	**14**	**8.3**	**2019**	**10.32**	**4.82**	**10.0**	**162**	**7.4**
Women	Up to 30	14	5.79	3.38	5.0	0	0.0	240	5.64	3.53	5.0	4	0.1
	31 to 40	50	5.60	3.88	4.5	0	0.0	433	7.01	4.04	6.0	6	0.1
	41 to 50	93	8.80	4.25	9.0	3	0.5	1398	9.54	4.47	9.0	15	0.2
	51 to 60	270	11.56	4.65	12.0	9	1.4	2601	11.41	4.50	11.0	66	1.0
	61 to 70	140	12.46	4.29	12.0	10	1.6	1169	12.39	4.29	12.0	105	1.6
	Over 70	53	13.38	4.67	13.0	5	0.8	569	12.91	4.28	13.0	71	1.1
	Total	**620**	**10.89**	**4.93**	**10.5**	**27**	**4.2**	**6410**	**10.80**	**4.73**	**11.0**	**267**	**4.0**
Total	Up to 30	23	4.96	3.17	4.0	0	0.0	332	5.23	3.50	5.0	5	0.1
	31 to 40	63	5.70	3.74	5.0	0	0.0	581	6.98	4.15	6.0	6	0.1
	41 to 50	112	8.75	4.43	9.0	5	0.6	1812	9.52	4.47	9.0	26	0.3
	51 to 60	330	11.41	4.77	11.0	13	1.6	3302	11.29	4.53	11.0	115	1.4
	61 to 70	183	11.84	4.47	11.0	14	1.7	1602	12.27	4.33	12.0	167	2.0
	Over 70	64	13.25	4.64	13.0	9	1.1	800	12.62	4.27	12.0	110	1.3
	Total	**775**	**10.62**	**5.00**	**10.0**	**41**	**5.0**	**8429**	**10.69**	**4.76**	**10.0**	**429**	**5.1**

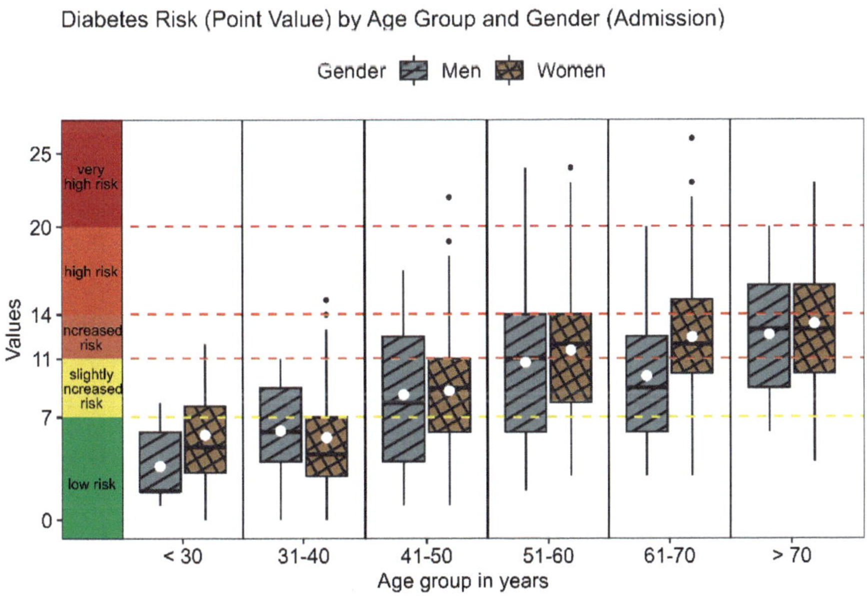

Fig. 5.101 Diabetes risk (FINDRISK point value); separated by gender and age in 2023 ($n = 775$); white circles indicate the mean, black lines the median; the coloured lines indicate the thresholds according to the traffic light system

Table 5.92 Frequency distribution of diabetes risk (categorised FINDRISK percentage value), broken down by gender and age in 2023 on admission

		Percentage risk 2023												Percentage risk previous years											
		< 1%		~ 4%		~ 17%		~ 33%		> 50%		Total		< 1%		~ 4%		~ 17%		~ 33%		> 50%		Total	
	Age group	*n*	%	*n*	%	*n*	%	*n*	%	*n*	%	*n*	%	*n*	%	*n*	%	*n*	%	*n*	%	*n*	%	*n*	%
Men	Up to 30	8	5.2	1	0.7	0	0.0	0	0.0	0	0.0	9	5.8	75	3.7	14	0.7	2	0.1	1	0.1	0	0.0	92	4.6
	31 to 40	7	4.5	6	3.9	0	0.0	0	0.0	0	0.0	13	8.4	80	4.0	41	2.0	21	1.0	4	0.2	2	0.1	148	7.3
	41 to 50	7	4.5	6	3.9	2	1.3	4	2.6	0	0.0	19	12.3	110	5.5	165	8.2	88	4.4	46	2.3	5	0.3	414	20.5
	51 to 60	16	10.3	19	12.3	11	7.1	11	7.1	3	1.9	60	38.7	131	6.5	284	14.1	136	6.7	131	6.5	19	0.9	701	34.7
	61 to 70	13	8.4	18	11.6	3	1.9	9	5.8	0	0.0	43	27.7	59	2.9	139	6.9	120	5.9	101	5.0	14	0.7	433	21.4
	Over 70	1	0.7	4	2.6	1	0.7	5	3.2	0	0.0	11	7.1	23	1.1	95	4.7	56	2.8	48	2.4	9	0.5	231	11.4
	Total	**52**	**33.5**	**54**	**34.8**	**17**	**11.0**	**29**	**18.7**	**3**	**1.9**	**155**	**100**	**478**	**23.7**	**738**	**36.6**	**423**	**21.0**	**331**	**16.4**	**49**	**2.4**	**2019**	**100**
Women	Up to 30	8	1.3	5	0.8	1	0.2	0	0.0	0	0.0	14	2.3	158	2.5	64	1.0	16	0.3	2	0.0	0	0.0	240	3.7
	31 to 40	34	5.5	10	1.6	5	0.8	1	0.2	0	0.0	50	8.1	220	3.4	151	2.4	39	0.6	23	0.4	0	0.0	433	6.8
	41 to 50	29	4.7	41	6.6	15	2.4	7	1.1	1	0.2	93	15.0	351	5.5	600	9.4	250	3.9	176	2.8	21	0.3	1398	21.8
	51 to 60	40	6.5	91	14.7	74	11.9	53	8.6	12	1.9	270	43.5	325	5.1	1077	16.8	567	8.8	556	8.7	76	1.2	2601	40.6
	61 to 70	9	1.5	56	9.0	33	5.3	35	5.7	7	1.1	140	22.6	98	1.5	421	6.6	302	4.7	302	4.7	46	0.7	1169	18.2
	Over 70	5	0.8	13	2.1	14	2.3	16	2.6	5	0.8	53	8.5	43	0.7	193	3.0	129	2.0	183	2.9	23	0.4	571	8.9
	Total	**125**	**20.2**	**216**	**34.8**	**142**	**22.9**	**112**	**18.1**	**25**	**4.0**	**620**	**100**	**1195**	**18.6**	**2506**	**39.1**	**1303**	**20.3**	**1242**	**19.4**	**166**	**2.6**	**6412**	**100**
Total	Up to 30	16	2.1	6	0.8	1	0.1	0	0.0	0	0.0	23	3.0	233	2.8	78	0.9	18	0.2	3	0.0	0	0.0	332	3.9
	31 to 40	41	5.3	16	2.1	5	0.7	1	0.1	0	0.0	63	8.1	300	3.6	192	2.3	60	0.7	27	0.3	2	0.0	581	6.9
	41 to 50	36	4.7	47	6.1	17	2.2	11	1.4	1	0.1	112	14.5	461	5.5	765	9.1	338	4.0	222	2.6	26	0.3	1812	21.5
	51 to 60	56	7.2	110	14.2	85	11.0	64	8.3	15	1.9	330	42.6	456	5.4	1361	16.1	703	8.3	687	8.2	95	1.1	3302	39.2
	61 to 70	22	2.8	74	9.6	36	4.7	44	5.7	7	0.9	183	23.6	157	1.9	560	6.6	422	5.0	403	4.8	60	0.7	1602	19.0
	Over 70	6	0.8	17	2.2	15	1.9	21	2.7	5	0.7	64	8.3	66	0.8	288	3.4	185	2.2	231	2.7	32	0.4	802	9.5
	Total	**177**	**22.8**	**270**	**34.8**	**159**	**20.5**	**141**	**18.2**	**28**	**3.6**	**775**	**100**	**1673**	**19.8**	**3244**	**38.5**	**1726**	**20.5**	**1573**	**18.7**	**215**	**2.6**	**8431**	**100**

Table 5.93 FINDRISK in the before/after comparison in 2023; t-test for paired samples; significance at $p < 0.05$; Cohen's d = effect measure ($d \geq 0.2$ = small, ≥ 0.5 = moderate, ≥ 0.8 = large effect); previous year's data since 2022

		2023								Previous year 2022			
FINDRISK		Cross-section: A/F			Course: A–F $n = 570$		Difference from admission: A–F $n = 570$			Course: A–F $n = 500$	Difference from admission: A–F $n = 500$		
		n	M	SD	M	SD	ΔM	p	d	M	ΔM	p	d
Points	**A**	776	10.63	5.00	10.78	5.06				10.96			
	F	570	10.53	5.18	10.53	5.18	−0.26	0.048	−0.05	10.70	−0.26	0.063	–

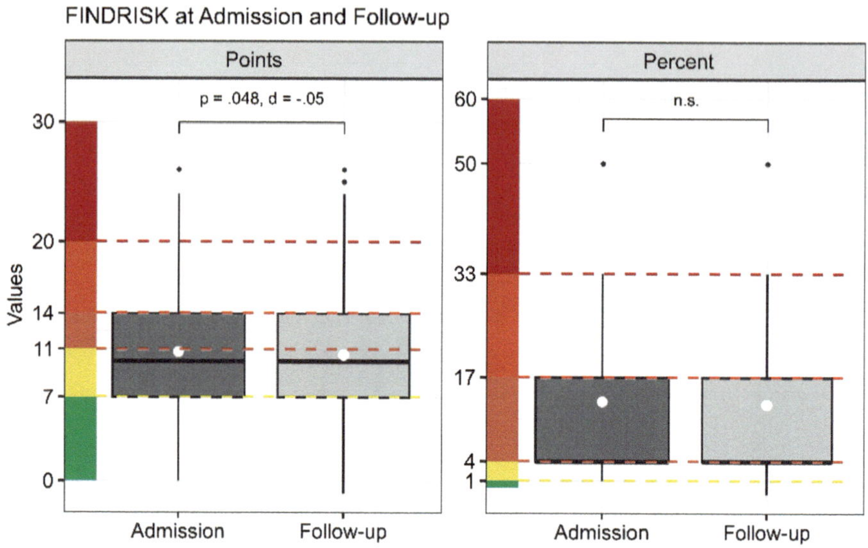

Fig. 5.102 FINDRISK over the course of the measurement points in 2023; *t*-test with paired samples; significance at $p < 0.05$; Cohen's d = effect measure ($d \geq 0.2$ = small, ≥ 0.5 = moderate, ≥ 0.8 = large effect); red segment and line indicate the critical area, yellow the improvable area, and green the desirable area

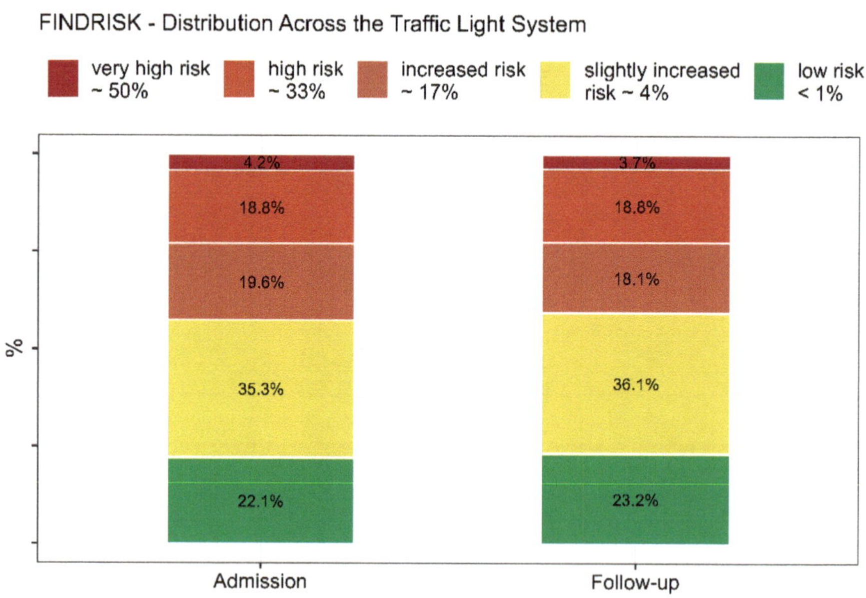

Fig. 5.103 Percentage distribution of the FINDRISK value across the levels of the traffic light system in 2023 (n = 570); risk of developing a diabetes mellitus disease within the next 10 years

Table 5.94 Measures of distribution for the 1-year hypertension risk score of developing high blood pressure, broken down by gender and age in 2023 and previous years; *M* mean, *SD* standard deviation, *Md* median; the distribution of patients who already have high blood pressure are presented in separated columns (already ill)

1-year risk													
		2023						Previous years					
						Alread ill						Already ill	
	Age group	*n*	M (in %)	SD	Md	*n*	%	*n*	M (in %)	SD	Md	*n*	%
Men	Up to 30	8	1.58	2.40	0.88	1	0.6	90	1.85	2.55	1.00	3	0.1
	31 to 40	13	2.21	2.03	1.39	0	0.0	139	2.93	3.18	2.00	9	0.4
	41 to 50	15	6.16	3.61	5.26	6	3.6	332	4.71	3.95	3.20	93	4.3
	51 to 60	47	6.08	4.37	5.26	17	10.1	488	6.39	4.86	5.00	262	12.0
	61 to 70	26	6.50	4.02	5.73	21	12.4	273	8.93	5.74	8.58	221	10.1
	Over 70	5	10.02	5.15	10.08	10	5.9	137	9.68	5.32	10.00	133	6.1
	Total	**114**	**5.60**	**4.28**	**4.46**	**55**	**32.5**	**1459**	**6.18**	**5.18**	**4.00**	**721**	**33.1**
Women	Up to 30	14	0.73	0.68	0.66	0	0.0	240	1.03	1.49	0.92	4	0.1
	31 to 40	49	2.02	3.09	0.84	1	0.2	425	1.72	2.41	1.00	14	0.2
	41 to 50	85	3.42	4.63	1.64	11	1.7	1248	3.45	4.07	2.00	165	2.5
	51 to 60	228	5.40	5.40	3.20	52	8.0	2038	5.45	5.25	4.00	629	9.4
	61 to 70	92	8.68	7.18	6.20	58	9.0	777	8.60	6.50	7.00	497	7.4
	Over 70	26	12.93	7.75	11.82	32	4.9	317	10.87	6.51	10.00	323	4.8
	Total	**494**	**5.60**	**6.16**	**3.20**	**154**	**23.8**	**5045**	**5.25**	**5.6**	**3.00**	**1632**	**24.4**
Total	Up to 30	22	1.04	1.54	0.66	1	0.1	330	1.26	1.87	1.00	7	0.1
	31 to 40	62	2.06	2.89	0.99	1	0.1	564	2.01	2.67	1.00	23	0.3
	41 to 50	100	3.83	4.58	2.12	17	2.1	1580	3.71	4.07	2.00	258	2.9
	51 to 60	275	5.51	5.24	3.78	69	8.5	2526	5.63	5.19	4.00	891	10.1
	61 to 70	118	8.20	6.66	6.20	79	9.7	1050	8.68	6.31	7.00	718	8.1
	Over 70	31	12.46	7.40	11.82	42	5.1	454	10.51	6.19	10.00	456	5.2
	Total	**608**	**5.60**	**5.85**	**3.20**	**209**	**25.6**	**6504**	**5.46**	**5.52**	**3.78**	**2353**	**26.6**

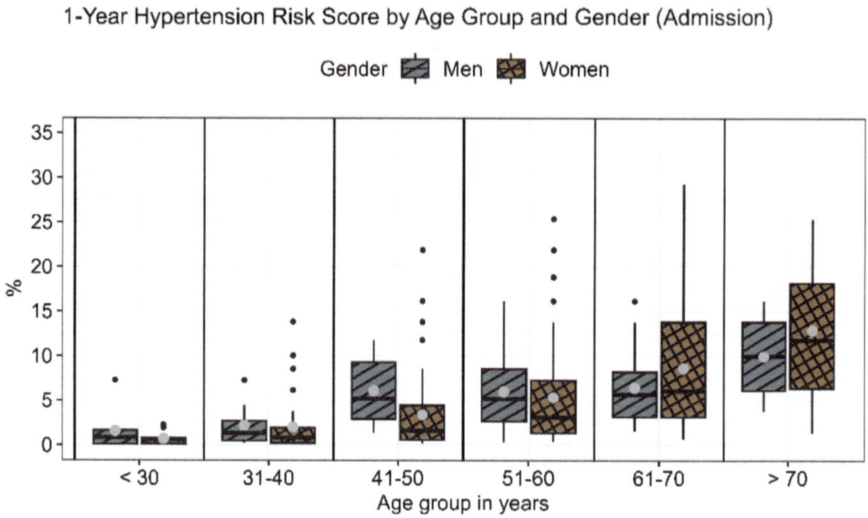

Fig. 5.104 Distribution of 1-year hypertension risk on admission in 2023, broken down by gender and age group; grey circles indicate the mean, black lines the median; the coloured lines indicate the thresholds according to the traffic light system

Table 5.95 Measures of distribution for the 2-year hypertension risk score of developing high blood pressure, broken down by gender and age in 2023 and previous years; *M* mean, *SD* standard deviation, *Md* median; the distribution of patients who already have high blood pressure are presented in separated columns (already ill)

2-year risk													
		2023						Previous years					
						Already ill						Already ill	
	Age group	*n*	M (in %)	SD	Md	*n*	%	*n*	M (in %)	SD	Md	*n*	%
Men	Up to 30	8	3.08	4.62	1.76	1	0.6	90	3.80	4.77	2.00	3	0.1
	31 to 40	13	4.33	3.92	2.75	0	0.0	139	5.62	6.01	4.00	9	0.4
	41 to 50	15	11.82	6.75	10.24	6	3.6	332	9.01	7.29	6.30	93	4.3
	51 to 60	47	11.61	8.08	10.24	17	10.1	488	12.12	8.82	10.00	262	12.0
	61 to 70	26	12.43	7.39	11.12	21	12.4	273	16.69	10.21	16.00	221	10.1
	Over 70	5	18.82	9.28	19.15	10	5.9	137	18.19	9.57	19.00	133	6.1
	Total	**114**	**10.71**	**7.95**	**8.72**	**55**	**32.5**	**1459**	**11.71**	**9.41**	**9.00**	**721**	**33.1**
Women	Up to 30	14	1.44	1.34	1.30	0	0.0	240	2.11	2.87	1.00	4	0.1
	31 to 40	49	3.91	5.84	1.67	1	0.2	425	3.42	4.53	2.00	14	0.2
	41 to 50	85	6.50	8.47	3.25	11	1.7	1248	6.62	7.45	4.00	165	2.5
	51 to 60	228	10.21	9.82	6.30	52	8.0	2038	10.32	9.52	7.00	629	9.4
	61 to 70	92	16.10	12.60	12.01	58	9.0	777	16.02	11.58	14.00	497	7.4
	Over 70	26	23.6	13.39	22.25	32	4.9	317	20.18	11.42	19.00	323	4.8
	Total	**494**	**10.50**	**11.08**	**6.30**	**154**	**23.8**	**5045**	**9.93**	**10.14**	**6.00**	**1632**	**24.4**
Total	Up to 30	22	2.04	2.98	1.30	1	0.1	330	2.57	3.57	1.00	7	0.1
	31 to 40	62	4.00	5.46	1.97	1	0.1	564	3.96	5.02	2.00	23	0.3
	41 to 50	100	7.30	8.42	4.19	17	2.1	1580	7.13	7.48	5.00	258	2.9
	51 to 60	275	10.45	9.55	7.41	69	8.5	2526	10.66	9.42	7.41	891	10.1
	61 to 70	118	15.29	11.73	12.01	79	9.7	1050	16.20	11.24	14.00	718	8.1
	Over 70	31	22.83	12.81	22.25	42	5.1	454	19.58	10.93	19.00	456	5.2
	Total	**608**	**10.54**	**10.56**	**6.30**	**209**	**25.6**	**6504**	**10.33**	**10.01**	**7.00**	**2353**	**26.6**

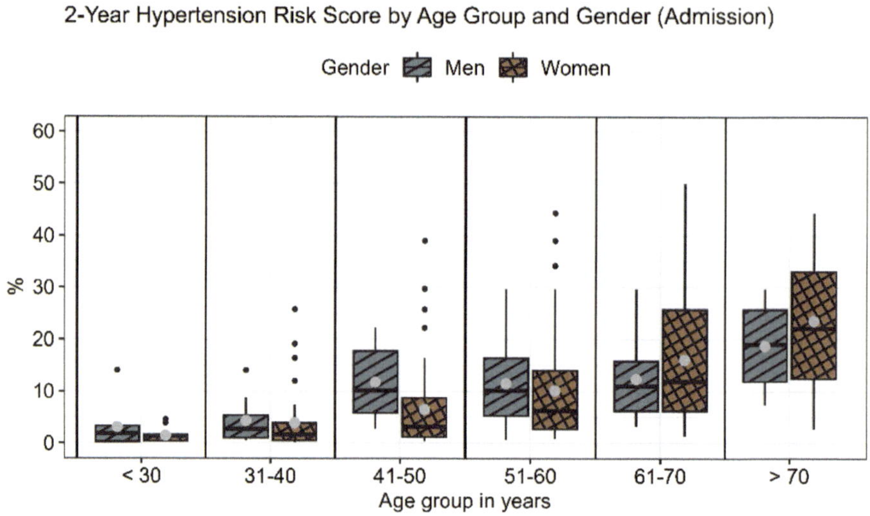

Fig. 5.105 Distribution of 2-year hypertension risk on admission in 2023, broken down by gender and age group; grey circles indicate the mean, black lines the median; the coloured lines indicate the thresholds according to the traffic light system

Table 5.96 Measures of distribution for the 4-year hypertension risk score of developing high blood pressure, broken down by gender and age in 2023 and previous years; *M* mean, *SD* standard deviation, *Md* median; the distribution of patients who already have high blood pressure are presented in separated columns (already ill)

4-year risk													
		2023						Previous years					
						Already ill						Already ill	
	Age group	*n*	M (in %)	SD	Md	*n*	%	n	M (in %)	SD	Md	*n*	%
Men	Up to 30	8	5.89	8.58	3.49	1	0.6	90	7.27	8.72	5.00	3	0.1
	31 to 40	13	8.33	7.33	5.43	0	0.0	139	10.62	10.76	8.00	9	0.4
	41 to 50	15	21.81	11.79	19.43	6	3.6	332	16.83	12.88	12.20	93	4.3
	51 to 60	47	21.23	13.93	19.43	17	10.1	488	22.16	14.98	19.00	262	12.0
	61 to 70	26	22.79	12.55	21.00	21	12.4	273	29.72	16.59	30.00	221	10.1
	Over 70	5	33.41	15.12	34.63	10	5.9	137	32.31	15.67	35.00	133	6.1
	Total	**114**	**19.65**	**13.78**	**16.68**	**55**	**32.5**	**1459**	**21.30**	**15.97**	**17.00**	**721**	**33.1**
Women	Up to 30	14	2.84	2.62	2.58	0	0.0	240	4.08	5.44	2.00	4	0.1
	31 to 40	49	7.34	10.47	3.31	1	0.2	425	6.59	8.25	3.00	14	0.2
	41 to 50	85	11.87	14.35	6.40	11	1.7	1248	12.32	13.06	8.00	165	2.5
	51 to 60	228	18.42	16.44	12.2	52	8.0	2038	18.78	16.03	14.00	629	9.4
	61 to 70	92	28.03	19.82	22.58	58	9.0	777	28.33	18.64	26.00	497	7.4
	Over 70	26	39.91	20.38	39.55	32	4.9	317	35.16	18.04	35.00	323	4.8
	Total	**494**	**18.67**	**18.22**	**12.20**	**154**	**23.8**	**5045**	**17.95**	**17.04**	**12.00**	**1632**	**24.4**
Total	Up to 30	22	3.95	5.57	2.58	1	0.1	330	4.95	6.64	2.00	7	0.1
	31 to 40	62	7.55	9.85	3.90	1	0.1	564	7.58	9.09	4.00	23	0.3
	41 to 50	100	13.37	14.39	8.20	17	2.1	1580	13.27	13.15	9.00	258	2.9
	51 to 60	275	18.90	16.05	14.28	69	8.5	2526	19.43	15.89	14.28	891	10.1
	61 to 70	118	26.88	18.55	22.58	79	9.7	1050	28.69	18.13	26.00	718	8.1
	Over 70	31	38.86	19.56	39.55	42	5.1	454	34.30	17.39	35.00	456	5.2
	Total	**608**	**18.86**	**17.47**	**12.20**	**209**	**25.6**	**6504**	**18.70**	**16.86**	**14.00**	**2353**	**26.6**

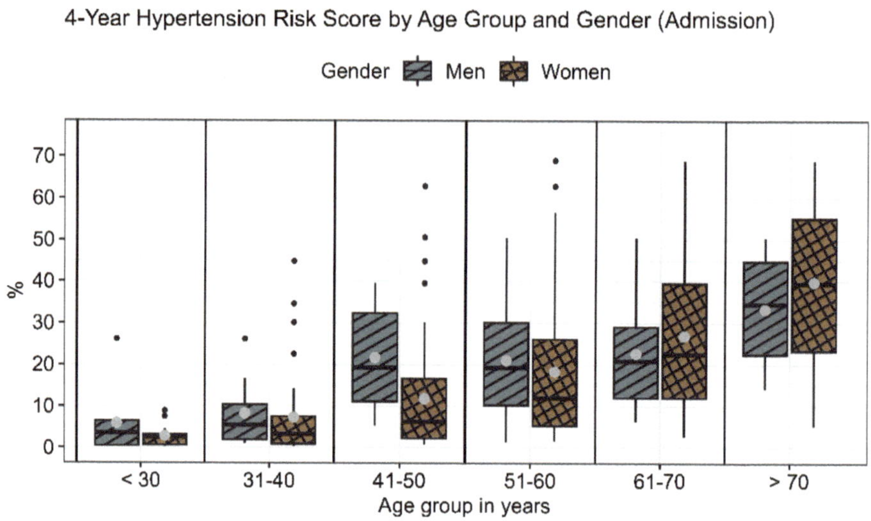

Fig. 5.106 Distribution of 4-year hypertension risk on admission in 2023, broken down by gender and age group; grey circles indicate the mean, black lines the median; the coloured lines indicate the thresholds according to the traffic light system

Table 5.97 Hypertension Risk in the before/after comparison in 2023; *t*-test for paired samples; significance at $p < 0.05$; Cohen's d = effect measure ($d \geq 0.2$ = small, ≥ 0.5 = moderate, ≥ 0.8 = large effect); previous year's data since 2022

		2023								Previous year 2022			
Hypertension risk		Cross-section: A/F			Course: A–F $n = 454$		Difference from admission: A–F $n = 454$			Course: A–F $n = 376$	Difference from admission: A–F $n = 376$		
		n	M	SD	M	SD	ΔM	p	d	M	ΔM	p	d
1-year risk	**A**	609	5.59	5.85	5.77	5.81				10.96			
	F	454	5.28	5.30	5.28	5.30	−0.49	0.024	−0.09	10.70	−0.40	0.140	–
2-year risk	**A**	609	10.53	10.55	10.87	10.47				10.96			
	F	454	10.04	9.58	10.04	9.58	−0.83	0.034	−0.08	10.70	−0.65	0.185	–
4-year risk	**A**	609	18.84	17.45	19.47	17.28				10.96			
	F	454	18.20	15.96	18.20	15.96	−1.27	0.052	–	10.70	−0.94	0.253	–

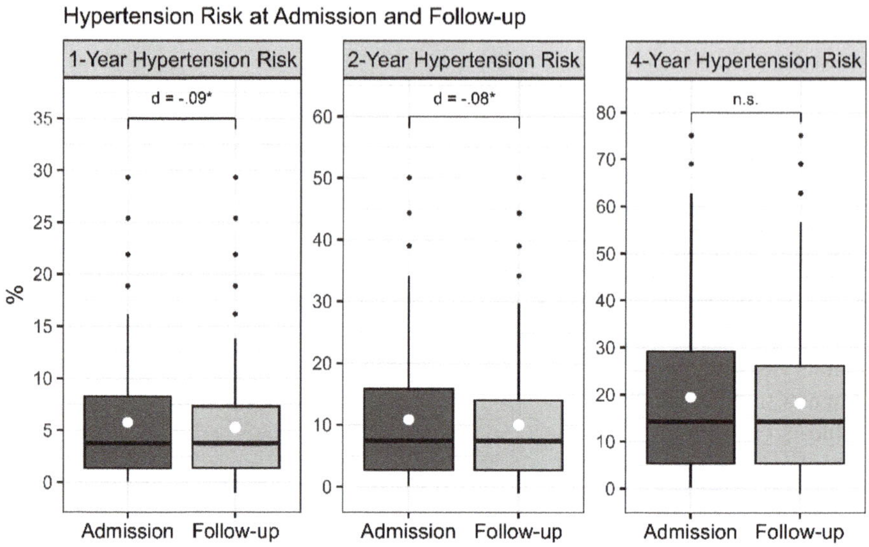

Fig. 5.107 Hypertension risk over the course of the measurement time points in 2023 ($n = 454$); t-test with paired samples; Cohen's d = effect measure ($d \geq 0.2$ = small, ≥ 0.5 = moderate, ≥ 0.8 = large effect); white circle indicates the mean, the black line the median

Table 5.98 Measures of distribution for the Metabolic Syndrome Index, broken down by gender and age in 2023 and previous years

Metabolic syndrome index									
		2023				Previous years			
	Age group	*n*	M	SD	Md	*n*	M	SD	Md
Men	Up to 30	8	0.75	0.71	1	106	0.95	1.01	1
	31 to 40	12	1.83	1.11	2	156	1.31	1.30	1
	41 to 50	19	1.79	1.18	2	441	2.00	1.39	2
	51 to 60	61	2.03	1.35	2	728	2.36	1.43	2
	61 to 70	42	2.31	1.32	2	464	2.65	1.32	3
	Over 70	14	2.86	1.35	3	303	2.53	1.26	3
	Total	**156**	**2.07**	**1.33**	**2**	**2198**	**2.23**	**1.42**	**2**
Women	Up to 30	14	1.00	0.88	1	281	1.00	0.99	1
	31 to 40	46	0.89	1.08	1	476	1.04	1.06	1
	41 to 50	87	1.52	1.32	1	1446	1.43	1.23	1
	51 to 60	253	1.89	1.25	2	2390	1.82	1.29	2
	61 to 70	138	2.10	1.17	2	1222	2.28	1.29	2
	Over 70	53	2.45	1.14	2	639	2.53	1.17	2
	Total	**591**	**1.84**	**1.27**	**2**	**6454**	**1.80**	**1.32**	**2**
Total	Up to 30	22	0.91	0.81	1	387	0.99	1.00	1
	31 to 40	58	1.09	1.14	1	632	1.11	1.13	1
	41 to 50	106	1.57	1.29	1	1887	1.56	1.29	1
	51 to 60	314	1.92	1.27	2	3118	1.94	1.35	2
	61 to 70	180	2.15	1.21	2	1686	2.38	1.31	2
	Over 70	67	2.54	1.18	2	942	2.53	1.20	2
	Total	**747**	**1.88**	**1.28**	**2**	**8652**	**1.91**	**1.36**	**2**

M mean, *SD* standard deviation, *Md* median

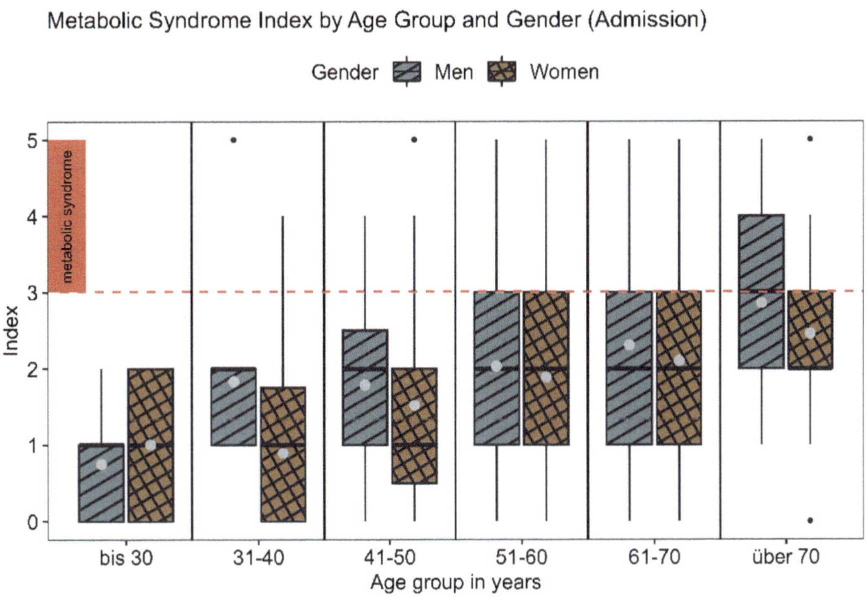

Fig. 5.108 Distribution of the Metabolic Syndrome Index on admission in 2023, broken down by gender and age group; grey circles indicate the mean, black lines the median; the red line indicates the thresholds at which a metabolic syndrome is present (i.e. three out of five criteria)

Table 5.99 Metabolic Syndrome Index before/after comparison in 2023; *t*-test for paired samples; significance at $p < 0.05$; Cohen's d = effect measure ($d \geq 0.2$ = small, ≥ 0.5 = moderate, ≥ 0.8 = large effect); previous year's data since 2022

		2023								Previous year 2022			
Metabolic syndrome index		Cross-section: A/D			Course: A–D $n = 690$		Difference from admission: A–D n 690			Course: A–D $n = 7533$	Difference from admission: A–D $n = 7533$		
		n	M	SD	M	SD	ΔM	p	d	M	ΔM	p	d
Index	**A**	747	1.88	1.28	1.87	1.29				1.87			
	D	701	1.83	1.29	1.82	1.29	−0.05	0.110	–	1.83	−0.04	<0.001	−0.03

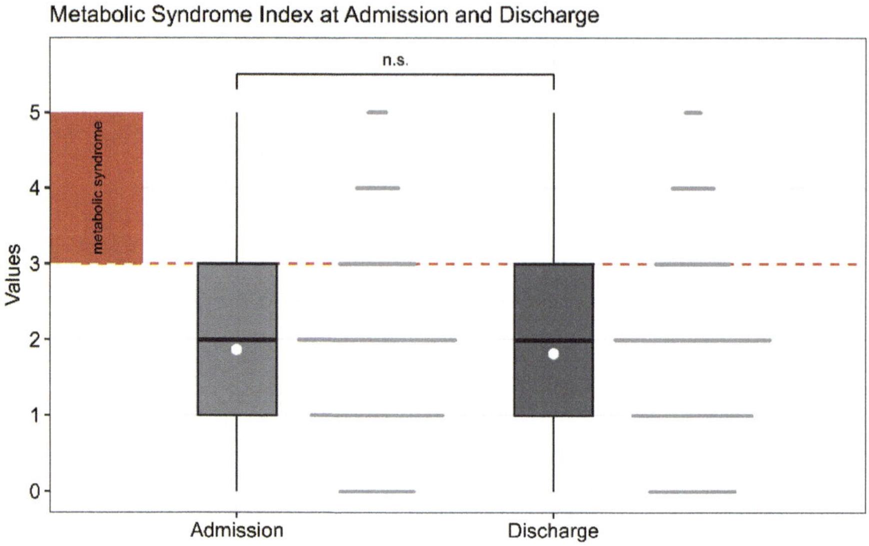

Fig. 5.109 Metabolic Syndrome Index over the course of the measurement time points in 2023; *t*-test with paired samples; *n.s.* not significant; white circle indicates the mean, the black line the median; the red line indicates the thresholds at which a metabolic syndrome is present (i.e. three out of five criteria)

Table 5.100 Measures of distribution for the Fatty Liver Index, broken down by gender and age in 2023 and previous years

Fatty liver index									
		2023				Previous years			
	Age group	*n*	M	SD	Md	*n*	M	SD	Md
Men	Up to 30	9	16.33	14.88	17.0	27	22.91	24.73	13.0
	31 to 40	13	30.54	19.77	31.0	55	40.88	32.56	24.0
	41 to 50	22	57.00	29.26	57.0	123	48.12	30.30	47.0
	51 to 60	62	53.03	30.03	52.0	309	53.91	28.73	55.0
	61 to 70	47	51.89	26.91	54.0	215	56.74	29.28	61.0
	Over 70	15	60.07	28.32	54.0	104	52.24	27.00	55.5
	Total	**168**	**50.15**	**29.21**	**49.5**	**833**	**51.71**	**29.73**	**53.0**
Women	Up to 30	14	19.86	25.94	7.0	75	20.71	25.35	9.0
	31 to 40	47	17.21	25.47	6.0	173	22.14	27.74	9.0
	41 to 50	93	27.23	29.22	14.0	534	27.68	27.41	15.0
	51 to 60	272	35.71	29.4	25.0	1294	34.94	29.21	24.0
	61 to 70	150	38.75	28.84	32.5	620	40.65	29.48	33.0
	Over 70	57	44.95	27.85	45.0	293	41.99	28.80	38.0
	Total	**633**	**34.29**	**29.50**	**23.0**	**2989**	**34.42**	**29.33**	**24.0**
Total	Up to 30	23	18.48	21.94	9.0	102	21.29	25.08	10.0
	31 to 40	60	20.10	24.81	7.0	228	26.66	30.00	12.3
	41 to 50	115	32.92	31.39	19.0	657	31.51	29.07	19.0
	51 to 60	334	38.93	30.23	29.0	1603	38.6	30.06	29.0
	61 to 70	197	41.88	28.88	37.0	835	44.79	30.24	41.0
	Over 70	72	48.10	28.43	46.5	397	44.68	28.67	42.0
	Total	**801**	**37.62**	**30.12**	**28.0**	**3825**	**38.19**	**30.27**	**29.0**

M mean, *SD* standard deviation, *Md* median

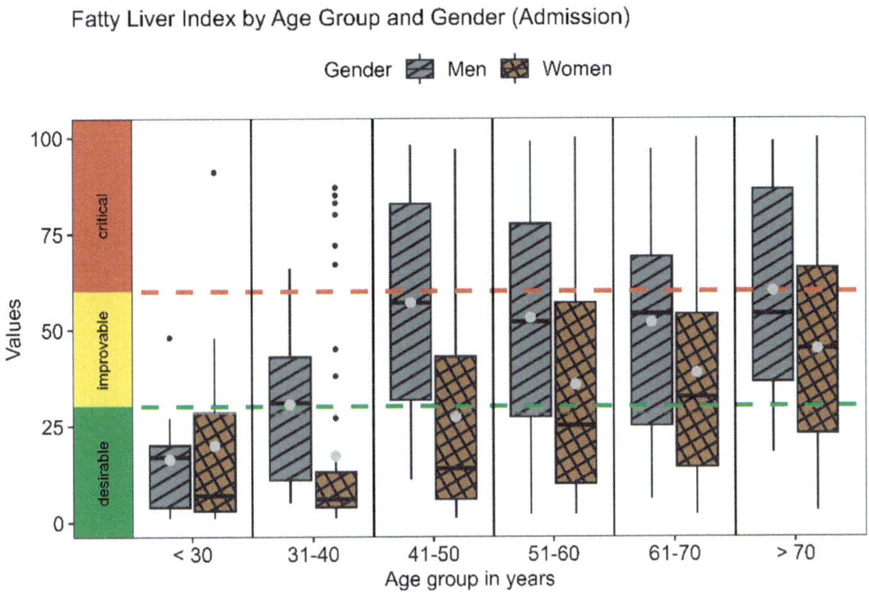

Fig. 5.110 Distribution measures of the Fatty Liver Index on admission in the 2023 reporting year ($n = 801$), broken down by gender and age group. Grey circles indicate the mean and black lines indicate the median. Coloured lines indicate the thresholds according to the traffic light system

Table 5.101 Fatty Liver Index before/after comparison in 2023; *t*-test for paired samples; significance at $p < 0.05$; Cohen's d = effect measure ($d \geq 0.2$ = small, ≥ 0.5 = moderate, ≥ 0.8 = large effect)

		2023								Previous years[a]			
Fatty liver index		Cross-section: A/D			Course: A–D $n = 788$		Difference from admission: A–D $n = 788$			Course: A–D $n = 2798$	Difference from admission: A–D $n = 2798$		
		n	M	SD	M	SD	ΔM	p	d	M	ΔM	p	d
Index	**A**	801	37.62	30.12	37.62	30.17				38.33			
	D	805	35.83	29.92	36.03	29.94	−1.60	<0.001	−0.05	34.80	−3.52	<0.001	−0.12

[a]Previous years without the year 2019

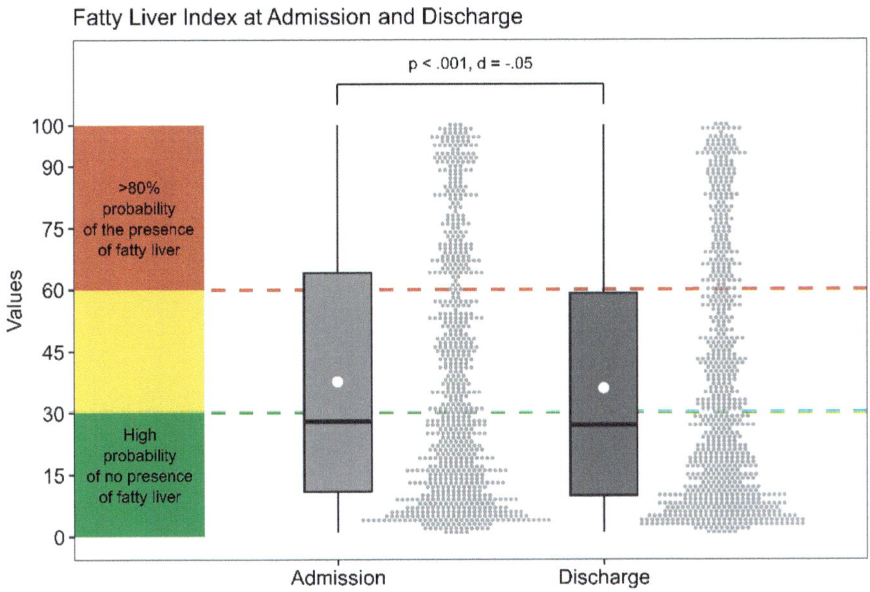

Fig. 5.111 Fatty Liver Index over the course of the measurement time points in 2023 ($n = 788$); t-test with paired samples; Cohen's d = effect measure ($d \geq 0.2$ = small, ≥ 0.5 = moderate, ≥ 0.8 = large effect); white circle indicates the mean, the black line the median

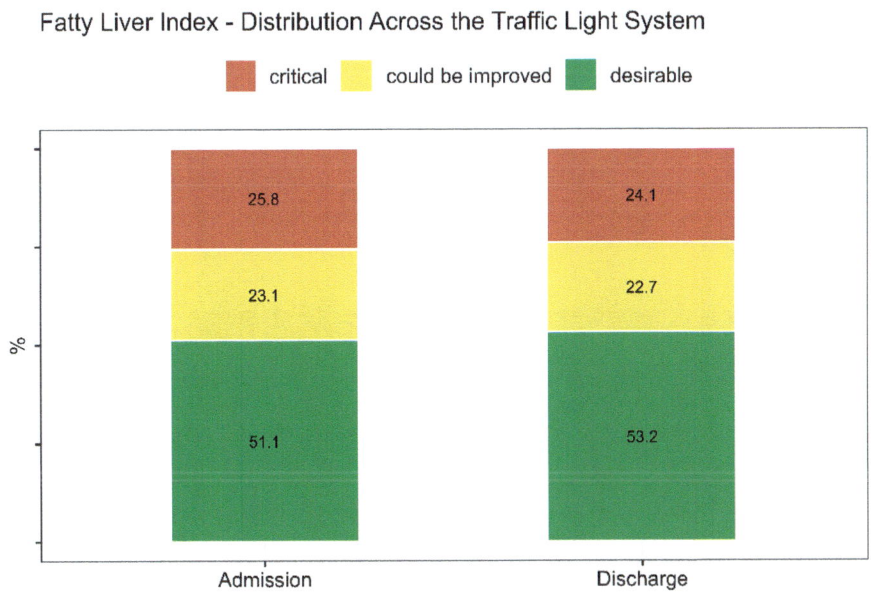

Fig. 5.112 Distribution of the Fatty Liver Index across the levels of the traffic light system in 2023 ($n = 788$)

Table 5.102 Change in cardiometabolic values for patients with a high blood pressure diagnosis I10 (admission—discharge); *t*-test for dependent samples; significance at $p < 0.05$; Cohen's d = effect measure ($d \geq 0.2$ = smaller, ≥ 0.5 = medium effect, ≥ 0.8 = strong effect)

	2023							Previous years			
High blood pressure diagnosis		Course admission–discharge			Difference from admission admission–discharge			A/D	Difference from admission A–D n = 2208		
		n	M	SD	M	*p*	*d*	M	ΔM	*p*	*d*
Systolic blood pressure	A	190	145.31	17.88	0.57	0.645	–	136.36	−2.78	**<0.001**	−0.14
	D	19	145.88	18.03				133.58			
Diastolic blood pressure	A	190	87.09	9.78	−0.17	0.826	–	82.27	−1.11	**0.004**	−0.07
	D	190	86.93	9.76				81.16			
Weight	A	192	83.40	19.57	−1.19	**<0.001**	−0.06	81.79	−1.32	**<0.001**	−0.08
	D	192	82.21	19.24				80.47			
Abdominal circumference	A	190	99.85	15.69	−1.33	**<0.001**	−0.09	99.28	−2.66	**<0.001**	−0.18
	D	190	98.51	15.02				96.62			
Total cholesterol	A	183	215.68	50.48	−14.58	**<0.001**	−0.30	226.27	−17.11	**<0.001**	−0.37
	D	183	201.10	47.49				209.17			
HDL	A	183	57.15	15.30	−3.85	**<0.001**	−0.26	55.56	−5.12	**<0.001**	−0.38
	D	183	53.30	13.99				50.43			
LDL	A	183	142.79	47.52	−9.87	**<0.001**	−0.21	147.85	−10.24	**<0.001**	−0.28
	D	183	132.92	43.88				137.61			
Triglycerides	A	183	132.15	61.33	−3.12	0.304	–	150.56	−7.95	**<0.001**	−0.11
	D	183	129.03	61.76				142.61			

5.3 Successful Therapy for Disease-Specific Psychological Diagnoses

The main diagnosis groups F45 (including all subcategories) and F32/F33, which are the most frequently represented, will be examined in more detail below. These groups are described using the corresponding WHO definitions and presented separately. Mental illnesses are associated with emotional, cognitive, and social impairments that can make participation in social, family, and professional life difficult. To gain a comprehensive understanding of patients with a primary mental health diagnosis from chapters F45 and F32/F33, a selection of patients was examined based on the severity of their main complaint, their ICD symptom rating, and all protective and risk factors at the time of admission, discharge, and follow-up.

5.3.1 Functional Somatic Disorders (FSD)—F45 (ICD-10)/ Somatoform Disorders (ICD-11)

Patients diagnosed with somatoform disorders (ICD-10 group F45) experienced significant improvements in their primary symptoms during inpatient treatment, with effect sizes of $d = -1.09$ and $d = -1.11$ at discharge and follow-up, respectively (both $p < 0.001$). On average, patients with an F45 diagnosis improved their main symptom severity by 22.74 points at discharge and by 23.19 points at follow-up (Table 5.103).

Table 5.103 Global assessments of treatment success for patients with a main F45 mental health diagnosis, surveyed at discharge ($n = 489$) and follow-up ($n = 392$) in 2023; *t*-test for paired samples; significance at $p < 0.05$; Cohen's d = effect measure ($d \geq 0.2$ = small, ≥ 0.5 = moderate, ≥ 0.8 = large effect)

F45 functional somatic disorders (FSD)	Course						Difference from admission			
	Admission (A)			Discharge (D)/ follow-up (F)			A–D/A–F		Significance	Effect size
	n	M	SD		M	SD	*n*	ΔM	*p*	*d*
Main complaint severity VAS	489	69.06	19.70	D	46.32	21.98	489	−22.74	<0.001	**−1.09**
	392	68.29	20.00	F	46.53	24.15	392	−23.19	<0.001	**−1.11**

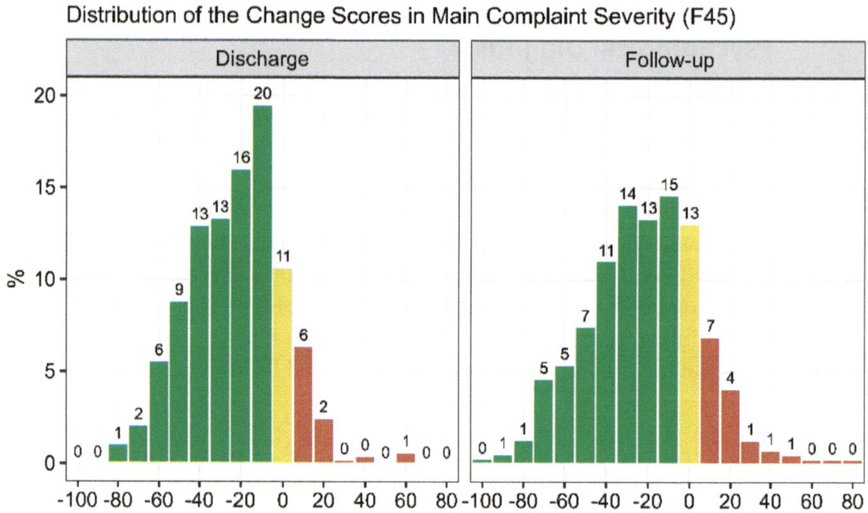

Fig. 5.113 Distribution of the change scores in main complaint severity between hospital admission and hospital discharge or hospital admission and follow-up for patients with a main diagnosis of F45 in 2023 (A–D n = 487; A–D–F n = 390); negative differences correspond to an improvement

Figure 5.113 depicts the distribution of differences. Values below zero indicate an improvement, zero means no change, and values above zero show deterioration. Overall, 79.3% of patients reported an improvement, 10.6% reported no change, and 13.0% reported deterioration. At follow-up, 72.5% still showed an improvement, 13.0% no change, and 14.5% a deterioration.

At discharge, 14.9% of patients rated the overall success of the treatment as 'very good' and 50.1% as 'good'. In response to the question 'From today's perspective, was the treatment worthwhile?', 40.5% answered 'very worthwhile' and 54.4% answered 'worthwhile' (Table 5.104, Fig. 5.114). The overall assessment was better at the time of the follow-up survey than at discharge.

Table 5.105 and Fig. 5.115 provide an overview of changes in subjective complaints, protective factors, and risk factors at discharge and after the six-month follow-up. For patients with functional somatic stress disorder, all overall parameter scores showed significant positive changes at hospital discharge, with effect sizes ranging from small to large. Notable improvements were seen in well-being (d = 1.17, p < 0.001), vitality (d = 0.93, p < 0.001), depressive symptoms (ISR: d = −0.96, p < 0.001), exhaustion (Tedium: d = −0.73, p < 0.001), the complaint index (d = 0.87, p < 0.001), generalised anxiety (GAD: d = −0.94, p < 0.001), health-related life satisfaction (d = 0.73, p < 0.001) and all dimensions of the Perceived Stress Questionnaire (total score: d = −0.97, p < 0.001).

Table 5.104 Global assessments of treatment success for patients with a main F45 mental health diagnosis, surveyed at discharge (n = 487) and follow-up (n = 393 and 394) in 2023

Overall success of the therapy		**Very good**		**Good**		**Moderate**		**No success**		**Total**	
		n	%	*n*	%	*n*	%	*n*	%	*n*	%
F45 patients	D	73	14.9	245	50.1	155	31.7	16	3.3	489	100
	F	115	29.1	164	41.5	102	25.8	14	3.5	395	100
Treatment worthwhile		**Very worthwhile**		**Worthwhile**		**Not worth it**		**Rather harmed**		**Total**	
		n	%	*n*	%	*n*	%	*n*	%	*n*	%
F45 patients	D	198	40.5	266	54.4	24	4.9	1	0.2	489	100
	F	213	53.8	157	39.6	25	6.3	1	0.3	396	100

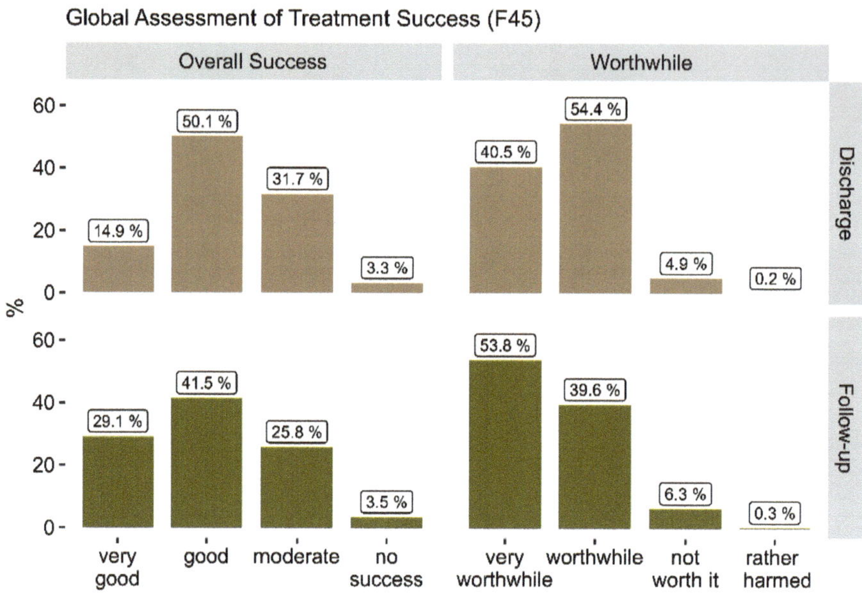

Fig. 5.114 Global assessments of treatment success for patients with a main F45 mental health diagnosis, surveyed at discharge (n = 487) and follow-up (n = 393 and 394) in 2023

Table 5.105 Changes in various parameters for patients with a main F45 diagnosis in 2023; t-test: Cohen's d = effect measure ($d \geq 0.2$ = small effect, ≥ 0.5 = moderate effect, ≥ 0.8 = large effect)

Main diagnosis F45	Course						Difference from admission			
		Admission (A)		Discharge (D)/ follow-up (F)			A–D/A–F		Significance	Effect size
	n	M	SD	D/F	M	SD	*n*	M	*p*	*d*
ICD symptom ratings (ISR)										
Total value	489	1.04	0.57	D	0.72	0.51	489	−0.32	< 0.001	**−0.58**
	387	1.01	0.57	F	0.70	0.52	387	−0.31	< 0.001	**−0.57**
Depression	489	1.87	0.87	D	1.06	0.81	489	−0.81	< 0.001	**−0.96**
	387	1.85	0.87	F	1.16	0.84	387	−0.69	< 0.001	**−0.80**
Anxiety	489	1.25	1.01	D	0.84	0.85	489	−0.41	< 0.001	−0.43
	387	1.22	1.01	F	0.80	0.86	387	−0.42	< 0.001	−0.44
Obsessive-compulsion	489	0.86	0.93	D	0.66	0.81	489	−0.20	< 0.001	−0.23
	387	0.83	0.92	F	0.61	0.81	387	−0.22	< 0.001	−0.25
Somatoform	489	0.85	0.90	D	0.59	0.76	489	−0.26	< 0.001	−0.31
	387	0.79	0.86	F	0.49	0.73	387	−0.30	< 0.001	−0.36
Eating disorder	489	0.58	0.82	D	0.49	0.76	489	−0.09	0.001	−0.11
	387	0.58	0.81	F	0.47	0.74	387	−0.11	< 0.001	−0.15

(continued)

Table 5.105 (continued)

Main diagnosis	Course						Difference from admission			
		Admission (A)		Discharge (D)/ follow-up (F)			A–D/A–F		Significance	Effect size
F45	*n*	M	SD	D/F	M	SD	*n*	M	*p*	*d*
Pain disability index										
Total index	482	29.86	15.11	D	24.85	14.44	482	−5.01	< 0.001	−0.34
	379	29.54	15.17	F	23.25	16.07	379	−6.29	< 0.001	−0.40
Family/domestic	482	5.03	2.75	D	4.22	2.74	482	−0.81	< 0.001	−0.30
obligations	379	5.01	2.76	F	4.04	2.89	379	−0.97	< 0.001	−0.34
Recreation	482	5.55	2.69	D	4.66	2.76	482	−0.89	< 0.001	−0.33
	379	5.50	2.67	F	4.30	2.90	379	−1.20	< 0.001	−0.43
Social activity	482	4.82	2.94	D	4.12	2.86	482	−0.70	< 0.001	−0.24
	379	4.72	2.93	F	3.78	2.96	379	−0.94	< 0.001	−0.32
Profession	482	5.42	3.17	D	4.90	3.09	482	−0.52	< 0.001	−0.16
	379	5.30	3.17	F	3.95	3.22	379	−1.35	< 0.001	−0.42
Sex life	482	4.58	3.61	D	3.73	3.37	482	−0.85	< 0.001	−0.24
	379	4.57	3.63	F	3.85	3.58	379	−0.72	< 0.001	−0.20
Self-sufficiency	482	2.34	2.60	D	1.84	2.33	482	−0.50	< 0.001	−0.20
	379	2.31	2.58	F	1.77	2.50	379	−0.54	< 0.001	−0.21
Essentials	482	2.13	2.57	D	1.37	2.03	482	−0.76	< 0.001	−0.32
Activities	379	2.15	2.59	F	1.57	2.31	379	−0.58	< 0.001	−0.24
Life satisfaction										
Total value	488	27.07	33.40	D	45.12	36.29	488	18.05	< 0.001	**0.52**
	392	28.83	31.84	F	44.46	32.80	392	15.63	< 0.001	0.48
Friends /	488	5.18	6.73	D	6.90	6.56	488	1.72	< 0.001	0.26
acquaintances	392	5.40	6.57	F	6.33	6.13	392	0.93	0.001	0.15
Leisure/hobbies	488	1.66	6.43	D	4.28	6.48	488	2.62	< 0.001	0.41
	392	1.68	6.24	F	4.14	5.61	392	2.46	< 0.001	0.41
Health	488	−5.34	5.94	D	−0.43	7.40	488	4.91	< 0.001	**0.73**
	392	−5.27	5.98	F	0.22	7.71	392	5.49	< 0.001	**0.79**
Income	488	3.27	6.78	D	4.72	6.63	488	1.45	< 0.001	0.22
	392	3.25	6.70	F	4.64	6.17	392	1.39	< 0.001	0.21
Profession	488	1.35	6.59	D	2.62	6.53	488	1.27	< 0.001	0.19
	392	1.49	6.48	F	3.32	6.25	392	1.83	< 0.001	0.29
Housing	488	6.92	7.31	D	8.19	7.39	488	1.27	< 0.001	0.17
situation	392	7.30	7.09	F	8.08	6.49	392	0.78	0.022	0.12
Family/children	488	7.78	8.27	D	10.19	7.86	488	2.41	< 0.001	0.30
	392	8.23	8.12	F	9.45	7.39	392	1.22	< 0.001	0.16
Partnership	488	6.23	9.35	D	8.64	9.37	488	2.41	< 0.001	0.26
	392	6.74	9.20	F	8.28	8.65	392	1.54	< 0.001	0.17
SOC										
Total value	484	59.79	12.02	D	64.24	12.25	484	4.45	< 0.001	0.37
	385	60.40	12.18	F	64.94	12.59	385	4.54	< 0.001	0.37
Meaningfulness	484	19.60	3.92	D	20.70	3.93	484	1.10	< 0.001	0.28
	385	19.74	3.93	F	20.75	4.13	385	1.01	< 0.001	0.25
Comprehen-sibility	484	22.37	5.51	D	24.15	5.52	484	1.78	< 0.001	0.32
	385	22.62	5.58	F	24.71	5.71	385	2.09	< 0.001	0.37
Manageability	484	17.79	4.66	D	19.40	4.68	484	1.61	< 0.001	0.35
	385	18.01	4.73	F	19.48	4.69	385	1.47	< 0.001	0.31

(continued)

Table 5.105 (continued)

Main diagnosis F45	Course						Difference from admission			
		Admission (A)		Discharge (D)/ follow-up (F)			A–D/A–F		Significance	Effect size
	n	M	SD	D/F	M	SD	*n*	M	*p*	*d*
WHO-5 Well-being and vitality										
Well-being	486	31.95	19.39	D	56.53	22.42	486	24.58	< 0.001	**1.17**
	387	32.22	19.18	F	48.40	24.06	387	16.18	< 0.001	**0.73**
Vitality	486	30.44	17.79	D	49.14	21.71	486	18.70	< 0.001	**0.93**
	387	30.99	17.64	F	45.76	22.83	387	14.77	< 0.001	**0.71**
SWOP										
Self-efficacy	485	12.84	2.80	D	13.76	2.67	485	0.92	< 0.001	0.34
	382	12.96	2.74	F	13.94	2.60	382	0.98	< 0.001	0.37
Optimism	485	5.19	1.43	D	5.84	1.40	485	0.65	< 0.001	0.46
	382	5.21	1.42	F	5.68	1.35	382	0.47	< 0.001	0.34
Pessimism	485	4.38	1.36	D	4.00	1.36	485	−0.38	< 0.001	−0.28
	382	4.31	1.38	F	4.07	1.44	382	−0.24	0.002	−0.17
SSS										
Total value	474	54.49	16.73	D	59.10	15.04	474	4.61	< 0.001	0.29
	370	55.57	16.29	F	57.19	15.56	370	1.62	0.003	0.10
Emotional	474	17.98	5.40	D	19.10	4.98	474	1.12	< 0.001	0.21
	370	18.34	5.25	F	18.48	5.14	370	0.14	0.470	–
Social interaction	474	10.83	3.71	D	11.88	3.37	474	1.05	< 0.001	0.29
	370	11.02	3.67	F	11.52	3.40	370	0.50	< 0.001	0.14
Material	474	11.65	4.45	D	12.90	3.75	474	1.25	< 0.001	0.30
	370	11.96	4.28	F	12.52	3.96	370	0.56	< 0.001	0.14
Affective	474	8.95	3.10	D	9.63	2.72	474	0.68	< 0.001	0.23
	370	9.13	3.05	F	9.34	2.84	370	0.21	0.051	–
Tedium measure (burnout)										
Total value	488	4.04	0.94	D	3.41	1.03	488	−0.63	< 0.001	**−0.64**
	393	3.98	0.93	F	3.43	1.04	393	−0.55	< 0.001	**−0.55**
Discouragement	488	3.56	1.13	D	2.99	1.14	488	−0.57	< 0.001	**−0.50**
	393	3.49	1.11	F	2.99	1.14	393	−0.50	< 0.001	−0.44
Exhaustion	488	4.82	1.08	D	3.99	1.20	488	−0.83	< 0.001	**−0.73**
	393	4.78	1.07	F	4.07	1.24	393	−0.71	< 0.001	**−0.60**
Loss of motivation	488	4.07	0.84	D	3.54	0.94	488	−0.53	< 0.001	**−0.58**
	393	4.01	0.83	F	3.55	0.96	393	−0.46	< 0.001	**−0.50**
PSQ										
Total value	486	54.46	18.50	D	36.55	18.33	486	−17.91	< 0.001	**−0.97**
	390	53.60	18.39	F	42.81	19.16	390	−10.79	< 0.001	**−0.57**
Worries	486	46.75	23.72	D	32.07	22.14	486	−14.68	< 0.001	**−0.64**
	391	45.49	23.57	F	34.00	22.89	391	−11.49	< 0.001	**−0.49**
Demands	486	45.17	25.28	D	23.32	20.62	486	−21.85	< 0.001	**−0.94**
	391	44.55	24.89	F	36.35	23.35	391	−8.20	< 0.001	−0.34
Joy	486	37.17	19.73	D	52.41	22.22	486	15.24	< 0.001	**0.72**
	391	38.07	19.93	F	48.47	22.87	391	10.40	< 0.001	0.48
Tension	486	63.11	22.02	D	43.22	23.67	486	−19.89	< 0.001	**−0.87**
	391	62.52	22.15	F	49.50	22.56	391	−13.02	< 0.001	**−0.58**
PSQI										
Total value	481	10.16	3.92	D	9.32	4.51	481	−0.84	< 0.001	−0.20
	386	10.10	3.94	F	8.47	4.14	386	−1.63	< 0.001	−0.40

(continued)

Table 5.105 (continued)

Main diagnosis F45	Course						Difference from admission			
		Admission (A)		Discharge (D)/ follow-up (F)			A–D/A–F		Significance	Effect size
	n	M	SD	D/F	M	SD	*n*	M	*p*	*d*
Sleep quality	481	1.76	0.67	D	1.42	0.71	481	−0.34	< 0.001	−0.48
	386	1.76	0.67	F	1.46	0.72	386	−0.30	< 0.001	−0.42
Sleep latency	481	1.68	1.05	D	1.41	1.04	481	−0.27	< 0.001	−0.26
	386	1.64	1.05	F	1.44	1.02	386	−0.20	< 0.001	−0.20
Sleep duration	481	1.53	0.90	D	1.47	0.92	481	−0.06	0.164	–
	386	1.51	0.93	F	1.28	0.90	386	−0.23	< 0.001	−0.25
Sleep efficiency	481	1.26	1.17	D	1.16	1.20	481	−0.10	0.065	–
	386	1.24	1.16	F	0.91	1.07	386	−0.33	< 0.001	−0.29
Sleep disorders	481	1.70	0.64	D	1.53	0.62	481	−0.17	< 0.001	−0.28
	386	1.72	0.64	F	1.52	0.63	386	−0.20	< 0.001	−0.31
Sleeping pills	481	0.52	1.01	D	1.25	1.40	481	0.73	< 0.001	**0.59**
	386	0.51	1.02	F	0.54	1.04	386	0.03	0.481	–
Daytime sleepiness	481	1.72	0.78	D	1.08	0.78	481	−0.64	< 0.001	**−0.82**
	386	1.72	0.77	F	1.32	0.82	386	−0.40	< 0.001	**−0.51**
GAD										
Total value	485	9.51	4.77	D	5.27	4.19	485	−4.24	< 0.001	**−0.94**
	376	9.30	4.72	F	5.95	4.34	376	−3.35	< 0.001	**−0.74**
Complaint complexes of psycho-vegetative stability										
Complaints index	487	0.34	0.55	D	0.95	0.78	487	0.61	< 0.001	**0.87**
	393	0.36	0.54	F	0.88	0.75	393	0.52	< 0.001	**0.78**
Total value	487	59.57	16.52	D	41.97	18.52	487	−17.6	< 0.001	**−1.00**
	393	59.11	16.43	F	46.49	18.90	393	−12.62	< 0.001	**−0.71**
Dizziness	487	3.25	2.20	D	2.22	2.19	487	−1.03	< 0.001	−0.47
	393	3.21	2.17	F	2.54	2.05	393	−0.67	< 0.001	−0.32
Sleep	487	6.84	2.26	D	5.25	2.53	487	−1.59	< 0.001	**−0.66**
	393	6.83	2.28	F	5.50	2.52	393	−1.33	< 0.001	**−0.55**
Heat balance	487	5.60	2.80	D	3.78	2.58	487	−1.82	< 0.001	**−0.67**
	393	5.58	2.82	F	4.40	2.56	393	−1.18	< 0.001	−0.43

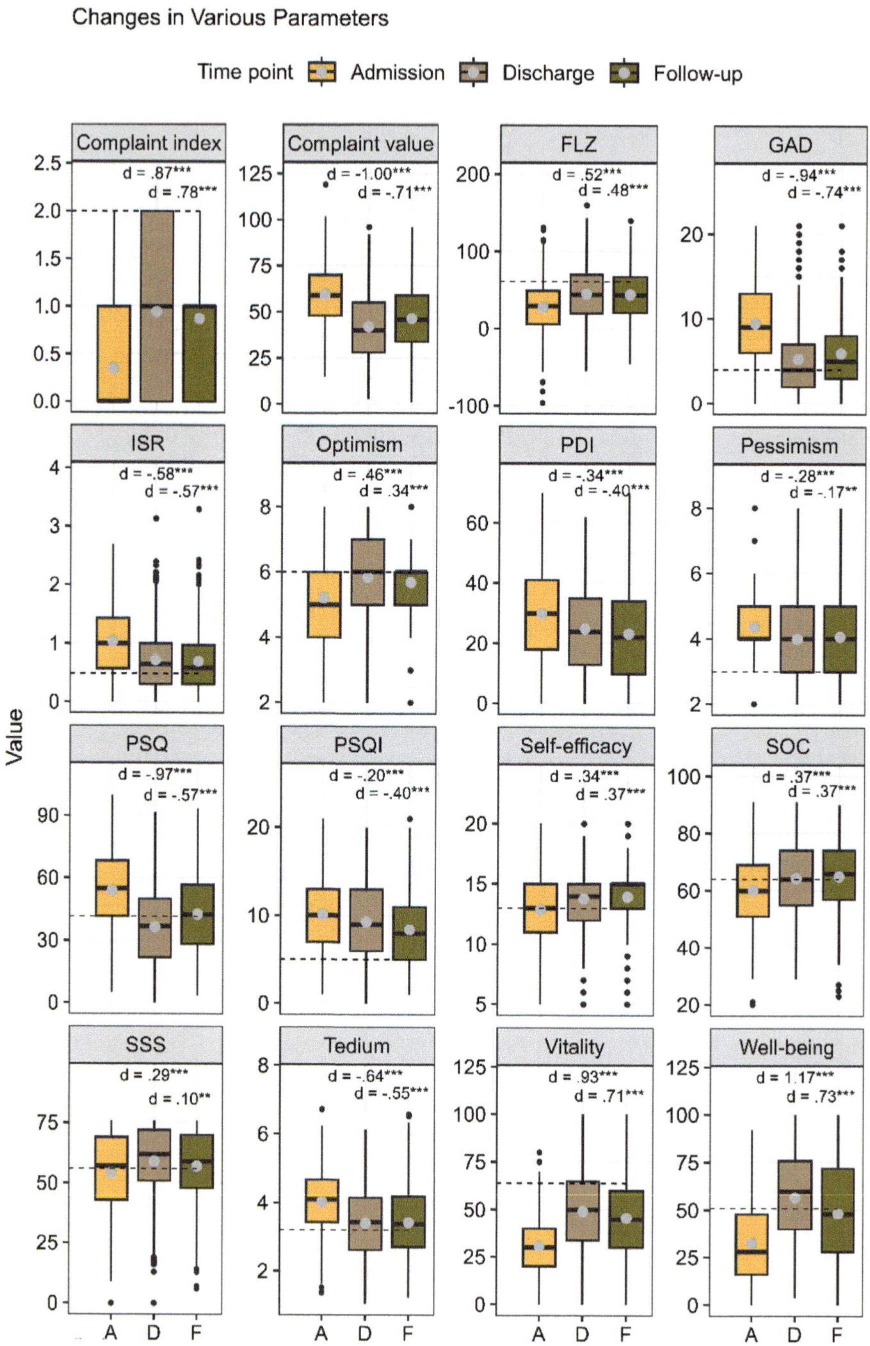

Fig. 5.115 Changes in various parameters for patients with a main F45 diagnosis in 2023; The dashed black lines indicate the desired target values; significance: $*p < 0.05$, $**p < 0.01$, $***p < 0.001$; Cohen's d = effect measure ($d \geq 0.2$ = small effect, ≥ 0.5 = moderate effect, ≥ 0.8 = large effect); the graph shows all available data, the effect sizes refer to the individual comparison (A–D/A–F)

At follow-up, the previously large effect sizes had decreased to predominantly moderate levels. However, positive changes remained stable for most parameters, with moderate and small effect sizes persisting over time. The most pronounced decline between discharge and follow-up was observed in the demand's subscale of the PSQ ($d = -0.94$, $p < 0.001$ vs. $d = -0.34$, $p < 0.001$).

According to guideline S3 functional somatic complaints (2018) [8], the current recommendation is under revision. An important diagnostic consideration involves taking a targeted case history for anxiety and/or depression. This includes asking the patient about their subjective model of illness and their beliefs about the cause of their symptoms, for example, 'What do you think is causing your symptoms?'. Allow enough time for the patient to fully describe and acknowledge their physical complaints.

In addition to revising the guideline, changes to the terminology have already been made in the DSM-5 and the ICD-11.

Functional somatic complaints are now referred to as somatic stress disorder (functional somatic disorder): DMS-5.

In the ICD-11, which came into force on 1 January 2022, the classification has also changed. In future, physical complaints can also have an organic correlation. There must be at least one somatic symptom. This is coded 6C20 in the ICD-11 and referred to as 'Bodily Distress Disorder'. It is essential that at least one of the following three mental abnormalities is also present:

These are:

- inappropriate and persistent thoughts about the seriousness of the symptoms.
- and/or.
- persistent, severe anxiety about health or the symptoms, or.
- excessive amounts of time and energy spent on the symptoms or health concerns [9–13].

The various functional somatic and affective complaints and symptoms are presented in the psycho-vegetative complaints questionnaire, which contains 42 individual items. Here, the individual symptoms are assigned to physical organs and functional systems, and the number of affected system areas and their respective degrees of severity are calculated in an index.

Table 5.106 presents how often the answers 'fairly/often' and 'strong/very frequently' were given for each complaint. On admission, 45.0% of responses for the total complaint score were rated as 'fairly/often' or 'strong/very frequently'. This proportion dropped to 27.2% at discharge and remained lower at 30.5% at follow-up. Table 5.107 summarises the mean number of these responses for each category and organ system.

Furthermore, statistical comparisons of the sum of 'fairly/often' and 'strong/very frequently' responses at admission, discharge and follow-up show significant improvements, especially for fatigue and sleep-related symptoms ($d = -0.78$, $p < 0.001$; $d = -0.66$, $p < 0.001$, respectively), as well as affective symptoms ($d = -0.93$, $p < 0.001$; $d = -0.74$, $p < 0.001$, respectively). Additionally, all other parameters indicating various functional somatic disorders in different organ

Table 5.106 Psycho-vegetative complaints; frequency distribution in % for patients with a main F45 mental health diagnosis in 2023; different symptom groups for different functional and organ systems (admission: $n = 512$, discharge: $n = 488$, follow-up: $n = 394$)

Category (number of subcategories)	Admission				Discharge				Follow-up			
	Fairly/ often		Strong/ very frequently		Fairly/ often		Strong/ very frequently		Fairly/ often		Strong/ very frequently	
	n	%	*n*	%	*n*	%	*n*	%	*n*	%	*n*	%
Immune system (1)	121	23.6	36	7.0	46	9.4	16	3.3	56	14.3	15	3.8
Gastrointestinal system (1)	184	35.9	139	27.1	149	30.5	83	17.0	123	31.4	57	14.5
Urogenital system (1)	167	32.6	76	14.8	170	34.8	60	12.3	111	28.3	43	11.0
Fatigue and sleep related symptoms (6)												
Dullness	267	52.1	137	26.8	176	36.1	45	9.2	166	42.1	40	10.2
Problems falling asleep	159	31.1	108	21.1	108	22.1	54	11.1	91	23.1	52	13.2
Restless sleep	223	43.6	149	29.1	150	30.7	84	17.2	128	32.5	60	15.2
Rapid fatigue	212	41.4	156	30.5	182	37.3	50	10.2	135	34.3	67	17.0
Memory of dreams	118	23.0	35	6.8	87	17.8	27	5.5	89	22.6	18	4.6
Unrested	194	37.9	190	37.1	155	31.8	86	17.6	124	31.5	66	16.8
Brain-related symptoms (4)												
Lack of concentration	237	46.3	74	14.5	144	29.5	29	5.9	117	29.7	31	7.9
Reduced ability to react	79	15.4	16	3.1	47	9.6	7	1.4	49	12.4	5	1.3
Memory disorders	147	28.7	52	10.2	79	16.2	29	5.9	90	22.8	15	3.8
Headaches and facial pain	159	31.1	109	21.3	94	19.3	57	11.7	90	22.8	36	9.1
Cardiovascular system (6)												
Shortness of breath	132	25.8	32	6.2	68	13.9	19	3.9	67	17.0	16	4.1
Irregular heartbeat	93	18.2	20	3.9	43	8.8	11	2.3	37	9.4	8	2.0
Heart and chest pain	73	14.3	22	4.3	32	6.6	8	1.6	27	6.9	8	2.0
Dizziness when standing up or bending down	136	26.6	52	10.2	79	16.2	30	6.1	83	21.1	14	3.6
Dizziness when looking into the depths	101	19.7	62	12.1	43	8.8	35	7.2	68	17.3	24	6.1
Dizziness when getting up in the morning	72	14.1	24	4.7	44	9.0	14	2.9	35	8.9	12	3.0

(continued)

Table 5.106 (continued)

Category (number of subcategories)	Admission				Discharge				Follow-up			
	Fairly/ often		Strong/ very frequently		Fairly/ often		Strong/ very frequently		Fairly/ often		Strong/ very frequently	
	n	%	*n*	%	*n*	%	*n*	%	*n*	%	*n*	%
Musculoskeletal system (3)												
Back pain	159	31.1	233	45.5	156	32.0	95	19.5	128	32.5	108	27.4
Joint problems	157	31.1	210	41.0	153	31.4	71	14.5	127	32.2	97	24.6
Muscle weakness in the legs	140	27.3	82	16.0	103	21.1	31	6.4	91	23.1	44	11.2
Affective symptoms (8)												
Restlessness	228	44.5	95	18.6	132	27.0	29	5.9	117	29.7	20	5.1
Irritability	204	39.8	57	11.1	59	12.1	10	2.0	86	21.8	16	4.1
Mood swings	204	39.8	67	13.1	94	19.3	23	4.7	97	24.6	20	5.1
Indecision	198	38.7	71	13.9	94	19.3	21	4.3	92	23.4	18	4.6
Sadness	200	39.1	58	11.3	99	20.3	23	4.7	78	19.8	20	5.1
Anxiety	178	34.8	66	12.9	87	17.8	28	5.7	77	19.5	22	5.6
Trembling (eyelid, tongue, mouth, hands)	77	15.0	18	3.5	43	8.8	5	1.0	23	5.8	13	3.3
Decreased sexual desire	151	29.5	131	25.6	100	20.5	65	13.3	105	26.6	66	16.8
(thermal) regulation-related symptoms (7)												
Cold hands/feet	146	28.5	152	29.7	130	26.6	60	12.3	117	29.7	50	12.7
Hypersensitivity to cold/wind	138	27.0	157	30.7	137	28.1	76	15.6	126	32.0	76	19.3
Heat or cold is poorly tolerated	186	36.3	92	18.0	100	20.5	46	9.4	110	27.9	46	11.7
Feeling hot	120	23.4	56	10.9	96	19.7	35	7.2	82	20.8	29	7.4
Excessive sweating	105	20.5	65	12.7	68	13.9	43	8.8	64	16.2	34	8.6
Shivering/ freezing	166	32.4	67	13.1	87	17.8	26	5.3	120	30.5	29	7.4
Delayed reheating after cold	153	29.9	49	9.6	86	17.6	27	5.5	82	20.8	23	5.8
Allergy related symptoms (5)												
Itchy skin	107	20.9	51	10.0	69	14.1	8	1.6	52	13.2	15	3.8
Dry mouth	117	22.9	44	8.6	90	18.4	37	7.6	65	16.5	23	5.8
Skin rashes/ changes	73	14.3	51	10.0	47	9.6	17	3.5	37	9.4	14	3.6
Severe thirst	112	21.9	33	6.4	56	11.5	24	4.9	59	15.0	8	2.0
Allergic reactions (including asthma)	52	10.2	19	3.7	26	5.3	7	1.4	35	8.9	6	1.5
Total number of responses	**6247**	**29.1**	**3415**	**15.9**	**4008**	**19.6**	**1551**	**7.6**	**3659**	**22.1**	**1384**	**8.4**

Table 5.107 Psycho-vegetative complaints; summary of the mean number of responses for 'fairly/often' and 'strong/very frequently' for patients with a main F45 mental health diagnosis; (admission: $n = 512$, discharge: $n = 488$, follow-up: $n = 394$); a value of 0 means that on average the respective response was not given (values between 0 and 8 are possible depending on the organ system)

Category (number of subcategories)	Admission		Discharge		Follow-up	
	Fairly/ often	Strong/very frequently	Fairly/ often	Strong/very frequently	Fairly/ often	Strong/very frequently
	M (SD)	M (SD)	M (SD)	M (SD)	M (SD)	M (SD)
Immune system (1)	0.24 (0.43)	0.07 (0.26)	0.09 (0.29)	0.03 (0.18)	0.14 (0.35)	0.04 (0.19)
Gastrointestinal system (1)	0.36 (0.48)	0.27 (0.45)	0.31 (0.46)	0.17 (0.38)	0.32 (0.47)	0.14 (0.35)
Urogenital system (1)	0.33 (0.47)	0.15 (0.36)	0.35 (0.48)	0.12 (0.33)	0.28 (0.45)	0.11 (0.31)
Fatigue and sleep related symptoms (6)	2.29 (1.38)	1.51 (1.47)	1.76 (1.43)	0.71 (1.19)	1.86 (1.51)	0.77 (1.33)
Brain-related symptoms (4)	1.21 (1.06)	0.49 (0.82)	0.75 (0.95)	0.25 (0.60)	0.88 (1.04)	0.22 (0.58)
Cardiovascular system (6)	1.19 (1.30)	0.41 (0.86)	0.63 (1.05)	0.24 (0.71)	0.80 (1.12)	0.21 (0.68)
Musculoskeletal system (3)	0.89 (0.88)	1.03 (0.98)	0.84 (0.87)	0.40 (0.69)	0.88 (0.90)	0.63 (0.92)
Affective symptoms (8)	2.81 (1.82)	1.10 (1.48)	1.45 (1.68)	0.42 (0.92)	1.71 (1.81)	0.49 (1.05)
(Thermal) regulation-related symptoms (7)	1.98 (1.53)	1.25 (1.54)	1.44 (1.50)	0.64 (1.21)	1.78 (1.68)	0.73 (1.31)
Allergy related symptoms (5)	0.90 (1.00)	0.39 (0.75)	0.59 (0.92)	0.19 (0.52)	0.63 (0.98)	0.17 (0.52)
Total (42)	**12.20 (5.04)**	**6.67 (5.27)**	**8.21 (5.46)**	**3.18 (4.08)**	**9.29 (5.88)**	**3.51 (4.53)**

systems (except urogenital symptoms) improved with small to moderate effect sizes. There was a significant improvement in total complaint value with a large effect size at discharge ($d = -0.97$, $p < 0.001$) and a moderate-to-large effect size at follow-up ($d = -0.74$, $p < 0.001$). Figure 5.116 illustrates the differences for each category graphically, while Table 5.108 presents the numerical data.

5.3.2 Depression (ICD-10 F32 and F33)—Depressive Episode and Recurrent Repressive Disorder

5.3.2.1 Definition According to ICD-10 of the WHO

The following definitions apply to depression diagnoses F32 and F33:

This group includes disorders characterised by a change in mood or affectivity, either towards depression (with or without accompanying anxiety) or towards elevated mood. This change in mood is usually accompanied by a change in general level of activity. Most of the other symptoms are based on this or can easily be

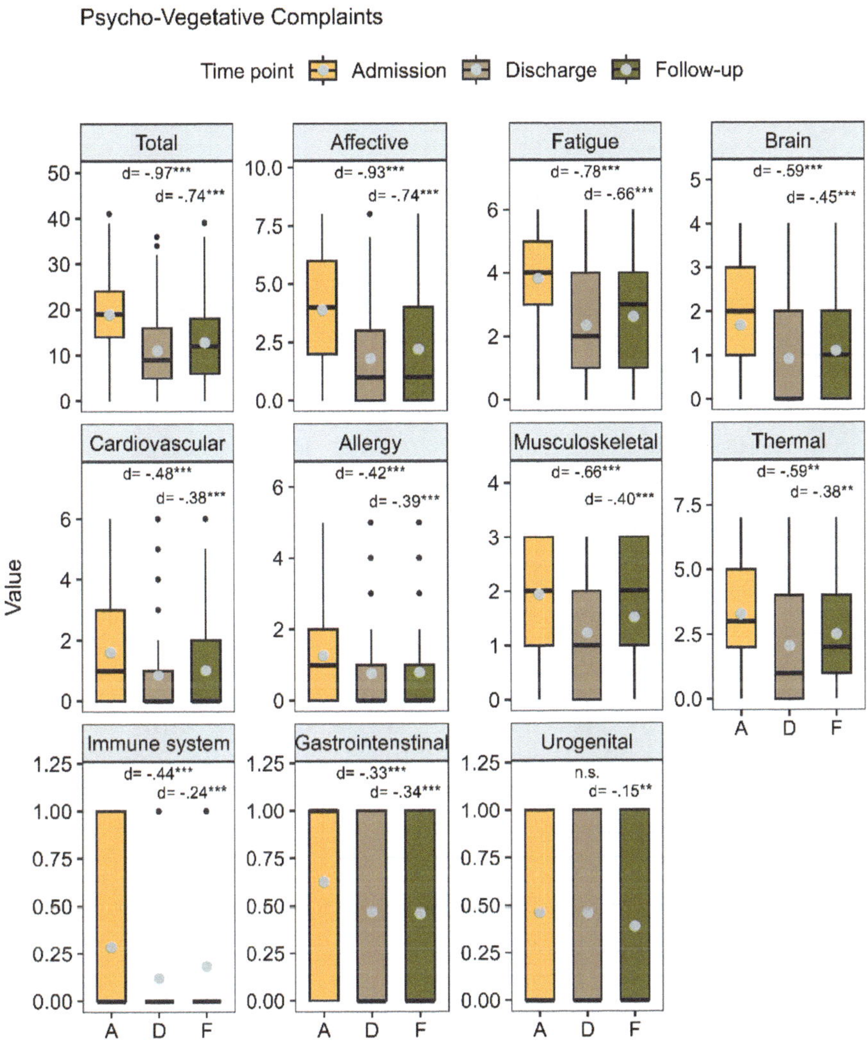

Fig. 5.116 Psycho-vegetative complaints; change in the total number of responses 'quite/often' and 'strong/very frequent' for patients with main mental health diagnosis F45 and complete data history (n = 388); 2023; significance: *$p < 0.05$, **$p < 0.01$, ***$p < 0.001$; Cohen's d = effect measure (d 0.2 = small effect, 0.5 = moderate effect, 0.8 = large effect)
Note: The graph shows data from the full follow-up sample (n = 388), the effect sizes refer to the individual comparison (A–D n = 487 or A–F n = 388)

Table 5.108 Psycho-vegetative complaints; change in the total number of responses 'fairly/often' and 'strong/very frequently' for patients with a main F45 mental health diagnosis in 2023; Cohen's $d \geq 0.2$ = small effect, ≥ 0.5 = moderate effect, ≥ 0.8 = large effect

Main diagnosis	Course						Difference from admission			
		Admission (A)		Discharge (D)/ follow-up (F)			A–D/A–F		Significance	Effect size
F45	*n*	M	SD	D/F	M	SD	*n*	M	*p*	*d*
Psycho-vegetative complaints: Sum of the answers 'fairly/often' and 'strongly/very frequently'										
Immune system	487	0.31	0.46	D	0.13	0.33	487	−0.18	<0.001	−0.44
	388	0.28	0.45	F	0.18	0.39	388	−0.10	<0.001	−0.24
Gastrointestinal	487	0.64	0.48	D	0.47	0.50	487	−0.16	<0.001	−0.33
system	388	0.62	0.49	F	0.46	0.50	388	−0.16	<0.001	−0.34
Urogenital system	487	0.47	0.50	D	0.47	0.50	487	0.00	0.874	–
	388	0.46	0.50	F	0.39	0.49	388	−0.07	0.007	−0.15
Fatigue/sleep-	487	3.81	1.59	D	2.47	1.82	487	−1.34	<0.001	**−0.78**
related symptoms	388	3.82	1.61	F	2.63	1.95	388	−1.19	<0.001	**−0.66**
Brain-related	487	1.71	1.26	D	0.99	1.18	487	−0.72	<0.001	**−0.59**
symptoms	388	1.68	1.27	F	1.11	1.25	388	−0.57	<0.001	−0.45
Cardiovascular	487	1.61	1.63	D	0.87	1.38	487	−0.74	<0.001	−0.48
system	388	1.60	1.62	F	1.01	1.40	388	−0.59	<0.001	−0.38
Musculoskeletal	487	1.92	0.97	D	1.25	1.05	487	−0.67	<0.001	**−0.66**
system	388	1.94	0.98	F	1.52	1.11	388	−0.42	<0.001	−0.40
Affective	487	3.93	2.30	D	1.87	2.09	487	−2.06	<0.001	**−0.93**
symptoms	388	3.87	2.30	F	2.21	2.16	388	−1.66	<0.001	**−0.74**
(Thermal)	487	3.26	1.99	D	2.08	1.99	487	−1.18	<0.001	**−0.59**
regulation-related symptoms	388	3.28	2.02	F	2.51	2.04	388	−0.77	<0.001	−0.38
Allergy-related	487	1.29	1.32	D	0.78	1.08	487	−0.51	<0.001	−0.42
symptoms	388	1.26	1.28	F	0.79	1.13	388	−0.47	<0.001	−0.39
Total	487	18.95	7.56	D	11.38	8.08	487	−7.57	<0.001	**−0.97**
	388	18.82	7.57	F	12.80	8.50	388	−6.02	<0.001	**−0.74**

understood in the context of the change in mood and activity. Most of these conditions tend to relapse. The onset of individual episodes can often be linked to stressful events or situations [14].

In typical mild (F32.0), moderate (F32.1) or severe (F32.2 and F32.3) episodes, the person suffers from a depressed mood, reduced energy levels, and decreased activity. Pleasure, interest, and concentration are reduced. Tiredness may occur after the slightest exertion. Sleep is usually disturbed and appetite is reduced. Self-esteem and self-confidence are almost always affected. Even in the mild form, feelings of guilt or worthlessness may be present [14].

The depressed mood changes little from day to day and remains unresponsive to life circumstances. This may be accompanied by so-called 'somatic' symptoms, such as loss of interest or pleasure, waking early, morning depression, marked psychomotor inhibition, agitation, loss of appetite, weight loss, and loss of libido. Depending on the number and severity of symptoms present, a depressive episode can be classified as mild, moderate or severe [14].

Recurrent depressive disorder is a disorder characterised by recurrent depressive episodes (F32). There are no independent episodes of elevated mood and in-creased energy (mania) in medical history. However, brief episodes of slightly elevated mood and hyperactivity (hypomania) may occur immediately after a depressive episode, sometimes as a result of antidepressant treatment. The more severe forms of recurrent depressive disorder (F33.2 and 0.3) have much in common with the earlier concepts of manic-depressive illness, melancholia, vital depression, and endogenous depression. The first episode may occur at any age from childhood to senility, the onset may be acute or gradual, and the duration may range from a few weeks to many months [14].

Patients with a main diagnosis of F32 or F33 'depressive episode' or 'recurrent depressive disorder' showed a highly significant improvement in their main complaint during their inpatient stay at the TCM-Klinik Bad Kötzting, both at discharge ($d = -1.35$, $p < 0.001$) as well as at follow-up ($d = -1.16$, $p < 0.001$; Table 5.109). Figure 5.117 shows the distribution of change intensity. At follow-up, 75.8% of

Table 5.109 Global assessments of treatment success for patients with a main F32/F33 mental health diagnosis, surveyed at discharge ($n = 246$) and follow-up ($n = 190$) in 2023; t-test for paired samples; significance at $p < 0.05$; Cohen's d = effect measure ($d \geq 0.2$ = small, ≥ 0.5 = moderate, ≥ 0.8 = large effect)

	Course						Difference from admission			
	Admission (A)			Discharge (D)/ follow-up (F)			A–D/A–F		Significance	Effect size
F32/F33	*n*	M	SD		M	SD	*n*	ΔM	*p*	*d*
Main complaint	246	74.92	16.65	D	48.01	22.45	246	−26.91	**< 0.001**	**−1.35**
severity VAS	190	74.47	16.67	F	50.37	23.85	190	−24.11	**<0.001**	**−1.16**

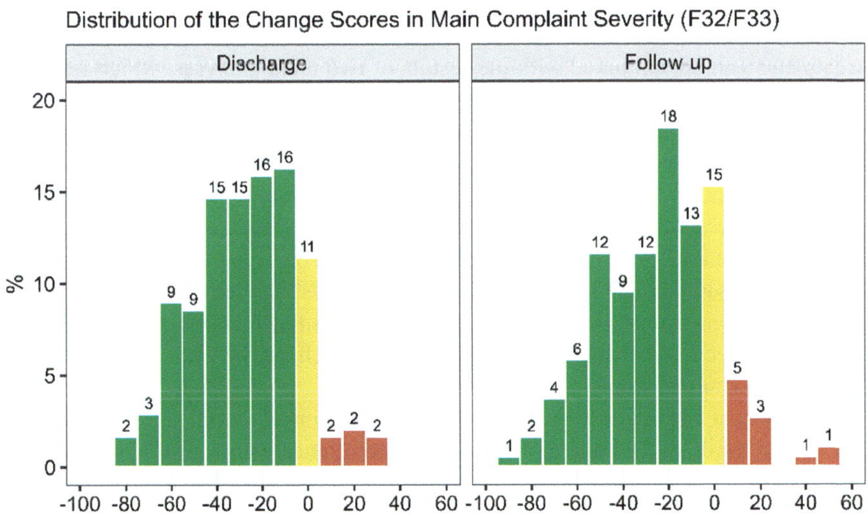

Fig. 5.117 Distribution of the change scores in main complaint severity between hospital admission and hospital discharge or hospital admission and follow-up for patients with a main diagnosis of F32/F33 in 2023 (A–D n = 246; A–D–F n = 190); negative differences correspond to an improvement

participants reported an improvement, 15.3% reported no change, and 8.9% reported a deterioration.

At the time of discharge, 15.0% of patients rated the treatment success as very good, 48.4% as good, 32.9% as moderate, and 3.7% reported no success. At follow-up, patients reported greater satisfaction, with 24.5% rating the success as very good, 49.0% as good, 24.0% as moderate, and 2.6% as none.

When asked, 'From today's point of view, was the treatment worthwhile?', 45.1% answered 'very worthwhile' and 47.6% answered 'worthwhile' at discharge. Again, patients were more satisfied at follow-up, with 55.2% rating the treatment as 'very worthwhile' and 39.1% as 'worthwhile'. Table 5.110 and Fig. 5.118 illustrate the results.

Overall, patients experiencing depressive episodes or recurrent depressive disorder showed significant improvements in protective and risk factors at discharge and at the 6-month follow-up.

Particularly high effect sizes were found for mental stress, including depression ($d = -1.02$, $p < 0.001$; F: $d = -0.93$, $p < 0.001$), well-being ($d = 1.16$, $p < 0.001$; F: $d = 0.78$, $p < 0.001$), vitality ($d = 0.97$, $p < 0.001$; F: $d = 0.81$, $p < 0.001$), Generalised Anxiety Disorder (GAD: $d = -1.09$, $p < 0.001$; F: $d = -0.80$, $p < 0.001$) and perceived stress (PSQ: $d = -1.07$, $p < 0.001$; F: $d = -0.80$, $p < 0.001$)0.1), burnout (D: $d = -0.70$, $p < 0.001$; F: $d = -0.77$, $p < 0.001$) and the complaint index (D: $d = 0.90$, $p < 0.001$; F: $d = 0.92$, $p < 0.001$) (Table 5.111, Fig. 5.119).

A closer look at the self-assessed symptom burden using the questionnaire on psycho-vegetative complaints reveals a dominance of fatigue and sleep-related complaints as well as affective symptoms. In addition, poor concentration and back pain are more pronounced in this patient group. When comparing measurement time points, affective symptoms in particular show an improvement, followed by the fatigue-related symptoms (Fig. 5.120).

Our own data on the effectiveness of inpatient psychosomatic-psychotherapeutic treatments can be compared with the results of two meta-analyses, which reported pre-post effect sizes of $d = 0.51$ for inpatient rehabilitation [15] and $d = 0.73$ for hospital treatment [16]. The indirect measure of change using the VAS (0–100) complaints scale showed strong effect sizes ($d > 0.80$; Cohen's d) for the follow-up times 'admission – discharge' for the three main diagnoses. The same was true for the ISR depression scores. For the ISR total score, however, only moderate effect sizes were obtained for the three indications. Effect sizes based on means say little about an individual patient's response to treatment, as they represent averaged values across large groups. For this reason, more differentiated presentations reflecting different aspects according to age, gender, and defined numbers of responders according to cut-off values are required.

Differential treatment response, as defined by clinical significance, shows that about two-thirds of all patients benefit from inpatient treatment [17]. Conversely, this also means that therapeutic interventions are unsuccessful in around one-third of patients [18].

Table 5.110 Global assessments of treatment success for patients with a main F32/F33 diagnosis, surveyed at discharge ($n = 246$) and follow-up ($n = 192$) in 2023

Overall success of the therapy		**Very good**		**Good**		**Moderate**		**No success**		**Total**	
		n	%	*n*	%	*n*	%	*n*	%	*n*	%
F32/F33 patients	D	37	15.0	119	48.4	81	32.9	9	3.7	246	100
	F	47	24.5	94	49.0	46	24.0	5	2.6	192	100
Treatment worthwhile		**Very worthwhile**		**Worthwhile**		**Not worth it**		**Rather harmed**		**Total**	
		n	%	*n*	%	*n*	%	*n*	%	*n*	%
F32/F33 patients	D	111	45.1	117	47.6	15	6.1	3	1.2	246	100
	F	106	55.2	75	39.1	11	5.7	0	–	192	100

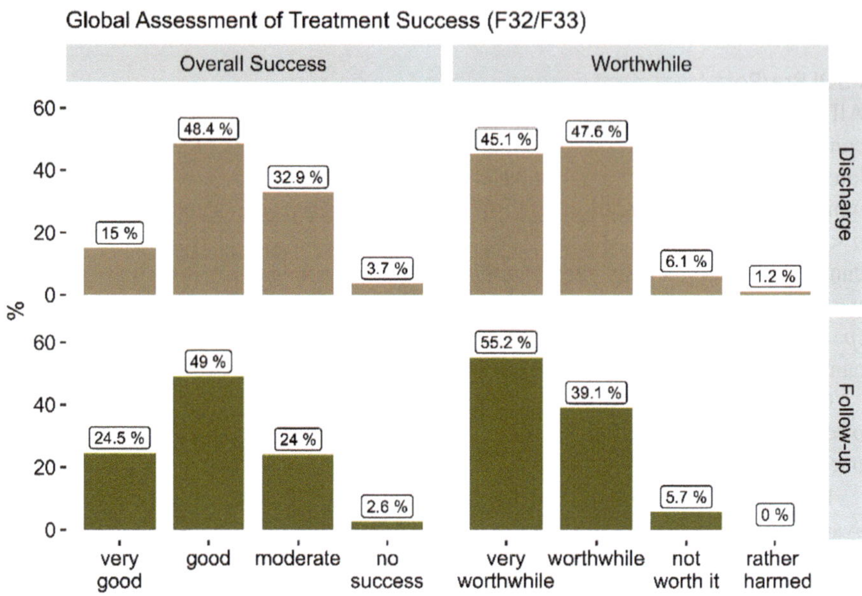

Fig. 5.118 Global assessments of treatment success for patients with a main F32/F33 diagnosis, surveyed at discharge (n = 246) and follow-up (n = 192) in 2023

Table 5.111 Changes in various parameters for patients with a main F32/F33 diagnosis in 2023; t-test: Cohen's d = effect measure ($d \geq 0.2$ = small effect, ≥ 0.5 = moderate effect, ≥ 0.8 = large effect)

Main diagnosis F32/F33	Course						Difference from admission			
		Admission (A)		Discharge (D)/ follow-up (F)			A–D/A–F		Significance	Effect size
	n	M	SD	D/F	M	SD	*n*	M	*p*	*d*
ICD symptom ratings (ISR)										
Total value	247	1.35	0.60	D	1.01	0.60	247	−0.34	< 0.001	**−0.57**
	187	1.37	0.60	F	0.94	0.58	187	−0.43	< 0.001	**−0.73**
Depression	247	2.47	0.87	D	1.54	0.96	247	−0.93	< 0.001	**−1.02**
	187	2.51	0.85	F	1.66	0.96	187	−0.85	< 0.001	**−0.93**
Anxiety	247	1.68	1.10	D	1.26	1.04	247	−0.42	< 0.001	−0.39
	187	1.67	1.09	F	1.13	0.94	187	−0.54	< 0.001	**−0.53**
Obsessive-compulsion	247	1.18	1.07	D	0.94	0.97	247	−0.24	< 0.001	−0.23
	187	1.24	1.08	F	0.80	0.86	187	−0.44	< 0.001	−0.45
Somatoform	247	0.95	0.90	D	0.71	0.81	247	−0.24	< 0.001	−0.27
	187	0.91	0.86	F	0.59	0.74	187	−0.32	< 0.001	−0.40
Eating disorder	247	0.64	0.84	D	0.59	0.80	247	−0.05	0.151	–
	187	0.68	0.87	F	0.60	0.82	187	−0.08	0.073	–
Pain disability index										
Total index	247	29.41	15.9	D	26.01	16.25	247	−3.40	< 0.001	−0.21
	184	29.96	16.21	F	26.70	16.91	184	−3.26	0.003	−0.20
Family/domestic obligations	247	4.80	2.89	D	4.29	2.90	247	−0.51	0.003	−0.18
	185	4.94	2.85	F	4.49	2.93	185	−0.45	0.031	−0.15

(continued)

Table 5.111 (continued)

Main diagnosis F32/F33	Course						Difference from admission			
		Admission (A)		Discharge (D)/ follow-up (F)			A–D/A–F		Significance	Effect size
	n	M	SD	D/F	M	SD	*n*	M	*p*	*d*
Recreation	247	5.39	2.83	D	4.57	2.92	247	−0.82	< 0.001	−0.28
	185	5.50	2.81	F	4.87	3.05	185	−0.63	0.003	−0.22
Social activity	247	4.60	3.07	D	4.09	3.00	247	−0.51	0.007	−0.17
	185	4.74	3.13	F	4.25	3.18	185	−0.49	0.030	−0.16
Profession	247	5.35	3.27	D	4.97	3.34	247	−0.38	0.048	−0.12
	184	5.47	3.27	F	4.67	3.48	184	−0.80	0.002	−0.24
Sex life	247	4.81	3.79	D	4.38	3.52	247	−0.43	0.041	−0.12
	184	4.87	3.78	F	4.62	3.66	184	−0.25	0.310	–
Self-sufficiency	247	2.29	2.59	D	2.09	2.67	247	−0.20	0.278	–
	184	2.34	2.59	F	2.27	2.66	184	−0.07	0.737	–
Essentials	247	2.17	2.64	D	1.62	2.40	247	−0.55	< 0.001	−0.22
activities	184	2.11	2.57	F	1.51	2.20	184	−0.60	0.002	−0.25
Life satisfaction										
Total value	246	16.52	35.68	D	34.79	38.28	246	18.27	< 0.001	0.49
	189	18.12	34.72	F	34.32	33.80	189	16.20	< 0.001	0.47
Friends/	246	3.71	6.71	D	5.70	6.74	246	1.99	< 0.001	0.30
acquaintances	189	3.67	6.46	F	5.28	6.14	189	1.61	< 0.001	0.25
Leisure/hobbies	246	0.41	5.47	D	2.95	6.02	246	2.54	< 0.001	0.44
	189	0.31	5.16	F	2.82	5.30	189	2.51	< 0.001	0.48
Health	246	−5.28	6.02	D	−0.62	7.63	246	4.66	< 0.001	**0.67**
	189	−5.21	6.23	F	−0.66	7.07	189	4.55	< 0.001	**0.68**
Income	246	2.05	7.60	D	3.30	7.37	246	1.25	< 0.001	0.17
	189	2.41	7.16	F	3.12	6.39	189	0.71	0.116	0.10
Profession	246	−0.38	6.68	D	0.39	6.29	246	0.77	0.048	0.12
	189	0.03	6.88	F	1.52	5.93	189	1.49	0.001	0.23
Housing	246	5.69	7.78	D	6.95	8.07	246	1.26	0.004	0.16
situation	189	5.82	7.53	F	7.40	7.11	189	1.58	0.004	0.22
Family/children	246	5.92	8.49	D	8.53	8.29	246	2.61	< 0.001	0.31
	189	6.21	8.66	F	8.02	8.13	189	1.81	0.003	0.22
Partnership	246	4.41	9.47	D	7.59	9.34	246	3.18	< 0.001	0.34
	189	4.88	9.45	F	6.83	9.05	189	1.95	0.003	0.21
SOC										
Total value	247	53.20	12.11	D	57.84	12.56	247	4.64	< 0.001	0.38
	187	53.43	11.52	F	58.11	12.56	187	4.68	< 0.001	0.39
Meaningfulness	247	17.91	4.16	D	19.35	4.29	247	1.44	< 0.001	0.34
	187	18.02	4.03	F	18.99	4.26	187	0.97	< 0.001	0.24
Comprehen-	247	19.29	5.57	D	21.51	5.57	247	2.22	< 0.001	0.40
sibility	187	19.32	5.41	F	21.79	5.70	187	2.47	< 0.001	0.44
Manageability	247	16.00	4.63	D	16.98	4.86	247	0.98	< 0.001	0.21
	187	16.10	4.58	F	17.33	4.72	187	1.23	< 0.001	0.27
WHO-5 well-being and vitality										
Well-being	247	22.32	16.48	D	47.26	24.18	247	24.94	< 0.001	**1.16**
	187	22.44	16.82	F	39.10	23.88	187	16.66	< 0.001	**0.78**
Vitality	247	21.62	14.99	D	39.94	21.12	247	18.32	< 0.001	**0.97**
	187	21.66	15.38	F	37.57	22.04	187	15.91	< 0.001	**0.81**

(continued)

Table 5.111 (continued)

Main diagnosis F32/F33	Course						Difference from admission			
		Admission (A)		Discharge (D)/ follow-up (F)			A–D/A–F		Significance	Effect size
	n	M	SD	D/F	M	SD	*n*	M	*p*	*d*
SWOP										
Self-efficacy	247	11.69	3.08	D	12.68	2.87	247	0.99	< 0.001	0.33
	187	11.72	2.93	F	12.75	2.80	187	1.03	< 0.001	0.36
Optimism	247	4.72	1.43	D	5.37	1.36	247	0.65	< 0.001	0.46
	187	4.72	1.41	F	5.26	1.41	187	0.54	< 0.001	0.39
Pessimism	247	4.60	1.44	D	4.44	1.43	247	−0.16	0.095	–
	187	4.63	1.43	F	4.53	1.35	187	−0.10	0.309	–
SSS										
Total value	241	50.36	17.53	D	55.46	15.54	241	5.10	< 0.001	0.30
	182	50.93	16.64	F	53.62	15.56	182	2.69	< 0.001	0.17
Emotional	241	17.06	5.93	D	18.07	5.31	241	1.01	< 0.001	0.18
	182	17.34	5.71	F	17.66	5.14	182	0.32	0.298	–
Social	241	9.86	3.73	D	11.08	3.34	241	1.22	< 0.001	0.34
interaction	182	9.86	3.55	F	10.70	3.49	182	0.84	< 0.001	0.24
Material	241	10.71	4.71	D	12.16	3.97	241	1.45	< 0.001	0.33
	182	10.96	4.56	F	11.74	4.17	182	0.78	< 0.001	0.18
Affective	241	8.27	3.24	D	9.06	2.91	241	0.79	< 0.001	0.25
	182	8.36	3.16	F	8.68	2.95	182	0.32	0.029	0.10
Tedium measure (burnout)										
Total value	246	4.63	0.82	D	3.97	1.02	246	−0.66	< 0.001	**−0.70**
	189	4.65	0.81	F	3.94	0.98	189	−0.71	< 0.001	**−0.77**
Discouragement	246	4.19	1.00	D	3.60	1.10	246	−0.59	< 0.001	**−0.56**
	189	4.21	1.00	F	3.56	1.11	189	−0.65	< 0.001	**−0.61**
Exhaustion	246	5.38	0.93	D	4.53	1.20	246	−0.85	< 0.001	**−0.78**
	189	5.40	0.92	F	4.52	1.14	189	−0.88	< 0.001	**−0.85**
Loss of	246	4.63	0.83	D	4.03	1.00	246	−0.60	< 0.001	**−0.63**
motivation	189	4.62	0.82	F	4.00	0.96	189	−0.62	< 0.001	**−0.69**
PSQ										
Total value	247	64.45	15.64	D	44.95	20.16	247	−19.50	< 0.001	**−1.07**
	189	64.71	15.62	F	51.26	17.72	189	−13.45	< 0.001	**−0.80**
Worries	247	58.00	21.99	D	42.56	24.40	247	−15.44	< 0.001	**−0.66**
	189	58.13	20.61	F	43.84	23.18	189	−14.29	< 0.001	**−0.65**
Demands	247	51.09	25.34	D	28.96	23.53	247	−22.13	< 0.001	**−0.90**
	189	51.96	25.26	F	40.78	22.28	189	−11.18	< 0.001	−0.47
Joy	247	26.83	17.01	D	43.86	21.72	247	17.03	< 0.001	**0.86**
	189	26.91	17.18	F	38.34	21.74	189	11.43	< 0.001	**0.57**
Tension	247	75.55	17.79	D	52.15	24.42	247	−23.40	< 0.001	**−1.08**
	189	75.66	17.78	F	58.77	22.17	189	−16.89	< 0.001	**−0.83**

(continued)

Table 5.111 (continued)

Main diagnosis F32/F33	Course						Difference from admission			
		Admission (A)		Discharge (D)/ follow-up (F)			A–D/A–F		Significance	Effect size
	n	M	SD	D/F	M	SD	*n*	M	*p*	*d*
PSQI										
Total value	245	11.14	4.03	D	10.06	4.27	245	−1.08	< 0.001	−0.26
	186	11.19	4.19	F	8.80	4.21	186	−2.39	< 0.001	**−0.57**
Sleep quality	245	1.84	0.68	D	1.47	0.67	245	−0.37	< 0.001	**−0.55**
	186	1.83	0.70	F	1.40	0.69	186	−0.43	< 0.001	**−0.62**
Sleep latency	245	1.87	1.07	D	1.63	1.01	245	−0.24	< 0.001	−0.23
	186	1.80	1.06	F	1.45	1.02	186	−0.35	< 0.001	−0.34
Sleep duration	245	1.52	0.95	D	1.49	0.86	245	−0.03	0.639	–
	186	1.53	0.96	F	1.29	0.89	186	−0.24	< 0.001	−0.26
Sleep efficiency	245	1.36	1.17	D	1.14	1.16	245	−0.22	0.010	−0.19
	186	1.39	1.19	F	0.89	1.14	186	−0.50	< 0.001	−0.43
Sleep disorders	245	1.82	0.63	D	1.62	0.58	245	−0.20	< 0.001	−0.32
	186	1.82	0.66	F	1.51	0.68	186	−0.31	< 0.001	−0.47
Sleeping pills	245	0.85	1.26	D	1.45	1.42	245	0.60	< 0.001	0.45
	186	0.90	1.29	F	0.74	1.18	186	−0.16	0.054	–
Daytime	245	1.88	0.69	D	1.24	0.82	245	−0.64	< 0.001	**−0.83**
sleepiness	186	1.92	0.69	F	1.53	0.82	186	−0.39	< 0.001	**−0.51**
GAD										
Total value	244	12.05	4.35	D	7.21	4.54	244	−4.84	< 0.001	**−1.09**
	182	12.08	4.38	F	8.38	4.86	182	−3.70	< 0.001	**−0.80**
Complaint complexes of psycho-vegetative stability										
Complaints	247	0.21	0.44	D	0.78	0.74	247	0.57	< 0.001	**0.90**
index	189	0.20	0.42	F	0.78	0.76	189	0.58	< 0.001	**0.92**
Total value	247	65.31	16.93	D	47.80	18.69	247	−17.51	< 0.001	**−0.98**
	189	66.30	16.46	F	51.28	19.85	189	−15.02	< 0.001	**−0.81**
Dizziness	247	3.66	2.25	D	2.42	2.21	247	−1.24	< 0.001	**−0.56**
	189	3.74	2.20	F	2.87	2.26	189	−0.87	< 0.001	−0.39
Sleep	247	7.47	2.06	D	5.83	2.59	247	−1.64	< 0.001	**−0.69**
	189	7.49	2.06	F	5.72	2.40	189	−1.77	< 0.001	**−0.79**
Heat balance	247	5.72	2.72	D	3.93	2.58	247	−1.79	< 0.001	**−0.68**
	189	5.84	2.74	F	4.62	2.58	189	−1.22	< 0.001	−0.45

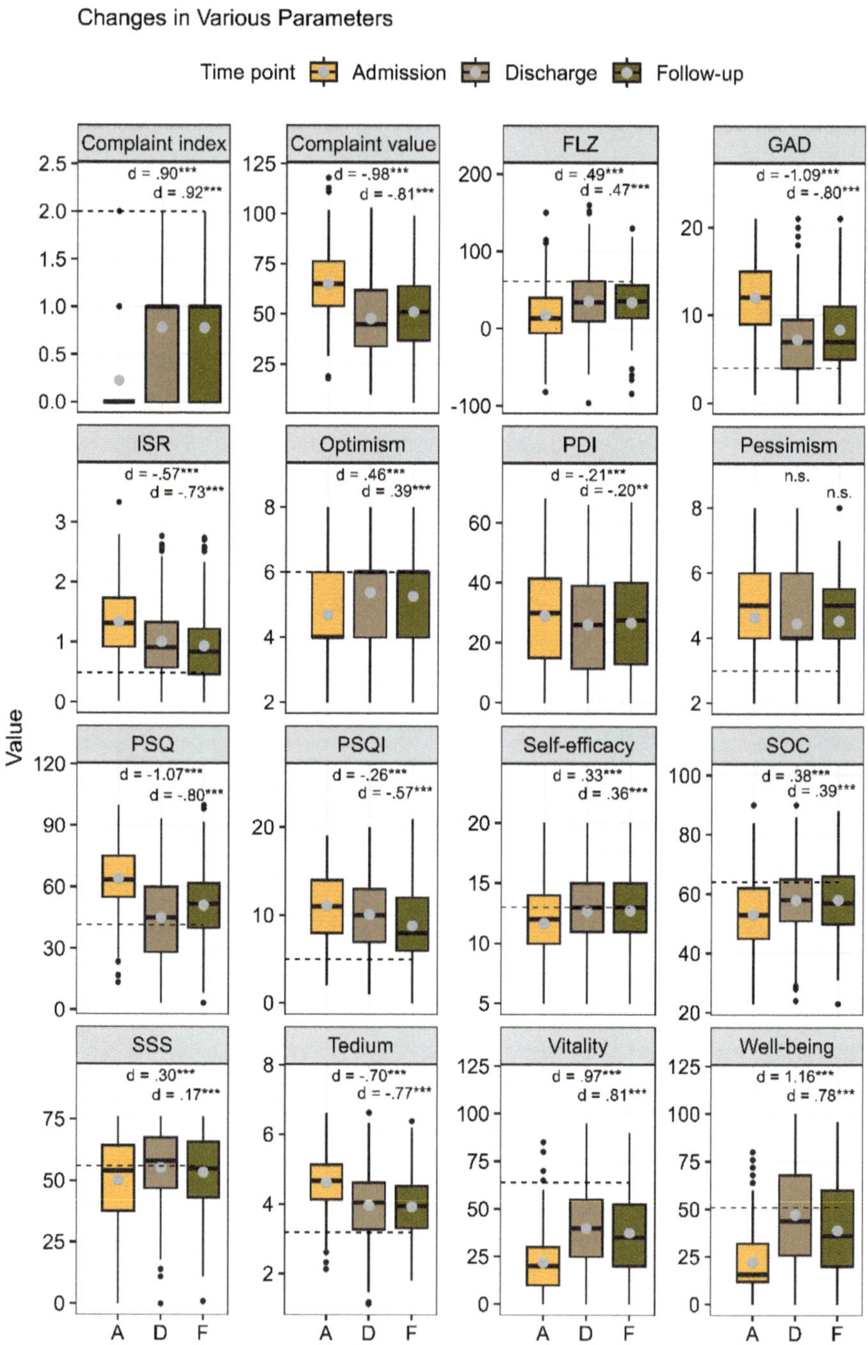

Fig. 5.119 Changes in various parameters for patients with a main F33/F32 diagnosis in 2023; the dashed black lines indicate the desired target values; significance: *$p < 0.05$, **$p < 0.01$, ***$p < 0.001$; Effect measure ($d \geq 0.2$ = small effect, ≥ 0.5 = moderate effect, ≥ 0.8 = large effect); the graph shows all available data, the effect sizes refer to the individual comparison (A–D/A–F)

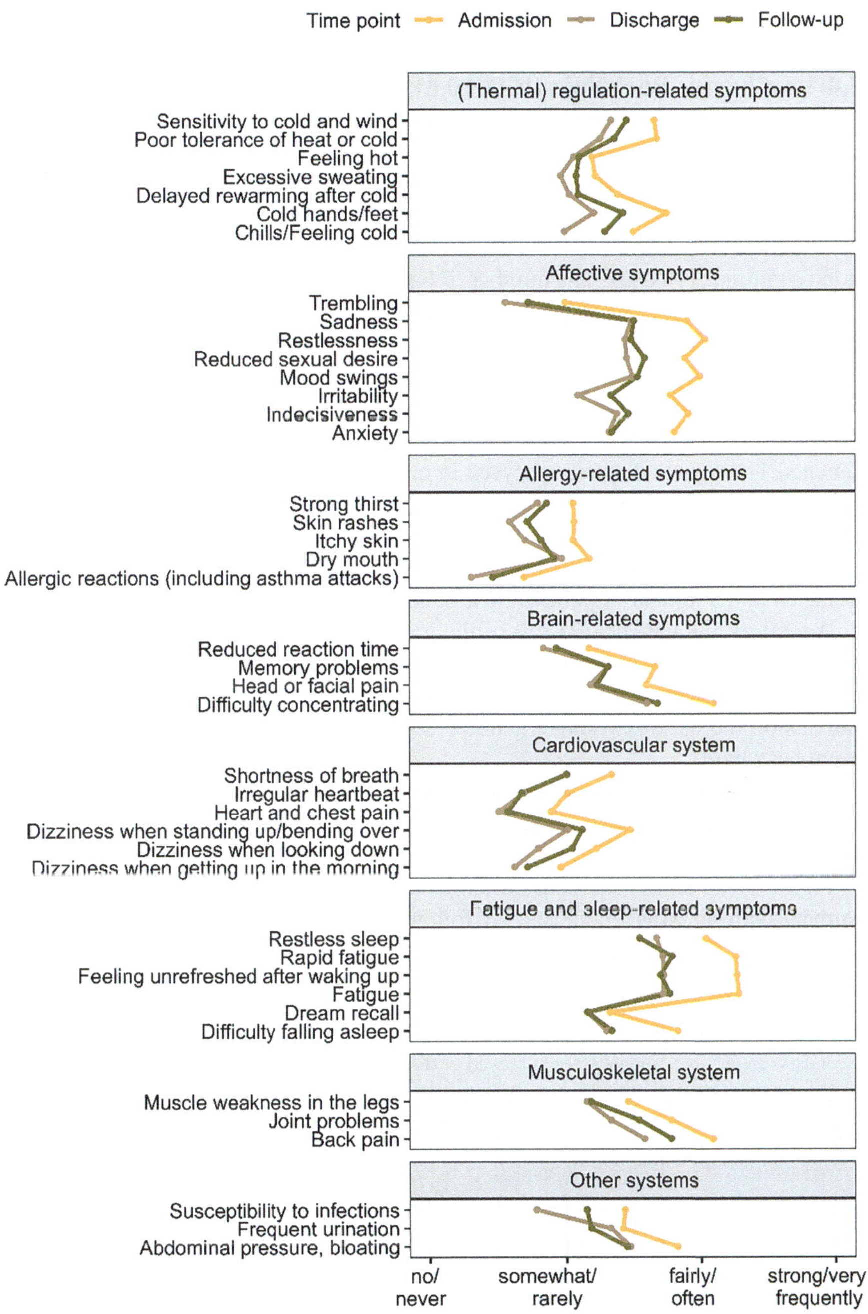

Fig. 5.120 Psycho-vegetative complaints; change in complaints for patients with a main F32/F33 mental health diagnosis; admission: $n = 267$, discharge: $n = 247$; follow-up: $n = 189$ in 2023

5.4 Therapeutic Success of Somatic Diagnoses

5.4.1 Chronic Back Pain (ICD-10 M54) and Other Diseases of the Spine (Back; ICD-10 M53)

Based solely on diagnoses of back pain, KKH—a German health insurance company—recorded an average of around 142 sick days per 100 insured members for the whole year in 2024 [19]. This figure is almost 20% higher than in 2019, when it stood at around 118 days. The number of back pain cases has also increased significantly over the past 5 years: in 2019, one in 13 people received a corresponding diagnosis, whereas last year, it was one in eight working people. Back pain is the second most common reason for taking sick leave. Extrapolated to the working population, this equates to around 35 million lost working days. Stress is a common trigger. Back pain was also the most common somatic complaint among TCM patients. These patients were analysed in more detail, and the results of their treatment are presented below.

Of the 825 patients admitted as inpatients in 2023, 425 were diagnosed with back pain or other spinal disorders. Of these patients, approximately 33.2% had pain localised in the lumbar region, while around 43.7% had pain in the cervical region.

A total of 588 patients (71.4% of the total) reported back pain in their medical history (Chap. 3); Of these, 191 (32.5%) were taking medication and 420 (71.4%) experienced additional limitations in their daily activities. Subjectively, 74.5% of all patients on the list of psycho-vegetative complaints reported frequent or very frequent back pain.

According to the VAS assessment, back pain (M54) had decreased significantly by the time of discharge (A–D, $d = -1.29$, $p < 0.001$). This positive effect was maintained until follow-up ($d = -1.12$, $p < 0.001$, Table 5.112).

Figure 5.121 shows the distribution of change scores for complaint severity in patients with an M54 diagnosis. At follow-up, 13% reported no change, 72.6% improvement, and 14.4% deterioration.

Table 5.112 Global assessments of treatment success for patients with a somatic M54 or M53 secondary diagnosis. Patients were surveyed at discharge (n = 367) and follow-up (n = 296). A t-test for paired samples was used, with significance set at $p < 0.05$. Cohen's d was used as the effect measure ($d \geq 0.2$ = small effect, $d \geq 0.5$ = moderate effect, $d \geq 0.8$ = large effect)

Main complaint severity	Course						Difference from admission			
	Admission (A)			Discharge (D)/ follow-up (F)			A–D/A–F		Significance	Effect size
	n	M	SD		M	SD	n	ΔM	p	d
M54 Back pain	367	72.45	16.94	D	47.77	21.05	367	−24.69	< 0.001	**−1.29**
	296	72.60	16.76	F	50.00	22.91	296	−22.60	< 0.001	**−1.12**
M53 other diseases of the spine	77	72.08	15.07	D	45.84	21.11	77	−26.23	< 0.001	**−1.41**
	62	71.94	14.91	F	48.06	23.81	62	−23.87	< 0.001	**−1.20**

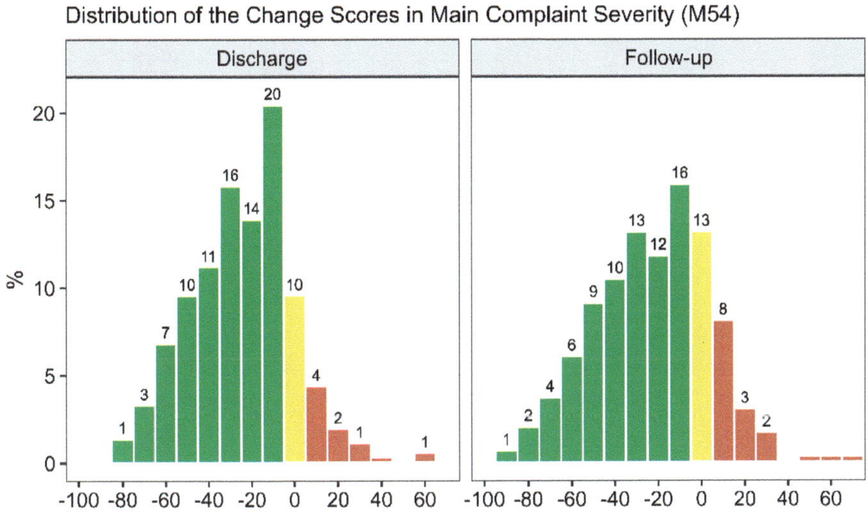

Fig. 5.121 Distribution of the change scores in main complaint severity between hospital admission and hospital discharge or hospital admission and follow-up for patients with a M54 diagnosis in 2023 (A–D $n = 367$; A–D–F $n = 296$); negative differences correspond to an improvement

From the patients' point of view, the following interventions contributed significantly to this overall success: physiotherapy (93.5%), acupuncture (93.2%), tuina (93.0%), individual qigong (90.1%), and group qigong (84.8%). This assessment of effectiveness is supported by evidence for TCM interventions in terms of pain relief.

The back pain category also encompasses M53, 'Other diseases of the spinal column'. Cervicobrachial syndromes are included within this group of indications. VAS ratings for these 77 patients also indicated a high level of clinical effectiveness, with an effect size of $d = -1.41$ ($p < 0.001$). At follow-up, effectiveness remained substantial, with $d = -1.20$ ($p < 0.001$, Table 5.112).

At discharge from hospital, 14.1% of the back pain patients M54 rated the overall success as very good and 49.7% as good, and at follow-up 26.8% rated it as very good and 45.2% as good. When asked, 'From today's perspective, was the treatment worthwhile?' 43.5% of patients rated it as 'very worthwhile' and 50.8% as 'worthwhile' at discharge. At follow-up, 53.0% considered it 'very worthwhile' and 40.3% 'worthwhile' (Table 5.113, Fig. 5.122).

The global treatment success for patients in the M53 indication group was rated as 'very good' by 11.7% and 'good' by 54.5% at discharge and as 'very good' by 27.7% and 'good' by 43.1% at follow-up. Whether the clinical stay was worthwhile was rated as 'very worthwhile' by 41.6% and as 'worthwhile' by 53.2% of all patients in this diagnosis group at discharge. At follow-up, 61.5% rated the stay as 'very worthwhile' and 30.8% rated it as 'worthwhile' (Table 5.113). Figure 5.123 illustrates these results.

Table 5.113 Global assessments of treatment success for patients with a somatic M54 or M53 secondary diagnosis, surveyed at discharge ($n = 367/n = 77$) and follow-up ($n = 297/n = 65$) in 2023

Overall success of the therapy		**Very good**		**Good**		**Moderate**		**No success**		**Total**	
		n	%	*n*	%	*n*	%	*n*	%	*n*	%
M54 Back pain	D	51	13.9	182	49.6	119	32.4	15	4.1	367	100
	F	79	26.6	134	45.1	74	24.9	10	3.4	297	100
M53 other diseases of the spine	D	9	11.7	42	54.5	23	29.9	3	3.9	77	100
	F	18	27.7	28	43.1	15	23.1	4	6.2	65	100
Treatment worthwhile		**Very worthwhile**		**Worthwhile**		**Not worth it**		**Rather harmed**		**Total**	
		n	%	*n*	%	*n*	%	*n*	%	*n*	%
M54 Back pain	D	159	43.3	187	51.0	19	5.2	2	0.5	367	100
	F	157	52.7	121	40.6	19	6.4	1	0.3	298	100
M53 other diseases of the spine	D	32	41.6	41	53.2	4	5.2	0	0.0	77	100
	F	40	61.5	20	30.8	5	7.7	0	0.0	65	100

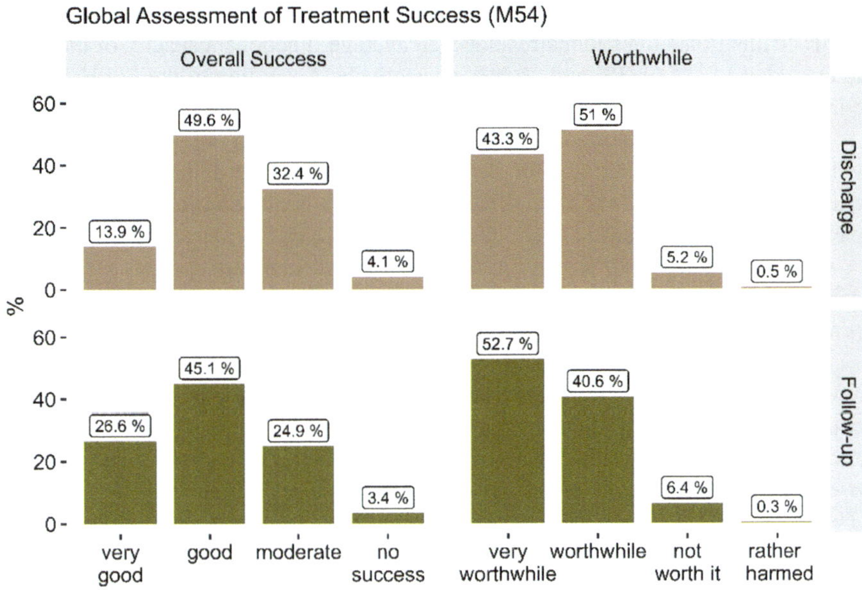

Fig. 5.122 Global assessments of treatment success for patients with a somatic secondary diagnosis of M54, surveyed at discharge ($n = 370$), follow-up ($n = 299$) in 2023

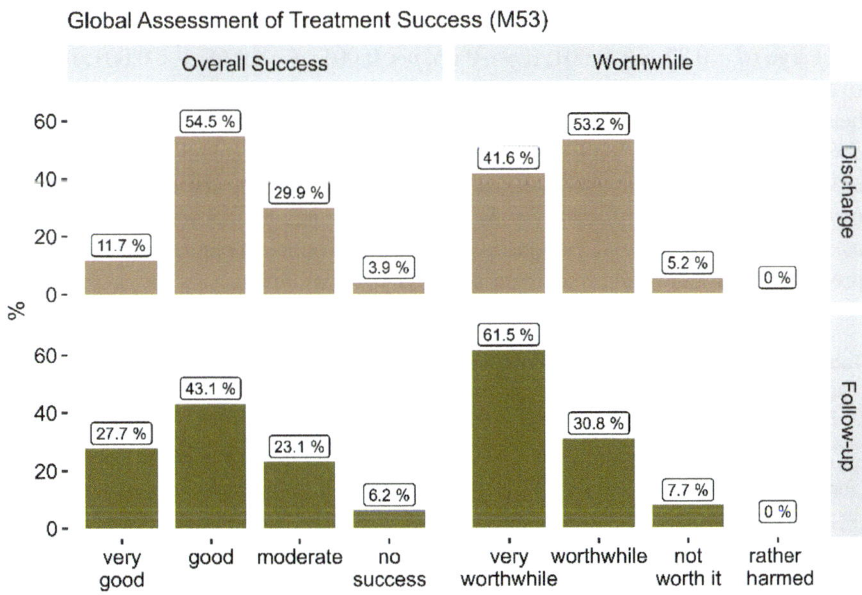

Fig. 5.123 Global assessments of treatment success for patients with a somatic secondary diagnosis of M53, surveyed at discharge ($n = 77$), follow-up ($n = 65$) in 2023

When analysing the data of patients diagnosed with M54 or M53, the Hannover FFbH-R functional questionnaire shows an average functional capacity of the back in everyday life of 68.3% and 70.6%, respectively. According to the FFbH-R, this corresponds to a moderate functional capacity.

At discharge, the functional capacity of the back only shows significant changes with a neglectable effect size for patients with the somatic diagnosis M54 ‘back pain’ (Table 5.114). At the time of follow-up, there is no significant change compared to before treatment.

For the results of the protective and risk factors, the indication groups M54 ‘Back pain“ and M53 “Other diseases of the spine” are evaluated together. Overall, there is a positive balance at discharge (Table 5.115).

Patients with chronic back pain or other diseases of the spine show moderate to strong benefit measures in the monitoring of mental stress until follow-up, especially for the symptoms of depression ($d = -0.95$, $p < 0.001$), well-being ($d = 1.14$, $p < 0.001$) and vitality ($d = 0.90$, $p < 0.001$), all PSQ scales (worries: $d = -0.62$, $p < 0.001$; demands: $d = -0.94$, $p < 0.001$; joy: $d = 0.71$, $p < 0.001$; tension: $d = -0.88$, $p < 0.001$), the burnout scales exhaustion ($d = -0.74$, $p < 0.001$) and loss of motivation ($d = -0.57$, $p < 0.001$), as well as for GAD ($d = -0.96$, $p < 0.001$) (Table 5.115). Until follow-up there were still moderate significant improvements for these factors. The largest decline was observed for the PSQ subscales demands ($d = -0.37$, $p < 0.001$) and joy ($d = 0.46$, $p < 0.001$). Figure 5.124 illustrates the results.

The complaint complexes of Psycho-Vegetative Stability (overall index, sleep, and heat balance) similarly improved with moderate to large effect sizes at hospital discharge ($d = 0.87$, $p < 0.001$; $d = -0.66$, $p < 0.001$; $d = -0.68$, $p < 0.001$; respectively). These positive changes remained until follow-up, only symptoms regarding heat balance slightly increased compared to discharge ($d = 0.83$, $p < 0.001$; $d = -0.70$, $p < 0.001$; $d = -0.47$, $p < 0.001$; respectively) (Table 5.115).

A closer look at the self-assessed symptom burden using the questionnaire on psycho-vegetative complaints reveals a clear dominance of back pain and joint pain as well as fatigue-related symptoms. In addition, poor concentration, abdominal pressure, cold hands/feet and hypersensitivity to cold/wind as well as almost all

Table 5.114 Functional capacity of the back for patients with a somatic M54/M53 secondary diagnosis; 2023; t-test for paired samples; significance at $p < 0.05$; Cohen’s d = effect measure ($d \geq 0.2$ = small, ≥ 0.5 = moderate, ≥ 0.8 = large effect)

Percentage value for the functional capacity despite back pain	Course						Difference from admission			
	Admission (A)			Discharge (D)/ follow-up (F)			A–D/A–F		Significance	Effect size
	n	M	SD		M	SD	n	ΔM	p	d
M54 Back pain	267	68.26	20.02	D	65.61	21.15	267	−2.65	<0.001	−0.13
	212	66.71	19.88	F	67.67	20.77	212	0.96	0.345	–
M53 other spine diseases	50	70.58	20.09	D	69.42	21.41	50	−1.17	0.435	–
	37	69.14	19.63	F	71.73	19.35	37	2.59	0.144	–

Table 5.115 Changes in various parameters for patients with a secondary M54/M53 diagnosis; 2023; *t*-test: Cohen's *d* = effect measure ($d \geq 0.2$ = small effect, ≥ 0.5 = moderate effect, ≥ 0.8 = large effect)

Somatic secondary diagnosis M54 and M53	Course						Difference from admission			
		Admission (A)		Discharge (D)/ follow-up (F)			A–D/A–F		Significance	Effect size
	n	M	SD	D/F	M	SD	*n*	M	*p*	*d*
ICD symptom ratings (ISR)										
Total value	401	1.16	0.59	D	0.84	0.56	401	−0.32	< 0.001	**−0.54**
	316	1.16	0.60	F	0.82	0.54	316	−0.34	< 0.001	**−0.59**
Depression	401	2.06	0.89	D	1.21	0.88	401	−0.85	< 0.001	**−0.95**
	316	2.07	0.89	F	1.39	0.91	316	−0.68	< 0.001	**−0.75**
Anxiety	401	1.47	1.06	D	1.07	0.95	401	−0.40	< 0.001	−0.40
	316	1.45	1.06	F	0.99	0.91	316	−0.46	< 0.001	−0.47
Obsessive-compulsion	401	0.96	0.98	D	0.77	0.89	401	−0.19	< 0.001	−0.20
	316	0.99	1.01	F	0.72	0.84	316	−0.27	< 0.001	−0.28
Somatoform	401	0.88	0.90	D	0.62	0.74	401	−0.26	< 0.001	−0.31
	316	0.84	0.89	F	0.54	0.75	316	−0.30	< 0.001	−0.36
Eating disorder	401	0.63	0.86	D	0.57	0.84	401	−0.06	0.024	−0.08
	316	0.66	0.86	F	0.57	0.83	316	−0.09	0.009	−0.11
Pain disability index										
Total index	399	30.53	14.85	D	25.72	14.62	399	−4.81	< 0.001	−0.33
	309	30.65	14.70	F	24.27	15.57	309	−6.38	< 0.001	−0.42
Family/domestic obligations	399	5.16	2.58	D	4.37	2.67	399	−0.79	< 0.001	−0.30
	310	5.14	2.55	F	4.19	2.72	310	−0.95	< 0.001	−0.36
Recreation	399	5.50	2.55	D	4.67	2.73	399	−0.83	< 0.001	−0.32
	310	5.53	2.52	F	4.58	2.86	310	−0.95	< 0.001	−0.35
Social activity	399	4.84	2.86	D	4.12	2.79	399	−0.72	< 0.001	−0.26
	310	4.85	2.87	F	3.93	2.96	310	−0.92	< 0.001	−0.32
Profession	399	5.53	3.07	D	5.02	3.02	399	−0.51	< 0.001	−0.17
	309	5.56	3.01	F	4.24	3.23	309	−1.32	< 0.001	−0.42
Sex life	399	4.74	3.63	D	4.03	3.41	399	−0.71	< 0.001	−0.20
	309	4.86	3.65	F	3.93	3.57	309	−0.93	< 0.001	−0.26
Self-sufficiency	399	2.46	2.50	D	1.97	2.41	399	−0.49	< 0.001	−0.20
	309	2.46	2.47	F	1.82	2.37	309	−0.64	< 0.001	−0.26
Essentials activities	399	2.29	2.53	D	1.54	2.19	399	−0.75	< 0.001	−0.32
	309	2.26	2.51	F	1.58	2.27	309	−0.68	< 0.001	−0.28
Life satisfaction										
Total value	400	24.05	34.7	D	40.37	36.40	400	16.32	< 0.001	0.46
	320	25.04	34.3	F	38.89	34.38	320	13.85	< 0.001	0.40
Friends/ acquaintances	400	4.64	6.70	D	6.25	6.60	400	1.61	< 0.001	0.24
	320	4.65	6.66	F	5.50	6.15	320	0.85	0.005	0.13
Leisure/hobbies	400	1.58	6.25	D	3.86	6.39	400	2.28	< 0.001	0.36
	320	1.43	6.09	F	3.65	5.19	320	2.22	< 0.001	0.39
Health	400	−5.25	6.10	D	−0.54	7.17	400	4.71	< 0.001	0.71
	320	−5.33	6.27	F	−0.27	7.59	320	5.06	< 0.001	0.72
Income	400	2.94	7.08	D	4.00	6.87	400	1.06	< 0.001	0.15
	320	3.08	6.89	F	3.78	6.48	320	0.70	0.031	0.11

(continued)

Table 5.115 (continued)

Somatic secondary diagnosis M54 and M53	Course						Difference from admission			
		Admission (A)		Discharge (D)/ follow-up (F)			A–D/A–F		Significance	Effect size
	n	M	SD	D/F	M	SD	*n*	M	*p*	*d*
Profession	400	0.87	6.89	D	1.77	6.35	400	0.90	< 0.001	0.14
	320	1.02	6.86	F	2.67	6.24	320	1.65	< 0.001	0.25
Housing situation	400	6.28	7.44	D	7.42	7.65	400	1.14	< 0.001	0.15
	320	6.52	7.41	F	6.94	7.12	320	0.42	0.294	–
Family/children	400	7.04	8.42	D	9.37	8.16	400	2.33	< 0.001	0.28
	320	7.38	8.61	F	8.79	8.14	320	1.41	< 0.001	0.17
Partnership	400	5.94	9.49	D	8.24	9.32	400	2.30	< 0.001	0.24
	320	6.29	9.55	F	7.83	8.96	320	1.54	< 0.001	0.17
SOC										
Total value	398	57.03	12.02	D	61.35	12.64	398	4.32	< 0.001	0.35
	315	57.44	11.97	F	61.99	13.19	315	4.55	< 0.001	0.36
Meaningfulness	398	18.82	4.01	D	20.10	4.02	398	1.28	< 0.001	0.32
	315	19.00	3.94	F	20.11	4.23	315	1.11	< 0.001	0.27
Comprehen-sibility	398	21.13	5.59	D	22.91	5.73	398	1.78	< 0.001	0.31
	315	21.23	5.66	F	23.44	5.94	315	2.21	< 0.001	0.38
Manageability	398	17.08	4.50	D	18.34	4.83	398	1.26	< 0.001	0.27
	315	17.21	4.56	F	18.44	5.01	315	1.23	< 0.001	0.26
WHO-5 well-being and vitality										
Well-being	400	28.67	18.38	D	52.96	23.35	400	24.29	< 0.001	**1.14**
	317	28.57	17.95	F	43.74	24.49	317	15.17	< 0.001	**0.68**
Vitality	400	28.05	17.05	D	46.11	21.96	400	18.06	< 0.001	**0.90**
	317	28.17	17.14	F	42.33	22.38	317	14.16	< 0.001	**0.70**
SWOP										
Self-efficacy	400	12.51	3.02	D	13.31	2.84	400	0.80	< 0.001	0.27
	314	12.53	2.98	F	13.41	2.81	314	0.88	< 0.001	0.30
Optimism	400	5.04	1.42	D	5.65	1.41	400	0.61	< 0.001	0.43
	314	5.03	1.43	F	5.47	1.40	314	0.44	< 0.001	0.32
Pessimism	400	4.48	1.35	D	4.18	1.42	400	–0.30	< 0.001	–0.22
	314	4.44	1.35	F	4.23	1.41	314	–0.21	0.014	–0.15
SSS										
Total value	389	52.91	17.27	D	57.05	16.13	389	4.14	< 0.001	0.25
	303	53.45	16.95	F	55.06	16.58	303	1.61	0.013	0.10
Emotional	389	17.54	5.60	D	18.41	5.42	389	0.87	< 0.001	0.16
	303	17.80	5.50	F	17.98	5.33	303	0.18	0.431	–
Social interaction	389	10.49	3.87	D	11.45	3.60	389	0.96	< 0.001	0.26
	303	10.55	3.82	F	10.94	3.75	303	0.39	0.014	0.10
Material	389	11.29	4.52	D	12.49	4.04	389	1.20	< 0.001	0.28
	303	11.46	4.48	F	12.06	4.23	303	0.60	< 0.001	0.14
Affective	389	8.71	3.19	D	9.40	2.87	389	0.69	< 0.001	0.22
	303	8.82	3.14	F	9.00	3.03	303	0.18	0.131	–
Tedium measure (burnout)										
Total value	400	4.24	0.92	D	3.62	1.04	400	–0.62	< 0.001	**–0.63**
	320	4.22	0.91	F	3.67	1.05	320	–0.55	< 0.001	**–0.56**
Discouragement	400	3.75	1.11	D	3.21	1.15	400	–0.54	< 0.001	–0.48
	320	3.72	1.11	F	3.24	1.15	320	–0.48	< 0.001	–0.42

(continued)

Table 5.115 (continued)

Somatic secondary diagnosis M54 and M53	Course						Difference from admission			
		Admission (A)		Discharge (D)/ follow-up (F)			A–D/A–F		Significance	Effect size
	n	M	SD	D/F	M	SD	*n*	M	*p*	*d*
Exhaustion	400	5.03	1.01	D	4.21	1.18	400	−0.82	< 0.001	**−0.74**
	320	5.02	1.01	F	4.29	1.22	320	−0.73	< 0.001	**−0.64**
Loss of motivation	400	4.26	0.84	D	3.73	0.99	400	−0.53	< 0.001	**−0.57**
	320	4.24	0.83	F	3.76	0.98	320	−0.48	< 0.001	**−0.52**
PSQ										
Total value	400	58.51	17.20	D	40.97	19.01	400	−17.54	< 0.001	**−0.96**
	319	58.34	17.21	F	47.52	18.69	319	−10.82	< 0.001	**−0.60**
Worries	400	50.62	23.17	D	36.48	23.07	400	−14.14	< 0.001	**−0.61**
	319	50.12	23.23	F	38.70	23.38	319	−11.42	< 0.001	−0.49
Demands	400	48.68	23.83	D	27.13	21.91	400	−21.55	< 0.001	**−0.94**
	319	48.74	23.97	F	40.19	23.09	319	−8.55	< 0.001	−0.36
Joy	400	33.52	18.83	D	48.25	21.95	400	14.73	< 0.001	**0.71**
	319	33.79	18.95	F	43.43	22.37	319	9.64	< 0.001	0.46
Tension	400	68.27	20.57	D	48.52	23.76	400	−19.75	< 0.001	**−0.88**
	319	68.32	20.25	F	54.61	22.39	319	−13.71	< 0.001	**−0.64**
PSQI										
Total value	394	10.75	3.92	D	9.92	4.37	394	−0.83	< 0.001	−0.20
	314	10.79	3.95	F	8.88	3.81	314	−1.91	< 0.001	−0.49
Sleep quality	394	1.82	0.66	D	1.48	0.69	394	−0.34	< 0.001	**−0.51**
	314	1.83	0.67	F	1.50	0.67	314	−0.33	< 0.001	−0.49
Sleep latency	394	1.75	1.03	D	1.51	1.02	394	−0.24	< 0.001	−0.24
	314	1.72	1.03	F	1.52	0.97	314	−0.20	< 0.001	−0.20
Sleep duration	394	1.55	0.93	D	1.52	0.91	394	−0.03	0.499	–
	314	1.53	0.95	F	1.32	0.88	314	−0.21	< 0.001	−0.23
Sleep efficiency	394	1.32	1.17	D	1.22	1.20	394	−0.10	0.099	–
	314	1.33	1.17	F	0.89	1.08	314	−0.44	< 0.001	−0.39
Sleep disorders	394	1.82	0.63	D	1.62	0.61	394	−0.20	< 0.001	−0.31
	314	1.83	0.64	F	1.60	0.65	314	−0.23	< 0.001	−0.36
Sleeping pills	394	0.68	1.15	D	1.41	1.42	394	0.73	< 0.001	**0.57**
	314	0.72	1.19	F	0.65	1.12	314	−0.07	0.201	–
Daytime sleepiness	394	1.81	0.75	D	1.15	0.80	394	−0.66	< 0.001	**−0.85**
	314	1.82	0.75	F	1.40	0.79	314	−0.42	< 0.001	**−0.56**
GAD										
Total value	399	10.53	4.59	D	6.25	4.27	399	−4.28	< 0.001	**−0.96**
	307	10.52	4.55	F	7.23	4.72	307	−3.29	< 0.001	**−0.71**
Complaint complexes of psycho-vegetative stability										
Complaints index	400	0.26	0.48	D	0.85	0.79	400	0.59	< 0.001	**0.87**
	320	0.26	0.47	F	0.79	0.73	320	0.53	< 0.001	**0.83**
Total value	400	62.58	15.72	D	45.85	19.14	400	−16.73	< 0.001	**−0.94**
	320	62.56	15.86	F	49.26	19.42	320	−13.30	< 0.001	**−0.74**
Dizziness	400	3.32	2.16	D	2.36	2.21	400	−0.96	< 0.001	−0.44
	320	3.27	2.11	F	2.54	2.13	320	−0.73	< 0.001	−0.34
Sleep	400	7.18	2.09	D	5.61	2.58	400	−1.57	< 0.001	**−0.66**
	320	7.18	2.10	F	5.61	2.38	320	−1.57	< 0.001	**−0.70**
Heat balance	400	5.74	2.74	D	3.93	2.58	400	−1.81	< 0.001	**−0.68**
	320	5.74	2.75	F	4.51	2.58	320	−1.23	< 0.001	−0.46

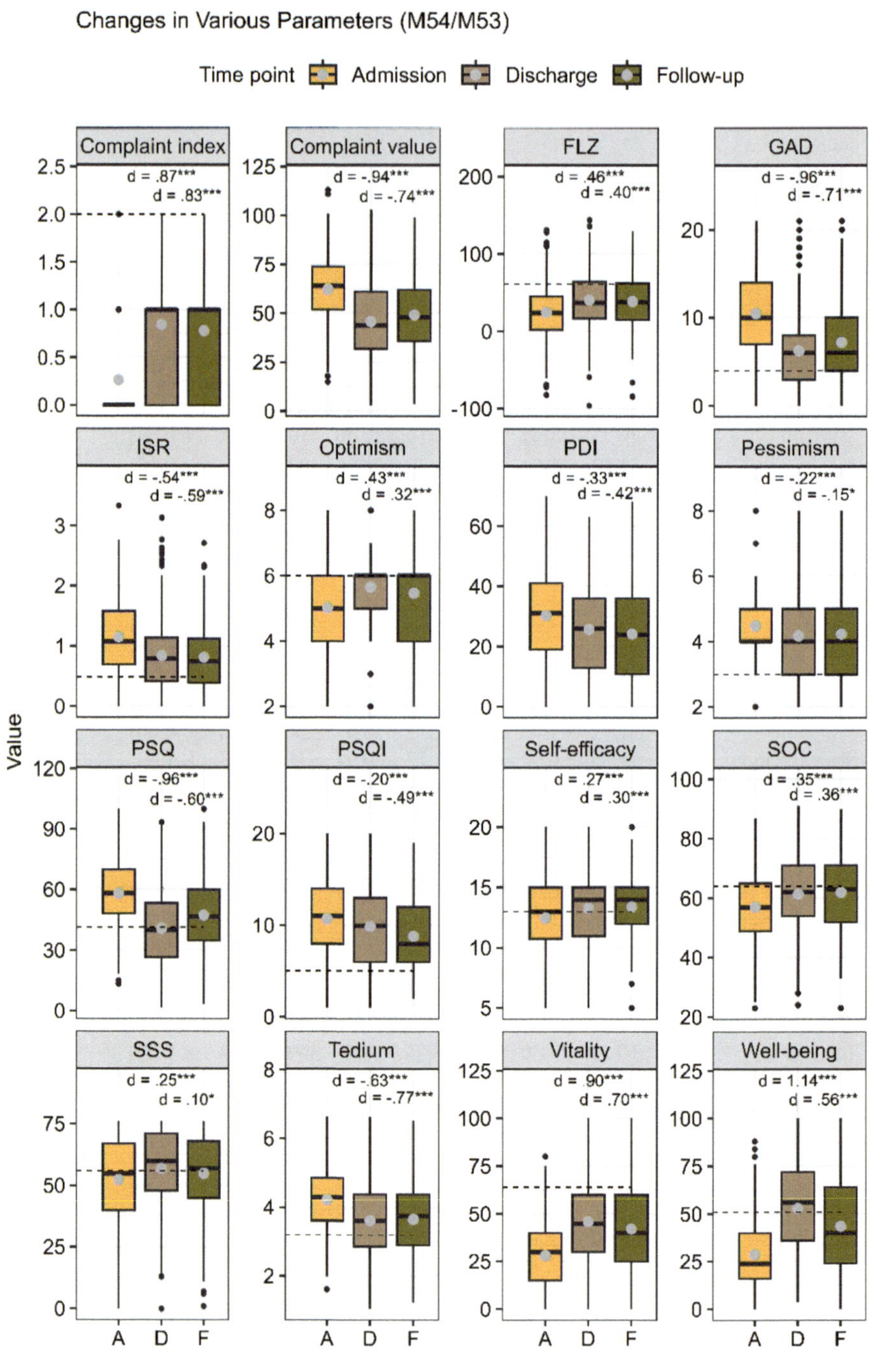

Fig. 5.124 Changes in various parameters for patients with a somatic diagnosis in 2023 (M54/M53). The dashed black lines show the desired target values. Significance: $*p < 0.05$, $**p < 0.01$, $***p < 0.001$. Effect measure ($d \geq 0.2$ = small effect, ≥ 0.5 = moderate effect, ≥ 0.8 = large effect). The graph shows all available data; the effect sizes refer to individual comparisons (A–D/A–F)

affective symptoms are pronounced in this group. When comparing the admission, discharge and follow-up examination values, improvements were seen particularly in affective symptoms, followed by fatigue-related symptoms and musculoskeletal symptoms (Fig. 5.125).

5.4.2 Sleep Disorders (ICD-10 G 47)

A diagnosis of insomnia (ICD-10 code G47) requires persistent difficulty falling asleep and staying asleep for at least 4 weeks, accompanied by daytime sleepiness. Chronic insomnia is defined as poor sleep occurring on more than three nights per week for over 1 month. Insomnia manifests as mental fatigue, depression, general malaise, or cognitive impairment during the day [20, 21].

According to the BARMER press release (2023), 7% of their insured members are affected by sleep disorders [22].

There are numerous remedies and methods for treating sleep disorders, but their effectiveness has not been sufficiently studied:

- Home remedies include taking a hot bath, drinking a glass of warm milk, or a cup of valerian tea before going to bed.
- Herbal sleeping pills and sedatives, such as valerian.
- Relaxation techniques such as progressive muscle relaxation and autogenic training.
- Physical activity: evening walks and quiet exercises such as yoga, tai chi, or qigong.
- Sleep hygiene: avoid heavy meals shortly before bedtime, reduce your alcohol and coffee intake, don't watch TV in bed, and only go to bed when you are tired.
- Cognitive behavioural therapy: This can be used to change thought patterns and behaviours that affect sleep. Combining it with relaxation techniques can be helpful.

Of the 255 patients diagnosed with sleep disorders, the majority (154) were coded as having difficulty falling or staying asleep, according to the ICD-10 classification system. Six patients had two different sleep diagnoses. Of all patients, 640 reported feeling 'sleepy after getting up' (77.8%), and 608 suffered from 'restless sleep' (73.9%).

At the end of their inpatient stay, 247 of the 255 patients diagnosed with sleep disorders reported that they had experienced a major clinical benefit from their stay. For patients with sleep disorders, there was a reduction in symptoms at discharge, with a large, significant effect size ($d = -1.29$, $p < 0.001$), as measured by the Visual Analogue Scale (VAS). At follow-up, this reduction continued to show a large effect size ($d = -1.16$, $p < 0.001$). Table 5.116 presents the statistical results and Fig. 5.126 illustrates the distribution of VAS score differences, indicating the degree of improvement.

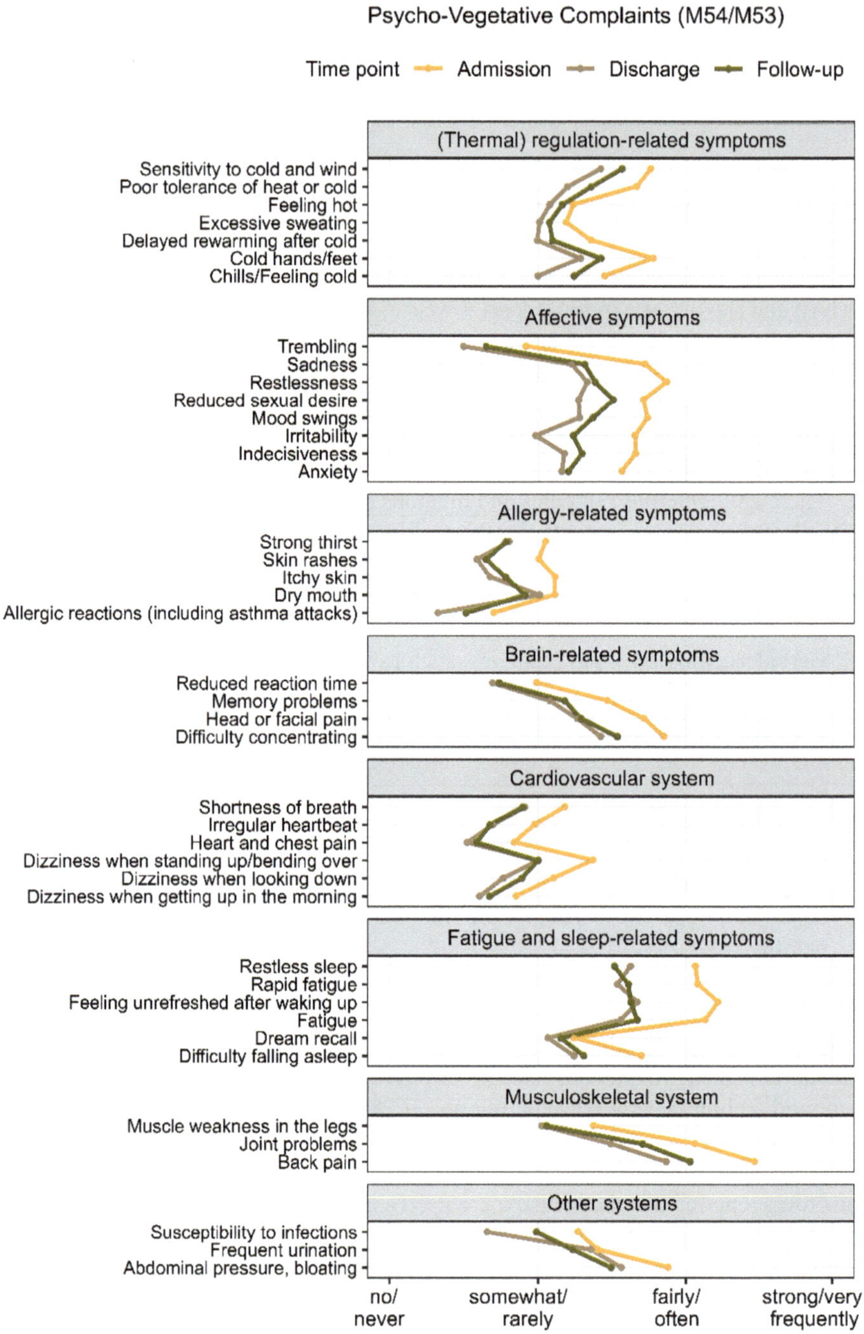

Fig. 5.125 Psycho-vegetative complaints; change in complaints for patients with a somatic M54/M;53 diagnosis in 2023; admission: $n = 425$, discharge: $n = 402$; follow-up: $n = 321$

Table 5.116 Global assessments of treatment success for patients with sleep disorder diagnosis, surveyed at discharge and follow-up in 2023; *t*-test for paired samples; significance at $p < 0.05$; Cohen's d = effect measure ($d \geq 0.2$ = small, ≥ 0.5 = moderate, ≥ 0.8 = large effect)

Main complaint severity (VAS)	Course						Difference from admission			
	Admission (A)			Discharge (D)/ follow-up (F)			A–D/A–F		Significance	Effect size
	n	M	SD		M	SD	*n*	ΔM	*p*	*d*
G47	247	72.87	17.57	D	48.79	19.78	247	−24.09	< 0.001	**−1.29**
	194	72.06	17.42	F	48.40	22.99	194	−23.66	<0.001	**−1.16**

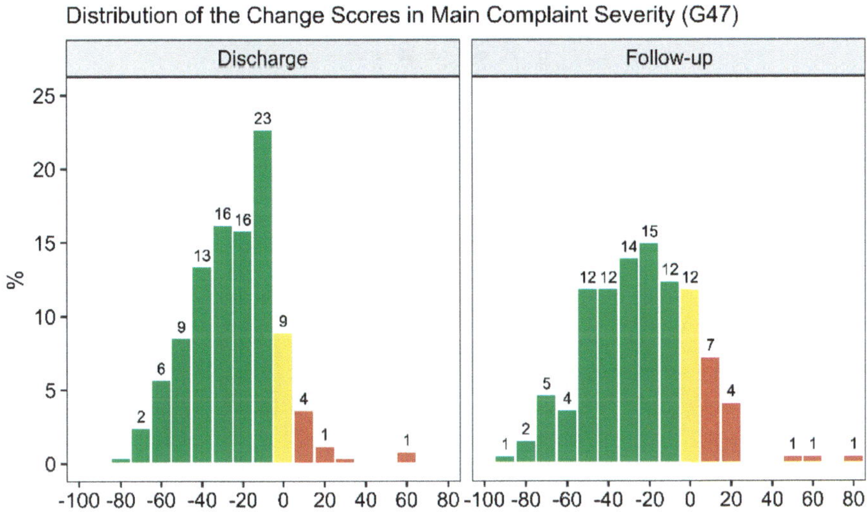

Fig. 5.126 Distribution of the change scores in main complaint severity between hospital admission and hospital discharge or hospital admission and follow-up for patients with a G47 sleep disorder diagnosis in 2023 (A–D $n = 247$; A–D–F $n = 194$); negative differences correspond to an improvement

In general, the assessment of treatment success upon discharge indicated good or very good outcomes for 65.1% of patients. More specifically, 11.3% rated the overall success of the treatment as 'very good', 53.8% as 'good', 30.8% as 'moderate', and 4.0% as 'no success'. At follow-up, these figures were 23.1%, 48.7%, 24.1% and 4.1%, respectively (Table 5.117, Fig. 5.127).

When asked at discharge whether the treatment had been worthwhile, 37.1% said it had been 'very worthwhile', 57.1% said it had been 'worthwhile', 5.3% said it had 'not been worthwhile', and nobody reported that the treatment had been 'rather harmful'. At follow-up, 54.9% said the treatment had been 'very worthwhile', 38.5% said it had been 'worthwhile', 6.2% said it had 'not been worthwhile', and one person said it had caused harm (Table 5.117, Fig. 5.127).

Table 5.117 Global assessments of treatment success for patients with a G47 diagnosis, surveyed at discharge and at follow-up in 2023

Overall success of the therapy		**Very good**		**Good**		**Moderate**		**No success**		**Total**	
		n	%	*n*	%	*n*	%	*n*	%	*n*	%
G47 sleep disorders	D	28	11.3	133	53.8	76	30.8	10	4.0	247	100
	F	45	23.1	95	48.7	47	24.1	8	4.1	195	100
Treatment worthwhile		**Very worthwhile**		**Worthwhile**		**Not worth it**		**Rather harmed**		**Total**	
		n	%	*n*	%	*n*	%	*n*	%	*n*	%
G47 sleep disorders	D	93	37.1	141	57.1	13	5.3	0	0.0	247	100
	F	107	54.9	75	38.5	12	6.2	1	0.5	195	100

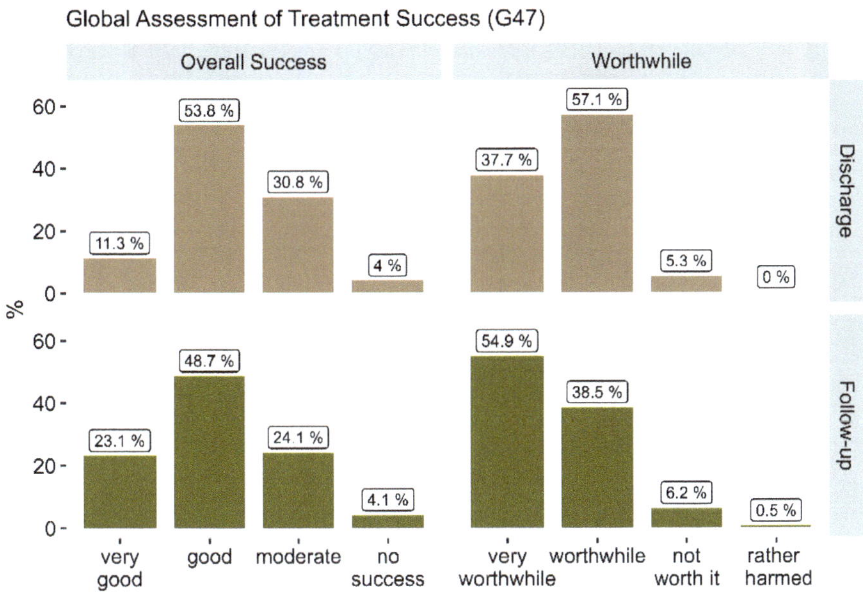

Fig. 5.127 Global assessments of treatment success for patients with a G47 diagnosis who were surveyed at discharge ($n = 247$) and at follow-up ($n = 195$) in 2023

Overall sleep quality (PSQI) showed significant improvement with a small effect size at hospital discharge ($d = -0.29$, $p < 0.001$). At the follow-up, the improvement was even more pronounced, with a moderate effect size ($d = -0.65$, $p < 0.001$). Examining the PSQI subscales more closely reveals that the largest effects were observed for sleep quality (D: $d = -0.67$; F: $d = -0.65$) and daytime sleepiness (D: $d = -0.89$; F: $d = -0.53$). At follow-up, sleep efficiency increased ($d = -0.54$), accompanied by a decrease in sleep duration ($d = -0.39$). Consumption of sleeping pills increased by the time of hospital discharge ($d = 0.69$) but dropped again to the pre-hospital admission level by follow-up (Figs. 5.128, 5.129).

Regarding protective and risk factors, the sleep clientele reported positive results at discharge and at the 6-month follow-up. In particular, positive changes were observed with moderate to large effect sizes in the following areas:

- ISR total score (D: $d = -0.59$, $p < 0.001$; F: $d = -0.65$, $p < 0.001$).
- Depression (D: $d = -0.99$, $p < 0.001$; F: $d = -0.83$, $p < 0.001$).
- Well-being (D: $d = 1.22$, $p < 0.001$; F: $d = 0.85$, $p < 0.001$).
- Vitality (D: $d = 0.95$, $p < 0.001$; F: $d = 0.83$, $p < 0.001$).
- Generalised Anxiety Disorder (D: $d = -1.01$, $p < 0.001$; F: $d = -$, $p < 0.001$).
- Perceived Stress Questionnaire (D: $d = -1.05$, $p < 0.001$; F: $d = -0.72$, $p < 0.001$).
- And burnout (D: $d = -0.70$, $p < 0.001$; F: $d = -0.68$, $p < 0.001$) (Table 5.118, Fig. 5.130).

Table 5.118 Changes in various parameters for patients with a secondary G47 diagnosis in 2023; t-test: Cohen's d = effect measure ($d \geq 0.2$ = small effect, ≥ 0.5 = moderate effect, ≥ 0.8 = large effect)

Sleep disorders G47	Course						Difference from admission			
		Admission (A)		Discharge (D)/ follow-up (F)			A–D/A–F		Significance	Effect size
	n	M	SD	D/F	M	SD	*n*	M	*p*	*d*
ICD symptom ratings (ISR)										
Total value	248	1.18	0.58	D	0.85	0.53	248	−0.33	<0.001	**−0.59**
	190	1.17	0.60	F	0.80	0.54	190	−0.37	<0.001	**−0.65**
Depression	248	2.15	0.88	D	1.29	0.85	248	−0.86	<0.001	**−0.99**
	190	2.12	0.89	F	1.37	0.91	190	−0.75	<0.001	**−0.83**
Anxiety	248	1.42	1.07	D	1.01	0.91	248	−0.41	<0.001	−0.41
	190	1.39	1.07	F	0.92	0.83	190	−0.47	<0.001	−0.47
Obsessive-compulsion	248	0.93	0.97	D	0.77	0.85	248	−0.15	0.004	−0.17
	190	0.96	0.99	F	0.65	0.78	190	−0.30	<0.001	−0.33
Somatoform	248	0.92	0.95	D	0.64	0.75	248	−0.28	<0.001	−0.33
	190	0.90	0.91	F	0.50	0.70	190	−0.40	<0.001	−0.48
Eating disorder	248	0.66	0.84	D	0.60	0.84	248	−0.06	0.170	–
	190	0.70	0.86	F	0.59	0.81	190	−0.11	0.018	−0.13
Pain disability index										
Total index	247	28.85	15.31	D	25.91	14.62	247	−2.94	<0.001	−0.20
	187	28.18	14.9	F	23.80	16.65	187	−4.38	<0.001	−0.28
Family/domestic obligations	247	4.73	2.85	D	4.20	2.75	247	−0.54	0.001	−0.19
	187	4.68	2.82	F	4.19	3.02	187	−0.49	0.029	−0.17
Recreation	247	5.27	2.80	D	4.63	2.86	247	−0.64	<0.001	−0.23
	187	5.21	2.73	F	4.37	2.96	187	−0.84	<0.001	−0.29
Social activity	247	4.67	2.99	D	4.31	2.84	247	−0.36	0.069	–
	187	4.60	2.95	F	3.87	3.02	187	−0.73	<0.001	−0.25
Profession	247	5.32	3.09	D	5.20	3.07	247	−0.12	0.543	–
	187	5.18	3.06	F	3.89	3.35	187	−1.29	<0.001	−0.40
Sex life	247	4.47	3.69	D	4.01	3.43	247	−0.46	0.026	−0.13
	187	4.33	3.60	F	4.01	3.64	187	−0.32	0.136	–
Self-sufficiency	247	2.18	2.45	D	1.93	2.39	247	−0.24	0.132	–
	187	2.04	2.33	F	1.86	2.47	187	−0.18	0.351	–
Essentials activities	247	2.24	2.60	D	1.62	2.25	247	−0.62	<0.001	−0.26
	187	2.18	2.48	F	1.61	2.32	187	−0.57	0.008	−0.34
Life satisfaction										
Total value	247	24.86	31.38	D	42.45	36.92	247	17.59	<0.001	**0.51**
	193	26.76	30.90	F	38.89	33.00	193	12.13	<0.001	0.38
Friends/ acquaintances	247	4.91	6.84	D	6.98	6.74	247	2.06	<0.001	0.30
	193	5.02	6.77	F	5.57	6.42	193	0.55	0.181	–
Leisure/hobbies	247	1.24	6.28	D	3.75	6.67	247	2.51	<0.001	0.39
	193	1.38	6.27	F	3.33	5.62	193	1.94	<0.001	0.33
Health	247	−5.17	5.85	D	−0.55	7.73	247	4.62	<0.001	**0.67**
	193	−4.93	5.94	F	−0.12	7.54	193	4.80	<0.001	**0.70**
Income	247	3.04	6.83	D	4.14	6.70	247	1.10	0.003	0.16
	193	3.28	6.59	F	4.13	6.00	193	0.85	0.037	0.14

(continued)

Table 5.118 (continued)

Sleep disorders G47	Course							Difference from admission			
		Admission (A)		Discharge (D)/ follow-up (F)				A–D/A–F		Significance	Effect size
	n	M	SD	D/F	M	SD		*n*	M	*p*	*d*
Profession	247	1.23	6.69	D	2.28	6.36		247	1.05	0.006	0.16
	193	1.57	6.68	F	2.99	6.42		193	1.42	0.006	0.22
Housing situation	247	6.68	7.34	D	7.62	7.38		247	0.94	0.025	0.13
	193	6.79	7.27	F	6.72	6.83		193	−0.07	0.885	–
Family/children	247	7.21	8.20	D	9.64	7.80		247	2.43	<0.001	0.30
	193	7.35	8.23	F	8.39	7.75		193	1.04	0.046	0.13
Partnership	247	5.71	9.05	D	8.62	9.11		247	2.90	<0.001	0.32
	193	6.28	9.11	F	7.89	8.81		193	1.61	0.004	0.18
SOC											
Total value	246	57.07	12.08	D	62.11	12.31		246	5.04	<0.001	0.41
	189	57.63	12.33	F	61.97	13.09		189	0.34	<0.001	0.34
Meaningfulness	246	19.12	3.95	D	20.39	3.86		246	1.27	<0.001	0.33
	189	19.16	4.07	F	20.07	4.44		189	0091	0.002	0.21
Comprehen-sibility	246	20.98	5.67	D	23.17	5.59		246	2.20	<0.001	0.39
	189	21.20	5.70	F	23.59	5.97		189	2.39	<0.001	0.41
Manageability	246	16.97	4.61	D	18.54	4.86		246	1.57	<0.001	0.33
	189	17.19	4.71	F	18.31	4.62		189	1.12	<0.001	0.24
WHO-5 well-being and vitality											
Well-being	247	26.49	16.69	D	51.01	22.64		247	24.52	<0.001	**1.22**
	189	26.05	16.10	F	43.64	23.18		189	17.59	<0.001	**0.85**
Vitality	247	25.16	16.43	D	43.70	21.64		247	18.54	<0.001	**0.95**
	189	25.48	16.24	F	42.35	22.91		189	16.88	<0.001	**0.83**
SWOP											
Self-efficacy	247	12.47	2.77	D	13.27	2.82		247	0.81	<0.001	0.29
	189	12.40	2.59	F	13.54	2.83		189	1.14	<0.001	0.42
Optimism	247	4.98	1.46	D	5.66	1.40		247	0.68	<0.001	0.47
	189	4.95	1.48	F	5.44	1.47		189	0.49	<0.001	0.33
Pessimism	247	4.51	1.40	D	4.23	1.38		247	−0.28	<0.001	−0.20
	189	4.49	1.41	F	4.12	1.39		189	−0.38	<0.001	−0.27
SSS											
Total value	245	53.82	15.92	D	58.28	14.72		245	4.47	<0.001	0.29
	187	54.60	15.55	F	56.90	14.29		187	2.30	0.002	0.15
Emotional	245	17.82	5.28	D	18.87	4.96		245	1.05	<0.001	0.21
	187	18.13	5.20	F	18.49	4.77		187	0.36	0.220	–
Social interaction	245	10.70	3.55	D	11.76	3.19		245	1.06	<0.001	0.31
	187	10.76	3.51	F	11.32	3.29		187	0.56	0.003	0.16
Material	245	11.47	4.29	D	12.67	3.66		245	1.21	<0.001	0.30
	187	11.69	4.12	F	12.62	3.72		187	0.93	<0.001	0.24
Affective	245	8.84	2.98	D	9.51	2.69		245	0.67	<0.001	0.23
	187	8.95	2.94	F	9.27	2.72		187	0.32	0.018	0.11
Tedium measure (burnout)											
Total value	247	4.33	0.87	D	3.67	1.01		247	−0.66	<0.001	**−0.70**
	193	4.28	0.86	F	3.66	0.98		193	−0.63	<0.001	**−0.68**
Discouragement	247	3.85	1.06	D	3.23	1.14		247	−0.63	<0.001	**−0.57**
	193	3.80	1.04	F	3.24	1.08		193	−0.56	<0.001	**−0.52**

(continued)

Table 5.118 (continued)

Sleep disorders G47	Course						Difference from admission			
		Admission (A)		Discharge (D)/ follow-up (F)			A–D/A–F		Significance	Effect size
	n	M	SD	D/F	M	SD	*n*	M	*p*	*d*
Exhaustion	247	5.13	1.01	D	4.32	1.14	247	−0.82	<0.001	**−0.75**
	193	5.11	1.01	F	4.27	1.17	193	−0.83	<0.001	**−0.76**
Loss of motivation	247	4.31	0.80	D	3.76	0.94	247	−0.56	<0.001	**−0.63**
	193	4.27	0.80	F	3.74	0.95	193	−0.52	<0.001	**−0.59**
PSQ										
Total value	247	60.90	16.43	D	42.07	19.11	247	−18.83	<0.001	**−1.05**
	192	60.56	16.32	F	47.86	18.57	192	−12.70	<0.001	**−0.72**
Worries	247	53.63	22.46	D	37.73	23.29	247	−15.90	<0.001	**−0.69**
	192	52.33	21.94	F	39.55	22.45	192	−12.78	<0.001	**−0.58**
Demands	247	49.82	24.99	D	28.39	22.96	247	−21.43	<0.001	**−0.89**
	192	49.86	24.95	F	39.55	23.41	192	−10.31	<0.001	−0.43
Joy	247	31.63	17.79	D	48.48	22.65	247	16.84	<0.001	**0.82**
	192	31.70	17.67	F	43.19	22.37	192	11.49	<0.001	**0.56**
Tension	247	71.79	19.17	D	50.63	23.02	247	−21.16	<0.001	**−0.99**
	192	71.74	19.54	F	55.52	22.22	192	−16.22	<0.001	**−0.77**
PSQI										
Total value	244	11.64	3.57	D	10.53	4.07	244	−1.11	<0.001	−0.29
	188	11.58	3.59	F	9.14	3.90	188	−2.44	<0.001	**−0.65**
Sleep quality	244	1.98	0.61	D	1.55	0.67	244	−0.43	<0.001	**−0.67**
	188	1.98	0.60	F	1.56	0.69	188	−0.42	<0.001	**−0.65**
Sleep latency	244	1.95	1.07	D	1.57	0.99	244	−0.38	<0.001	−0.37
	188	1.88	1.08	F	1.50	1.04	188	−0.38	<0.001	**−0.36**
Sleep duration	244	1.73	0.84	D	1.65	0.90	244	−0.09	0.119	–
	188	1.72	0.83	F	1.38	0.89	188	−0.34	<0.001	**−0.39**
Sleep efficiency	244	1.57	1.12	D	1.36	1.22	244	−0.22	0.007	−0.19
	188	1.58	1.12	F	0.97	1.13	188	−0.61	<0.001	**−0.54**
Sleep disorders	244	1.85	0.60	D	1.61	0.62	244	−0.24	<0.001	−0.39
	188	1.84	0.62	F	1.54	0.62	188	−0.30	<0.001	−0.48
Sleeping pills	244	0.70	1.17	D	1.61	1.42	244	0.91	<0.001	**0.69**
	188	0.72	1.21	F	0.71	1.18	188	−0.01	0.946	–
Daytime sleepiness	244	1.84	0.72	D	1.18	0.76	244	−0.66	<0.001	**−0.89**
	188	1.86	0.72	F	1.47	0.76	188	−0.39	<0.001	**−0.53**
GAD										
Total value	245	10.81	4.68	D	6.28	4.28	245	−4.53	<0.001	**−1.01**
	185	10.62	4.64	F	7.28	4.98	185	−3.35	<0.001	**−0.69**
Complaint complexes of psycho-vegetative stability										
Complaints index	248	0.25	0.49	D	0.90	0.79	247	0.65	<0.001	**0.96**
	193	0.26	0.50	F	0.85	0.79	193	0.59	<0.001	**0.86**
Total value	247	62.86	16.44	D	45.24	18.42	247	−17.63	<0.001	**−1.00**
	193	62.44	16.37	F	4862	19.55	193	−13.82	<0.001	**−0.76**
Dizziness	247	3.36	2.36	D	2.33	2.28	247	−1.03	<0.001	−0.44
	193	3.24	2.26	F	2.66	2.16	193	−0.58	<0.001	−0.26
Sleep	247	7.69	1.90	D	5.91	2.44	247	−1.78	<0.001	**−0.80**
	193	7.65	1.91	F	5.94	2.48	193	−1.72	<0.001	**−0.77**
Heat balance	247	5.68	2.75	D	3.66	2.52	247	−2.02	<0.001	**−0.76**
	193	5.74	2.80	F	4.49	2.58	193	−1.24	<0.001	−0.46

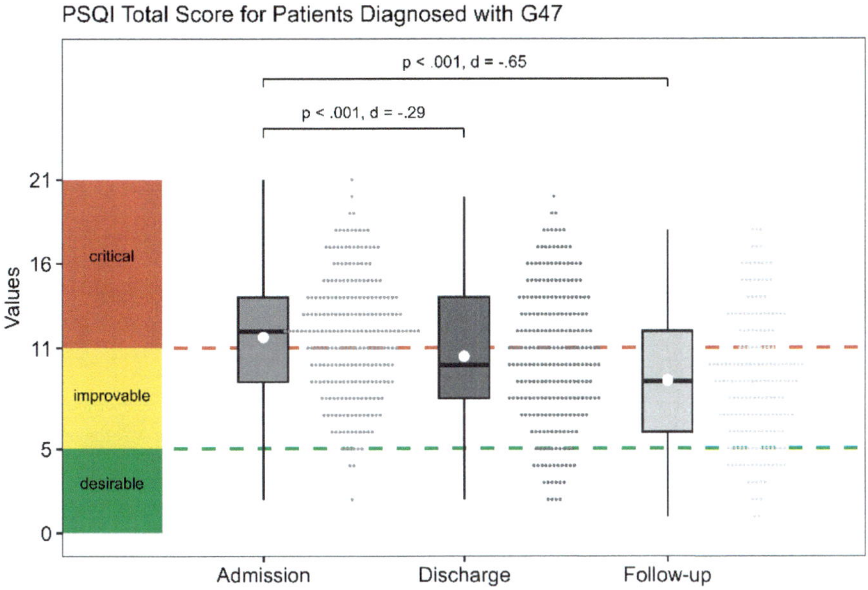

Fig. 5.128 PSQI total score for patients diagnosed with a sleep disorder G47, measured at discharge (n = 244) and at follow-up (n = 188) in 2023; Note: Graph shows all available data, the effect sizes refer to the individual comparison (A–D/A–F)

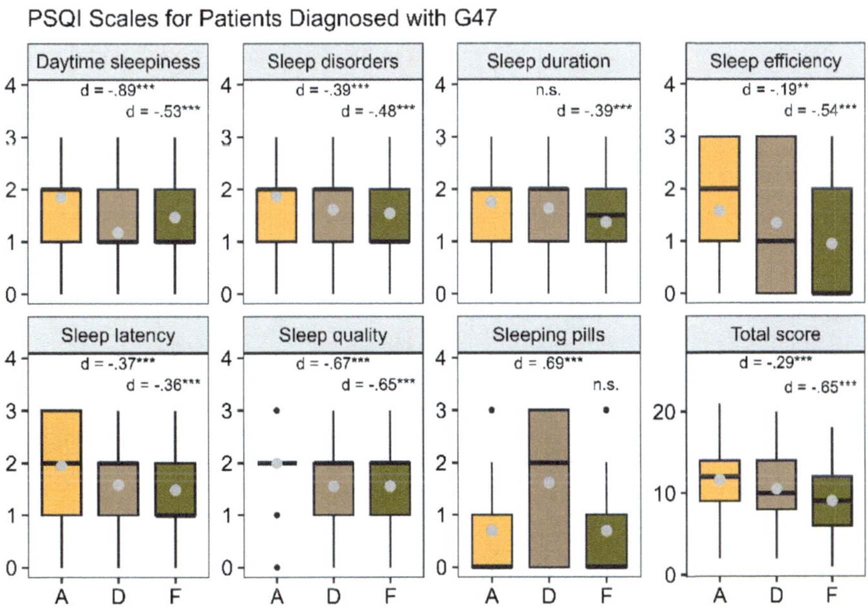

Fig. 5.129 PSQI scales for patients diagnosed with sleep disorder G47, measured at discharge (D: n = 244) and at follow-up (F: n = 188) in 2023; Note: Graph shows all available data, the effect sizes refer to the individual comparison from admission (A) (A–D/A–F)

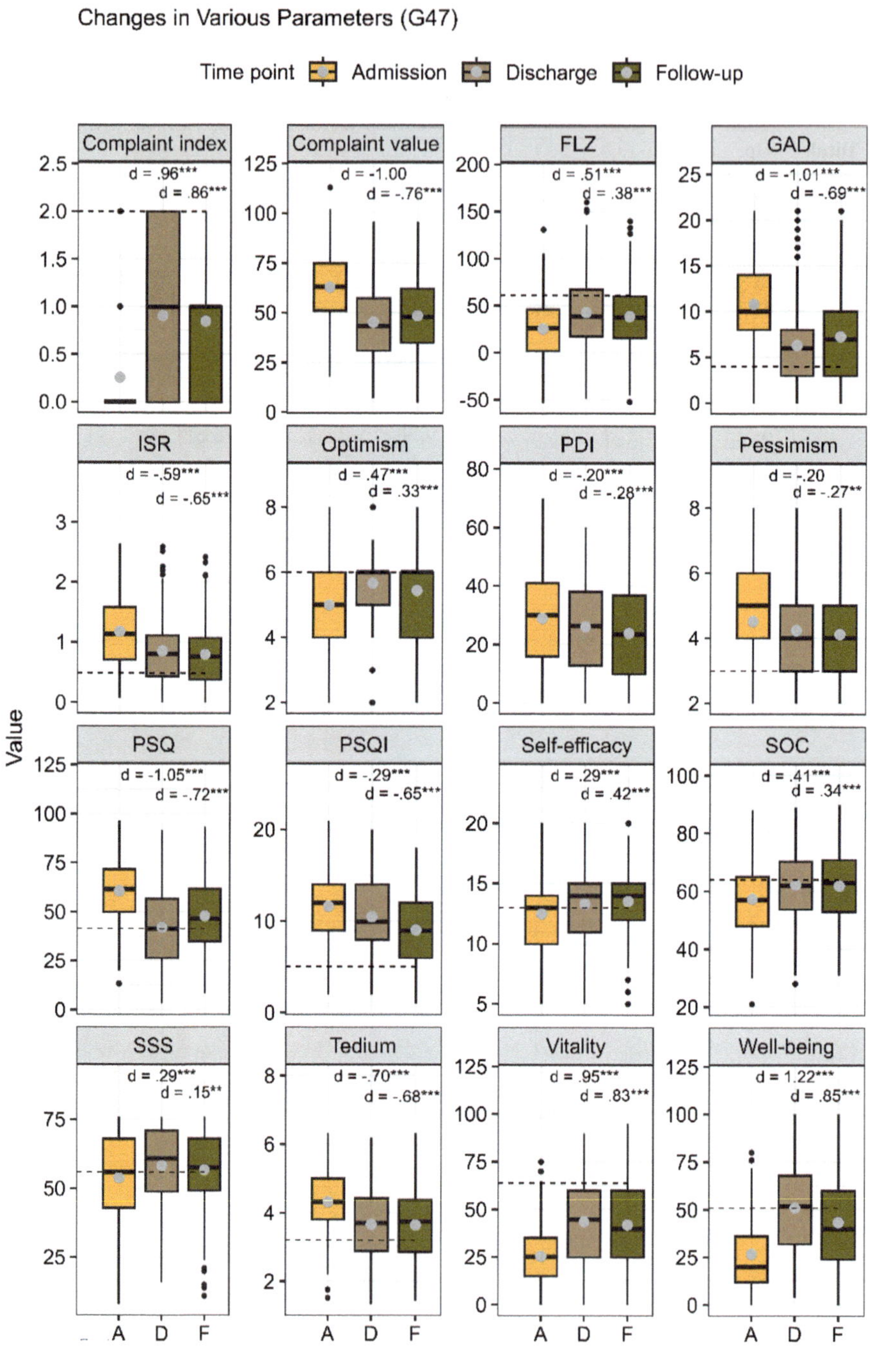

Fig. 5.130 Changes in various parameters for patients with a G47 diagnosis in 2023; the dashed black lines indicate the desired target values; significance: $*p < 0.05$, $**p < 0.01$, $***p < 0.001$; Cohen's d = effect measure ($d \geq 0.2$ = small effect, ≥ 0.5 = moderate effect, ≥ 0.8 = large effect); the graph shows all available data, the effect sizes refer to the individual comparison (A–D/A–F)

Complaints relating to Psycho-Vegetative Stability (overall index) significantly improved at hospital discharge and at follow-up, with large effect sizes observed ($d = 0.96, p < 0.001$; $d = 0.86, p < 0.001$, respectively). This improvement was particularly evident in sleep symptoms ($d = -0.80, p < 0.001$ at discharge and $d = -0.77, p < 0.001$ at follow-up).

Examining the self-assessed symptom burden using the psycho-vegetative complaint questionnaire reveals a clear dominance of fatigue, sleep-related complaints, back pain, and joint pain. This group is also characterised by poor concentration, a feeling of pressure in the stomach, cold hands and feet, and almost all affective symptoms. When comparing admission, discharge, and follow-up values, it is particularly notable that affective symptoms and fatigue-related symptoms show improvements (Fig. 5.131).

5.4.3 Other Diseases of the Soft Tissue: Fibromyalgia and Pain in the Extremities and Joint Diseases (M79 and M25)

The third most common somatic diagnosis is M79 "other soft tissue diseases", with 222 patients. This group includes individuals with fibromyalgia (42.9%), myalgia (6.6%), and pain localised to the extremities. Two or more different 'soft tissue diseases' were diagnosed in 42 people. Additionally, this group includes 82 people with the indication 'other joint diseases (M25)'. Most of these patients suffer from osteoarthritis of the knee, shoulder, and hip. Five people have two different joint diseases and one person has three. According to their self-reported medical histories, 550 patients reported joint complaints, accounting for 66.8% of the total clientele.

Fibromyalgia syndrome (FMS) is defined by the American College of Rheumatology's criteria and is classified as a functional somatic syndrome. FMS is diagnosed based on a typical pattern of symptoms, after excluding inflammatory and metabolic diseases that can lead to similar symptoms. In 40–70% of patients, relevant emotional or psychosocial conflicts can be identified as occurring in temporal connection with the manifestation or intensification of pain symptoms [23]. Sixty percent of patients report experiencing relevant emotional or psychosocial conflicts in temporal connection with the manifestation or intensification of pain symptoms [24].

According to the GEDA 2019/2020-EHIS survey, 17.1% of adults reported having osteoarthritis in the previous 12 months (95% CI: 16.4–17.8%), with the condition affecting women significantly more often than men (21.6% vs. 12.4%) [25]. Osteoarthritis and other joint diseases considerably impair quality of life, primarily due to pain and restricted mobility. The most common complaints are caused by wear and tear or joint inflammation. Pain can occur at a specific point or radiate from the primary affected area to the surrounding area. In most cases, joint pain is caused by inflammation and swelling of the tissue. Around half of all people over the age of 45 complain of aching joints, particularly knee pain.

The following risk factors for joint diseases are known:

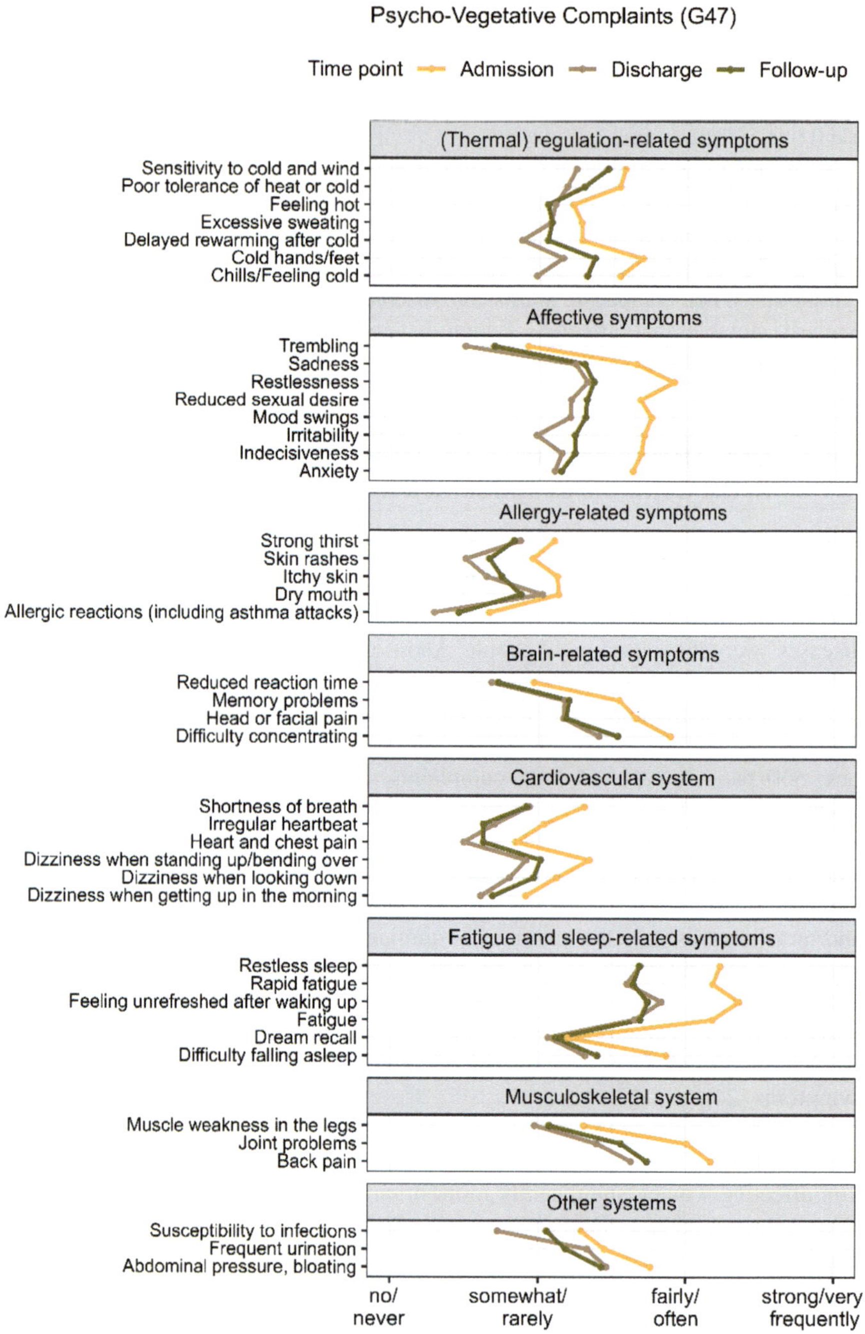

Fig. 5.131 Psycho-vegetative complaints; change in complaints for patients with a G47 diagnosis at admission: $n = 254$, discharge: $n = 248$ and follow-up: $n = 193$ in 2023

- Overweight [26].
- Chronic poor posture [27].
- Low-nutrient diet [28–30].
- Lack of physical activity [31].
- Smoking [32, 33].
- Alcohol and drugs [33].
- Sports that strain the joints such as tennis, soccer, basketball [34].

For both diagnostic groups (M79 and M25), TCM patients show a large, significant effect size for change in main complaint severity at discharge (M79: $d = -1.25$, $p < 0.001$; M25: $d = -1.41$, $p < 0.001$), which is maintained at follow-up (M79: $d = -1.03$, $p < 0.001$; M25: $d = -1.13$, $p < 0.001$) (Table 5.119). Figure 5.132 illustrates the differences in measurement times between the two indication groups.

Patients with soft tissue muscle pain rated the global assessment of treatment success as 'very good' in 13.8% of cases at discharge and 27.1% at follow-up, and as 'good' in 50.0% of cases at discharge and 44.1% at follow-up. No success was indicated by 3.8% of patients at discharge and only 1.7% at follow-up.

Patients with arthrosis (joint disease) rated treatment success as 'very good' in 24.0% of cases (follow-up: 40.4%) and 'good' in 53.3% of cases (follow-up: 42.1%). No patients reported having gained no benefit from the treatment at either discharge or follow-up. Furthermore, 42.9% of patients with muscle pain and 52.0% of patients with arthrosis rated the question of a worthwhile stay as 'very worthwhile' (follow-up: 56.5% and 75.4%, respectively) (Table 5.120, Figs. 5.133 and 5.134).

Patients with fibromyalgia, pain in the extremities, and joint diseases showed significant improvements with moderate to large effect sizes at discharge in the monitoring of mental stress, especially for depression ($d = -0.94$, $p < 0.001$), as well as for well-being ($d = 1.14$, $p < 0.001$) and vitality ($d = 0.99$, $p < 0.001$). Such improvements were also observed across all PSQ scales: worries ($d = -0.65$, $p < 0.001$), demands ($d = -1.10$, $p < 0.001$), joy ($d = 0.82$, $p < 0.001$), and tension

Table 5.119 Global assessments of treatment success for patients with a somatic M79 or M25 secondary diagnosis, surveyed at discharge (n = 210/*n* = 75) and follow-up (*n* = 175/*n* = 57) in 2023; *t*-test for paired samples; significance at $p < 0.05$; Cohen's d = effect measure ($d \geq 0.2$ = small, ≥ 0.5 = moderate, ≥ 0.8 = large effect)

Main complaint severity	Course						Difference from admission			
	Admission (A)			Discharge (D)/ follow-up (F)			A–D/A–F		Significance	Effect size
	n	M	SD		M	SD	*n*	ΔM	*p*	*d*
M79 other diseases of soft tissue	210	74.00	17.48	D	49.62	21.11	210	−24.38	< 0.001	**−1.25**
	175	73.60	18.01	F	51.49	23.97	175	−22.11	< 0.001	**−1.03**
M25 other diseases of the spine	75	70.93	17.72	D	42.80	21.84	75	−28.13	< 0.001	**−1.41**
	57	70.70	15.57	F	47.02	25.28	57	−23.68	< 0.001	**−1.13**

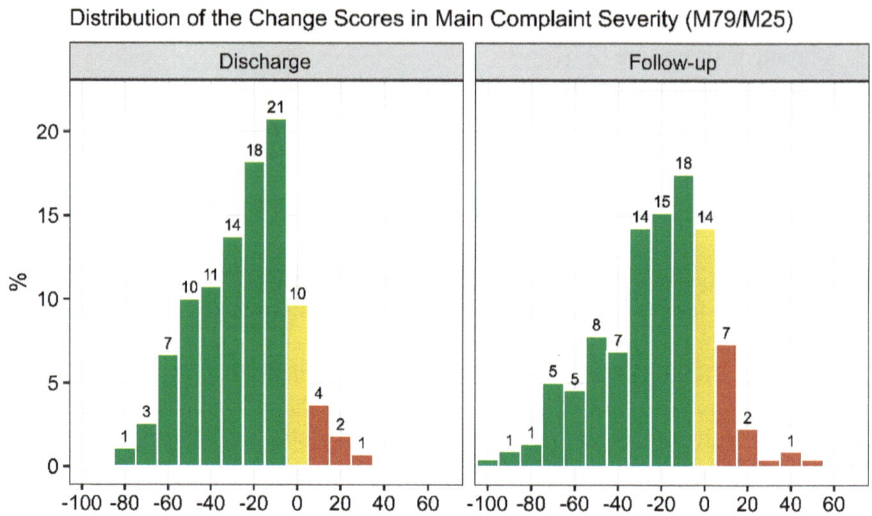

Fig. 5.132 Distribution of the change scores in main complaint severity between hospital admission and hospital discharge or at hospital admission and at follow-up for patients with a M79 and/or M25 diagnosis in 2023 (A–D $n = 269$; A–D–F $n = 217$); negative differences correspond to an improvement

($d = -1.00$, $p < 0.001$); and the burnout scales: exhaustion ($d = -0.72$, $p < 0.001$) and loss of motivation ($d = -0.51$, $p < 0.001$), and the GAD scale ($d = -0.99$, $p < 0.001$). These positive effects persisted with a moderate to large magnitude until follow-up, except for the PSQ subscale 'Demands', for which only a small to moderate effect remained ($d = -0.47$, $p < 0.001$).

Complaint complexes relating to Psycho-Vegetative Stability (overall index, dizziness, sleep, and heat balance) were also found to have significantly improved, with moderate to large effect sizes, at hospital discharge ($d = 0.88$, $p < 0.001$; $d = -0.50$, $p < 0.001$; $d = -0.70$, $p < 0.001$; $d = -0.69$, $p < 0.001$, respectively). The results at follow-up were particularly evident for sleep quality ($d = -0.57$, $p < 0.001$). Table 5.121 and Fig. 5.135 present the results in more detail.

An analysis of self-assessed symptom burden using the psycho-vegetative complaint questionnaire shows a clear predominance of sleep-related complaints, as well as back and joint pain. In addition, affective symptoms, poor concentration, abdominal pressure, and some thermoregulatory symptoms are more pronounced in this diagnostic group. Across admission, discharge, and follow-up values, there was a particular improvement in affective and fatigue-related symptoms (Fig. 5.136).

5.4.4 Chronic Headaches G43 and G44

The most significant headache syndromes are migraine and tension headaches. These are mostly covered by the two ICD-10 codes, G43 and G44. Many people in Germany suffer from chronic headaches. Around 54 million people in

Table 5.120 Global assessments of treatment success for patients with a somatic M79 or M25 secondary diagnosis, surveyed at discharge ($n = 210/n = 75$) and at follow-up ($n = 177/n = 57$) in 2023

Overall success of the therapy		**Very good**		**Good**		**Moderate**		**No success**		**Total**	
		n	%	*n*	%	*n*	%	*n*	%	*n*	%
M54 Back pain	D	29	13.8	105	50.0	68	32.4	8	3.8	210	100
	F	48	27.1	78	44.1	48	27.1	3	1.7	177	100
M53 other diseases of the spine	D	18	24.0	40	53.3	17	22.7	0	0.0	75	100
	F	23	40.4	24	42.1	10	17.5	0	0.0	57	100
Treatment worthwhile		**Very worthwhile**		**Worthwhile**		**Not worth it**		**Rather harmed**		**Total**	
		n	%	*n*	%	*n*	%	*n*	%	*n*	%
M54 Back pain	D	90	42.9	108	51.4	9	4.3	3	1.4	210	100
	F	100	56.5	68	38.4	9	5.1	0	0.0	177	100
M53 other diseases of the spine	D	39	52.0	34	45.3	2	2.7	0	0.0	75	100
	F	43	75.4	13	22.8	1	1.8	0	0.0	57	100

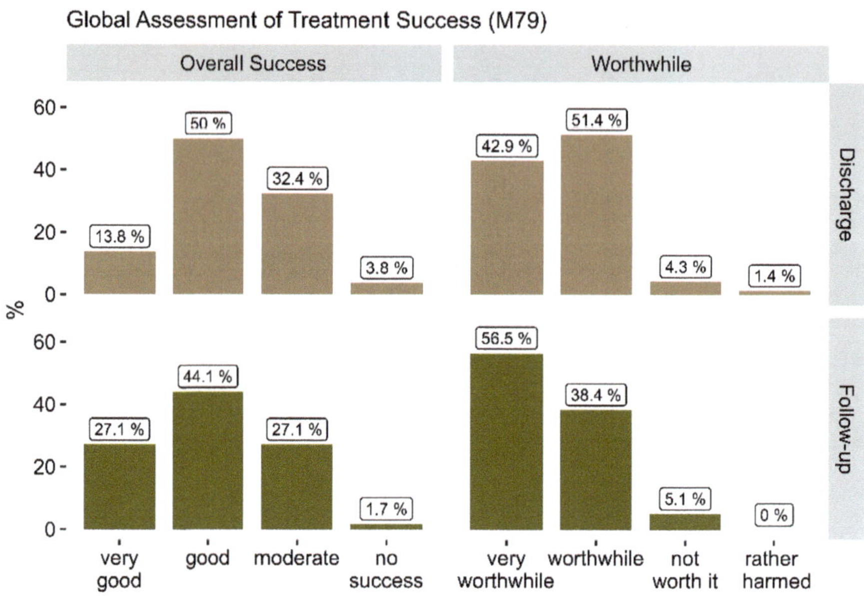

Fig. 5.133 Global assessments of treatment success for patients with a somatic secondary diagnosis of M79, surveyed at discharge ($n = 210$) and at follow-up ($n = 177$) in 2023

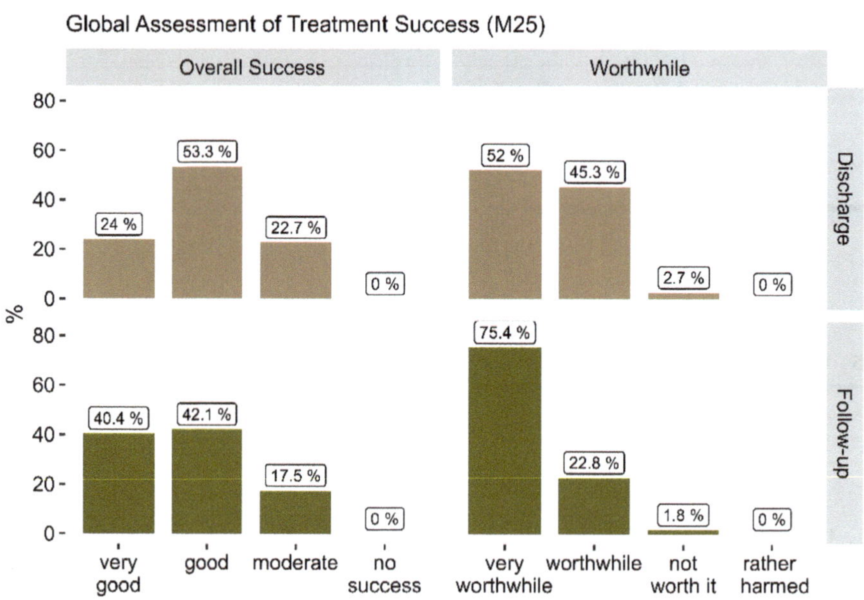

Fig. 5.134 Global assessments of treatment success for patients with a somatic secondary diagnosis of M25, surveyed at discharge ($n = 75$), and follow-up ($n = 57$) in 2023

Table 5.121 Changes in various parameters for patients with a secondary M79 and/or M25 diagnosis in 2023; *t*-test: Cohen's *d* = effect measure ($d \geq 0.2$ = small effect, ≥ 0.5 = moderate effect, ≥ 0.8 = large effect)

Somatic diagnosis M79 and/or M25	Course						Difference from admission			
		Admission (A)		Discharge (D)/ follow-up (F)			A–D/A–F		Significance	Effect size
	n	M	SD	D/F	M	SD	*n*	M	*p*	*d*
ICD symptom ratings (ISR)										
Total value	269	1.23	0.59	D	0.90	0.55	269	−0.34	<0.001	**−0.59**
	212	1.22	0.59	F	0.87	0.59	212	−0.35	<0.001	**−0.59**
Depression	269	2.17	0.89	D	1.33	0.89	269	−0.84	<0.001	**−0.94**
	212	2.17	0.91	F	1.41	0.93	212	−0.76	<0.001	**−0.82**
Anxiety	269	1.49	1.08	D	1.09	0.96	269	−0.40	<0.001	**−0.39**
	212	1.44	1.09	F	1.03	1.00	212	−0.41	<0.001	−0.39
Obsessive-compulsion	269	1.05	1.05	D	0.83	0.91	269	−0.22	<0.001	−0.22
	212	1.03	1.04	F	0.78	0.89	212	−0.25	<0.001	−0.26
Somatoform	269	0.92	0.90	D	0.67	0.82	269	−0.25	<0.001	−0.29
	212	0.88	0.89	F	0.57	0.78	212	−0.31	<0.001	−0.37
Eating disorder	269	0.71	0.91	D	0.59	0.78	269	−0.12	<0.001	−0.14
	212	0.75	0.93	F	0.62	0.82	212	−0.13	0.006	−0.15
Pain disability index										
Total index	266	32.17	15.10	D	27.92	15.35	266	−4.25	<0.001	−0.28
	209	32.11	15.21	F	27.30	16.81	209	−4.80	<0.001	−0.30
Family/domestic obligations	266	5.42	2.69	D	4.73	2.77	266	−0.69	<0.001	−0.25
	209	5.48	2.70	F	4.62	2.94	209	−0.86	<0.001	−0.30
Recreation	266	6.03	2.57	D	5.08	2.76	266	−0.96	<0.001	−0.36
	209	6.04	2.56	F	4.99	2.95	209	−1.05	<0.001	−0.38
Social activity	266	5.11	2.96	D	4.56	3.02	266	−0.55	0.002	−0.18
	209	5.00	3.03	F	4.26	3.13	209	−0.74	<0.001	−0.24
Profession	266	5.77	3.06	D	5.49	3.05	266	−0.28	0.110	–
	209	5.72	3.06	F	4.87	3.37	209	−0.85	<0.001	−0.26
Sex life	266	4.92	3.60	D	4.22	3.49	266	−0.70	<0.001	−0.20
	209	4.99	3.63	F	4.55	3.65	209	−0.44	0.056	–
Self-sufficiency	266	2.58	2.55	D	2.17	2.50	266	−0.40	0.011	−0.16
	209	2.53	2.48	F	2.16	2.57	209	−0.36	0.027	−0.14
Essentials activities	266	2.34	2.65	D	1.67	2.33	266	−0.67	<0.001	−0.27
	209	2.35	2.62	F	1.84	2.45	209	−0.51	0.005	−0.20
Life satisfaction										
Total value	268	20.81	34.77	D	37.55	37.28	268	16.74	<0.001	0.46
	215	22.48	33.35	F	37.02	35.77	215	14.54	<0.001	0.42
Friends/acquaintances	268	4.62	7.19	D	6.19	6.58	268	1.56	<0.001	0.23
	215	4.64	7.11	F	5.01	6.22	215	0.37	0.377	–
Leisure/hobbies	268	0.79	6.45	D	2.90	6.13	268	2.10	<0.001	0.33
	215	0.76	6.24	F	2.65	5.12	215	1.89	<0.001	0.33
Health	268	−5.78	5.38	D	−0.96	7.21	268	4.82	<0.001	**0.75**
	215	−5.68	5.30	F	−0.87	7.65	215	4.82	<0.001	**0.72**
Income	268	2.55	7.12	D	3.79	6.80	268	1.24	<0.001	0.18
	215	2.60	6.79	F	3.71	6.62	215	1.11	0.004	0.17
Profession	268	0.43	7.21	D	1.24	6.86	268	0.82	0.015	0.12
	215	0.58	7.17	F	2.51	6.73	215	1.93	<0.001	0.28

(continued)

Table 5.121 (continued)

Somatic diagnosis M79 and/or M25	Course						Difference from admission			
		Admission (A)		Discharge (D)/ follow-up (F)			A–D/A–F		Significance	Effect size
	n	M	SD	D/F	M	SD	*n*	M	*p*	*d*
Housing situation	268	6.30	7.59	D	6.99	7.90	268	0.69	0.067	–
	215	6.53	7.50	F	7.31	7.09	215	0.79	0.102	0.11
Family/children	268	6.81	8.55	D	9.35	8.06	268	2.54	<0.001	0.31
	215	7.35	8.64	F	8.75	7.89	215	1.40	0.008	0.17
Partnership	268	5.08	9.64	D	8.05	9.51	268	2.97	<0.001	0.31
	215	5.68	9.63	F	7.94	8.55	215	2.26	<0.001	0.25
SOC										
Total value	267	56.08	12.29	D	61.30	12.95	267	5.22	<0.001	0.41
	212	56.56	11.86	F	60.97	13.27	212	4.42	<0.001	0.35
Meaningfulness	267	18.93	4.06	D	20.19	4.15	267	1.26	<0.001	0.31
	212	18.99	3.97	F	20.00	4.43	212	1.00	<0.001	0.24
Comprehensi-bility	267	20.63	5.62	D	22.94	5.82	267	2.31	<0.001	0.40
	212	20.86	5.62	F	22.92	5.88	212	2.06	<0.001	0.36
Manageability	267	16.52	4.71	D	18.18	4.87	267	1.66	<0.001	0.35
	212	16.71	4.53	F	18.06	4.83	212	1.35	<0.001	0.29
WHO-5 well-being and vitality										
Well-being	268	26.66	17.76	D	50.97	23.82	268	24.31	<0.001	**1.14**
	212	26.91	17.43	F	42.34	24.27	212	15.43	<0.001	0.71
Vitality	268	24.03	16.19	D	43.25	21.41	268	19.22	<0.001	**0.99**
	212	24.72	16.00	F	40.33	22.67	212	15.61	<0.001	0.78
SWOP										
Self-efficacy	267	12.25	2.98	D	13.30	2.95	267	1.05	<0.001	0.35
	210	12.47	2.96	F	13.48	2.96	210	1.01	<0.001	0.34
Optimism	267	4.92	1.48	D	5.53	1.49	267	0.61	<0.001	0.41
	210	4.96	1.49	F	5.41	1.47	210	0.45	<0.001	0.31
Pessimism	267	4.52	1.38	D	4.20	1.39	267	−0.32	<0.001	−0.23
	210	4.51	1.39	F	4.30	1.43	210	−0.21	0.057	–
SSS										
Total value	264	51.94	17.68	D	56.55	15.77	264	4.61	<0.001	0.27
	205	52.95	17.32	F	55.03	16.24	205	2.08	0.010	0.12
Emotional	264	17.11	5.71	D	18.27	5.25	264	1.17	<0.001	0.21
	205	17.41	5.57	F	17.87	5.37	205	0.46	0.126	–
Social interaction	264	10.26	3.91	D	11.18	3.53	264	0.92	<0.001	0.24
	205	10.40	3.84	F	10.85	3.64	205	0.45	0.016	0.12
Material	264	11.24	4.59	D	12.56	3.88	264	1.32	<0.001	0.31
	205	11.61	4.36	F	12.29	3.99	205	0.67	0.001	0.16
Affective	264	8.58	3.23	D	9.27	2.87	264	0.69	<0.001	0.22
	205	8.79	3.25	F	9.00	3.03	205	0.21	0.155	–
Tedium measure (burnout)										
Total value	268	4.38	0.88	D	3.80	1.03	268	−0.58	<0.001	**−0.60**
	216	4.34	0.85	F	3.74	1.07	216	−0.60	<0.001	**−0.60**
Discouragement	268	3.89	1.10	D	3.37	1.15	268	−0.53	<0.001	−0.47
	216	3.85	1.08	F	3.28	1.20	216	−0.57	<0.001	**−0.50**
Exhaustion	268	5.23	0.90	D	4.47	1.14	268	−0.76	<0.001	**−0.72**
	216	5.19	0.89	F	4.45	1.22	216	−0.73	<0.001	**−0.67**

(continued)

Table 5.121 (continued)

Somatic diagnosis M79 and/or M25	Course						Difference from admission			
		Admission (A)		Discharge (D)/ follow-up (F)			A–D/A–F		Significance	Effect size
	n	M	SD	D/F	M	SD	*n*	M	*p*	*d*
Loss of motivation	268	4.34	0.87	D	3.85	1.02	268	−0.49	<0.001	**−0.51**
	216	4.29	0.82	F	3.80	1.03	216	−0.49	<0.001	**−0.51**
PSQ										
Total value	268	61.16	16.31	D	41.49	19.52	268	−19.66	<0.001	**−1.09**
	214	60.93	16.08	F	48.81	19.31	214	−12.12	<0.001	**−0.67**
Worries	268	52.96	22.12	D	38.11	23.55	268	−14.85	<0.001	**−0.65**
	214	52.55	21.25	F	40.47	23.53	214	−12.09	<0.001	**−0.54**
Demands	268	51.59	22.52	D	27.26	21.74	268	−24.33	<0.001	**−1.10**
	214	51.65	22.41	F	41.09	22.37	214	−10.56	<0.001	−0.47
Joy	268	30.85	18.42	D	48.36	23.47	268	17.51	<0.001	**0.82**
	214	31.40	18.54	F	42.27	24.02	214	10.87	<0.001	**0.50**
Tension	268	70.92	19.46	D	48.96	23.79	268	−21.97	<0.001	**−1.00**
	214	70.90	19.11	F	55.95	23.31	214	−14.95	<0.001	**−0.70**
PSQI										
Total value	264	11.12	3.91	D	10.10	4.49	264	−1.02	<0.001	−0.24
	211	11.18	3.95	F	9.40	4.42	211	−1.78	<0.001	−0.42
Sleep quality	264	1.84	0.64	D	1.48	0.70	264	−0.37	<0.001	**−0.55**
	211	1.87	0.65	F	1.56	0.74	211	−0.31	<0.001	−0.45
Sleep latency	264	1.80	1.08	D	1.49	1.06	264	−0.31	<0.001	−0.29
	211	1.75	1.09	F	1.55	1.06	211	−0.19	0.004	**−0.18**
Sleep duration	264	1.66	0.89	D	1.52	0.91	264	−0.14	0.012	−0.16
	211	1.68	0.89	F	1.41	0.90	211	−0.27	<0.001	**−0.30**
Sleep efficiency	264	1.47	1.19	D	1.20	1.20	264	−0.27	<0.001	−0.23
	211	1.48	1.19	F	1.06	1.15	211	−0.42	<0.001	−0.36
Sleep disorders	264	1.80	0.65	D	1.63	0.61	264	−0.17	<0.001	−0.27
	211	1.81	0.66	F	1.65	0.68	211	−0.16	0.001	−0.23
Sleeping pills	264	0.66	1.15	D	1.54	1.42	264	0.88	<0.001	**0.68**
	211	0.69	1.18	F	0.0.65	1.14	211	−0.04	0.633	–
Daytime sleepiness	264	1.89	0.71	D	1.25	0.82	264	−0.64	<0.001	**−0.83**
	211	1.91	0.70	F	1.51	0.87	211	−0.39	<0.001	−0.49
GAD										
Total value	266	11.04	4.95	D	6.44	4.28	266	−4.60	<0.001	**−0.99**
	207	11.02	4.87	F	7.43	4.99	207	−3.58	<0.001	**−0.73**
Complaint complexes of psycho-vegetative stability										
Complaints index	269	0.21	0.43	D	0.77	0.75	269	0.56	<0.001	**0.88**
	216	0.19	0.40	F	0.69	0.74	216	0.50	<0.001	**0.79**
Total value	269	66.17	15.84	D	48.26	19.32	269	−17.91	<0.001	**−1.00**
	216	66.25	15.41	F	53.44	19.82	216	−12.82	<0.001	**−0.71**
Dizziness	269	3.64	2.15	D	2.54	2.25	269	−1.10	<0.001	**−0.50**
	216	3.63	2.17	F	2.89	2.35	216	−0.74	<0.001	−0.33
Sleep	269	7.38	2.09	D	5.70	2.64	269	−1.69	<0.001	**−0.70**
	216	7.39	2.09	F	6.05	2.54	216	−1.34	<0.001	**−0.57**
Heat balance	269	6.08	2.70	D	4.20	2.74	269	−1.88	<0.001	**−0.69**
	216	6.10	2.70	F	4.94	2.61	216	−1.16	<0.001	−0.44

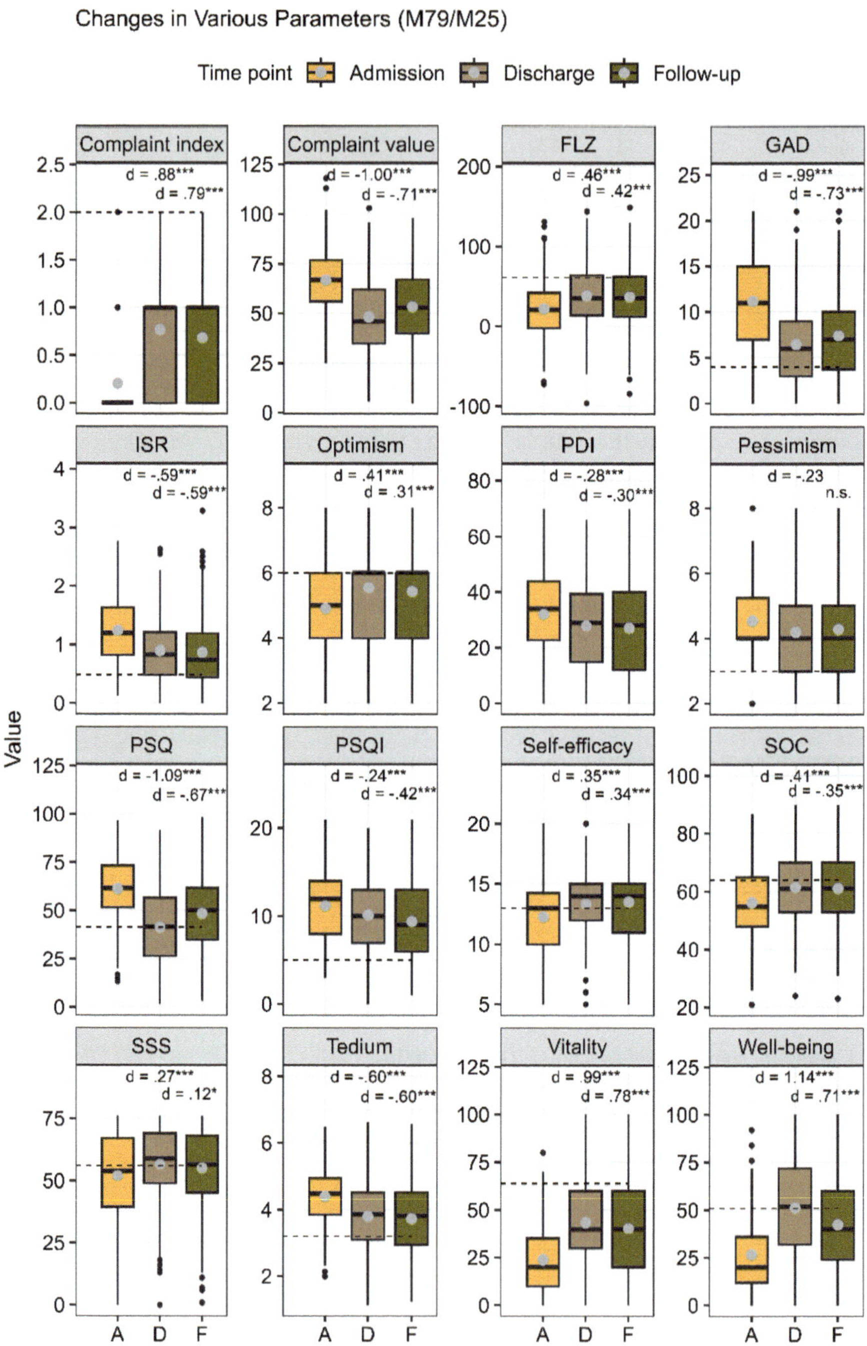

Fig. 5.135 Changes in various parameters for patients with a M79/M25 diagnosis in 2023; the dashed black lines indicate the desired target values; significance: $*p < 0.05$, $**p < 0.01$, $***p < 0.001$; Cohen's d = effect measure ($d \geq 0.2$ = small effect, ≥ 0.5 = moderate effect, ≥ 0.8 = large effect); the graph shows all available data, the effect sizes refer to the individual comparison (A–D/A–F)

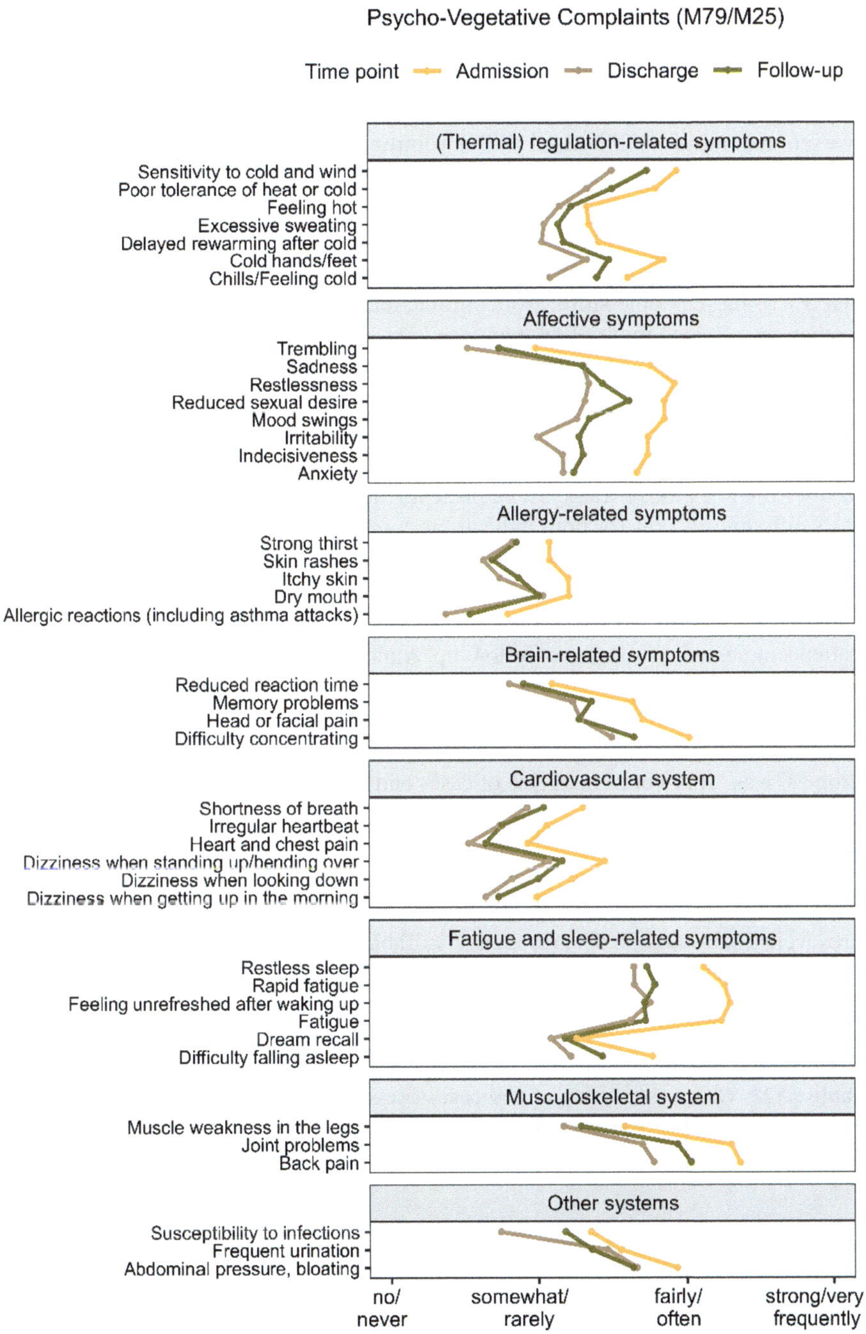

Fig. 5.136 Psycho-vegetative complaints; change in complaints for patients with a M79/M25 diagnosis at admission: $n = 286$. at discharge: $n = 269$ and at follow-up: $n = 216$ in 2023

Germany—about 70% of the population—experience temporary or persistent headaches. Tension headaches affect 53.6% of all patients with headaches, while migraines account for 38.4% of diagnoses.

Symptoms include pulsating or throbbing headaches, usually on one side, which worsen with movement. Nausea and/or vomiting, sensitivity to light and noise, and visual and speech disturbances are common. Tension headaches are accompanied by a pressing or pulling sensation, rather than a pulsating one. The pain intensity is mild to moderate. Unlike migraines, nausea and vomiting are not present. Around a third of the German population experiences tension headaches at least once a month, and 3% of these people suffer from chronic tension headaches. As with migraines, women are affected more often than men [35].

For patients with tension headaches (G44), the VAS showed a very high effect size at discharge ($d = -1.35$, $p < 0.001$) and at follow-up ($d = -1.22$, $p < 0.001$). Similar positive effects that were maintained until follow-up were found for patients suffering from migraine (G43): discharge ($d = -1.07$, $p < 0.001$); follow-up ($d = -1.05$, $p < 0.001$). Table 5.122 presents the data, and Fig. 5.137 illustrates the VAS difference scores for both indications combined.

At hospital discharge, half of the migraine patients (49.5%) reported a 'good' outcome, while 12.9% rated it as 'very good'. At follow-up, the assessment was slightly better, with 29.3% rating it as 'very good' and 40.2% as 'good'. 6.1% of patients indicated no success at follow-up. Almost all patients thought the treatment was 'worthwhile' or 'very worthwhile' (91.0% at discharge and 93.9% at follow-up) (Fig. 5.138).

Similarly, the global treatment success rate at discharge for 'other headache syndromes' was 'very good' in 12.1% of cases and 'good' in 52.5% of cases. Moderate success was reported by 31.9% of patients. At follow-up, success was rated slightly higher than at discharge, with 27.0% answering 'very good' and 41.7% answering 'good'. At discharge, 40.4% of patients answered that the hospital stay was 'very worthwhile' and 51.8% answered that it was 'worthwhile'. At follow-up, these figures were 56.5% and 36.5%, respectively (Table 5.123, Fig. 5.139).

Changes in protective and risk factors, including mental load, are comparable to those observed in patients with other somatic secondary diagnoses. Significant,

Table 5.122 Global assessments of treatment success for patients with a somatic G43 or G44 secondary diagnosis, surveyed at discharge ($n = 101/n = 141$) and at follow-up ($n = 83/n = 114$) in 2023; t-test for paired samples; significance at $p < 0.05$; Cohen's d = effect measure ($d \geq 0.2$ = small, ≥ 0.5 = moderate, ≥ 0.8 = large effect)

Main complaint severity	Course						Difference from admission			
	Admission (A)			Discharge (D)/ follow-up (F)			A–D/A–F		Significance	Effect size
	n	M	SD		M	SD	*n*	ΔM	*p*	*d*
G43 migraine	101	72.67	17.54	D	50.59	22.97	101	−22.08	<0.001	**−1.07**
	83	71.45	17.61	F	49.04	24.53	83	−22.41	<0.001	**−1.05**
G44 other headache	141	73.97	16.64	D	47.16	22.43	141	−26.81	<0.001	**−1.35**
	114	74.21	16.66	F	48.68	24.44	114	−25.53	<0.001	**−1.22**

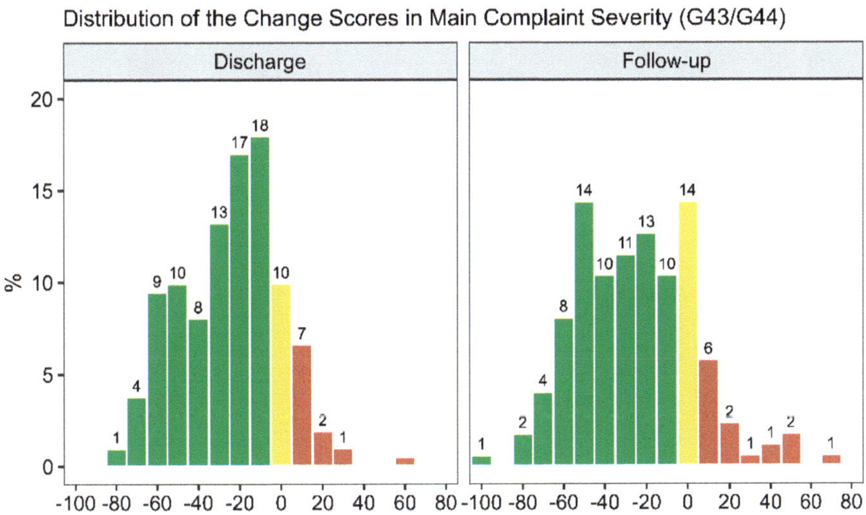

Fig. 5.137 Distribution of the change scores in main complaint severity between hospital admission and hospital discharge or hospital admission and follow-up for patients with a G43 and/or G44 diagnosis in 2023 (A–D n = 212; A–D–F n = 174); negative differences correspond to an improvement

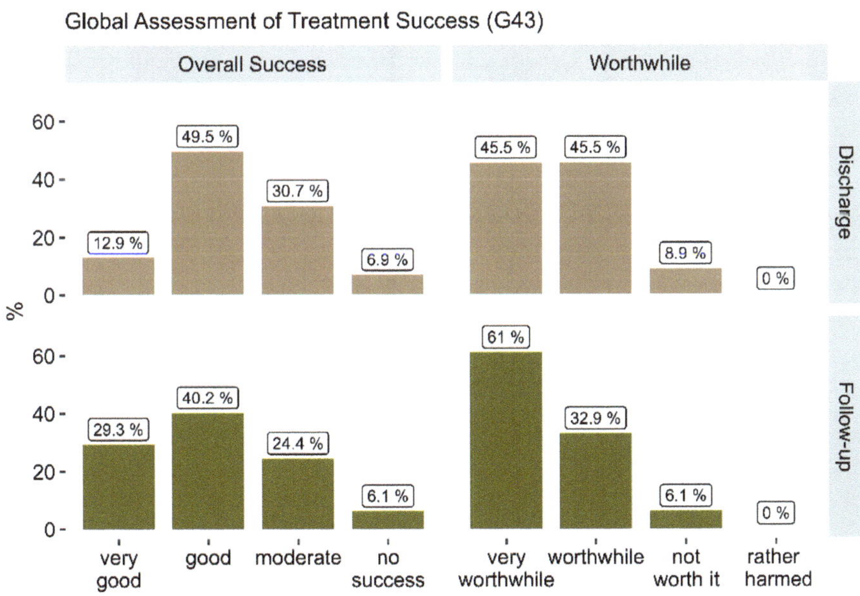

Fig. 5.138 Global assessments of treatment success for patients with a somatic secondary diagnosis G43, surveyed at discharge (n = 101) and at follow-up (n = 82) in 2023

Table 5.123 Global assessments of treatment success for patients with a somatic G43 or G44 secondary diagnosis, surveyed at discharge ($n = 101/n = 141$) and at follow-up ($n = 82/n = 115$) in 2023

Overall success of the therapy		**Very good**		**Good**		**Moderate**		**No success**		**Total**	
		n	%	*n*	%	*n*	%	*n*	%	*n*	%
G43 migraine	D	13	12.9	50	49.5	31	30.7	7	6.9	101	100
	F	24	29.3	33	40.2	20	24.4	5	6.1	82	100
G44 other headache syndromes	D	17	12.1	74	52.5	45	31.9	5	3.5	141	100
	F	31	27.0	48	41.7	30	26.1	6	5.2	115	100
Treatment worthwhile		**Very worthwhile**		**Worthwhile**		**Not worth it**		**Rather harmed**		**Total**	
		n	%	*n*	%	*n*	%	*n*	%	*n*	%
G43 migraine	D	46	45.5	46	45.5	9	8.9	0	0.0	101	100
	F	50	61.0	27	32.9	5	6.1	0	0.0	82	100
G44 other headache syndromes	D	57	40.4	73	51.8	10	7.1	1	0.7	141	100
	F	65	56.5	42	36.5	8	7.0	0	0.0	115	100

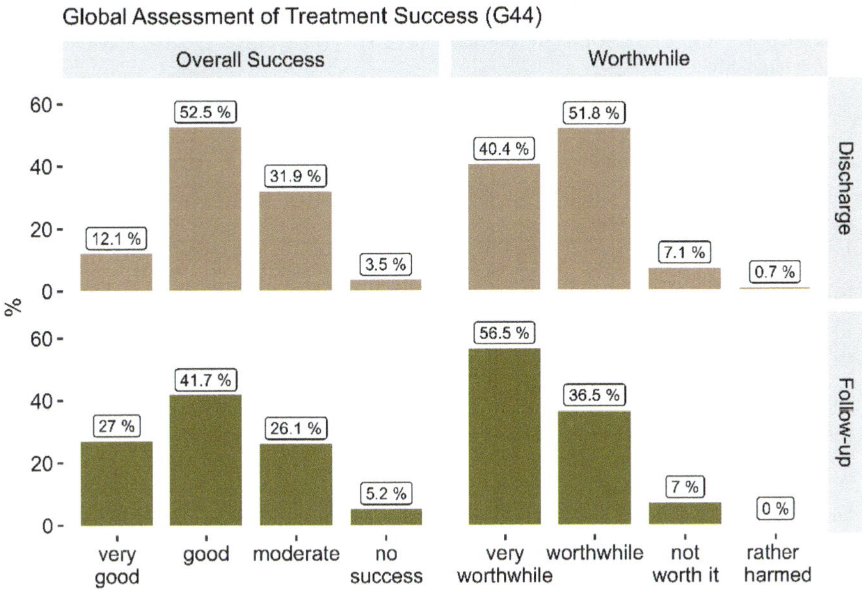

Fig. 5.139 Global assessments of treatment success for patients with a somatic secondary diagnosis G44, surveyed at discharge (n = 141) and at follow-up (n = 101) in 2023

moderate-to-large improvements were found in particular for ISR depression (D: $d = -0.98$, $p < 0.001$; F: $d = -0.77$, $p < 0.001$), well-being (D: $d = 1.25$, $p < 0.001$; F: $d = 0.79$, $p < 0.001$), vitality (D: $d = 0.94$, $p < 0.001$; F: $d = 0.76$, $p < 0.001$), Generalised Anxiety Disorder (D: $d = -0.95$, $p < 0.001$; F: $d = -0.72$, $p < 0.001$) and burnout (D: $d = -0.67$, $p < 0.001$; F: $d = -0.59$, $p < 0.001$). Regarding perceived stress, the largest effects were found for the 'Tension' subscale ($d = -1.10$ for D, $p < 0.001$; $d = -0.65$ for F, $p < 0.001$).

The overall complaint index of Psycho-Vegetative Stability decreased significantly at discharge ($d = 0.97$, $p < 0.001$), and the positive effects remained until the follow-up ($d = 0.94$, $p < 0.001$). Sleep-related difficulties in particular showed significant improvement at discharge ($d = -0.67$, $p < 0.001$) and at follow-up ($d = -0.70$, $p < 0.001$). These positive effects on sleep were reflected in the 'sleep quality' subscale of the PSQI questionnaire (D: $d = -0.56$, $p < 0.001$; F: $d = -0.50$, $p < 0.001$). Table 5.124 and Fig. 5.140 provide an overview of the results of the protective and risk factors.

Taking a closer glance at the self-reported symptom burden using the questionnaire on psycho-vegetative complaints, it is evident that headaches, back pain, and fatigue- or sleep-related issues were the most prevalent upon admission. These symptoms were all less frequently reported at discharge and follow-up (Fig. 5.141).

Table 5.124 Changes in various parameters for patients with a secondary G43 and/or G44 diagnosis in 2023; *t*-test: Cohen's d = effect measure ($d \geq 0.2$ = small effect, ≥ 0.5 = moderate effect, ≥ 0.8 = large effect)

Somatic diagnosis G43 and/or G44	Course			Discharge (D)/ follow-up (F)			Difference from admission A–D/A–F		Significance	Effect size
		Admission (A)								
	n	M	SD	D/F	M	SD	*n*	M	*p*	*d*
ICD symptom ratings (ISR)										
Total value	213	1.28	0.61	D	0.94	0.58	213	−0.34	<0.001	**−0.57**
	170	1.26	0.62	F	0.88	0.58	170	−0.38	<0.001	**−0.63**
Depression	213	2.22	0.88	D	1.36	0.89	213	−0.87	<0.001	**−0.98**
	170	2.18	0.89	F	1.47	0.97	170	−0.71	<0.001	**−0.77**
Anxiety	213	1.61	1.09	D	1.20	0.98	213	−0.42	<0.001	−0.40
	170	1.60	1.09	F	1.12	0.97	170	−0.48	<0.001	−0.46
Obsessive-compulsion	213	1.07	1.05	D	0.87	0.97	213	−0.20	<0.001	−0.20
	170	1.06	1.05	F	0.79	0.92	170	−0.27	<0.001	−0.27
Somatoform	213	0.98	0.90	D	0.70	0.81	213	−0.29	<0.001	−0.33
	170	0.93	0.86	F	0.59	0.77	170	−0.34	<0.001	−0.41
Eating disorder	213	0.70	0.89	D	0.62	0.82	213	−0.08	0.042	−0.10
	170	0.74	0.91	F	0.58	0.83	170	−0.16	0.003	−0.19
Pain disability index										
Total index	212	32.50	15.45	D	28.56	15.82	212	−3.94	<0.001	−0.25
	164	32.87	15.69	F	26.32	17.08	164	−6.55	<0.001	−0.40
Family/domestic obligations	212	5.30	2.73	D	4.78	2.73	212	−0.52	<0.001	−0.19
	164	5.41	2.72	F	4.47	2.95	164	−0.94	<0.001	−0.33
Recreation	212	5.81	2.74	D	5.16	2.84	212	−0.65	<0.001	−0.23
	164	5.90	2.77	F	4.82	3.01	164	−1.09	<0.001	−0.37
Social activity	212	5.42	2.91	D	4.85	2.89	212	−0.57	0.002	−0.20
	164	5.54	2.93	F	4.60	3.09	164	−0.93	<0.001	−0.31
Profession	212	6.19	2.97	D	5.57	3.27	212	−0.62	0.001	−0.20
	164	6.14	2.99	F	4.82	3.38	164	−1.32	<0.001	−0.41
Sex life	212	4.82	3.63	D	4.14	3.45	212	−0.68	0.002	−0.19
	164	4.84	3.68	F	3.87	3.62	164	−0.97	<0.001	−0.27
Self-sufficiency	212	2.60	2.76	D	2.34	2.71	212	−0.26	0.178	–
	164	2.66	2.72	F	2.02	2.52	164	−0.63	0.006	−0.24
Essentials activities	212	2.38	2.69	D	1.73	2.43	212	−0.65	<0.001	−0.25
	164	2.43	2.72	F	1.71	2.43	164	−0.71	<0.001	−0.28
Life satisfaction										
Total value	212	16.89	33.91	D	36.73	36.35	212	19.84	<0.001	**0.56**
	171	19.04	33.59	F	36.94	34.55	171	17.89	<0.001	**0.53**
Friends/ acquaintances	212	3.82	6.71	D	6.31	6.82	212	2.50	<0.001	0.37
	171	3.90	6.29	F	5.32	6.32	171	1.42	0.001	0.23
Leisure/hobbies	212	0.19	5.66	D	3.00	6.35	212	2.81	<0.001	0.47
	171	0.46	5.68	F	2.90	5.65	171	2.44	<0.001	0.43
Health	212	−6.41	5.37	D	−1.56	7.44	212	4.85	<0.001	**0.73**
	171	−6.14	5.62	F	−0.63	7.82	171	5.51	<0.001	**0.80**
Income	212	1.45	7.55	D	3.02	7.03	212	1.57	<0.001	0.21
	171	1.71	7.39	F	2.86	6.38	171	1.15	0.004	0.16

(continued)

Table 5.124 (continued)

Somatic diagnosis G43 and/or G44	Course						Difference from admission			
		Admission (A)		Discharge (D)/ follow-up (F)			A–D/A–F		Significance	Effect size
	n	M	SD	D/F	M	SD	*n*	M	*p*	*d*
Profession	212	−0.41	6.90	D	0.97	6.77	212	1.37	<0.001	0.20
	171	−0.13	6.97	F	2.53	6.99	171	2.67	<0.001	0.38
Housing situation	212	6.01	7.76	D	7.43	7.71	212	1.42	<0.001	0.18
	171	6.15	7.58	F	7.36	6.83	171	1.20	0.057	–
Family/children	212	6.52	8.23	D	9.42	7.77	212	2.89	<0.001	0.36
	171	6.87	8.43	F	8.56	7.97	171	1.69	0.001	0.21
Partnership	212	5.71	9.81	D	8.15	9.22	212	2.43	<0.001	0.25
	171	6.23	9.68	F	8.04	8.96	171	1.80	0.002	0.19
SOC										
Total value	212	56.17	12.31	D	60.21	12.04	212	4.04	<0.001	0.33
	168	57.13	12.68	F	61.88	12.67	168	4.75	<0.001	0.37
Meaningfulness	212	18.71	4.02	D	19.71	4.02	212	1.01	<0.001	0.25
	168	18.88	4.02	F	20.12	4.32	168	1.24	<0.001	0.30
Comprehensibility	212	20.83	5.70	D	22.52	5.36	212	1.70	<0.001	0.31
	168	21.27	5.87	F	23.40	5.87	168	2.14	<0.001	0.36
Manageability	212	16.64	4.84	D	17.98	4.91	212	1.34	<0.001	0.27
	168	16.90	4.93	F	18.36	4.77	168	1.46	<0.001	0.30
WHO-5 well-being and vitality										
Well-being	212	24.53	16.05	D	50.00	22.99	212	25.47	<0.001	**1.25**
	169	24.71	15.67	F	41.75	24.41	169	17.04	<0.001	**0.79**
Vitality	212	24.06	15.99	D	42.38	21.76	212	18.33	<0.001	**0.94**
	169	25.06	16.06	F	40.00	21.94	169	14.94	<0.001	**0.76**
SWOP										
Self-efficacy	212	12.06	2.86	D	12.94	2.83	212	0.88	<0.001	0.31
	167	12.19	2.75	F	13.28	2.95	167	1.10	<0.001	0.38
Optimism	212	4.95	1.42	D	5.53	1.41	212	0.58	<0.001	0.41
	167	4.99	1.44	F	5.50	1.46	167	0.51	<0.001	0.35
Pessimism	212	4.62	1.49	D	4.33	1.43	212	−0.29	0.002	−0.20
	167	4.57	1.48	F	4.34	1.46	167	−0.23	0.055	–
SSS										
Total value	210	51.98	16.92	D	57.05	15.02	210	5.07	<0.001	0.31
	164	52.35	16.94	F	54.91	16.88	164	2.55	0.004	0.15
Emotional	210	17.31	5.69	D	18.45	5.15	210	1.14	<0.001	0.21
	164	17.42	5.69	F	17.82	5.56	164	0.40	0.232	–
Social interaction	210	10.31	3.69	D	11.49	3.23	210	1.18	<0.001	0.34
	164	10.34	3.73	F	10.99	3.78	164	0.65	0.004	0.17
Material	210	10.96	4.62	D	12.35	3.94	210	1.39	<0.001	0.32
	164	11.28	4.49	F	12.09	4.30	164	0.81	<0.001	0.18
Affective	210	8.68	3.08	D	9.47	2.63	210	0.79	<0.001	0.27
	164	8.70	3.14	F	8.98	2.99	164	0.29	0.080	–
Tedium measure (burnout)										
Total value	212	4.42	0.88	D	3.76	1.04	212	−0.66	<0.001	**−0.67**
	171	4.37	0.88	F	3.75	1.12	171	−0.61	<0.001	**−0.59**
Discouragement	212	3.93	1.09	D	3.33	1.14	212	−0.60	<0.001	**−0.53**
	171	3.87	1.09	F	3.33	1.26	171	−0.55	<0.001	−0.46

(continued)

Table 5.124 (continued)

Somatic diagnosis G43 and/or G44	Course						Difference from admission			
		Admission (A)		Discharge (D)/ follow-up (F)			A–D/A–F		Significance	Effect size
	n	M	SD	D/F	M	SD	*n*	M	*p*	*d*
Exhaustion	212	5.22	0.96	D	4.40	1.20	212	−0.83	<0.001	**−0.75**
	171	5.18	0.96	F	4.41	1.23	171	−0.77	<0.001	**−0.69**
Loss of motivation	212	4.43	0.81	D	3.86	1.00	212	−0.57	<0.001	**−0.61**
	171	4.37	0.80	F	3.82	1.06	171	−0.55	<0.001	**−0.57**
PSQ										
Total value	212	61.84	17.58	D	41.33	19.60	212	−20.51	<0.001	**−1.10**
	170	60.65	17.88	F	48.27	20.08	170	−12.37	<0.001	**−0.65**
Worries	212	55.35	24.25	D	38.71	25.23	212	−16.64	<0.001	**−0.67**
	170	53.10	24.06	F	40.82	25.93	170	−12.27	<0.001	−0.49
Demands	212	51.13	26.78	D	24.50	21.48	212	−26.64	<0.001	**−1.09**
	170	50.67	27.15	F	40.08	25.28	170	−10.59	<0.001	−0.40
Joy	212	30.72	17.05	D	47.33	22.22	212	16.60	<0.001	**0.82**
	170	31.65	17.59	F	42.90	23.99	170	11.25	<0.001	**0.52**
Tension	212	71.60	19.63	D	49.43	24.22	212	−22.17	<0.001	**−1.00**
	170	70.47	19.74	F	55.10	22.50	170	−15.37	<0.001	**−0.72**
PSQI										
Total value	211	10.86	4.16	D	10.21	4.70	211	−0.65	0.010	−0.14
	168	10.90	4.17	F	9.25	4.49	168	−1.65	<0.001	−0.38
Sleep quality	211	1.90	0.67	D	1.50	0.75	211	−0.40	<0.001	**−0.56**
	168	1.92	0.67	F	1.57	0.70	168	−0.35	<0.001	**−0.50**
Sleep latency	211	1.75	1.05	D	1.56	1.06	211	−0.20	0.009	−0.18
	168	1.70	1.04	F	1.50	1.05	168	−0.20	0.003	−0.19
Sleep duration	211	1.50	0.92	D	1.49	0.93	211	−0.01	0.939	–
	168	1.52	0.94	F	1.38	0.90	168	−0.14	0.039	−0.16
Sleep efficiency	211	1.31	1.18	D	1.27	1.21	211	−0.04	0.595	–
	168	1.33	1.18	F	1.04	1.17	168	−0.29	0.002	−0.25
Sleep disorders	211	1.83	0.62	D	1.62	0.64	211	−0.21	<0.001	−0.33
	168	1.86	0.63	F	1.61	0.65	168	−0.25	<0.001	−0.39
Sleeping pills	211	0.71	1.18	D	1.52	1.42	211	0.81	<0.001	**0.61**
	168	0.71	1.19	F	0.73	1.16	168	0.01	0.881	–
Daytime sleepiness	211	1.86	0.71	D	1.26	0.85	211	−0.61	<0.001	**−0.77**
	168	1.86	0.73	F	1.43	0.86	168	−0.43	<0.001	**−0.54**
GAD										
Total value	212	11.24	4.91	D	6.76	4.47	212	−4.48	<0.001	**−0.95**
	163	11.03	4.81	F	7.58	4.82	163	−3.45	<0.001	**−0.72**
Complaint complexes of psycho-vegetative stability										
Complaints index	213	0.17	0.39	D	0.80	0.79	213	0.63	<0.001	**0.97**
	171	0.19	0.41	F	0.80	0.77	171	0.60	<0.001	**0.94**
Total value	213	66.47	16.18	D	48.45	19.66	213	−18.02	<0.001	**−0.99**
	171	65.89	16.66	F	51.25	20.06	171	−14.65	<0.001	**−0.78**
Dizziness	213	3.59	2.21	D	2.49	2.39	213	−1.09	<0.001	−0.47
	171	3.48	2.13	F	2.73	2.09	171	−0.75	<0.001	−0.35
Sleep	213	7.63	2.03	D	6.04	2.63	213	−1.59	<0.001	**−0.67**
	171	7.64	2.03	F	6.07	2.37	171	−1.57	<0.001	**−0.70**
Heat balance	213	6.31	2.78	D	4.31	2.71	213	2.00	<0.001	**−0.73**
	171	6.23	2.80	F	4.95	2.63	171	−1.28	<0.001	−0.47

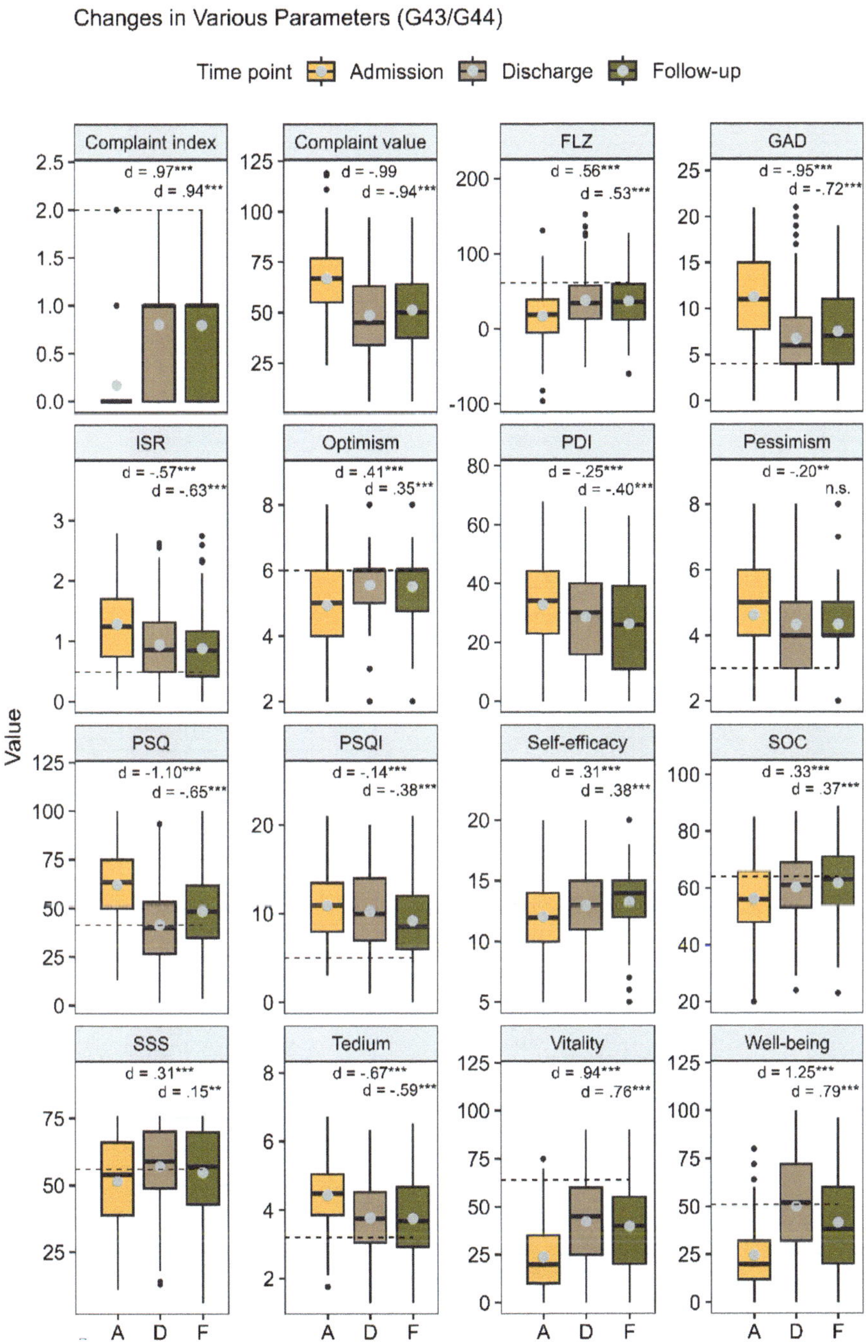

Fig. 5.140 Changes in various parameters for patients with a G43/G44 diagnosis in 2023; the dashed black lines indicate the desired target values; significance: $*p < 0.05$, $**p < 0.01$, $***p < 0.001$; Cohen's d = effect measure ($d \geq 0.2$ = small effect, ≥ 0.5 = moderate effect, ≥ 0.8 = large effect); the graph shows all available data, the effect sizes refer to the individual comparison (A–D/A–F)

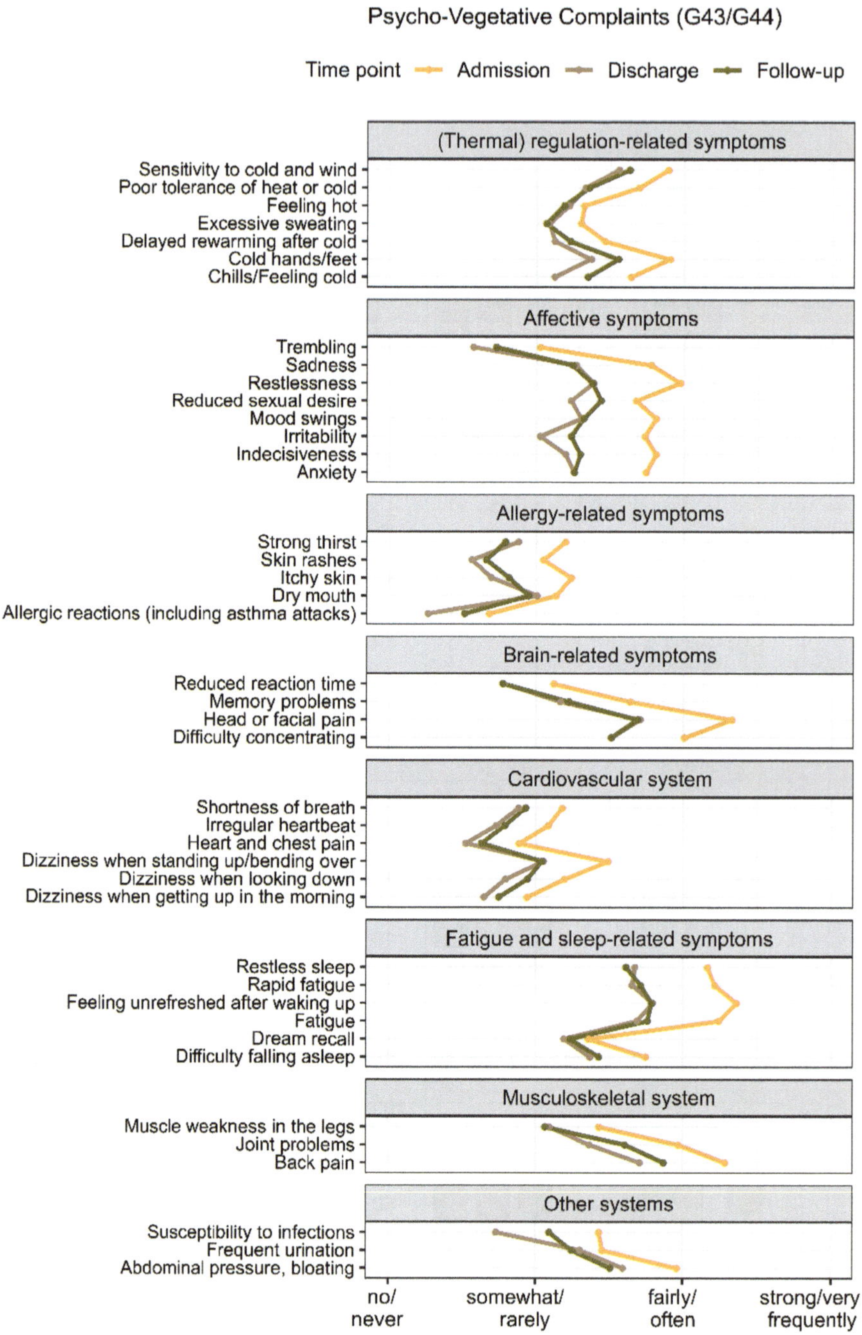

Fig. 5.141 Psycho-vegetative complaints; change in complaints for patients with a G43/G44 diagnosis at admission: $n = 221$, at discharge: $n = 213$, and at follow-up: $n = 171$ in 2023

5.4.5 Other Pain Indications, Such as G62 Polyneuropathy

Patients with other pain indications, such as G62 polyneuropathies, show equally strong effect sizes in treatment results. For example, the main complaint severity at discharge was $d = -0.98$ ($p < 0.001$), and at follow-up it was $d = -0.84$ ($p < 0.001$) (Table 5.125; Fig. 5.142). Compared to other somatic diagnoses, the proportion of patients who rate the treatment as 'very worthwhile' falls by the time of the follow-up. However, the number of patients rating the treatment as 'very worthwhile' or 'worthwhile' combined increased slightly until follow-up (92.3% at discharge vs. 94.6% at follow-up) (Table 5.126, Fig. 5.143).

Patients with other pain indications (G62) showed positive changes with moderate to large effect sizes at hospital discharge, particularly with regard to.

Table 5.125 Global assessments of treatment success for patients with a G62 diagnosis, surveyed at discharge and at follow-up in 2023; *t*-test for paired samples; significance at $p < 0.05$; Cohen's d = effect measure ($d \geq 0.2$ = small, ≥ 0.5 = moderate, ≥ 0.8 = large effect)

	Course						Difference from admission			
Main complaint severity (VAS)	Admission (A)			Discharge (D)/ follow-up (F)			A–D/A–F		Significance	Effect size
	n	M	SD		M	SD	*n*	ΔM	*p*	*d*
G62 other polyneuropathies	52	71.73	18.55	D	51.54	22.35	52	−20.19	<0.001	**−0.98**
	37	69.46	19.71	F	52.97	19.70	37	−16.49	<0.001	**−0.84**

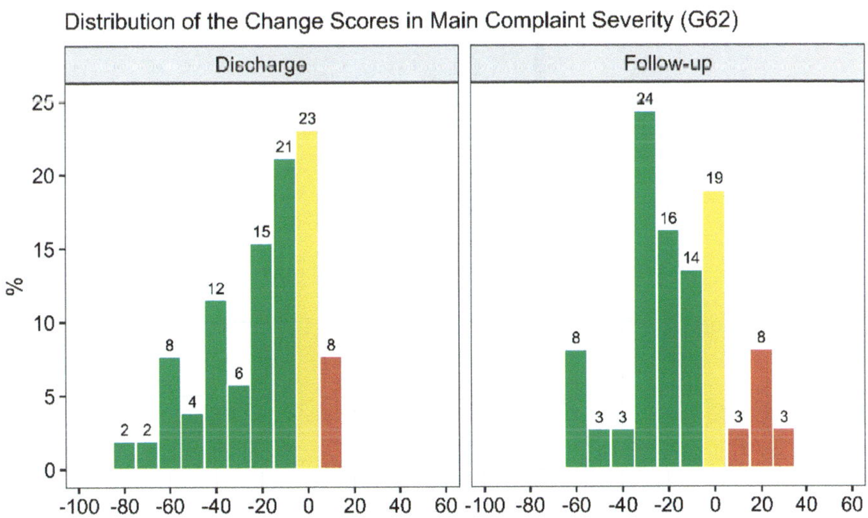

Fig. 5.142 Distribution of the change scores in main complaint severity between hospital admission and hospital discharge or hospital admission and follow-up for patients with a somatic G62 diagnosis in 2023 (A–D $n = 52$; A–D–F $n = 37$); negative differences correspond to an improvement

Table 5.126 Global assessments of treatment success for patients with a G62 diagnosis, surveyed at discharge and at follow-up in 2023

Overall success of the therapy		**Very good**		**Good**		**Moderate**		**No success**		**Total**	
		n	%	*n*	%	*n*	%	*n*	%	*n*	%
G62 other polyneuropathies	D	8	15.4	25	48.1	17	32.7	2	3.8	52	100
	F	8	21.6	14	37.8	14	37.8	1	2.7	37	100
Treatment worthwhile		**Very worthwhile**		**Worthwhile**		**Not worth it**		**Rather harmed**		**Total**	
		n	%	*n*	%	*n*	%	*n*	%	*n*	%
G62 other polyneuropathies	D	25	48.1	23	44.2	4	7.7	0	0.0	52	100
	F	15	40.5	20	54.1	2	5.4	0	0.0	37	100

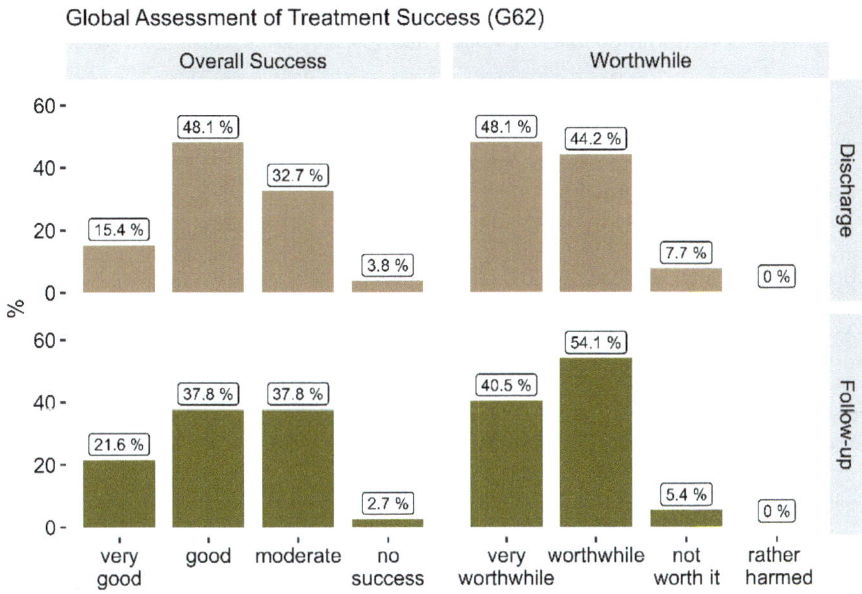

Fig. 5.143 Global assessments of treatment success for patients with a G62 diagnosis, surveyed at discharge ($n = 52$) and at follow-up ($n = 37$) in 2023

- Depression symptoms ($d = -0.86$, $p < 0.001$).
- Recreation due to pain disability ($d = -0.73$, $p < 0.001$).
- Well-being ($d = 1.06$, $p < 0.001$), vitality ($d = 1.11$, $p < 0.001$).
- Exhaustion ($d = -0.77$, $p < 0.001$).
- Generalised Anxiety Disorder ($d = -0.92$, $p < 0.001$).
- Psycho-vegetative complaint index ($d = 0.87$, $p < 0.001$).

Similar results were found at follow-up, albeit somewhat weaker. The strongest improvements until follow-up were seen in depression ($d = -0.75$, $p < 0.001$), recreation ($d = -0.70$, $p < 0.001$), well-being ($d = 0.52$, $p < 0.001$), vitality ($d = 0.62$, $p < 0.001$), Generalised Anxiety Disorder ($d = -0.80$, $p < 0.001$) and the psycho-vegetative complaint index ($d = 0.81$, $p < 0.001$).

Overall, the results for this clientele are comparatively less positive than for the other indications (Table 5.127, Fig. 5.144).

The most common psycho-vegetative symptoms reported by patients with a G62 diagnosis are fatigue, sleep disturbances, back pain, and joint pain, followed by other symptoms. Interestingly, all symptoms improved slightly until the follow-up, except for 'feeling hot' and 'excessive sweating' (Fig. 5.145).

Table 5.127 Changes in various parameters for patients with a secondary G62 diagnosis in 2023; *t*-test: Cohen's d = effect measure ($d \geq 0.2$ = small effect, ≥ 0.5 = moderate effect, ≥ 0.8 = large effect)

Somatic secondary diagnosis G62	Course			Discharge (D)/ follow-up (F)			Difference from admission			
		Admission (A)					A–D/A–F		Significance	Effect size
	n	M	SD	D/F	M	SD	*n*	M	*p*	*d*
ICD symptom ratings (ISR)										
Total value	51	1.06	0.57	D	0.77	0.54	51	−0.29	<0.001	**−0.52**
	37	0.97	0.58	F	0.69	0.41	37	−0.29	<0.001	**−0.53**
Depression	51	1.98	1.00	D	1.15	0.92	51	−0.83	<0.001	**−0.86**
	37	1.82	1.03	F	1.11	0.80	37	−0.71	<0.001	**−0.75**
Anxiety	51	1.17	1.09	D	0.84	0.88	51	−0.32	<0.001	−0.31
	37	0.95	0.94	F	0.76	0.84	37	−0.20	0.066	–
Obsessive-compulsion	51	0.71	0.79	D	0.63	0.77	51	−0.08	0.414	–
	37	0.61	0.75	F	0.41	0.64	37	−0.20	0.028	−0.28
Somatoform	51	079	0.76	D	0.62	0.72	51	−0.17	0.129	–
	37	0.74	0.78	F	0.40	0.55	37	−0.34	<0.001	−0.47
Eating disorder	51	0.66	0.71	D	0.55	0.65	51	−0.11	0.195	–
	37	0.68	0.66	F	0.59	0.72	37	−0.08	0.419	–
Pain disability index										
Total index	50	34.00	15.59	D	25.68	15.06	50	−8.32	<0.001	**−0.54**
	36	31.69	14.71	F	25.39	13.71	36	−6.31	0.004	−0.44
Family/domestic obligations	50	5.78	2.45	D	4.60	2.66	50	−1.18	0.001	−0.46
	36	5.42	2.38	F	4.42	2.50	36	−1.00	0.024	−0.41
Recreation	50	6.50	2.37	D	4.62	2.77	50	−1.88	<0.001	**−0.73**
	36	6.36	2.28	F	4.56	2.80	36	−1.81	<0.001	**−0.70**
Social activity	50	5.02	2.64	D	3.82	2.71	50	−1.20	<0.001	−0.45
	36	4.47	2.63	F	3.50	270	36	−0.97	0.016	−0.36
Profession	50	4.92	3.38	D	4.16	3.03	50	−0.76	0.091	–
	36	4.44	3.41	F	3.14	2.74	36	−1.31	0.027	−0.42
Sex life	50	5.88	3.88	D	4.30	3.93	50	−1.58	0.005	−0.40
	36	5.78	4.02	F	5.58	3.83	36	−0.19	0.704	–
Self-sufficiency	50	3.10	2.92	D	2.00	2.34	50	−1.10	0.004	−0.41
	36	2.69	2.74	F	2.17	2.30	36	−0.53	0.092	–
Essentials activities	50	2.80	3.04	D	2.18	2.70	50	−0.62	0.146	–
	36	2.53	2.72	F	2.03	2.56	36	−0.50	0.193	–
Life satisfaction										
Total value	50	36.66	39.28	D	55.82	36.40	50	19.16	<0.001	**0.50**
	37	37.05	41.57	F	48.76	34.37	37	11.70	0.042	0.30
Friends/ acquaintances	50	5.44	7.28	D	7.66	7.37	50	2.22	0.021	0.30
	37	4.43	6.34	F	6.68	5.43	37	2.24	0.047	0.38
Leisure/hobbies	50	3.06	7.09	D	5.22	5.92	50	2.16	0.019	0.33
	37	1.95	5.92	F	4.35	5.09	37	2.41	0.015	0.43
Health	50	−4.54	6.91	D	0.06	7.08	50	4.60	<0.001	**0.66**
	37	−3.54	7.27	F	0.38	7.96	37	3.92	**0.003**	**0.51**
Income	50	5.24	6.53	D	6.74	6.61	50	1.50	0.084	–
	37	5.24	6.64	F	5.68	6.23	37	0.43	0.566	–

(continued)

Table 5.127 (continued)

Somatic secondary diagnosis G62	Course						Difference from admission			
	Admission (A)			Discharge (D)/ follow-up (F)			A–D/A–F		Significance	Effect size
	n	M	SD	D/F	M	SD	*n*	M	*p*	*d*
Profession	50	1.84	6.72	D	4.04	6.13	50	2.20	0.026	0.34
	37	2.43	6.37	F	3.89	6.29	37	1.46	0.151	–
Housing situation	50	9.00	8.07	D	10.78	7.65	50	1.78	0.064	–
	37	9.27	8.11	F	9.30	6.28	37	0.03	0.981	–
Family/children	50	9.84	8.56	D	11.32	7.31	50	1.48	0.084	–
	37	10.38	8.19	F	10.27	7.01	37	−0.11	0.927	–
Partnership	50	6.78	10.64	D	10.10	9.05	50	3.22	0.001	0.32
	37	6.89	11.09	F	8.22	9.40	37	1.32	0.255	–
SOC										
Total value	50	60.74	13.09	D	64.40	12.61	50	3.66	0.012	0.29
	37	62.51	13.04	F	64.84	11.25	37	2.32	0.178	–
Meaningfulness	50	19.88	4.91	D	20.72	4.13	50	0.84	0.097	–
	37	20.43	4.66	F	20.46	4.07	37	0.03	0.966	–
Comprehensibility	50	22.66	5.81	D	24.32	5.20	50	1.66	0.014	0.30
	37	23.38	6.15	F	24.68	4.56	37	1.30	0.091	–
Manageability	50	18.20	4.43	D	19.36	4.72	50	1.16	0.054	–
	37	18.70	4.48	F	19.70	4.58	37	1.00	0.152	–
WHO-5 well-being and vitality										
Well-being	51	30.12	22.56	D	55.16	24.64	51	25.02	<0.001	**1.06**
	38	34.11	23.80	F	46.00	21.16	38	11.89	<0.001	**0.52**
Vitality	51	28.33	16.84	D	49.22	20.28	51	20.88	<0.001	**1.11**
	38	32.24	17.03	F	44.34	20.99	38	12.11	<0.001	**0.62**
SWOP										
Self-efficacy	51	12.41	3.07	D	13.65	2.94	51	1.24	0.003	0.41
	37	12.81	2.81	F	14.11	2.37	37	1.30	<0.001	0.49
Optimism	51	5.20	1.55	D	5.78	1.55	51	0.59	<0.001	0.38
	37	5.35	1.51	F	5.73	1.30	37	0.38	0.042	0.26
Pessimism	51	4.67	1.47	D	4.31	1.67	51	−0.35	0.063	–
	37	4.51	1.59	F	4.32	1.70	37	−0.19	0.361	–
SSS										
Total value	51	50.71	19.49	D	56.88	16.02	51	6.18	<0.001	0.33
	37	51.11	21.39	F	54.32	17.72	37	3.22	0.035	0.15
Emotional	51	16.61	6.11	D	18.31	5.00	51	1.71	0.005	0.30
	37	16.54	6.78	F	17.59	5.37	37	1.05	0.098	–
Social interaction	51	10.20	3.96	D	11.61	3.23	51	1.41	0.001	0.38
	37	10.70	4.13	F	11.5	3.48	37	0.65	0.065	–
Material	51	11.22	5.17	D	12.61	4.73	51	1.39	0.002	0.28
	37	11.19	5.58	F	11.84	5.03	37	0.65	0.173	–
Affective	51	8.41	3.64	D	9.10	3.20	51	0.69	0.040	0.20
	37	8.51	3.80	F	8.76	3.43	37	0.24	0.292	–
Tedium measure (burnout)										
Total value	50	3.99	1.04	D	3.39	1.11	50	−0.60	<0.001	**−0.55**
	37	3.83	1.10	F	3.35	1.01	37	−0.48	<0.001	−0.45
Discouragement	50	3.51	1.12	D	3.04	1.25	50	−0.47	0.001	−0.37
	37	3.31	1.30	F	2.90	1.07	37	−0.41	0.008	−0.34

(continued)

Table 5.127 (continued)

Somatic secondary diagnosis G62	Course						Difference from admission			
		Admission (A)		Discharge (D)/ follow-up (F)			A–D/A–F		Significance	Effect size
	n	M	SD	D/F	M	SD	*n*	M	*p*	*d*
Exhaustion	50	4.76	1.05	D	3.87	1.24	50	−0.89	<0.001	**−0.77**
	37	4.64	1.09	F	3.99	1.22	37	−0.64	<0.001	**−0.56**
Loss of motivation	50	4.01	0.96	D	3.52	1.01	50	−0.50	<0.001	**−0.50**
	37	3.91	1.01	F	3.50	1.04	37	−0.41	0.005	−0.40
PSQ										
Total value	51	50.69	21.74	D	37.09	20.03	51	−13.60	<0.001	**−0.65**
	37	46.08	20.40	F	38.11	16.88	37	−7.97	0.003	−0.42
Worries	51	44.84	27.43	D	32.03	21.95	51	−12.81	<0.001	**−0.51**
	37	38.20	24.38	F	30.81	20.21	37	−7.39	0.007	−0.32
Demands	51	36.60	24.81	D	23.92	19.69	51	−12.68	<0.001	**−0.56**
	37	32.61	21.53	F	25.05	18.28	37	−7.57	0.006	−0.37
Joy	51	38.04	25.90	D	52.16	25.43	51	14.12	<0.001	**0.55**
	37	41.62	26.87	F	50.45	24.12	37	8.83	0.018	0.34
Tension	51	59.35	25.66	D	44.57	23.76	51	−14.77	<0.001	**−0.60**
	37	55.14	25.66	F	47.03	20.18	37	−8.11	0.022	−0.34
PSQI										
Total value	50	10.96	4.21	D	10.02	4.89	50	−0.94	0.100	–
	38	10.82	4.35	F	7.87	3.62	38	−1.95	0.004	−0.48
Sleep quality	50	1.86	0.76	D	1.44	0.70	50	−0.42	<0.001	**−0.57**
	38	1.89	0.73	F	1.61	0.68	38	−0.29	0.020	−0.41
Sleep latency	50	1.94	1.10	D	1.64	1.06	50	−0.30	0.087	–
	38	1.95	1.01	F	1.82	0.90	38	−0.13	0.376	–
Sleep duration	50	1.58	0.86	D	1.64	0.83	50	0.06	0.595	–
	38	1.55	0.92	F	1.32	0.81	38	−0.24	0.071	–
Sleep efficiency	50	1.38	1.14	D	1.18	1.21	50	−0.20	0.222	–
	38	1.39	1.22	F	0.87	0.99	38	−0.53	0.012	−0.47
Sleep disorders	50	1.84	0.68	D	1.62	0.64	50	−0.22	0.033	−0.33
	38	1.79	0.70	F	1.53	0.60	38	−0.26	0.023	−0.40
Sleeping pills	50	0.64	1.08	D	1.40	1.44	50	−0.76	<0.001	**0.58**
	38	0.58	1.06	F	0.47	0.98	38	−0.11	0.554	–
Daytime sleepiness	50	1.72	0.78	D	1.10	0.86	50	−0.62	<0.001	**−0.75**
	38	1.66	0.81	F	1.26	0.86	38	−0.39	<0.001	−0.47
GAD										
Total value	50	10.00	5.16	D	5.58	4.32	50	−4.42	<0.001	**−0.92**
	36	9.28	4.55	F	6.00	3.44	36	−3.28	<0.001	**−0.80**
Complaint complexes of psycho-vegetative stability										
Complaints index	51	0.27	0.45	D	0.84	0.76	51	0.57	<0.001	**0.87**
	38	0.32	0.47	F	0.79	0.66	38	0.47	<0.001	**0.81**
Total value	51	61.27	16.38	D	45.00	18.29	51	−16.28	<0.001	**−0.93**
	38	60.13	15.62	F	48.63	16.54	38	−11.50	<0.001	**−0.71**
Dizziness	51	4.12	2.28	D	3.00	2.12	51	−1.12	<0.001	**−0.51**
	38	3.97	1.99	F	3.08	2.08	38	−0.89	<0.001	−0.43
Sleep	51	7.27	2.14	D	5.49	2.72	51	−1.78	<0.001	**−0.72**
	38	7.18	2.24	F	5.53	2.04	38	−1.66	<0.001	**−0.77**
Heat balance	51	5.47	2.79	D	4.02	2.84	51	−1.45	<0.001	**−0.52**
	38	5.61	2.94	F	4.34	2.53	38	−1.26	0.002	−0.46

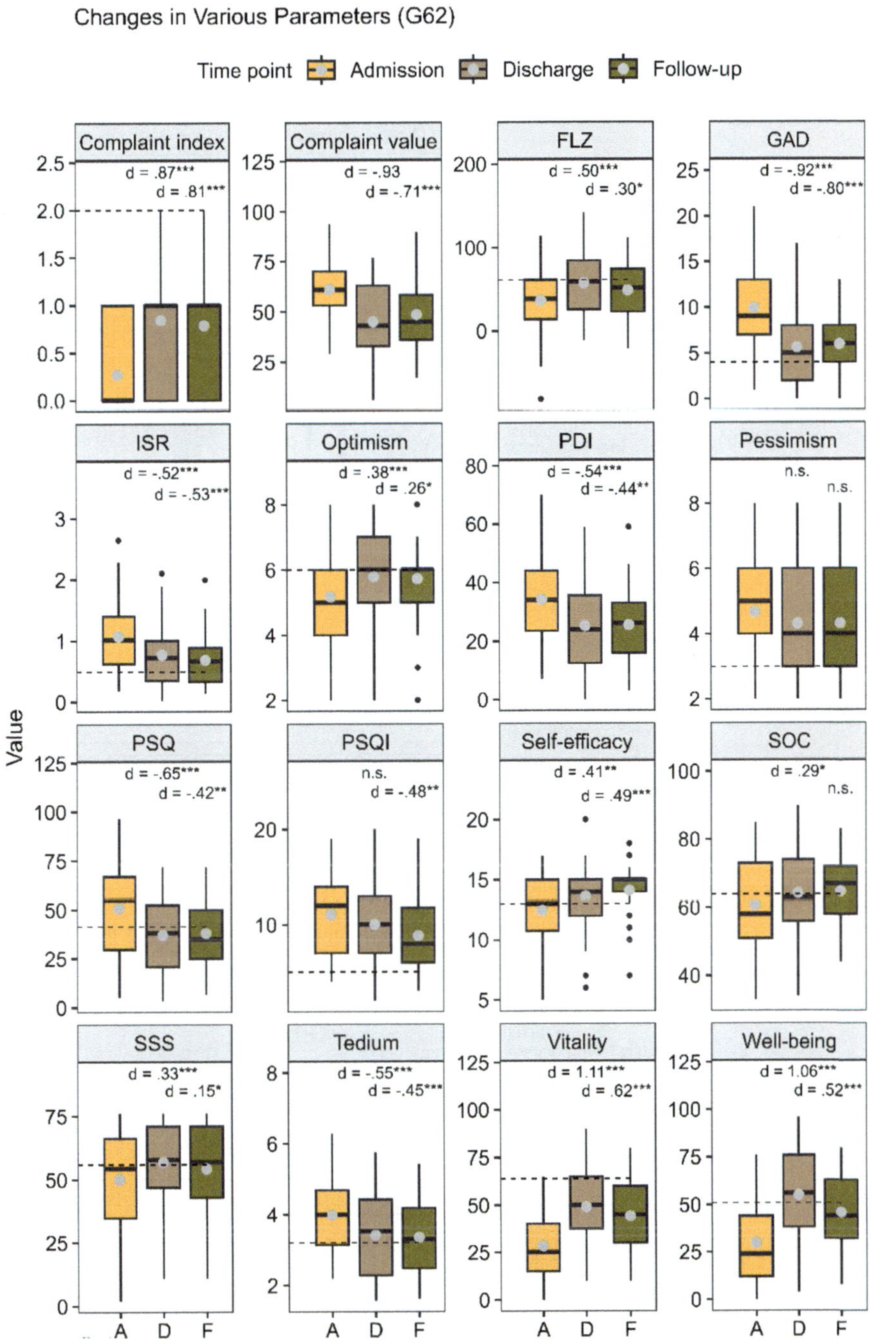

Fig. 5.144 Changes in various parameters for patients with a G62 diagnosis in 2023; the dashed black lines indicate the desired target values; significance: $*p < 0.05$, $**p < 0.01$, $***p < 0.001$; Cohen's d = effect measure ($d \geq 0.2$ = small effect, ≥ 0.5 = moderate effect, ≥ 0.8 = large effect); the graph shows all available data, the effect sizes refer to the individual comparison (A–D/A–F)

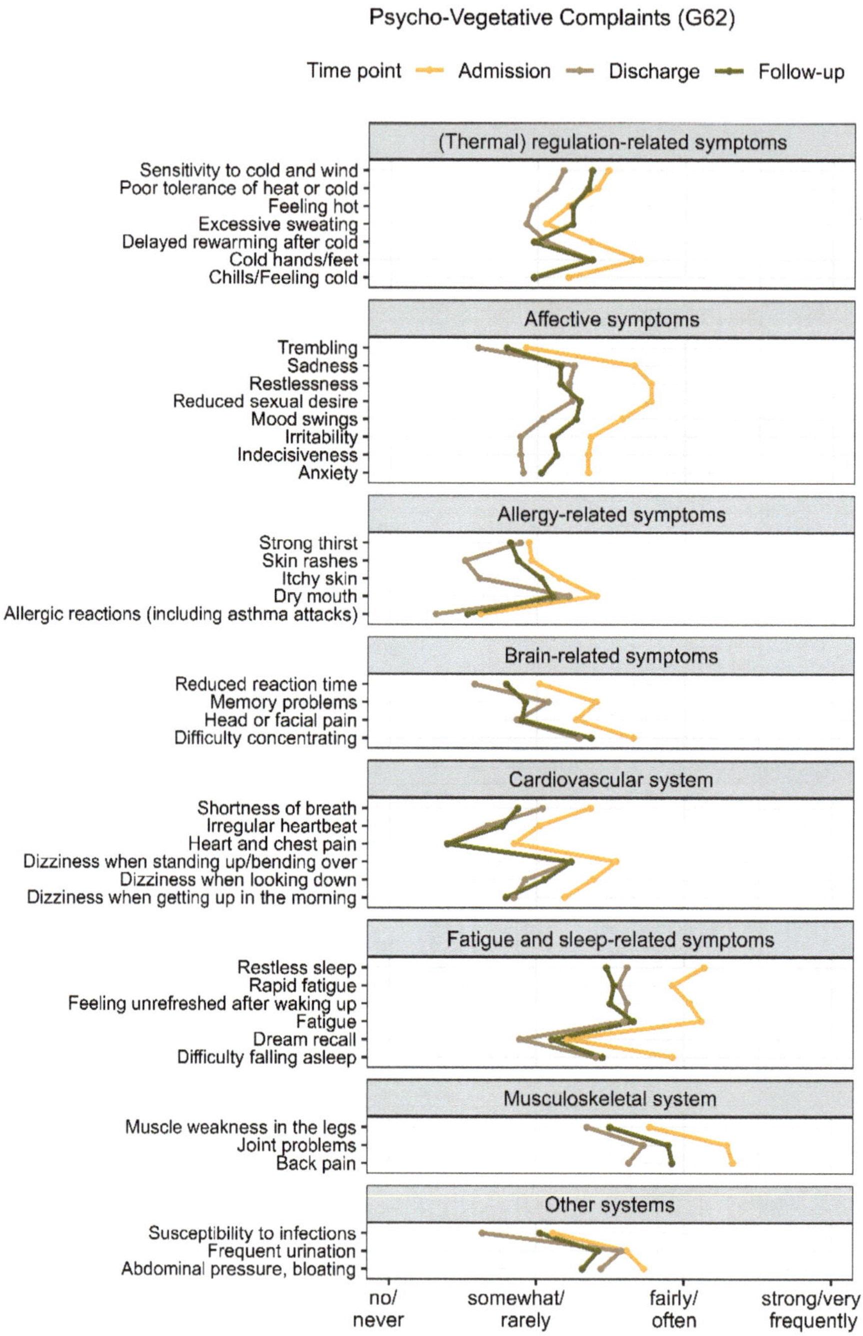

Fig. 5.145 Psycho-vegetative complaints; change in complaints for patients with a G62 diagnosis at admission: $n = 52$ at discharge: $n = 52$ and at follow-up: $n = 38$ in 2023

5.5 Routine Laboratory and Liver Value Screening

5.5.1 Routine Laboratory

Values determined in the external laboratory are fed directly into the central database via a digital interface and assigned to individual cases using the central PIN number. The system considers a full laboratory determination upon admission to hospital and a routine laboratory analysis of selected parameters at the time of discharge. Further control tests are performed on the laboratory data if necessary.

Within the scope of the laboratory analyses, measured values are available for 823 patients at the time of hospital admission (up to a maximum of 7 days into their stay). Depending on the measured value, discharge values are available for between 779 and 788 patients, which, in most cases, were collected up to 7 days before hospital discharge. For the following evaluations, only patients with valid admission and discharge values for the corresponding parameters are considered. As the number of valid values varies depending on the parameter, the exact case numbers can be found in Table 5.128.

T-tests showed statistically significant reductions in cholesterol levels for both men ($d = -0.37$, $p < 0.001$) and women ($d = -0.17$, $p < 0.001$) during their hospital stay. On average, the men's total cholesterol decreased from 204 mg/dl to 187 mg/dl. In women, total cholesterol decreased from 217 to 210 mg/dL. Average values for both LDL (men: $d = -0.29$, $p < 0.001$; women: $d = -0.07$, $p = 0.003$) and HDL (men: $d = -0.28$, $p < 0.001$; women: $d = -0.29$, $p < 0.001$) showed a statistically significant decrease in both sexes. However, this cannot be explained for HDL cholesterol, given that the objective of the inpatient programme is to encourage health-promoting behaviour, which is generally associated with increased HDL levels. According to Cohen, these changes correspond to a minimal to small effect. Mean triglyceride values only showed a significant reduction in men ($d = -0.11$, $p = 0.049$). In women, the glucose value decreased ($d = -0.14$, $p < 0.001$), but this showed no significant difference in men. There is a slight decrease in average uric acid values for both sexes (men: $d = -0.21$, $p < 0.001$; women: $d = -0.17$, $p < 0.001$). Regarding the liver-relevant laboratory parameters (ALT, GOT, and gamma-GT), significant changes in GOT values (men: $d = -0.18$, $p = 0.002$; women: $d = -0.07$, $p = 0.025$) and gamma-GT values (men: $d = -0.14$, $p = 0.001$; women: $d = -0.07$, $p = 0.003$) were observed in both sexes. According to Cohen's d, only a negligible effect can be demonstrated for these results. The AP values only changed significantly in men, with a minimal effect ($d = -0.09$, $p = 0.029$).

Further statistically significant changes in laboratory values and their respective effect sizes can be found in Table 5.128. The values given for Cohen's d are based on the effect sizes calculated by RStudio for dependent *t*-tests. Table 5.129 presents the results from previous years.

Table 5.128 Laboratory values in pre-post comparison in 2023, separated by gender; $^*p \leq .05$, $^{**}p \leq .01$, $^{***}p \leq .001$; n.s. (not significant); Cohen's d = effect measure ($d \geq 0.2$ = small, ≥ 0.5 = moderate, ≥ 0.8 = large effect)

		Laboratory parameters 2023									
		Men					Woman				
		n	M	SD	MD	*d*	*n*	M	SD	MD	*d*
Cholesterol	A	164	204.24	47.71	202.00	**–.37*** **	615	217.30	43.19	214.00	–.17***
mg/dl	D	164	186.65	47.64	178.00		615	209.98	41.15	207.00	
LDL	A	164	138.90	44.97	140.00	**–.29*** **	616	140.14	41.13	136.00	–.07**
mg/dl	D	164	125.93	43.51	121.00		616	137.28	38.49	133.00	
HDL	A	164	51.45	12.44	50.50	**–.28*** **	616	64.14	14.63	62.80	**–.29*** **
mg/dl	D	164	48.06	11.61	47.15		616	60.02	13.29	59.00	
Chol/HDL	A	164	4.14	1.20	3.92	–.09*	615	3.53	0.97	3.37	.11***
mg/dl	D	164	4.03	1.15	3.94		615	3.63	0.94	3.49	
LDL/HDL	A	164	2.84	1.10	2.73	–.10*	616	2.31	0.90	2.20	.10***
mg/dl	D	164	2.73	1.05	2.68		616	2.40	0.87	2.30	
Triglycerides mg/dl	A	164	125.17	65.08	109.50	–.11*	616	106.38	50.30	92.90	n.s.
	D	164	118.33	65.34	99.50		616	105.32	51.89	92.70	
Glucose	A	164	93.67	17.03	91.15	n.s.	616	90.95	14.20	88.50	–.14***
mg/dl	D	164	92.74	20.56	89.10		616	89.15	10.76	87.60	
Total		**779/780**									
Sodium	A	164	140.29	2.18	140.00	.20*	618	140.56	2.04	141.00	.08*
mmol/l	D	164	140.70	2.01	141.00		618	140.73	2.10	141.00	
Calcium	A	164	2.34	0.09	2.34	.17*	618	2.33	0.09	2.33	**.24*** **
mmol/l	D	164	2.35	0.09	2.34		618	2.35	0.09	2.35	
Iron	A	164	130.90	46.28	128.50	**–.44*** **	618	116.32	42.25	113.00	**–.48*** **
µg/dl	D	164	112.30	36.66	111.00		618	98.16	32.84	94.60	
Potassium	A	164	4.34	0.32	4.31	n.s.	618	4.27	0.33	4.27	.09*
mmol/l	D	164	4.34	0.32	4.36		618	4.30	0.32	4.29	
Total		**782**									

Uric acid	A	164	5.86	1.20	5.98	**–.21*** **	617	4.59	1.18	4.43	–.17***
mg/dl	D	164	5.61	1.17	5.57		617	4.40	1.08	4.25	
Creatine	A	164	0.96	0.13	0.94	–.11*	617	0.79	0.12	0.78	–.08***
mg/dl	D	164	0.95	0.14	0.93		617	0.78	0.12	0.77	
Total		**781**									
Erythrocytes mio/µl	A	163	4.97	0.39	4.98	n.s.	616	4.53	0.35	4.52	.11***
	D	163	4.97	0.38	4.98		616	4.57	0.35	4.57	
Leukocytes	A	163	6.67	1.98	6.42	**–.25*** **	616	6.22	1.84	5.96	**–.21*** **
1000/µl	D	163	6.18	1.96	5.83		616	5.84	1.74	5.60	
Thrombocyte 1000/µl	A	163	260.68	78.32	245.00	–.12***	616	278.92	77.78	272.00	–.13***
	D	163	251.72	77.09	234.00		616	268.90	78.90	264.00	
Hematocrit	A	163	46.11	3.24	46.00	n.s.	616	42.25	2.85	42.00	.07**
%	D	163	46.06	3.25	47.00		616	42.56	2.86	42.00	
Hemoglobin	A	163	15.15	1.23	15.30	n.s.	616	13.65	0.98	13.60	.11***
g/dl	D	163	15.16	1.20	15.30		616	13.76	0.97	13.80	
HbE (MCH)	A	163	30.48	1.47	30.40	n.s.	616	30.16	1.67	30.30	n.s.
pg	D	163	30.50	1.37	30.40		616	30.15	1.66	30.20	
MCHC	A	163	32.86	1.06	32.90	n.s.	616	32.34	0.98	32.40	.11**
g/dl	D	163	32.94	1.11	32.90		616	32.44	0.92	32.50	
MCV	A	163	92.83	4.10	93.00	n.s.	616	93.29	4.33	93.00	–.07***
Fl	D	163	92.67	3.88	93.00		616	93.00	4.37	93.00	
Total		**779**									

(continued)

Table 5.128 (continued)

		Laboratory parameters 2023									
		Men					Woman				
		n	M	SD	MD	*d*	*n*	M	SD	MD	*d*
GOT	A	166	26.97	7.48	25.75	–.18**	620	23.72	6.85	22.50	–.07*
U/l	D	166	25.64	7.75	24.40		620	23.23	6.12	22.30	
ALT	A	166	31.51	15.69	28.10	n.s.	621	22.60	11.74	19.80	n.s.
U/l	D	166	31.68	18.93	27.70		621	22.96	11.40	20.00	
Gamma-GT	A	166	40.51	46.99	25.90	–.14**	622	25.96	33.64	17.90	–.07**
U/l	D	166	33.87	33.71	23.55		622	23.72	25.67	17.20	
AP	A	164	69.32	20.24	67.85	–.09*	619	73.06	24.15	69.90	n.s.
U/l	D	164	67.54	19.47	67.55		619	72.55	25.45	69.80	
Total		**783–788**									
Metabol. S.	A	148	2.02	1.31	2.00	n.s.	542	1.82	1.28	2.00	n.s.
Index	D	148	1.94	1.38	2.00		542	1.78	1.27	2.00	
Fatty Liver	A	161	50.27	29.69	49.00	–.13***	604	34.27	30.02	23.00	–.08***
Index	D	161	46.58	29.12	40.00		604	32.04	29.13	20.00	

Table 5.129 Laboratory values in pre-post comparison (previous years), separated by gender; *$p \leq .05$, **$p \leq .01$, ***$p \leq .001$; *n.s.* not significant; Cohen's d = effect measure ($d \geq 0.2$ = small, ≥0.5 = moderate, ≥0.8 = large effect)

		Laboratory parameters previous years									
		Men					Woman				
		n	M	SD	MD	*d*	*n*	M	SD	MD	*d*
Cholesterol	A	2892	216.03	46.73	213.50	**–.43*** **	8327	226.38	45.43	224.00	**–.24*** **
mg/dl	D	2892	196.42	43.29	194.50		8327	215.76	43.09	213.00	
LDL	A	2892	142.64	37.73	140.00	**–.35*** **	8327	142.89	36.69	140.00	–.12***
mg/dl	D	2892	129.77	34.86	129.00		8327	138.44	34.61	136.00	
HDL	A	2892	49.45	11.57	48.00	**–.38*** **	8327	62.44	14.24	61.00	**–.39*** **
mg/dl	D	2892	45.27	10.02	44.10		8327	57.05	12.83	55.80	
Chol/HDL	A	2892	4.53	1.20	4.38	–.04***	8327	3.77	0.99	3.60	.15***
mg/dl	D	2892	4.48	1.17	4.34		8327	3.92	0.99	3.77	
LDL/HDL	A	2892	3.02	0.98	2.91	–.04***	8327	2.41	0.83	2.28	.16***
mg/dl	D	2892	2.98	0.96	2.89		8327	2.54	0.82	2.43	
Triglycerides mg/dl	A	2892	152.94	90.61	131.00	–.15***	8327	120.01	58.38	106.00	–.04***
	D	2892	139.98	79.07	119.00		8327	117.69	55.40	104.00	
Glucose	A	2892	100.32	20.14	95.90	**–.24*** **	8327	94.78	15.30	92.30	–.18***
mg/dl	D	2892	95.86	16.40	92.60		8327	92.12	16.60	90.10	
Total		**11219**									
Sodium	A	2251	139.82	1.95	140.00	.10***	6605	139.81	2.05	140.00	n.s.
mmol/l	D	2251	140.02	1.97	140.00		6605	139.83	2.13	140.00	
Calcium	A	2251	2.38	0.10	2.40	.04*	6605	2.37	0.10	2.40	.16***
mmol/l	D	2251	2.38	0.10	2.40		6605	2.39	0.10	2.40	
Iron	A	2251	126.18	44.79	124.00	**–.67*** **	6605	113.75	40.33	111.00	**–.66*** **
µg/dl	D	2251	99.15	34.50	97.82		6605	89.59	31.50	88.20	
Potassium	A	2251	4.31	0.32	4.29	n.s.	6605	4.25	0.32	4.23	.06***
mmol/l	D	2251	4.32	0.32	4.30		6605	4.27	0.32	4.25	
Total		**8856**									

(continued)

Table 5.129 (continued)

		Laboratory parameters previous years									
		Men					Woman				
		n	M	SD	MD	*d*	*n*	M	SD	MD	*d*
Uric acid	A	2252	6.22	1.24	6.10	−.16***	6612	4.77	1.16	4.63	−.16***
mg/dl	D	2252	6.03	1.15	5.89		6612	4.59	1.08	4.47	
Creatine	A	2252	0.96	0.33	0.92	−.04***	6612	0.75	0.15	0.74	−.03***
mg/dl	D	2252	0.95	0.33	0.92		6612	0.75	0.14	0.74	
Total		**8864**									
Erythrocytes mio/µl	A	2224	4.96	0.44	4.98	−.05***	6542	4.55	0.35	4.55	.04***
	D	2224	4.94	0.44	4.95		6542	4.57	0.35	4.57	
Leukocytes	A	2224	6.72	2.72	6.37	−.13***	6542	6.33	2.20	6.05	−.15***
1000/µl	D	2224	6.39	2.34	5.99		6542	6.00	2.15	5.73	
Thrombocyte 1000/µl	A	2224	247.69	68.38	241.00	n.s.	6542	278.51	69.35	270.00	−.12***
	D	2224	246.71	71.42	238.50		6542	270.49	69.43	262.00	
Hematocrit	A	2224	45.37	3.57	46.00	−.08***	6542	41.58	2.95	42.00	n.s.
%	D	2224	45.08	3.55	45.00		6542	41.59	2.92	42.00	
Hemoglobin	A	2224	15.04	2.16	15.10	−.07***	6542	13.58	1.00	13.60	.03***
g/dl	D	2224	14.91	1.23	15.00		6542	13.61	0.99	13.70	
HbE (MCH)	A	2224	30.36	1.81	30.20	−.04**	6542	29.90	1.75	30.00	−.02**
pg	D	2224	30.30	1.88	30.10		6542	29.88	1.71	30.00	
MCHC	A	2224	33.16	1.06	33.00	−.05*	6542	32.75	1.14	33.00	n.s.
g/dl	D	2224	33.11	1.00	33.10		6542	32.77	0.99	32.80	
MCV	A	2224	91.65	4.92	92.00	−.03***	6542	91.38	4.65	91.00	−.06***
Fl	D	2224	91.47	5.05	91.00		6542	91.13	4.53	91.00	
Total		**8766**									
GOT	A	2943	27.32	12.30	25.00	−.12***	8437	23.38	10.58	21.60	−.03**
U/l	D	2943	25.96	10.48	24.00		8437	23.08	10.56	21.20	
ALT	A	2944	31.80	19.94	26.80	n.s.	8439	22.27	15.17	18.90	.09***
U/l	D	2944	31.91	21.72	26.50		8439	23.85	19.42	19.30	

Gamma-GT	A	2945	42.57	56.83	28.50	−.12***	8439	25.42	33.36	17.20	−.05***
U/l	D	2945	35.87	40.35	24.90		8439	23.86	30.65	16.10	
AP	A	1066	71.38	21.20	69.00	−.03*	3621	71.74	22.90	69.00	n.s.
U/l	D	1066	70.65	21.40	67.80		3621	71.76	25.59	69.00	
Total		**4687–11384**									
Metabol. S.	A	1891	2.21	1.42	2.00	−.09***	5642	1.76	1.31	2.00	n.s.
Index	D	1891	2.08	1.41	2.00		5642	1.75	1.32	2.00	
Fatty Liver	A	807	51.62	29.73	52.00	.12***	2927	34.49	29.32	24.00	**.22*** **
Index	D	807	55.27	32.44	56.00		2927	41.56	34.98	28.00	

5.5.2 Screening for Liver Values as Part of the Complication Screening Programme (CSP)

As mentioned above, statistically significant changes in liver enzyme values were observed between the two measurement points. However, it is not possible to identify clinically relevant increases in individual cases as a consequence of Chinese drug therapy by comparing mean values alone. Additional liver enzyme tests are carried out if clinical symptoms indicative of liver problems are present. If the values are elevated, the TCM medication formula is adjusted. Individual RUCAM (Roussel Uclaf Causality Assessment Method) assessments are only initiated as part of the CSP if the ALT measurement is five times higher than normal or the AP measurement is more than twice as high [36]. These values indicate liver toxicity. ALT increases of 2–5 ULN are interpreted by clinicians as disorders of adaptive liver metabolism.

In addition to promptly carrying out liver value screening in the clinic at the end of the inpatient stay, another way of depicting conspicuous individual changes in liver values as part of a Complication Screening Programme is to statistically process the laboratory values collected over a year in the form of graphical scatter diagrams. Each person is represented by a point in a coordinate system showing their admission and discharge values. To provide orientation, a diagonal line is used to indicate where no changes (on the line) or only minor changes (in the immediate vicinity of the line) have occurred. ALT (alanine aminotransferase) values in 2023 are used as an example of the most important indicator of liver metabolism in Fig. 5.146. ALT is a synonym for GPT. The gender-specific normal limits (or the twofold normal limit) are indicated by the dashed lines. For women, the limit value is 35 U/l and for men, it is 50 U/l. This makes it easy to identify patients whose ALT values are below the standard limit on admission and above twice the standard limit at a later stage of their hospital stay. Cases >5 ULN should be analysed more closely to determine the possible cause of the deviation, which may be related to the intake of certain traditional Chinese medicine (TCM) substances.

A total of 792 patients had admission and follow-up ALT values, and 739 patients had admission and follow-up alkaline phosphatase (AP) values. Six categories for ALT and seven for AP were formed to assess the underlying admission and follow-up values. These represent the values as multiples of the upper normal value ('upper limit normal' ULN; two-, three-, four-, and over fivefold) and can be found in Table 5.130.

Regarding AP, it should be noted that normal values are 40–129 U/l for men and 35–104 U/l for women. This results in an additional category below the normal value: 1× < ULN.

The next step was to select only those patients from the above-described group who had an ALT or AP value within the normal range at admission, in order to identify value increases associated with the inpatient hospital stay (Table 5.131, left column). This results in 712 patients with valid ALT values and 677 patients with valid AP values. For ALT, four cases with a twofold increase in the upper normal value were identified in 2023, which apparently only developed during the inpatient course. This can be considered an example of the adaptation phenomenon. Similarly,

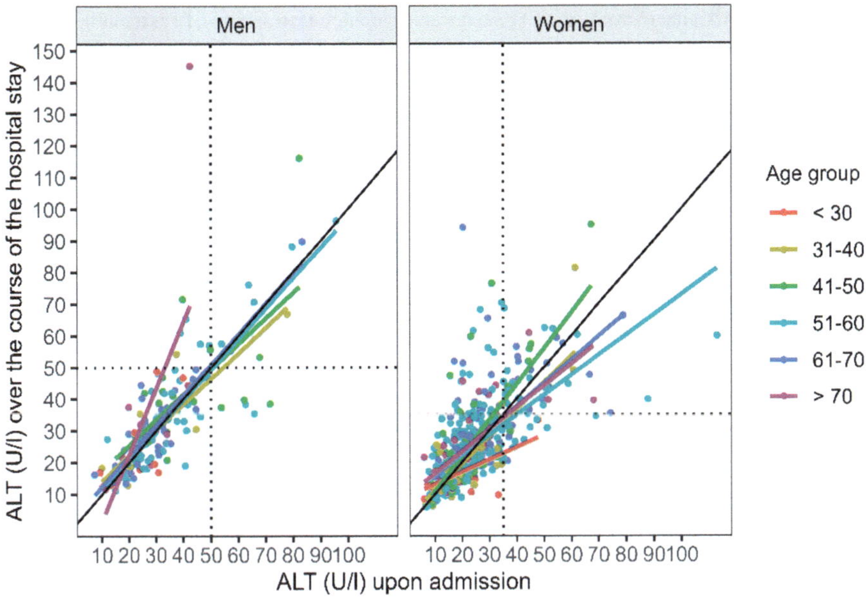

Fig. 5.146 This graph shows a comparison of the measured values for ALT (U/l) at hospital admission and over the course of 2023 (*n* = 794). The dashed lines represent the standard limits: onefold at admission and twofold over the course of 2023

Table 5.130 Alanine aminotransferase (ALT) and alkaline phosphatase (AP) as a multiple of the upper normal limit on admission and during the further course of hospitalisation in 2023

	2023				**Previous years**			
Alanine aminotransferase (ALT) as a multiple of the upper limit normal (ULN)	**ALT on admission**		**ALT in the further course**		**ALT on admission**		**ALT in the further course**	
	n	**%**	***n***	**%**	***n***	**%**	***n***	**%**
1 × ULN	712	89.9	685	86.5	10.254	90.1	9933	87.3
1 × ULN < 2 × ULN	76	9.6	100	12.6	965	8.5	1250	11.0
> = 2 × ULN < 3 × ULN	3	0.4	7	0.9	122	1.1	131	1.2
> = 3 × ULN < 4 × ULN	1	0.1	–	–	26	0.2	32	0.3
> = 4 × ULN < 5 × ULN	–	–	–	–	7	0.1	15	0.1
> = 5 × ULN	–	–	–	–	9	0.1	22	0.2
Total	**792**	**100%**	**792**	**100%**	**11,383**	**100%**	**11,383**	**100%**
Alkaline phosphatase (AP) as a multiple of the upper normal limit (ULN)	**AP on admission**		**AP in the further course**		**AP on admission**		**AP in the further course**	
	n	**%**	***n***	**%**	***n***	**%**	***n***	**%**
< 1 × ULN	9	1.2	13	1.8	83	1.8	80	1.7
1 × ULN	677	91.6	670	90.7	4309	91.9	4323	92.2
1 × ULN < 2 × ULN	52	7.0	55	7.4	290	6.2	272	5.8
> = 2 × ULN < 3 × ULN	1	0.1	1	0.1	4	0.1	10	0.2
> = 3 × ULN < 4 × ULN	–	–	–	–	1	0.0	1	0.0
> = 4 × ULN < 5 × ULN	–	–	–	–	–	–	1	0.0
> = 5 × ULN	–	–	–	–	–	–	–	–
Total	**739**	**100%**	**739**	**100%**	**4687**	**100%**	**4687**	**100%**

Table 5.131 Alkaline phosphatase (AP) and alanine aminotransferase (ALT) as a multiple of the upper normal value in the further course of hospitalisation in 2023; separated according to patients with admission values in the normal range and patients with already increased admission values

	2023				**Previous years**			
Alanine aminotransferase (ALT) as a multiple of the upper limit normal (ULN)	**Patients with baseline value in the normal range; ALT in the subsequent course**		**Patients with already elevated baseline value; ALT in the subsequent course**		**Patients with baseline value in the normal range; ALT in the subsequent course**		**Patients with already elevated baseline value; ALT in the subsequent course**	
	n	**%**	***n***	**%**	***n***	**%**	***n***	**%**
1 × ULN	665	93.4	20	25.0	9536	93.0	397	35.2
1 × ULN < 2 × ULN.	43	6.0	57	71.2	638	6.2	612	54.2
> = 2 × ULN < 3 × ULN	**4**	**0.6**	3	3.8	46	0.4	85	7.5
> = 3 × ULN < 4 × ULN	–	–	–	–	14	0.1	18	1.6
> = 4 × ULN < 5 × ULN	–	–	–	–	6	0.1	9	0.8
> = 5 × ULN	–	–	–	–	14	0.1	8	0.7
Total	**712**	**100%**	**80**	**100%**	**10,254**	**100%**	**1129**	**100%**
Alkaline phosphatase (AP) as a multiple of the upper normal limit (ULN)	**Patients with baseline value in the normal range; AP in the subsequent course**		**Patients with already elevated/ decreased baseline value; AP in the subsequent course**		**Patients with baseline value in the normal range; AP in the subsequent course**		**Patients with already elevated/ decreased baseline value; AP in the subsequent course**	
	n	**%**	***n***	**%**	***n***	**%**	***n***	**%**
< 1 × ULN	8	1.2	–	–	27	0.6	102	34.6
1 × ULN	655	96.8	11	20.8	4192	97.3	186	63.1
1 × ULN < 2 × ULN.	14	2.1	41	77.4	85	2.0	6	2.0
> = 2 × ULN < 3 × ULN	–	–	–	–	4	0.1	1	0.3
> = 3 × ULN < 4 × ULN	–	–	1	1.9	1	0.0	–	–
> = 4 × ULN < 5 × ULN	–	–	–	–	–	–	–	–
> = 5 × ULN	–	–	–	–	–	–	–	–
Total	**677**	**100%**	**53**	**100%**	**4309**	**100%**	**295**	**100%**

for AP, an abnormality is classified as such if there is a twofold increase in the upper normal limit, which could not be detected in any patient during the follow-up examination in 2023.

Patients with normal values of ALT as a diagnostic marker for ruling out pre-existing liver disease were enrolled in a former prospective study of a safety programme from 1994 to 2015 [36]. In 26 (0.12%) of 21,470 patients treated with herbal TCM, liver injury with ALT values of ≥5 × ULN was found, which normalised shortly following treatment cessation, also substantiating causality.

For the current reporting year (2023), the reference patients included those from 2008 to 2022.

In 2023, there were no patients with ALT values above 5xULN at the beginning or end of their inpatient stay, indicating that there were no suspected cases of hepatotoxicity. By contrast, during the reference period, 8 patients with elevated ALT values were admitted and 14 were discharged with elevated ALT values.

5.5.3 Vital Parameters

Patients at the TCM-Klinik Bad Kötzting are encouraged to record certain vital signs on the VITERIO® health portal before and during their inpatient stay. There are no fixed measurement intervals. Patients can make entries at any time and as often as they like. The recorded values include blood pressure, pulse rate, waist circumference, and body weight. To improve the comparability of vital data and reduce the probability of measurement and input errors, health coaches at the clinic also carry out and document examinations in addition to patient self-input.

The measured values collected by hospital staff at a comparable time point were extracted from the resulting irregular data pattern. For baseline and discharge values, the interval was defined as ±7 days around the date of admission or discharge.

The statistical comparison of admission and discharge values only included patients with values in both defined measurement intervals. The exact number of cases is shown in Tables 5.132 (2023) and 5.133 (previous years). Tests for statistical significance revealed minimal reductions in body weight and waist circumference for both men and women in 2023 (Table 5.132). On average, weight decreased by 0.8 kg for women and 1 kg for men during the observation period of around 4 weeks, while abdominal circumference decreased by approximately 1.1 cm for men and 1.3 cm for women. Patients whose BMI was over 25 upon admission experienced slightly higher weight loss. No statistically significant decrease in pulse rate was observed for either women or men in 2023. Systolic and diastolic blood pressure decreased minimally for women at hospital discharge.

When analysing the entire dataset from previous years, statistically significant changes were observed for all vital parameters except pulse rate in men and BMI in women (Table 5.133).

To enable the vital signs 'body weight' and 'BMI' to be classified more accurately at hospital admission and discharge, these values were grouped into weight categories and presented in Table 5.134 for 2023 and Table 5.135 for previous years.

Table 5.132 Vital signs in the pre-/post comparison in 2023; separated by gender; *$p < .05$, **$p < .01$, ***$p < .001$

	Vital signs 2023										
		Men					Woman				
		n	M	SD	MD	*d*	*n*	M	SD	MD	*d*
Pulse rate	A	165	66.71	10.10	65.00	n.s.	630	70.63	10.19	70.00	n.s.
beats/min	D	165	66.52	10.70	65.00		630	70.44	10.81	70.00	
RR systolic	A	165	135.62	18.07	133.00	n.s.	630	131.69	19.14	129.00	–.06*
mmHg	D	165	134.41	16.35	132.00		630	130.47	19.09	130.00	
RR diastolic	A	165	84.62	11.64	83.00	n.s.	630	82.37	10.39	82.00	–.08*
mmHg	D	165	83.32	9.49	84.00		630	81.53	10.44	80.00	
Body weight	A	165	86.81	16.79	85.00	–.06**	636	71.82	16.51	68.55	–.05***
KgDOUBLEHYPHEN-all	D	165	85.78	16.57	84.00		636	70.94	16.54	67.75	
Body weight	A	100	95.98	14.24	92.90	–.12***	293	83.82	13.46	82.10	–.10***
Kg BMI>25	D	100	94.26	13.79	91.50		293	82.43	13.11	80.70	
BMI	A	165	26.48	4.47	25.90	n.s.	633	25.56	5.39	24.70	–.02**
	D	165	26.46	4.39	25.80		633	25.45	5.35	24.70	
Waist circumference	A	163	97.98	13.88	96.00	–.08***	627	89.63	14.87	88.00	–.09***
	D	163	96.88	13.56	96.00		627	88.32	14.05	87.00	

n.s. not significant, *A* admission, *D* discharge

Table 5.133 Vital signs in the pre-/post comparison (previous years); separated by gender; *$p <. 05$, **$p < .01$, ***$p < .001$

		Vital signs previous years									
		Men					Woman				
		n	M	SD	MD	*d*	*n*	M	SD	MD	*d*
Pulse rate	A	2855	69.74	10.57	69.00	n.s.	8457	72.79	10.04	72.00	–.05***
beats/min	D	2855	69.51	15.10	68.00		8457	72.23	10.69	71.00	
RR systolic	A	2910	126.64	17.69	125.75	–.17***	8589	121.27	19.25	120.00	–.11***
mmHg	D	2910	123.52	18.81	121.00		8589	119.10	21.12	118.00	
RR diastolic	A	2910	79.24	10.60	80.00	–.18***	8589	76.16	10.81	76.00	–.07***
mmHg	D	2910	77.35	10.71	79.00		8589	75.32	14.08	75.00	
Body weight	A	2914	85.88	15.75	84.00	–.09***	8618	70.21	14.86	67.30	–.06***
KgDOUBLEHYPHEN-all	D	2914	84.44	15.41	83.15		8618	69.39	14.44	66.70	
Body weight	A	1872	93.38	13.71	91.05	–.15***	3898	81.96	13.12	79.62	–.11***
Kg BMI>25	D	1872	91.38	13.79	89.70		3898	80.54	12.92	78.30	
BMI	A	2870	27.00	4.94	26.45	–.06***	8494	25.53	5.33	24.44	n.s.
	D	2870	26.72	4.69	26.15		8494	25.65	27.96	24.30	
Waist circumference	A	2889	99.21	14.00	98.90	–.15***	8563	88.50	14.18	87.00	–.14***
	D	2889	97.10	14.26	97.00		8563	86.54	14.05	85.00	

n.s. not significant, *A* admission, *D* discharge

Table 5.134 Comparison of the categorisation of body weight and BMI at hospital admission and discharge in 2023; separated by gender

Weight classes	2023											
	On hospital admission						**At discharge from hospital**					
	Men $n = 169$		**Women $n = 650$**		**Total $n = 819$**		**Men $n = 165$**		**Women $n = 636$**		**Total $n = 801$**	
	n	%	n	%	n	%	n	%	n	%	n	%
<55 kg	1	0.6	80	12.3	81	9.9	1	0.6	92	14.5	93	11.6
56–60 kg	4	2.4	89	13.7	93	11.4	5	3.0	85	13.4	90	11.2
61–65 kg	8	4.7	86	13.2	94	11.5	7	4.2	94	14.8	101	12.6
66–70 kg	13	7.7	91	14.0	104	12.7	14	8.5	79	12.4	93	11.6
71–75 kg	18	10.7	77	11.8	95	11.6	19	11.5	73	11.5	92	11.5
76–80 kg	21	12.4	57	8.8	78	9.5	19	11.5	55	8.6	74	9.2
81–85 kg	20	11.8	48	7.4	68	8.3	23	13.9	51	8.0	74	9.2
86–90 kg	23	13.6	35	5.4	58	7.1	19	11.5	31	4.9	50	6.2
91–95 kg	18	10.7	30	4.6	48	5.9	17	10.3	26	4.1	43	5.4
96–100 kg	7	4.1	22	3.4	29	3.5	9	5.5	19	3.0	28	3.5
>100 kg	36	21.3	35	5.4	71	8.7	32	19.4	31	4.9	63	7.9
BMI	**Men $n = 170$**		**Women $n = 647$**		**Total $n = 817$**		**Men $n = 165$**		**Women $n = 633$**		**Total $n = 798$**	
	n	%	n	%	n	%	n	%	n	%	n	%
Underweight	3	1.8	30	4.6	33	4.0	3	1.8	32	5.1	35	4.4
Normal weight	63	37.1	313	48.4	376	46.0	64	38.8	302	47.7	366	45.9
Overweight	71	41.8	176	27.2	247	30.2	66	40.0	181	28.6	247	31.0
Grade I obesity	25	14.7	91	14.1	116	14.2	24	14.5	79	12.5	103	12.9
Grade II obesity	8	4.7	27	4.2	35	4.3	7	4.2	28	4.4	35	4.4
Grade III obesity	–	–	10	1.5	10	1.2	1	0.6	11	1.7	12	1.5

Table 5.135 Comparison of the categorisation of body weight and BMI at hospital admission and discharge in previous years; separated by gender

Weight classes	Previous years On hospital admission						At discharge from hospital					
	Men n = 3390		**Women n = 9608**		**Total n = 13,000**		**Men n = 2918**		**Women n = 8629**		**Total n = 11,548**	
	n	%	n	%	n	%	n	%	n	%	n	%
<55 kg	35	1.0	1265	13.2	1300	10.0	44	1.5	1154	13.4	1198	10.4
56–60 kg	61	1.8	1328	13.8	1389	10.7	55	1.9	1260	14.6	1315	11.4
61–65 kg	141	4.2	1547	16.1	1688	13.0	142	4.9	1463	17.0	1605	13.9
66–70 kg	254	7.5	1413	14.7	1667	12.8	250	8.6	1243	14.4	1493	12.9
71–75 kg	377	11.1	1116	11.6	1495	11.5	334	11.4	987	11.4	1322	11.4
76–80 kg	430	12.7	805	8.4	1235	9.5	397	13.6	755	8.7	1152	10.0
81–85 kg	505	14.9	671	7.0	1176	9.0	389	13.3	591	6.8	980	8.5
86–90 kg	420	12.4	479	5.0	899	6.9	392	13.4	410	4.8	802	6.9
91–95 kg	368	10.9	344	3.6	712	5.5	286	9.8	292	3.4	579	5.0
96–100 kg	249	7.3	252	2.6	501	3.9	200	6.9	160	1.9	360	3.1
>100 kg	550	16.2	388	4.0	938	7.2	429	14.7	314	3.6	743	6.4
BMI	**Men n = 3383**		**Women n = 9579**		**Total n = 12,963**		**Men n = 2870**		**Women n = 8494**		**Total n = 11,365**	
	n	%	n	%	n	%	n	%	n	%	n	%
Underweight	54	1.6	365	3.8	419	3.2	46	1.6	334	3.9	380	3.3
Normal weight	1134	33.5	4848	50.6	5983	46.2	1037	36.1	4379	51.6	5417	47.7
Overweight	1452	42.9	2611	27.3	4063	31.3	1174	40.9	2302	27.1	3476	30.6
Grade I obesity	567	16.8	1188	12.4	1755	13.5	478	16.7	1019	12.0	1497	13.2
Grade II obesity	126	3.7	410	4.3	536	4.1	104	3.6	340	4.0	44	3.9
Grade III obesity	50	1.5	157	1.6	207	1.6	31	1.1	120	1.4	151	1.3

Conflicts of Interest The corresponding author declare no conflicts of interest

References

1. Dunlap WP, Cortina JM, Vaslow JB, Burke MJ. Meta-analysis of experiments with matched groups or repeated measures designs. Psychol Methods. 1996;1(2):170–7.
2. Cohen J. Statistical power analysis for the behavioral sciences. 2nd ed. Hillsdale: Lawrence Erlbaum Associates; 1988.
3. Chibnall JT, Tait RC. The pain disability index: factor structure and normative data. Arch Phys Med Rehabil. 1994;75(11):1082–6.
4. Dillmann U, Nilges P, Saile H, Gerbershagen HU. Behinderungseinschätzung bei chronischen Schmerzpatienten [Pain Disability Index – German version]. Schmerz. 1994;8(2):100–10.
5. Beemster T, van Bennekom C, van Velzen J, Reneman M, Frings-Dresen M. The interpretation of change score of the pain disability index after vocational rehabilitation is baseline dependent. Health Qual Life Outcomes. 2018;16:182. https://doi.org/10.1186/s12955-018-1000-1.
6. Tritt K, von Heymann F, Zaudig M, Söllner W, Klapp B, Loew T. Der Fragebogen ICD-10-Symptom-Rating (ISR): Kurzdarstellung der Normierung. Bamberg: Institut für Qualitätsentwicklung in der Psychotherapie und Psychosomatik (IQP); 2010. p. 22.
7. Fischer HF, Tritt K, Klapp BF, Fliege H. Retest-reliability and sensitivity to change of the ICD-10-symptom-rating (ISR) in different samples. Psychother Psychosom Med Psychol. 2011;61(3–4):162–9. https://doi.org/10.1055/s-0030-1263144.
8. Techniker Krankenkasse. Kann Ausdauersport den Blutdruck senken? Hamburg: TK; [updated 2024; cited 2025 Nov 28]. Available from: https://www.tk.de/techniker/krankheit-und-behandlungen/erkrankungen/behandlungen-und-medizin/herz-kreislauf-erkrankungen/kann-ausdauersport-den-blutdruck-senken-2015830
9. Arbeitsgemeinschaft der Wissenschaftlichen Medizinischen Fachgesellschaften e. V. (AWMF). S3-Leitlinie Funktionelle Körperbeschwerden [S3 Guideline Functional Somatic Symptoms]. AWMF-Registernummer 051–001. Published 2018. Accessed March 12, 2025. Available from: https://register.awmf.org/de/leitlinien/detail/051-001
10. American Psychiatric Association. Diagnostic and statistical manual of mental disorders. 5th ed. Arlington (VA): American Psychiatric Association; 2013. Somatic symptom and related disorders. Available from: https://doi.org/10.1176/appi.books.9780890425596.
11. D'Souza RS, Hooten WM. Somatic syndrome disorders. [Updated 2021 Mar 21]. In: StatPearls [Internet]. Treasure Island (FL): StatPearls Publishing; 2021. Available from: https://www.ncbi.nlm.nih.gov/books/NBK532253/
12. Henningsen P. Management of somatic symptom disorder. Dialogues Clin Neurosci. 2018;20(1):23–31.
13. Association of the Scientific Medical Societies in Germany (AWMF). S3 guideline "Functional body complaints" [S3-Leitlinie Funktionelle Körperbeschwerden]; 2018. Accessed 2022 Jan 24. Available from: https://www.awmf.org/leitlinien/leitlinien-suche.html#result-list
14. World Health Organization. ICD-11: 6C20 Bodily Distress Disorder. Geneva: World Health Organization; 2020. Accessed 2022 Jan 24. Available from: https://icd.who.int/browse11/l-m/en#/http%3a%2f%2fid.who.int%2ficd%2fentity%2f767044268
15. World Health Organization. The ICD-10 classification of mental and behavioural disorders: clinical descriptions and diagnostic guidelines. Geneva: World Health Organization; 1992. p. 112–28. Available from: https://apps.who.int/iris/handle/10665/37958
16. Steffanowski A, Löschmann C, Schmidt J, Wittmann WW, Nübling R. Die MESTA-Studie: Methodische standards für Therapieergebnisse in der ambulanten Psychotherapie [the MESTA study: methodological standards for therapy outcomes in outpatient psychotherapy]. Psychotherapeut. 2007;52(2):112–21. https://doi.org/10.1007/s00278-007-0524-1.

17. Liebherz S, Rabung S. Wirksamkeit psychotherapeutischer Krankenhausbehandlung im deutschsprachigen Raum: Eine meta-analyse [effectiveness of psychotherapeutic hospital treatment in German-speaking countries: a meta-analysis]. Psychother Psychosom Med Psychol. 2013;63(9–10):355–64.
18. Hildenbrand G, Janssen PL. Current problems of hospital planning in psychosomatic medicine and psychotherapy. Psychotherapeut. 2005;50:229–35.
19. Rückenschmerzen. Hauptgrund für Fehlzeiten im Job. KHK-Pressemitteilung. Available from: https://www.kkh.de/presse/pressemeldungen/haeufigstediagnosenjob; 2024
20. Riemann D, Baum E, Cohrs S, et al. S3- Leitlinie Nicht erholsamer Schlaf/Schlafstörungen (AWMFRegisternummer 063-003). Somnologie. 2017;21:2–44.
21. Heidbreder A, Kunz D, Young P, et al. Insomnia in Germany – massively inadequate care? Somnologie. 2024; https://doi.org/10.1007/s11818-024-00460-9.
22. BARMER Pressemitteilungen. Available from: https://www.barmer.de/presse/presseinformationen/pressearchiv/barmer-analyse-schlafstoerungen-nehmen-weiter-zu%2D%2D1243652#:~:text=Berlin%2C%2025.%20Oktober%202023%20%E2%80%93,leitende%20Medizinerin%20bei%20der%20Barmer; 2023
23. Häuser W, Bernardy K, Arnold B. Fibromyalgia syndrome – a somatoform pain disorder? Schmerz. 2006;20(2):128–39. https://doi.org/10.1007/s00482-005-0391-1.
24. Häuser WC, Zimmer E, Felde E, Köllner V. What are the core symptoms of fibromyalgia syndrome? Survey results of the German fibromyalgia association. Schmerz. 2008;22(2):176–83. https://doi.org/10.1007/s00482-007-0602-z.
25. Heidemann C, Scheidt-Nave C, Beyer A-K, Baumert J, Thamm R, Maier B, Neuhauser H, Fuchs J, Kuhnert R, Hapke U. Gesundheitliche Lage von Erwachsenen in Deutschland – Ergebnisse zu ausgewählten Indikatoren der Studie GEDA 2019/2020-EHIS [Health status of adults in Germany – Results for selected indicators from the GEDA 2019/2020-EHIS study]. J Health Monit. 2021;6(3)
26. Reyes C, Leyland KM, Peat G, Cooper C, Arden NK, Prieto-Alhambra D. Association between overweight and obesity and risk of clinically diagnosed knee, hip, and hand osteoarthritis: a population-based cohort study. Arthritis Rheumatol. 2016;68(8):1869–75. https://doi.org/10.1002/art.39707.
27. World Health Organization; International Labour Organization. Working conditions and work-related musculoskeletal disorders: WHO/ILO joint estimates. Geneva: WHO; 2021.
28. Dominguez LJ, et al. Nutrition and physical activity in musculoskeletal health. Endocrine. 2025;6(1):10. https://doi.org/10.3390/endocrines6010010.
29. Xu C, Zeng Z, Wang P, et al. Dietary patterns and risk of knee osteoarthritis: a systematic review and meta-analysis. PLoS One. 2021;16(5):e0251496. https://doi.org/10.1371/journal.pone.0251496.
30. Veronese N, Shivappa N, Stubbs B, Smith T, Hébert JR, Cooper C, Maggi S. The relationship between the dietary inflammatory index and prevalence of radiographic symptomatic osteoarthritis: data from the osteoarthritis initiative. Eur J Nutr. 2017;56(1):207–14. https://doi.org/10.1007/s00394-017-1589-6.
31. Dominguez LJ, et al. Nutrition and physical activity in musculoskeletal health. Endocrine. 2025;6(1):10. https://doi.org/10.3390/endocrines6010010.9.
32. Dai Y, et al. Association of Cigarette Smoking with risk of chronic musculoskeletal pain: a meta-analysis. Pain Physician. 2021;24:495–506.
33. Wieczorek M, et al. Smoking, alcohol consumption and disease-specific outcomes in rheumatic and musculoskeletal diseases (RMDs): systematic reviews informing the 2021 EULAR recommendations. RMD Open. 2022;8:e002170. https://doi.org/10.1136/rmdopen-2021-002170.
34. Buckwalter JA. Sports, joint injury, and posttraumatic osteoarthritis. J Orthop Sports Phys Ther. 2003;33(10):578–88. https://doi.org/10.2519/jospt.2003.33.10.578.

35. Techniker Krankenkasse. Kopfschmerzen: So häufig ist die Volkskrankheit [Headaches: How common is this widespread condition] [Internet]. Hamburg: Techniker Krankenkasse; 2024 Jan 23 [cited 2025 Nov 25]. Available from: https://www.tk.de/techniker/krankheit-und-behandlungen/erkrankungen/behandlungen-und-medizin/kopfschmerzen-und-migraene/kopfschmerzen-so-haeufig-ist-die-volkskrankheit-2016918
36. Melchart D, Hager S, Albrecht S, Dai J, Weidenhammer W, Teschke R. Herbal traditional Chinese medicine and suspected liver injury: a prospective study. World J Hepatol. 2017;9(29):1141–57. https://doi.org/10.4254/wjh.v9.i29.1141.

Evaluation and Quality Assurance Profile of the TCM-Klinik Bad Kötzting

6

Dieter Melchart, Erich Wühr, and Lara Isabel Jötten

The evaluation and quality assurance profile of the TCM-Klinik Bad Kötzting outlines all activities relating to clinical studies, publications and quality improvement projects conducted in 2023. It also summarizes previous research results. The Competence Centre for Lifestyle Medicine and Naturopathy at Deggendorf Institute of Technology (DIT) provided significant support with these matters, as well as with the ongoing audit and peer review processes.

6.1 Finalisation of a Model Project on Obesity and Chronic Stress in an Outpatient Setting of the TCM-Klinik Bad Kötzting

A study on obesity and chronic stress, conducted by TCM-Klinik Bad Kötzting as part of a model project with AOK Bayern, was completed on 25 April 2023.

This multi-year model project was carried out to test clinical efficacy in the indications of stress-related damage and obesity grades 1 and 2. The project was scientifically supported by universities and co-financed by the Bavarian State Ministry of

D. Melchart (✉)
Former Head of Competence Centre for Lifestyle Medicine and Naturopathy (CoCoNat), Faculty of Applied Healthcare Sciences, Deggendorf Institute of Technology (DIT), Deggendorf, Germany
e-mail: dieter.melchart@th-deg.de

E. Wühr
Member of the Faculty of Applied Healthcare Sciences, Deggendorf Institute of Technology (DIT), Deggendorf, Germany
e-mail: erich.wuehr@th-deg.de

L. I. Jötten
Competence Centre for Lifestyle Medicine and Naturopathy (CoCoNat), Faculty of Applied Healthcare Sciences, Deggendorf Institute of Technology (DIT), Deggendorf, Germany
e-mail: lara.joetten@th-deg.de

D. Melchart et al. (eds.), *TCM-Klinik Bad Kötzting*,
https://doi.org/10.1007/978-3-032-23307-3_6

Health and Care and the Erich Rothenfußer—Foundation in Munich. The TCM-Klinik Bad Kötzting had already gained experience of treating obesity as part of a programme entitled 'Measures to improve medical quality in Bavaria's highly rated health resorts, spas, and recognized mineral spring and mud bath establishments'. The programme ran from 2013 to 2016 and was funded by the Bavarian State Ministry of Health and Care to the tune of €1.2 million.

In 2023, a final report was prepared for AOK Bayern in collaboration with the TCM-Klinik Bad Kötzting. Here is a summary:

Recruitment and Pre-screening

From May 2017 to April 2023, the statutory health insurance company AOK Bayern sent three letters by post to regionally insured persons, contacting a total of 84,134 people. The standard letter contained a link to the pilot project website, where individuals could assess their suitability and health risks. A total of 2684 individuals (3.2% of those contacted) took advantage of this offer. Of these, 1952 (72.8%) completed a comprehensive digital report on possible stress-related illnesses, obesity, and the risk of developing type 2 diabetes mellitus. Identifying individuals at high risk for a preventive pilot project by a statutory health insurance fund is an innovative approach that, to our knowledge, was implemented for the first time in Bavaria. Of the two main indications, 45.0% of users showed signs of stress (pre-burnout), 24.8% showed signs of obesity (grades I and II), and 38.9% showed signs of developing type 2 diabetes (prediabetes).

A total of 826 people registered with the TCM clinic to receive more detailed information about the pilot project. Over the course of the pilot project, 250 people underwent a medical suitability examination for the controlled randomized studies. Successful randomisation and recruitment were achieved for both clinical studies, with 101 participants (38 for stress management and 23 for obesity management with a diabetes risk) being included, as well as a further 250 individuals who participated exclusively in the pilot project designed as an observational study. Thus, a total of 351 individuals were included in the AOK pilot project.

Problems with recruitment between 2017 and 2019 were mainly caused by unfortunate timing between recruitment and the start of the project, due to a delayed ethics committee decision. In some cases, interested participants had to wait up to three months before being invited to the clinic, resulting in many losing interests. Between 2020 and early 2023, recruitment issues were primarily caused by organisational contact losses or bans due to the pandemic. However, it should be noted that a high proportion of potentially eligible patients were not interested in participating in randomisation since access to the pilot project remained possible as a health insurance benefit.

Results by Indication Group

When all participants are categorized according to their baseline values at the start of the study (M0) into various indications of obesity, diabetes risk, stress, and mental health disorders, some individuals exhibit multiple indications.

Participants: Of the 311 participants examined, 72.1% were female and 27.9% were male. This 'feminisation' is not unusual for naturopathic and preventive services. The average age is 49.29 years (SD = 11.57), ranging from 18 to 78 years. 64.7% of participants are employed, just under 10% are retired, and 20% did not provide information about their employment status. Academic qualifications are not overrepresented: 5.4% of participants have a university degree, and 7.1% have a degree from a technical college or engineering school.

The number of valid values in all subsequent results presentations fluctuates considerably, particularly for the parameters of diabetes and high blood pressure risk, as well as for the Perceived Stress Questionnaire (PSQ) and the International Classification of Diseases Symptom Rating (ISR). With regard to information on diabetes and hypertension risk, this can be explained by the fact that participants were excluded from the corresponding analyses because they already had a known diabetes or hypertension condition. The PSQ and ISR questionnaires, on the other hand, are only made available to participants after they have exceeded a certain maximum value on the Tedium Measure (burnout), so they cannot be answered by all participants regularly. Additionally, the results for all indicators demonstrate a decline in valid values throughout the measurement periods, which unfortunately cannot be prevented within the framework of scientific monitoring over the one-year programme duration.

Stress Indication Group

The primary target parameters for assessing the effectiveness of the lifestyle programme in reducing stress for pre-burnout and burnout indications are changes in total Tedium Measure (TM) scores (TM ≥3.20, ≤4.50 and ≥4.50, respectively) and Perceived Stress Questionnaire (PSQ) scores.

Both progression parameters (TM and PSQ), as well as most secondary indicators (WHO-5 Wellbeing, SOC-13, psycho-vegetative stability, social support, etc.), show significant mean improvements over 0, 3 and 6 months for pre-burnout and burnout. There are high significance values between M0 and M6 in complete samples. On average, the total Tedium Measure value can be reduced by 1.12 points (SD = 0.90; $p < .001$; $d = 1.53$), and the PSQ value by 24.46 points (SD = 16.71; $p < .001$; $d = 1.70$), in participants with high stress levels.

Comparing these values with those obtained for the main parameter (the Perceived Stress Questionnaire, or PSQ) in the controlled randomized clinical study 'TALENT Study Stress' confirms the positive results.

The clientele of the IGM (=IHM) group (the inclusion criterion for the model project) suffers from self-perceived stress that has persisted for at least three months, with a minimum PSQ total score of over 41 points. The IHM group achieved a statistically significant difference with a large clinical effect ($p < .001$, $d = 1.70$; $p < .001$, $d = 2.13$) when comparing the PSQ total score from months 0 and 6, and from months 0 and 12 respectively. Missing values for month 6 due to study discontinuation are imputed using a conservative and realistic regression estimate. The estimate is made separately for each group. "'Conservative' estimation means that the values of the IGM group are replaced by regression estimation of the comparison group and vice versa. The result of the variance analysis testing the differences between the groups again shows a highly significant difference ($F(1,75) = 16.31$, $p < .001$) between the groups and no significant influence ($F(1,75) = 0.03$, $p = .869$) of the covariate PSQ total value at month 0.

Further exploratory analyses of changes in secondary parameters (e.g. Tedium Measure, 5-WHO Wellbeing; ICD-10 symptom rating) between the IHM group and the comparison group CG up to month 6, as well as within the IHM group up to month 12, show statistically significant, clinically relevant and sustainable (up to month 12) results with predominantly high effect sizes, as demonstrated by the example of the total Tedium Measure value (comparison M0–M6 INTER IGM/VG: $p < .001$, $d = 1.09$; comparison M0–M12 IGM $p < .001$, $d = 2.04$).

Since the randomized stress study was originally planned with 136 participants, but only 78 participants could be recruited, a cross-over evaluation of the waiting list group was carried out in addition to the study protocol to supplement the evidence data. After 6 months of intervention (see Table 6.1), the participants on the waiting list showed comparably good results in stress reduction. The main target variable, the PSQ total score, also changed statistically significantly between months 6 and 12 and months 6 and 18, with a large clinical effect ($t(29) = -5.4$, $p < .001$, $d = 0.96$; $t(24) = -7.8$, $p < .001$, $d = 1.22$; respectively).

This clinical benefit remained even after statistical correction using various imputation methods.

Mental Disorders Indication Group

The ISR total score for measuring psychological symptoms such as anxiety, compulsion, depression and somatisation disorders showed a significant difference between the IHM test group and the comparison group ($t(34) = -2.6$, $p = .004$; $d = 0.76$). The analyses of all stress groups confirmed the reduction in psychological disorders between 0 and 6 months, particularly on the basis of high significance values of the ISR (ICD symptom rating) in the subdimensions of anxiety, depression, and somatisation. Comparable positive results were also found in the WHO-5 Wellbeing Index as an early indicator of depression.

Pre-obesity and Obesity Indication Group

In the pre-obesity group (BMI ≥25, <30), consisting of 99 individuals, the primary outcome parameter of BMI showed an average reduction of 0.93 BMI points (SD = 1.82), with $p = .004$. According to Cohen, this can be portrayed as a medium effect ($d = 0.51$). The obesity group (BMI ≥30, <40) showed a significant reduction of 2.95 BMI points on average (SD = 2.44) after 12 months ($n = 59$), which, according to Cohen, is considered a large clinical effect ($d = 1.21$). On average, participants' initial weight decreased by at least 10% after 12 months. Most secondary

Table 6.1 Comparison of the PSQ total score within the cross-over group

	IHM test group							Comparison group						
	n	M	SD	df	*t*	*p*	*d*	*n*	M	SD	df	*t*	*p*	*d*
M0	30	57.44	16.55	29	−5.44	**<.001**	**.96**	35	62.62	13.17	34	2.60	.014	.34
M6	30	38.33	22.08					35	57.57	16.06				
M0	25	56.07	17.47	24	−7.75	**<.001**	**1.22**							
M12	25	34.47	18.07											

df degrees of freedom, *t* t-value of the t-test

Table 6.2 Comparison of BMI values between M0 and M12 in the nested RCT-trial

	M0 $n = 22$	M3 $n = 22$	M6 $n = 21$	M9 $n = 21$	M12 $n = 19$	Comparison M12–M0 $n = 19$			
	M (SD)	M (SD)	M (SD)	M (SD)	M (SD)	M (SD)	ΔM (SD)	p	d
BMI	33.97 (2.37)	32.32 (2.74)	31.40 (3.10)	31.44 (3.34)	31.56 (3.68)	33.74 (2.18)	−2.18 (2.46)	.001	.61

parameters improved significantly after 12 months. Even in the nested RCT clinical study with a smaller number of cases ($n = 22$) but with stricter inclusion and exclusion criteria, comparable effects on body weight were observed between M0 and M12 with $p = .001$ and a moderate effect size of $d = 0.61$ (Table 6.2).

Pre-diabetes Indication Group

A significant reduction in the diabetes risk score was observed after 12 months in the pre-obesity participant group (1.29, SD = 3.36, $p = .030$), although the effect size was small ($d = 0.38$). In the obesity group, the diabetes risk score decreased significantly by 3.20 points (SD = 3.72) with a large effect size ($d = 0.86$) at $p < .001$. When the group with an exclusively increased diabetes risk (33%; 15–20 points; $n = 43$) is shown separately, the effects are confirmed again, with an effect size of $d = 0.89$ and a reduction of 3.70 points (SD = 4.14) at $p < .001$. These results confirm the success of the IHM lifestyle programme in reducing weight in people at high risk of diabetes and corroborate the findings of the controlled randomized TALENT study of 2017 [1].

Health Economic Considerations

Due to the failure to achieve the required number of cases in the controlled studies, the economic parameters should be based on the percentage reduction in diabetes risk and in the development of depression. Intangible benefits, such as improved life satisfaction and reduced general mental stress (see secondary analysis), can be demonstrated and generally lead to greater participation and higher consumption behaviour. Additionally, it should be determined jointly with AOK Bayern whether the change in sick days should be compared between 12 months before and 12 months after the start of the intervention. However, separate data protection requirements would be necessary for this, so these assessments are still optional.

6.2 Application for Recognition as a Supplementary Rehabilitation Service in Accordance with Section 43 of the German Social Code, Book V (SGB V)—IGM® SINOCUR® Lifestyle Programme

For the clinic to offer the IGM = IHM-Sinocur lifestyle programme as an intensive lifestyle intervention (ILI) for grade 1 and 2 obesity to state health insurance funds, an application for coverage of the costs was submitted in accordance with Section 43 of the Social Code (SGB) Book V. The prerequisite for this is proof of sufficient scientific evidence and fulfilment of all requirements of a recommendation for action by the Central Association of German Health Insurance Funds. On 15 October 2023, the application was submitted for review for the purpose of gaining recognition as a measure for patient education. The content of the application is briefly outlined below.

Target Group

The target patient group consists of individuals with grade 1 and 2 obesity requiring treatment who have been under medical treatment or supervision for at least 12 months and have had contact with their doctor at least once every 3 months during this period. Obesity is generally divided into primary obesity (obesity without an underlying disease) and secondary obesity (underlying somatic disease such as hypothyroidism or underlying mental illness such as eating disorders). The patient education concept described here will focus exclusively on primary obesity. Participants aged between 18 and 65 are accepted into the programme and are primarily divided into groups aged 18–40 and 41–65. In exceptional cases, participants aged 65 and over are also included. Participants often have no previous experience with patient education.

Group size: Group sizes of 10 to a maximum of 15 people are planned.

Group Composition

Patient training services are generally provided in closed groups, which go through certain programme phases together. Individual support may only be provided in exceptional cases in consultation with the coach or background physician. Life partners may also be involved on specific days for practical instruction such as teaching kitchen or exercise training.

Timetable and Structure of Lessons

The timetables with planned scheduling for the individual phases I–IV are portrayed in Figure 6.1. In principle, the planned schedule is based on the time available to the participants. The first three health days, each consisting of five full-time hours (on Saturdays) at weekly intervals, and phase 3 as a 10-week evening event (each lasting one hour) can be offered to local interested parties. However, afterwork training sessions can also be organized in the form of two health days. In addition, it should be possible to organize phases 1–3 at weekly intervals as health days or as a compact week. The respective closed group will decide on this at the beginning of the programme.

Phase I: Screening Programme

In the screening programme (Phase I), the TCM health portal is used to determine health data, cardio-metabolic risk factors, psychosomatic stress levels, motivation to change health behaviour and life satisfaction as an important protective factor for health. A personal health report and training measures are designed to increase risk awareness and promote motivation to adopt more health-promoting behaviours. The data provided by the attending physician in the medical necessity certificate is evaluated by the core team physician during the first team meeting and explained to the participant during the initial examination, if necessary. Between the health days, insured persons conduct seven days of self-observation of their lifestyle in terms of nutrition and exercise behaviour and measure their own health data several times. An optional time-mood analysis is designed to help them perceive their own emotion regulation in everyday life. The insured person receives the necessary materials in a starter kit. They are trained and encouraged to enter their relevant data in the TCM health portal and to repeat this daily or quarterly, if necessary. The amount of documentation required will depend on the programme section and the individual agreement with the coach and the insured person.

Phase II: Introductory Programme

In the introductory programme (Phase II), the TCM health portal is used to determine the insured person's life demands, individual responses to these demands, and resources and protective factors. The insured persons carry out self-observation over a period of seven days. The TCM health portal is then completed by the insured person and evaluated together with the coach. Data from the last health check (at the age of 35) should be documented by participants in the health portal. If there is a legal entitlement to a health check and this has not yet been carried out, participants are encouraged to have this done and to enter the data into the portal as part of their personal responsibility for their own health. An initial assessment of the individual's general state of health is then carried out, based on the values from the 'screening programme'. Based on this, the training packages in the areas of nutrition, exercise and stress management/relaxation (including a package of remedies and natural remedies, if applicable) are determined with the coach. The introductory programme is carried out over a total of two days. Based on this evaluation, the insured person receives their health values in the TCM health portal and is then able to determine the intensity of the programme themselves at any time. The insured person enters their vital parameters (weight, waist circumference, walking test, nutrition and satisfaction check) into the TCM health portal on a daily/weekly basis in order to determine the progression of their personal risk factors. The documentation interval in the TCM health portal depends on the programme section and individual agreements between the coach and the insured person.

Phase III: Everyday Programme

The everyday programme (Phase III) lasts 3 months and consists of ten weekly after-work practical seminars (after-work training sessions) and twelve indication-dependent individual weekly training plans, according to which the insured person practises their health behaviour. In the after-work training sessions, the insured persons are trained and practised by the coaches for 1 h. In addition, training materials are made available via the health portal.

Phase IV: Maintenance Programme

The maintenance programme (Phase IV) lasts nine months and includes refresher meetings and virtual visits. During this time, four refresher meetings lasting 3 h each are held. Throughout the 9 months, participants are monitored weekly by coaches on the basis of their documentation in the TCM health portal, and data on individual and group progress is generated. Group participants receive corresponding feedback from the coaches via email, text message or, if necessary, telephone call. *The core of the remote support (distant lifestyle counselling) initially consists of weekly (always on Wednesdays) virtual group visits lasting 15 min*. These are held weekly in the 2nd and 3rd quarters of the maintenance phase and every 14 days in the 4th quarter. At the end of the maintenance programme, a final assessment of the goals achieved is carried out. Alternatively, the 10 after-work seminars can also be arranged in the form of two 5-h health days and/or together with phases 1 and 2 as a compact week. The refresher times are adjusted.

Figures 6.1 illustrate the individual phases and training packages of the IHM that cover a period of 12 months (M0–M12), with the first 3 months (M3) characterized by intensive lifestyle intervention (ILI). Phases 1 and 2 of the IHM comprise screening and assessment and the introductory programme with a total of three

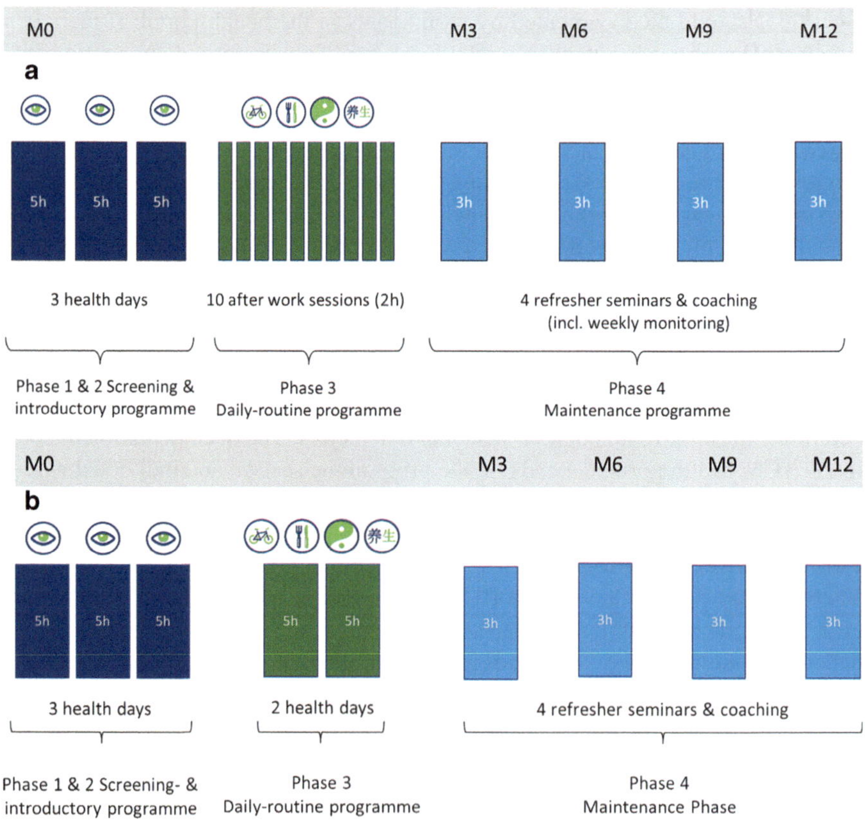

Fig. 6.1 (**a**) IHM individual phases and training packages with 10 after-work seminars in phase 3, (**b**) IHM individual phases and training packages with two health days in phase 3

health days (5 h each). This is followed by the everyday programme (phase 3) with 10 after-work seminars (2 h each) and the optional intensive training week (Fig. 6.1a), which participants complete themselves. Phase 3 can also be carried out in the form of 2 additional health days (5 h each) (Fig. 6.1b). The maintenance programme consists of four refresher events (3 h each) and online visits (15 min each), which are provided as '"distant lifestyle counselling' by the IGM health coaches

Methodological Approach (Methods Used)
Instruction is provided in closed groups by specially trained IHM coaches. In addition to traditional learning and experience in the face-to-face group and the principle of self-observation, self-perception and self-assessment through an individual health portal, online meetings with group visits are also held weekly as e-health contacts during the maintenance phase. The combination of face-to-face teaching and the use of an e-health tool (VITERIO® health portal—TCM health portal) is referred to as 'blended learning BL'. The concept of *blended* learning has proven to be an effective method of imparting knowledge and skills [2]. It successfully combines various teaching methods such as the internet, paper and personal support in the form of coaching, which is designed to enable course participants to make independent and autonomous changes to their health behaviour and attitudes. The working group led by Al-Badri M et al. [3] confirms, among other things, the benefits of the hybrid use of personal and internet-based media in patient education for obese adults in need of treatment.

Teaching and Learning Media
The entire lifestyle programme is based on systematic self-observation, self-awareness and self-reflection on one's own health behaviour, which participants are expected to acquire as basic skills. In addition to theoretical classroom teaching in groups (health days, after-work or day seminars), which are conducted face-to-face or in a circle of chairs using various media such as PowerPoint presentations, handouts, flipcharts and moderator's case-based materials, practical instruction is also provided in the teaching kitchen (followed by consumption of the food), movement exercises in the exercise room or spa gardens, or training in the form of an excursion (food shopping). The use of the web-based health portal enables individual, self-organized or self-directed learning in everyday life, mainly outside of face-to-face teaching. In addition, online visits and online meetings for the groups are organized and made possible.

The individual components of the teaching and learning media are therefore face-to-face events (health days, after-work seminars), activities such as 'distant lifestyle counselling' (online) and the web-based e-health portal VITERIO (TCM health portal), which also serves as a documentation medium for digital self-observation and as a learning medium via multimodal techniques such as videos, audio files and PDF info@cepts as counselling prescriptions, as well as via an appointment planner.

The Original Concept Is Individual Health Management (IHM)

The central element of IHM is self-management, which enables individuals to maintain and optimize their so-called basic physiological functions (exercise, nutrition, vegetative balance, immune system, heat balance, sleep, rhythm) as well as psychosocial and cognitive basic skills (self-competence, social competence) in everyday life in order to sustainably increase, maintain or restore personal quality of life and life satisfaction through a healthy lifestyle. Individual health management (IHM) encompasses both a pathogenetic perspective, which focuses on chronic disease and its risks, consequential damage and prevention, and a salutogenic perspective, which includes protective factors and resources for strengthening health. This not only complements a scientific-theoretical perspective but also opens up an additional course of action in treatment that emphasizes cross-disease, i.e. health-oriented aspects, and can thus have an additive effect.

The rationality of the programme lies primarily in strengthening self-awareness and self-reflection of maladaptive behaviours and inadequate emotional-cognitive assessments and their correction, as well as optimizing the functioning of the autonomic nervous system [4]. The central focus of the programme is to strengthen self-reflection and self-awareness through digital self-measurement and life logging, as well as group support and individual coaching. This enables participants to correct health-threatening behavioural components in their exercise and eating habits themselves, identify maladaptive cognitive evaluation patterns and improve them themselves. The background theories include Becker's systemic requirements and resources model, Boessmann & Peseschkian's balance and conflict model, M. Berking's emotional skills training, and Ellis' rational emotive behaviour therapy [5–8].

Inclusion Criteria

- $30\ \text{kg/m}^2 \geq \text{BMI} < 40\ \text{kg/m}^2$
- Waist-to-hip ratio (WHR = waist circumference in cm/hip circumference in cm) in women > 0.85 resp. in men > 1.0
- and obesity-associated comorbidities:
  - E66.0 Obesity due to excessive calorie intake; body mass index [BMI] of 30 to less than 40 in patients aged 18 years and older
  - I10 Essential (primary) hypertension grade I-2 with or without medication
  - E11 Diabetes mellitus, type 2
  - E68 Consequences of overeating
  - E78 Disorders of lipoprotein metabolism
  - G47.3 Sleep apnoea syndrome
  - I25 Chronic ischaemic heart disease
  - I50 Heart failure
  - R73 Elevated blood glucose level
  - R73.0 Abnormal glucose tolerance test
    R73.9 Hyperglycaemia, unspecified

Patients in Whom

- Despite personal initiative and medical treatment, no weight reduction could be achieved, whereby it must be ensured that hormonal disorders were treated in advance
- Secondary obesity has been ruled out
- A medical certificate of necessity is available
  - Height, weight, BMI, WHR and any existing risk factors
  - Obesity-associated diseases
  - Laboratory tests performed to date (including fasting blood sugar, HbA1c, oral glucose tolerance test if applicable, total, HDL and LDL cholesterol, triglycerides, uric acid, creatinine, electrolytes, TSH)
  - Further diagnostics performed to date (e.g. ECG, ergometry, echocardiography, 24-h blood pressure measurement, sleep apnoea screening, abdominal sonography, Doppler sonography)
  - Measures taken to date within the scope of statutory health insurance
  - As well as measures taken independently to date to reduce weight
  - Ability to participate in group activities and training (in particular, sufficient physical fitness to participate in all training modules)
  - Possible mental disorders and exclusion of manifest eating disorders
    Exclusion of secondary and syndromic obesity resulting from other diseases (e.g. Prader-Willi syndrome, Cushing's syndrome)

In addition to the need for training, the ability to participate in training must also be present. This includes:

- Language skills
- Ability to work in a group
- Physical and psychological suitability
- Willingness to actively participate

Exclusion Criteria

Participation in a training programme is not possible if any of the following criteria are met:

- Mental disorders or illnesses that impair active participation
- Manifest eating disorder/bulimia
- Lack of motivation on the part of the patient
- Insufficient mental resilience
- Insufficient cardiopulmonary fitness to participate in the exercise component
- Unstable angina pectoris, severe cardiac arrhythmia
- Pregnancy/breastfeeding
- Insufficient ability to work in a group

- Lack of ability to learn
- Secondary obesity caused by a disease or hormonal disorder (e.g. Prader-Willi syndrome, MC 4 receptor gene defect, Cushing's syndrome)
- Condition following obesity surgery

Disqualification Criteria

- No regular attendance at training sessions (at least 80% of training sessions must have been attended)
- Occurrence of one of the above exclusion criteria or other serious health problems that make regular attendance no longer possible.
- The discontinuation will be documented with reasons, and the health insurance company will be informed of the discontinuation.

Internal/External Quality Management
The internal quality management of the TCM-Klinik Bad Kötzting comprises:

- Compliance with and further development of the structured training concept
- Regular team meetings of the training team (IHM health coaches and core medical team)
- Continuous training of team members (train-the-trainer) and quality circles

All lecturers involved in patient training have a basic qualification in the form of a state-recognized vocational qualification in a healthcare profession and further training as an IHM health coach at the Deggendorf Institute of Technology (the healthcare profession is a prerequisite for obtaining the IHM health coach certificate). The IHM Health Coach certification training qualifies participants to conduct training courses in the areas of stress management, nutrition and lack of exercise for people who are overweight, stressed and at risk of secondary diseases, as well as those at risk of diabetes, cardiovascular disease or metabolic syndrome.

The concept of external quality management originates from the university and academic environment (Technical University of Munich, Deggendorf Institute of Technology). It is continuously adapted to the current state of research and technology. Participation in the health insurance fund's quality assurance measures is not necessary in the case of IGM, as scientific proof of effectiveness is available in the form of a randomized controlled clinical study (TALENT Study Adipositas [1, 9, 10]).

Accompanying Evaluation
Screening is based on scientifically validated questionnaires; contraindications are ruled out by a medical certificate of necessity. The duration and frequency of the individual patient education interventions in the IHM® lifestyle programme correspond to an *intensive lifestyle intervention (ILI)* which, according to a review by Navneet Singh et al. [11], involves *at least 28 individual interventions per year.*

According to Singh, the clinical results of an ILI can be further improved by increasing the frequency of interventions per year beyond this minimum number. In terms of *result quality*, all current health data and changes therein are documented in the VITERIO health portal and can be accessed and evaluated by all IHM participants (participants, coaches and doctors) and are available as case report forms (CRFs) or health reports. A minimum requirement for the quality of results can also be demonstrated offline by means of a 7-day self-observation protocol.

Efficacy

The clinical success of the programme has already been scientifically proven in the cardiometabolic field with the implementation and evaluation of a modern overweight and obesity management programme in the form of a randomized clinical study called TALENT (Tailored Lifestyle Intervention Study) [1]. In the TALENT study, after 12 months, the intervention group showed a reduction in body weight of 8.7 kg (SD = 6.1; n = 109) compared to their initial weight. In contrast, the body weight of participants in the control group receiving standard medical care (without the IGM lifestyle programme) was reduced by only 4.2 kg (SD = 5; n = 57) [1]. Compared to other guideline-compliant obesity studies conducted in Germany during this period, the TALENT study achieved the best results of all clinical studies conducted without a formula diet. In addition to the main variable '"body weight reduction', the secondary variables 'blood pressure', 'fasting blood sugar' and 'LDL' were also significantly reduced compared to the control group [1]. Similarly, evidence of the benefits of the 'IHM® SINOCUR® lifestyle programme' is available from a clinical study with a pre-post design. This study was conducted as part of a model project with AOK Bayern from 2017 to 2023 (see Sect. 6.1).

Result of the Request for Review

The social medical report by the Bavarian Medical Service, dated 27 February 2024 and bearing ID number 359999093, concluded that the structured and comprehensive concept meets all the criteria required by the joint recommendations for patient education measures, as set out in Section 43(1)(2) of the German Social Code, Book V (SGB V).

6.3 Supervision of Doctoral Theses Carried Out at the TCM-Klinik Bad Kötzting

6.3.1 Therapeutic Application and Effects of Astragali Radix (Huángqí) and Rehmanniae Radix (ShēnDìhuáng)/ Rehmanniae Radix Praeparatae (Shú Dìhuáng) in Type 2 Diabetes Mellitus. A Review

Title of dissertation: see 6.3.1
Doctoral candidate: Ulrike Wallauer
Date of acceptance: 20 December 2023

Degree-awarding institution: TUM (Technical University of Munich) School of Medicine and Health
Target doctorate: Dr. med. (M.D.)

Dissertation Abstract

Background: Diabetes mellitus refers to a group of metabolic diseases characterized by chronic hyperglycaemia. The cause is either impaired insulin secretion, impaired insulin action, or both. The spread of modern, sedentary lifestyles and changes in dietary habits are contributing to the steady increase in type 2 diabetes mellitus (T2DM) worldwide and posing an increasing challenge to global health. According to the IDF-Atlas (10th edition, 2021), the global diabetes prevalence of adults (20–79 years) was approximately 537 million (10.5%) in 2021. China is among the countries with the highest rates of diabetes in the world (140 million (13%) in 2021). To treat T2DM, many Chinese hospitals use a combination of Western medicine and traditional Chinese medicine. The drugs Astragali radix (Huangqi) and Rehmanniae radix (Sheng Dihuang and Shu Dihuang, respectively) are widely used in Chinese herbal medicine to treat T2DM. The aim of this review is to find out whether there is any scientific work available for these TCM drugs regarding a preventive or therapeutic use in T2DM. Of further interest is the level of knowledge and level of evidence of these studies as well as the suitability of Astragali radix and Rehmanniae radix for preventive or therapeutic use from a Western perspective in T2DM.

Search methods: With the help of a systematic literature search, the research question was investigated in the period 2000–2022 in the databases PubMed, Cochrane Library, Google Scholar, DIMI, Embase, Web of Science, Biomedcentral and Wiley Online Library. Selection criteria: there were no restrictions on study type and duration. Clinical and preclinical studies were included. Study participants were patients with T2DM, IGT or IFG without other restrictions. All galenic forms of the two Chinese drugs, their ingredients and herbal formulations containing one or both drugs were approved as interventions and compared with placebo, pharmacological or non-pharmacological interventions. All endpoints that could indicate an improvement in the pre-diabetic or diabetic metabolic situation were approved. The effects on diabetic complications were not the subject of this review. Regarding the publication language, Chinese publications with an English abstract were excluded. Data collection and analysis: all relevant data were systematically collected, arranged according to descending level of evidence and summarized in tables.

Main results: 140 relevant publications were identified. The evaluation of meta-analyses and systematic reviews showed that only a few studies on this topic are accessible due to language barriers and difficult access to Chinese databases. It also became apparent that the research question is being studied scientifically worldwide. The main focus (approx. 81,4%) of the studies is in the preclinical area and mostly examines single herbs, their main ingredients and less frequently herbal formulas. All basic research studies, except for one cell culture study, demonstrate multiple direct and/or indirect antidiabetic effects for both drugs. Multiple ingredients of Astragali radix and Rehmanniae radix have an antidiabetic, anti-inflammatory, antioxidant, immunomodulatory, tissue and organ protective effect via multiple pharmacological pathways and goals. In the area of clinical studies, all included meta-analyses (8), systematic reviews (3), RCTs (9), prospective (1) and retrospective (2) observational studies and individual case studies (3) show antidiabetic effects. TCM phyto-therapeutics showed additional benefit in T2DM as well as reduced T2DM incidence in impaired glucose tolerance. The use of herbal formulas, not single herbals, is characteristic of TCM. As expected, Astragali radix and Rehmanniae radix were predominantly found in herbal formulas in the clinical area. Analysis of the components of 30 antidiabetic herbal TCM formulas approved by the Chinese SDA (State Drug Administration) for T2DM therapy revealed that the most commonly used antidiabetic TCM herb is Astragali radix, followed by Rehmanniae radix in second place. However, due to lack of methodological information or insufficient methodological quality, a large proportion of the clinical studies show a methodological risk of bias.

In numerous animal experiments, experimental studies and clinical studies Astragali radix and Rehmanniae radix demonstrate multiple direct and indirect antidiabetic effects. These studies strongly suggest a possible additional benefit of Astragali radix and Rehmanniae radix in preventive and therapeutic use for T2DM. However, due to the methodological shortcomings of the existing studies, there is an urgent need for more methodologically excellent clinical controlled trials, both in formulas, single drugs and main ingredients, to draw definite conclusions.

Doctorate Completed
Availability: https://mediatum.ub.tum.de/doc/1688538/1688538.pdf.

6.3.2 Acceptance and Compliance with the Use of Traditional Chinese Medicine at the TCM Clinic in Bad Kötzting and Its Possible Side Effects

Title of dissertation: see 6.3.2
Doctoral candidate: Martin Rößner
Date of acceptance: unknown
Degree-awarding institution: TUM School of Medicine and Health
Target doctorate: Dr. med. (M.D.)

Dissertation Abstract

Objectives

The aim of the project is to record subjective assessments of TCM drug therapy in terms of acceptance, compliance and self-reported side effects by patients at the TCM clinic in the form of a semi-structured interview. In addition, the results of safety parameters from liver enzyme diagnostics carried out by the clinic laboratory and routine information provided by patients on side effects as part of the TCM clinic's 'complication screening programme' will be evaluated and compared with the results of our own survey. Causality assessment of liver damage should be performed using RUCAM (Roussel Uclaf Causality Assessment Method).

Primary/Secondary Endpoints

Primary: Gastrointestinal symptoms, vegetative symptoms, other symptoms and assessments; liver transaminases (GPT, AP), bilirubin from routine laboratory tests.

Secondary: compliance with taking the decoctions; continuity of drug therapy after hospitalisation, well-being during therapy, drugs taken or prescribed, diagnoses (Chinese/Western).

Study Population

1. Inclusion and exclusion criteria: A prerequisite for the study is a hospital stay of at least 2 weeks under TCM drug therapy.
2. Number of study participants: 120 patients who will be interviewed in a semi-structured interview, as well as approximately 1000 anonymous questionnaires from patients during their inpatient stay in the same time phase (via the VITERIO health portal) and a follow-up survey approximately three months after discharge
3. Recruitment: Recruitment takes place at the TCM Clinic in Bad Kötzting at specific times (prior information and explanation of participation by the clinic's TCM doctors).

During the exploratory year, around 1000 patients completed anonymous questionnaires about side effects via the VITERIO® health portal. They are due to complete a follow-up survey around 6 months after discharge.

Biometrics

Descriptive analysis of the side effects and compliance questionnaire.

Determination of mean liver values and subgroup analysis of patients with abnormal values. Analysis of prescribed medicines (TCM and conventional medicines) for the collective.

Progress of the Dissertation
Progress on the work has been very slow since November 2016. After taking a year out, the doctoral candidate is set to make a final attempt to finish his dissertation.

6.3.3 The Impact of Beliefs and Mental States on Treatment Success in a Psychosomatic Hospital Including Traditional Chinese Medicine

Title of dissertation: see 6.3.3
Doctoral candidate: Lara Isabel Jötten M.Sc.
Date of acceptance: unknown
Degree-awarding institution: LMU School of Medicine and Health
Target doctorate: Dr. rer. biol. Hum. (Ph.D. in Human Biology)

Summary

Background: The primary healthcare system in psychosomatic rehabilitation aims to improve or cure existing symptoms through various effective treatments that target biological, psychological and social aspects. There are therefore many factors that play a role and can lead to people responding well, less well or not at all to treatment. Understanding the interaction of biological, psychological, and social factors is crucial for predicting treatment outcomes and enhancing patient care.

Aim: The aim of this study is the classification of modifiable characteristics that influence the success of inpatient treatment at a complementary psychosomatic hospital. Identified influencing factors can help to customize treatment in order to achieve better results for patients.

Method: The study leverages patient registry data from the TCM Klinik Bad Kötzting and study-specific questionnaires distributed to randomly selected patients within the clinic. An exploratory approach is employed, using preliminary correlation analyses and regression analyses to identify and compare the predictive value of disease, personal, mental, and belief-based factors on treatment success. Additionally, a responder analysis will validate subgroup identification by assessing medium-term outcomes six months post-treatment.

Discussion: The findings from this research could significantly enhance our understanding of the underlying mechanisms at work and contribute to the improvement of clinical treatments.

Progress of the Dissertation
The questionnaires were first adapted on the basis of a preliminary study. The main study is currently running according to plan at the clinic. Overall, the process has been successful so far.

6.4 Quality Testing of Medicinal Products for Identity, Purity and Content, as Well as for Harmful Residues

While Chinese herbal remedies appear to be relatively safe, they are not free of risks, and a number of severe adverse events have been reported. Although hepatotoxic effects associated with Chinese drugs have been described, it is unclear how often such adverse effects occur.

The clinic maintains its own special pharmacy for TCM medicines. Before the tea mixtures are processed into decoctions and used in patient care, the drugs are subjected to the quality assurance program described below. Various institutions and laboratories under the responsibility of the clinic are involved in this process. In previous years, the Institute of Pharmacy at the Center for Pharmaceutical Research at the University of Munich assumed technical responsibility for this (Univ.Prof. Dr. Dr.h.c. H. Wagner). The Institute of Pharmaceutical Biology at the University of Düsseldorf (Univ.Prof. Dr. R. Bauer—later University of Graz) was commissioned to compile the scientific monograph. During this period, various books on monographs of the most important TCM drugs were published in collaboration with Prof. Wagner and Prof. Bauer, with the support of the clinic and the scientific advisory board [12–16].

Meanwhile, commercial companies have been carrying out these laboratory tests on behalf of the clinic for many years (e.g. SinoMed GmbH and Phyto-Chem).

The overall quality assurance programme for TCM medicines focuses on the following areas:

- Quality testing of medicines for identity, purity, and content of selected ingredients
- Testing of medicines for toxic loads and contamination

Drug Investigations Between 2003 and 2025—An Overview

The quality tests were primarily conducted on the basis of the German Pharmacopoeia (DAB 1996 and 1999), a 'collection of recognized pharmaceutical rules on the quality, testing, storage, labeling, and designation of medicinal products (§55 Medicinal Products Act)'. Since only a very small proportion of Chinese medicinal plants are mentioned in the DAB 1999 (e.g., Rhizoma Rhei, Radix Ginseng, Herba Ephedrae, Zingiberis radix), pharmacopoeias from other member states of the European Community were initially consulted. Only then were other reference books and sources from third countries used.

Here, the 'Pharmacopoeia of Chinese Medicine' (1985, 1990, and 1995 editions) formed a very important basis for the prescribed tests. Other official Chinese books with illustrations of drugs, individual regulations from the Japanese Pharmacopoeia, and supplementary regulations from Chinese monographs were also used for precise drug identification. In addition, special drug monographs were used to obtain clear identification through special analysis methods. In isolated cases, it was necessary to draw up additional test regulations.

The overall quality assurance program for TCM medicines focuses on the following areas:

- Quality testing of medicines for identity, purity, and content of selected ingredients
- Testing of medicines for toxic loads and contamination ("Drug Monitoring Program")

The *identification* of drugs by testing their morphology and identity was carried out by means of:

- Macroscopic (organoleptic)
- Microscopic determination
- Chemical reactions to substance groups
- Thin-layer chromatography (in approx. 25% of the batches examined in full)

In order to determine the quality of the drugs, the *purity test* in individual cases specified the quantification of foreign components and loss on drying.

The *content determinations* (specified in approx. 34% of the batches examined in full) primarily involved the following tests (listed in descending order of frequency):

- Extract content using various extraction agents
- Determination of the essential oil content in the drug
- Substance content of mineral substances
- Specific drug constituents (HPLC, UV spectroscopy, titration, gravimetry)

Acceptance criteria for foreign substances, ash and hydrochloric acid-insoluble ash, and drying losses were determined for the purity tests.

In accordance with the regulations of the German Pharmacopoeia, the drug batches were sent to specialized laboratories for testing for *microbial purity* and *pesticide residues*, as well as for *heavy metal residues* and *contamination with aflatoxins*.

The results were evaluated in accordance with the 1996 DAB limits for herbal medicinal products to which boiling water is added prior to use (microbial purity max. 10^7/g aerobic bacteria, max. 10^5/g fungi, max. 10^2/g *Escherichia coli*), the Maximum Residue Limits Regulation or DAB 1996 (pesticides according to the specifications of the individual substances of the DAB), the BGM recommendation (heavy metals max. 0.1 mg/kg mercury, max. 0.2 mg/kg cadmium, max. 5.0 mg/kg lead) and the 'Contaminant Recommendation Aflatoxins' of April 3, 1995 (aflatoxins max. 2 mg/kg aflatoxin B_1, max. 4 mg/kg total aflatoxins B_1, B_2, G_1, G_2).

Table 6.3 shows an overview of the test results for the various batches of drugs purchased between 2000 and 2025. A total of 781 batches of TCM medicines were purchased from China by the TCM Clinic in Bad Kötzting during this period. Of these, 131 batches—equivalent to 16.8% of all drugs—were rejected due to poor

Table 6.3 This is an overview of the test results for quality issues of TCM drugs between 2000 and 2025

					Reasons for poor quality			
Year	Delivery	Quantity of batches	of which were blocked	in %	Identity	Quality	Content	Purity
2000	August 30, 2000	45	7	15.56	2		2	2
	October 5, 2000	29	4	13.79	2		1	1
	10/30/2000	37	15	40.51			1	3
	12/20/2000	40	15	37.50			6	3
2001	March 14, 2001	47	17	36.17	2		4	4
2003	01/07/2003	55	6	10.91				
	Dec 30, 2003	29	2	6.90			1	
2004	April 26, 2004	36	2	5.56				
	Sep 24, 2004	45	6	13.36				
	11/03/2004	23	13	56.52			2	
2005	09/01/2005	24	3	12.50			2	
2006	01.08.2006	8	0	0.00				
2007	January 29, 2007	6	0	0.00				
	02.04.2007	6	0	0.00				
	07/09/2007	1	0	0				
	12/01/2007	30	8	26.67	1			
2008	January 1, 2008	16	0	0.00				
	04/01/2008	1	0	0.00				
2010	July 21, 2010	19	0	0.00				
2011	January 10, 2011	27	2	7.41				
	January 17, 2011	26	6	23.08				
2012	August 16, 2012	14	0	0.00				
2014	January 7, 2014	15	4	26.67				
	January 15, 2014	8	1	12.50				
2015	March 1, 2015	13	2	15.38	2			
2016	Jan 25, 2016	16	0	0.00				
	Feb 15, 2016	2	0	0.00				
	Sep 15, 2016	5	0	0.00				
2017	Feb 23, 2017	10	0	0.00				
2018	Jan. 11, 2018	22	2	9.09	1			
	August 23, 2018	12	0	0.00				
2019	06/06/2019	17	4	23.53				
2020	06/08/2020	22	1	4.55				
2021	June 25, 2021	10	1	10.00				

(continued)

Table 6.3 (continued)

					Reasons for poor quality			
Year	Delivery	Quantity of batches	of which were blocked	in %	Identity	Quality	Content	Purity
2022	14.11.2022	12	3	25.00				
2023	May 17, 2023	14	3	21.43				
2024	March 5, 2024	10	1	10.00				
	09/01/2024	9	1	11.11				
2025	02/01/2025	10	1	10.10				
	06/05/2025	10	1	10.00				
Total		**781**	**131**	**16.77**	**10**	**0**	**19**	**13**

quality or contamination. This means that these drugs were not approved for distribution or for patient care.

When looking at the individual reasons for the qualitative rejection of the various batches, it is striking that there were significantly more quality defects in the years 2000–2004 than in the period thereafter. In particular, the content and purity of the drugs improved significantly. However, isolated identity problems were observed until 2018.

Testing for toxic loads and contamination, Cadmium played the most frequent role in the early years from 2000 to 2004 (Table 6.4). For example, in a delivery on November 3, 2004, a total of 13 out of 23 batches (56.5%) had to be rejected, 10 of which were contaminated with excessive cadmium levels. Lead is the second most common issue associated with heavy metal contamination. These findings cannot currently be dismissed and continue to be observed in examinations conducted up to 2021.

Contamination by microbial organisms and exposure to insecticides is another highly relevant issue in the context of TCM drug safety and underlines the importance of such investigations. Insecticides are the third most common cause of rejection of TCM drugs within the TCM-Klinik Bad Kötzting.

Figure 6.2 shows an example of a test certificate from 2025 for the traditional Chinese medicine (TCM) drug Ligustici chuanxiong rhizome.

The medicinal plant was tested for identity and authenticity using macroscopic testing, TLC and HPLC fingerprint analysis.

The test results were found to comply with the specifications. Safety testing for possible contamination showed that microbial contaminants, heavy metals, pesticides and aflatoxins were within regulatory limits.

Table 6.4 An overview of toxic substances and contamination in TCM medicines between 2000 and 2025

					Impurities*						
Year	Delivery	Quantity of batches	of which were blocked	In %	Arsenic	Lead	Cadmium	Mercury	Pesticides	Aflatoxins	Microbiology
2000	Aug 30, 2000	45	7	15.56			1				
	10/05/2000	29	4	13.79			1				
	10/30/2000	37	15	40.51		3	8				1
	Dec 20, 2000	40	15	37.50			4			2	
2001	Mar 14, 2001	47	17	36.17	1	2	1	1			1
2003	07.01.2003	55	6	10.91			3		1	1	
	Dec 30, 2003	29	2	6.90			1				
2004	April 26, 2004	36	2	5.56		2	1				
	Sep 24, 2004	45	6	13.36		2	3			1	
	Nov 3, 2004	23	13	56.52		6	10	1			2
2005	Sep 1, 2005	24	3	12.50				1	1		
2006	01.08.2006	8	0	0.00							
2007	Jan. 29, 2007	6	0	0.00							
	02.04.2007	6	0	0.00							
	07/09/2007	1	0	0							
	12/01/2007	30	8	26.67		1	5		1		
2008	01/01/2008	16	0	0.00							
	04/01/2008	1	0	0.00							
2010	July 21, 2010	19	0	0.00							
2011	Jan. 10, 2011	27	2	7.41							2
	Jan 17, 2011	26	6	23.08			1		1		5
2012	Aug 16, 2012	14	0	0.00							
2014	Jan 7, 2014	15	4	26.67		1			2		2
	Jan 15, 2014	8	1	12.50					1		
2015	March 1, 2015	13	2	15.38							
2016	Jan 25, 2016	16	0	0.00							
	Feb 15, 2016	2	0	0.00							
	Sep 15, 2016	5	0	0.00							

2017	Feb 23, 2017	10	0	0.00							
2018	Jan. 11, 2018	22	2	9.09		1					
	Aug 23, 2018	12	0	0.00							
2019	06/06/2019	17	4	23.53		1			1	1	1
2020	June 8, 2020	22	1	4.55					1		
2021	June 25, 2021	10	1	10.00		1					
2022	14.11.2022	12	3	25.00					1		2
2023	May 17, 2023	14	3	21.43							3
2024	03/05/2024	10	1	10.00							
	09/01/2024	9	1	11.11					1		
2025	02/01/2025	10	1	10.10							
	06/05/2025	10	1	10.00					1		
Total		**781**	**131**	**16.77**	**1**	**20**	**39**	**3**	**12**	**5**	**19**

Dienstleistungsanalytik – Analysenbericht TCM Drogenfreigabe Phytochem

Certificate of Analysis

CoA acc. ApBetrO § 6 and § 11			
Test sample	Ligustici chuanxiong rhizhoma		
specification	IDN 236		
PC-code	CH 0197	No. of analysis	25004-9
Lot	236CX241211		
client	Sinomed GmbH		

Testing of the Identity and Authenticity of the Herbal / animal Product		
According to	Generelle Prüfvorschrift zur Freigabe von Drogen	
Testing parameter	**Specification**	**Test result**
Macroscopic testing	Prüfvorschrift Ligustici chuanxiong rhizhoma	**conforms**
TLC Fingerprint Analysis	Prüfvorschrift Ligustici chuanxiong rhizhoma	**conforms**
HPLC Fingerprint Analysis	Prüfvorschrift Ligustici chuanxiong rhizhoma	**conforms**

Testing of the Safety regarding to Contaminants of the Herbal Product contracted		
Testing parameter	**Specification**	**Test result**
Microbial contaminants	Ph. Eur. 5.1.8 Kat. A	**conforms**
Heavy metals	DIN EN 15763 (Hg, Pb, Cd)	**conforms**
Pesticides	§ 64 LFGB L 00.00-115	**conforms**
Aflatoxins	Aflatoxin-Verbots-VO 2000 / 2004	**conforms**

The reported Tests above confirm the Identity/Authenticity and the Safety regarding to Contaminants of the analysed Product

The test results relate only to the items tested.
The report shall not be reproduced except in full without the written approval of the testing laboratory.

Neu-Ulm, March 06, 2025

Fig. 6.2 Original certificate of analysis from 2025

6.5 A Case Report Form (CRF) for Hospital Therapists and a Health Report for Patients

To ensure continuous quality assurance and transparency, a case report form (CRF) is created for each patient on the VITERIO web portal, which is only made available to the clinic's psychologists and doctors. This comprehensive reporting system was developed by CoCoNat at the DIT in collaboration with the clinic. The following section uses the example of a patient with functional somatic disorders to illustrate the content and information that is compiled about the patient. In addition, a health report is generated for the patients themselves, which contains a summary of the completed evaluation questionnaires as well as diagnosis and therapy data.

The content of the individual case report form is presented in its original form on the following pages.

1. *General Information*

General note on the tables on all subsequent pages: Column entries marked with "–" indicate that no survey has been/is being conducted or that there are no target values.

Section 1.01 Sociodemographic Data

Gender	Female
Age	58

Section 1.02 Self-Motivation and Willingness to Change

In future, I would like to pay much more attention to my health	Yes, absolutely
I am prepared to maintain or improve my health by changing my behaviour in the following areas	Yes, absolutely
Change your daily routine (in terms of diet, exercise or relaxation)	
I am prepared to use an internet-based health portal to implement a lifestyle programme	Yes, absolutely
I have a PC with internet access at home	Yes, absolutely

Section 1.03 Anthropometric Data/Blood Pressure

	First measurement		Last measurement	
Height (cm)	168	06.09.2023	168	06.09.2023
Body weight (kg)	65.5	06.09.2023	64.8	27 September 2023
Body mass index	23.4	06.09.2023	23	27 September 2023
Waist circumference (cm)	81	06.09.2023	84	27 September 2023
Systolic blood pressure (mmHg)	103	06.09.2023	123	27
Diastolic blood pressure (mmHg)	73	06.09.2023	80	27
Heart rate (pulse)	63	06.09.2023	62	27

Period of inpatient stay: 5 September 2023–3 October 2023

Section 1.04 Laboratory Data

Parameter	Normal value	Unit	06/09/2023	27.09.2023
Thrombocytes	150–370	thousand/μl	227	217
Leukocytes	3.90–10.2	thousand/μl	3.6	4.9
Erythrocytes	3.90–5.20	million/μl	4.75	4.73
Haemoglobin	12.0–15.6	(g/dl)	14	13.9
Haematocrit	35.5–45.5	%	43	44
Mean corpuscular volume (MCV)	80–99	fl	90	93
HbE (MCH)	27.0–33.5	pg/ery	29.5	29.4
MCHC	31.5–36.0	g/dl	32.8	31.4
Sodium	136–145	mmol/l	141	145
Potassium	3.50–5.10	mmol/l	4.15	3.94
Calcium	2.15–2.58	mmol/l	2.25	2.33
Serum glucose/fasting	<100	mg/dl	79.9	79.1
Uric acid	2.60–6.00	mg/dl	4.73	4.78
Triglycerides (blood lipid levels)	<150	mg/dl	99.6	80.6
Cholesterol	<200	mg/dl	184	183
HDL cholesterol	40.0–60.0	mg/dl	77.7	74.3
LDL cholesterol	<115	mg/dl	91.7	95.4
Iron	37.0–145	μg/dl	52.8	91.5
Creatinine	0.45–1.00	mg/dl	0.77	0.73
GOT	<35	U/l	23.6	18.6
GPT	<35	U/l	18.2	15.5
Gamma-GT	< 40	U/l	21.8	19.1
Alkaline phosphatase	55.0–105	U/l	81.7	81

Section 1.05 Self-Reported Information on Previous Illnesses from 7 September 2023

Key ● = yes ○ = no blank field = not known

Health problems	Yes/No	Medication use	Activity Limited
High blood pressure	○		
Vascular diseases	○		
Stroke or cerebral haemorrhage	○		
Cardiac arrhythmia	●	○	○
Other cardiovascular diseases	○		
Respiratory diseases	○		
Stomach/intestinal diseases	○	○	○
Liver and bile duct disorders	○		
Thyroid disorders			
Diabetes			
Lipid metabolism disorders			
Other metabolic disorders			
Kidney and reproductive disorders	○		
Nervous system and mental disorders	○		
Eye diseases	○		
Mouth, throat, nose and ear disorders	○		
Dental diseases	○		
Skin diseases	○		
Allergies/intolerances	●	○	○
Joint and muscle disorders	●	○	○
Bone disorders	○		
Back problems	●	○	○
Anaemia and other blood disorders			
Paediatric and infectious diseases	○		
Cancer	○		
Addictions	○		
Family history of disease (e.g. diabetes, high blood lipid levels, cancer, obesity)	●	-	-

Section 1.06 Current ICD-10 Diagnoses

Admission	Discharge
F45.41	F45.41
F51.0	F51.0
G43.3	G43.3
G44.2	G44.2
G93.3	G93.3
I47.1	I47.1
I47.9	I47.9
J30.1	J30.1
K59.09	K59.09
R10.3	R10.3
R61.9	R61.9

Section 1.07 Previous Medical-Psychological Use of Services

Doctor visits in the past year	4
If yes,	partially successful
Hospital visits in the past year	No hospitalisation
Already in psychotherapy?	Yes
If yes, total number of psychotherapy sessions to date?	26–160 h
If yes, treated by how many psychotherapists/psychiatrists?	1
Currently undergoing psychotherapy?	No

Section 1.08 Subjective Causes of Illness

Stress/work	Yes
Stressful life events	Yes
Heredity/predisposition	No
Fate/chance	Yes
Environment	No
Lifestyle	No
Third-party fault	No
Other	No

Section 1.09 Change Due to the Condition

Self-esteem	Deteriorated
Relationship with one's own body	Very worsened
Assertiveness	Deteriorated
Appreciation by others	Significantly worsened

2. *Mental Health*

Section 2.01 IGM Resource Profile (Mental Health)

Indicator	Admission	Discharge	Follow-Up	Target
FLZ Overall life satisfaction score[a]	30	53	35	>60
FLZ Friends/acquaintances	−1	2	2	>8
FLZ Leisure/Hobbies	2	9	9	>6
FLZ Health	−4	4	3	>8

Indicator	Admission	Discharge	Follow-Up	Target
FLZ Income	3	9	3	>7
FLZ Occupation	6	3	9	>5
FLZ Living situation	9	15	9	>8
FLZ Family/children	6	2	3	>9
FLZ Partnership	9	9	–3	>7
WHO-5 Well-being[b]	52	56	36	>50
SOC Sense of coherence total score[c]	56	61	56	>64
SOC Significance	20	18	19	–
SOC Comprehensibility	20	24	21	–
SOC Manageability	18	19	16	–
SWOP Self-efficacy	9	11	6	≥13
SWOP Optimism	6	8	6	≥6
Vitality	50	60	45	>63
SSS social support total score	57	56	35	>55
SSS emotional/informative factor	18	17	12	≥25
SSS social interaction	12	12	8	≥14
SSS material factor	12	12	8	≥14
SSS affective factor	9	9	5	≥11
SSS Number of supporting persons	1	1	2	–

[a]Key: <= 29: critical value

[b]Key: 50: Well-being, no depressive symptoms 29–50: Mild depressive symptoms, <= 40: indication for depression diagnosis, Changes of 12 points or more are clinically relevant, <= 28: moderate to severe depressive symptoms

[c]Key: <= 51: critical value (low resilience)

Section 2.02 IGM Stress Profile (Mental Health)

Indicator	Admission	Discharge	Follow-up	Target value
Tedium total value[a]	3.7	3.6	4.1	≤3.2
Discouragement	3.4	3.4	4.1	≤2.5
Exhaustion	4.2	3.8	4.2	≤3.5
Loss of motivation	3.8	3.6	4	≤3
PSQ total value[b]	45	30	58.3	≤41.5
Concern	33.3	20	33.3	≤24
Tension	53.3	46.7	73.3	≤49
Joy	40	60	13.3	≥41
Requirement	33.3	13.3	40	≤24
3-level stress test[c]	5		2	
Cognitive-emotional level	16		18	<16
Vegetative level	22		16	<16
Motor level	22		26	<16
Internal stressors total value[d]	2	–	2	0

[a]Key: From 3.2 Pre-burnout with critical stress levels, From 4.5 Clear signs of burnout

[b]Key: >58.5 is the critical value

[c]Key: 0–48 points possible per level. The highest score indicates the preferred stress response level. The following applies per level: <16 (green), 16–20 (yellow), >20 (red)

[d]Key: 2 = red zone, i.e. always or frequently exposed to various stressors, 1 = yellow zone, i.e. only moderate stress from stressors that occur occasionally, 0 = green zone, i.e. no stressors present that cause stress

Section 2.03 Internal Stressors

Indicator	Admission	Discharge	Follow-up	Target value
Work-related stress				
Double burden of work and household	3	–	1	–
Hectic pace at work	3	–	2	–
Poor working atmosphere	2	–	1	–
Shift work	0	–	0	–
Unemployment	0	–	0	–
Becoming self-employed	0	–	0	–
Problems with your boss	1	–	1	–
Promotion	0	–	0	–
Change of workplace	0	–	0	–
Working overtime	1	–	1	–
Travelling a lot/business trips	0	–	0	–
Problems with colleagues	1	–	1	–
At home/in everyday life				
Arguments with your partner	1	–	2	–
Building a house	0	–	0	–
Raising children	0	–	0	–
Noisy neighbourhood	1	–	1	–
Difficulties with parents/parents-in-law	1	–	1	–
Illness of a family member	1	–	1	–
Illness/hospitalisation	0	–	0	–
Relocation	0	–	0	–
social obligations	0	–	0	–
Holiday preparations	0	–	0	–
Weekend/leisure hustle and bustle	0	–	0	–
Financial burdens				
Mortgages/loans	0	–	0	–
Legal disputes	0	–	0	–
Life-changing events				
Accident	0	–	0	–
Bereavement in the family	1	–	1	–
Separation/divorce from partner	0	–	1	–
Family disputes	1	–	1	–
Bankruptcy	0	–	0	–
Loss of job	0	–	0	–
Violence	0	–	0	–

Key to response options
Work-related stress and at home/in everyday life: 0 = never, 1 = sometimes, 2 = often, 3 = always
financial burdens: 0 = none/little, 1 = moderate, 2 = severe
Significant life events: 0 = none, 1 = one, 2 = more than one

Section 2.04 Mental Health

Indicator (total score)	Admission	Discharge	Follow-up	Target value
PHQ-9 Depression[a] *(in the planning phase)*				< 5
WHO-5 Wellbeing Index[b]	16	17	11	> 50
Generalized Anxiety Disorder Scale (GAD)-7[c]		8	9	< 5
PHQ-15 Somatic Symptom Severity[d] *(in the planning phase)*				< 5

Indicator (total score)	Admission	Discharge	Follow-up	Target value
ISR ICD symptom rating total score[c]	1.6	1.5	1.4	< 0.5
ISR Depression	1.5	1	1.5	< 0.8
ISR Anxiety	1.5	1.5	1	< 0.8
ISR Compulsion	1	0.7	1	< 0.7
ISR Somatisation	1.3	1.7	0.3	<0.3
ISR Eating disorder	4	4	4	<0.3

[a]Key to PHQ-9: <= 4: Minimal depressive symptoms, 5–9: Mild depressive symptoms, 10–14: Moderate symptoms of depression, 15–19: Severe symptoms of depression, ≥20: Severe depressive symptoms

[b]Key to WHO-5 Wellbeing: >50: Well-being, no depressive symptoms, 29–50: Mild depressive symptoms, <= 40: Indication for depression diagnosis, <= 28: moderate to severe depressive symptoms Changes of 12 points or more are clinically relevant

[c]Key to Generalized Anxiety Disorder Scale-7: <= 4: minimal anxiety symptoms, 5–9: mild anxiety symptoms, 10–14: moderate anxiety symptoms, >= 15: severe anxiety symptoms, With a cut-off of > 10 points, generalized anxiety disorder is possible; with a cut-off of > 15 points, it is probable

[d]Key to PHQ-15: <= 4: minimal symptom severity, 5–9: mild symptom severity, 10–14: Moderate symptom severity, ≥ 15: Severe symptom severity

PHQ-9 answers *(in the planning phase)*	**Admission**	**Discharge**	**Follow-up**

GAD-7 responses *(in the start-up phase)*	Admission	Discharge	Follow-up
Nervousness, anxiety or tension		1	1
Inability to stop or control worrying		1	1
Excessive worry about various matters		1	1
Difficulty relaxing		2	3
Restlessness, making it difficult to sit still		1	1
Quick to become annoyed or irritable		1	1
Feeling of anxiety, as if something bad were about to happen		1	1

PHQ-15 responses *(in the planning phase)*

ISR Additional questions	Admission	Discharge	Follow-up
I have difficulty concentrating.	2	1	2
I am considering taking my own life	0	0	0
I have trouble sleeping	4	4	4
I have a poor appetite	0	0	0
I am forgetful	1	1	1
I suffer from recurring dreams or memories of terrible experiences	0	0	0
I have psychological problems due to severe everyday stress (e.g. serious illness, loss of work or separation from a partner)	0	1	2
Suddenly, I no longer feel that my feelings and experiences are my own	0	0	1
People and my surroundings suddenly seem unreal to me, distant, lifeless	0	0	0
I feel impaired in the exercise of my sexuality	3	2	4

ISR Additional questions	Admission	Discharge	Follow-up
In recent years, I have changed permanently after experiencing extreme stress (e.g. traumatic brain injury, war experiences or abuse)	0	0	0
My sexual preferences are a burden to me	0	0	0

Key to possible answers
0 = does not apply, 1 = hardly applies, 2 = applies somewhat, 3 = applies significantly, 4 = applies extremely

3. *Somatic Health*

Section 3.1 IGM Resource Profile (Body)

Indicator	Admission	Discharge	Follow-up	Target
Total sleep score (PSQI)[a]	15	13	17	≤5
PSQI sleep quality	3	2	3	0
PSQI sleep latency	2	0	2	0
PSQI sleep duration	2	2	2	0
PSQI sleep efficiency	2	2	3	0
PSQI sleep efficiency %	71	67	56	100
PSQI sleep disturbances	2	2	2	0
PSQI sleep medication use	3	3	3	0
PSQI daytime sleepiness	1	2	2	0
Nutritional index[b]	7	–	10	>10
Exercise index[c]	5	–	6	≥6

[a]Key to sleep total score (PSQI): A maximum of 21 points can be calculated for a total of 7 sleep components. Each of the following sleep components can be scored from 0 to 3 points. The higher the score, the worse the sleep quality. A total score of up to 5 points is considered normal, scores between 6 and 10 points indicate sleep disturbances, and scores above 10 points are clear signs of a sleep disorder!
[b]Evaluation of responses to the nutrition index

	Admission		Follow-up	
Question	Answer	Points	Answer	Points
1. Do you eat a varied diet? Does your diet include plant-based foods such as vegetables, fruit, grains and potatoes, vegetable oils and nuts?	Yes	1/1	Yes	1/1
Is it supplemented with animal-based foods such as milk, dairy products, fish, meat and eggs?	Yes	1/1	Yes	1/1
Do you eat a small handful of (unsalted) nuts every day or do you eat legumes such as lentils, chickpeas and beans at least once a week?		/1		/1
2. How many portions of fruit and vegetables do you eat at least per day?	Not every day	0/2	Not every day	0/2
3. Do you eat cereal products such as bread, pasta, rice and flour, including whole grain varieties?—How often have you eaten whole grain bread, brown bread, whole grain pasta or whole grain rice in the last week?	1–2 times per week	0/2	5–6 times a week	1/2

	Admission		Follow-up	
Question	Answer	Points	Answer	Points
4. How often have you eaten fish or seafood in the last week?	1–2 times per week	1/1	1–2 times per week	1/1
5. How often have you eaten meat (pork, beef, poultry, sausage) in the last week?	1–2 times per week	1/1	1–2 times per week	1/1
7. Which oils do you consciously use in your cooking? Rapeseed oil Linseed oil Olive oil Walnut oil I consciously look for oils with unsaturated fatty acids	Yes No Yes No No	0/2	Yes Yes Yes No Yes	2/2
8. Sugar, salt and fluids. Which statements apply to me?		1/1		1/1
I avoid or use sugar-sweetened drinks or foods sparingly	Yes		Yes	
I rarely or never add extra salt to my food at the table	No		No	
I drink about 1.5 l of water or unsweetened beverages every day	Yes		Yes	
I do not drink alcohol regularly or frequently, e.g. in the form of beer, wine or other alcoholic beverages	Yes		Yes	
I avoid burning food when frying, grilling, baking and deep-frying	Yes		Yes	
9. How much time do you allow for your main meal?	Up to 10 min	0/2	Approximately 10–20 min	0/2
10. Watch your weight and regularly?	Yes	1/1	Yes	1/1
Total points		7/15		10/15

[c]Evaluation of responses to the movement index

Your total score is 6 points. Well done! You are actively exercising.

Evaluation of your answers regarding your general level of physical activity and sitting time.

Question	Answer	Points
How much active exercise do you do?	3 times a week for 30–45 min	2/3
		/6
Physical activity during working hours or in everyday life if no longer working	sitting, occasionally walking/ standing	2/6
Evaluation of your answers regarding your average sitting time per day		/1
	Hours	
	Hrs	
	Hrs	
	Hrs	
	Hours	

Question	Answer	Points
Total sitting time:	hours	
Movement index Total points		6/16
Physical activity index METmin value: No survey conducted		

Section 3.2 IGM Risk Profile (Body)

Indicator	Admission	Discharge	Follow-up	Target value
Diabetes risk in points[a]	10	–	9	<7
Diabetes risk in %[a]	4	–	4	<4
Risk of hypertension at age 4[a]	4.6	–	3.9	<10
Total cardiovascular risk ESC in %[b]	3	3	–	
Fatty liver[c]	18	18	–	<30
Smoking status	0	–	–	0
Alcohol status	0	–	–	0

[a] –1 = Diabetes or high blood pressure is already present
[b]An individual overall risk of heart attack, stroke or sudden cardiac death within the next 10 years is determined for men and women between the ages of 40 and 69 and separately for those over 70. For more details, see the table on the following page
[c]A value above 60 indicates an 80% probability of fatty liver disease. A value below 30 indicates a high probability that fatty liver disease is not present

4. *Neurovegetative Regulation—Symptom Profile*

Symptoms related to the cardiovascular system

Fatigue and sleep-related symptoms	A	D	**FUP 6 months**
Feeling unrested after getting up	2	2	2
Restless sleep	3	3	3
Difficulty falling asleep	3	1	3
Remembering dreams	1	1	1

Irregular heartbeat	2	1	3
Dizziness when standing up/bending over	2	1	1
Dizziness when looking down	2	1	2
Dizziness when getting up in the morning	1	1	2

(Thermo-)regulation-related symptoms

Key to possible answers
0 = no/never, 1 = somewhat/rarely, 2 = quite often/often, 3 = strongly/very often
For each symptom group, the following applies: <3 (green), 3–5 (yellow), >5 (red) and total points <9 (green), 9–15 (yellow), >15 (red)

Cold hands/feet	2	2	1
Shivering, feeling cold	1	2	1
Hypersensitive to cold/wind	1	2	1
Poor tolerance to heat/cold	2	1	1
Total points	22	18	21

Section 4.1 Psycho-vegetative Complaint Index

Indicator	Admission	Discharge	Follow-up
Neurovegetative regulation	22	18	21
3-level stress test Vegetative level	22		16
GAD-7		8	9
Total[a]	71	49	63

[a]Overall rating: <27: green zone; 27–55: yellow zone; 55: red zone

5. *Patient's Self-Perceived Benefit*

Section 5.1 VAS Main Complaint and Therapy Expectations

Indicator	Admission	Discharge	Follow-up	Target value
Main complaint	Migraine		Sleep disorder	–
VAS[a]	40	10	80	<30 (0–100)
Therapy expectations VAS[a]	20	–	–	–
Subjective assessment of state of health[b]	Not so good	Good	Poor	–

Key: [a]Clinical interpretation of changes on a 0–100 point scale Minor effects of change 5–10 points Moderate effects of change 10–20 points Significant effects of change >20 points Key to possible answers, [b]Excellent, very good, good, less good, poor

Section 5.2 PDI (Pain Disability Index)

Indicator	Admission	Discharge	Follow-up	Target value
PDI total value[a]	19	18	23	–
PDI Family commitments	2	2	2	–
PDI Recreation	3	2	2	–
PDI Social Activity	2	2	3	–
PDI Occupation	2	2	3	–
PDI Sex life	8	8	10	–
PDI Self-sufficiency	1	1	1	–
PDI Essential activities	1	1	2	–

[a]Values >= 33 are considered a significant impairment
At least 8.5–9 points reduction represent a relevant clinical improvement

Section 5.3 Change in Symptoms and Patient Expectations

Indicator	Admission	Discharge	Follow-up	Target value
Change in symptoms compared to admission[a]	–	Slightly weaker	Unchanged	No longer present
Expectations met?[b]	–	Completely	Largely	Completely

[a]Key to possible answers: No longer present, significantly weaker, slightly weaker, unchanged, slightly stronger, significantly stronger
[b]Key to response options: Completely, largely, partially, moderately, somewhat, not at all

Section 5.4 Benefits of the Types of Therapy

What helped you most from a personal perspective?

Indicator	Admission	Discharge	Follow-up
Acupuncture	–	Yes	Yes
Tuina	–	yes	Yes

Indicator	Admission	Discharge	Follow-up
TCM medicine/Chinese herbs	–	Yes	Yes
Group qigong	–	Yes	No
Individual qigong	–	I did not receive it	I did not receive
Physical therapy/physiotherapy	–	Yes	I did not receive
Dietary changes	–	Yes	Yes
Nutritional therapy/lectures	–	Yes	No
Individual Health Management IGM	–	Yes	No
psychological support	–	Yes	Yes
Hydrotherapy/foot baths/wraps	–	I did not receive	I did not receive
Medication therapy/medicines	–	Yes	Yes
Matrix rhythm therapy	–	yes	Yes
Atmosphere of the clinic	–	Yes	Yes
Distance from everyday life	–	Yes	Yes
Other	–	Yes	No hospital stay

Section 5.5 Patient Assessment of Success

Indicator	Admission	Discharge	Follow-up	Target value
How would you rate the overall success of the therapy today?[a]	–	Good success	Good success	–
From today's perspective, was this treatment?[b]	–	Very worthwhile	Very worthwhile	–

[a]Key to answer options: Very good success, good success, moderate success, no success
[b]Key to answer options: Very worthwhile, worthwhile, not worthwhile, rather harmful

6. *Interventions*

Chinese medication (see health portal PROFI page: Health dossier—Treatment—TCM medication)

Acupuncture (see health portal PROFI page: Health dossier—Treatment—Acupuncture)

7. *Side Effects*

Indicator	Discharge	Target
Have you noticed any side effects?	No	No

A health report is created for all patients at the clinic, recording data at the time of admission, discharge and follow-up. Patients who wish to use the VITERIO health portal for more than 6 months can pay an annual fee to access all portal features and receive an updated report. The health portal shows the progression of various risk and protective factors for health and is intended for documenting pain and well-being as well as other findings.

Figures 6.3 and 6.4 provide an overview of the health report. Due to space limitations, the health report is only as a supplement for download available.

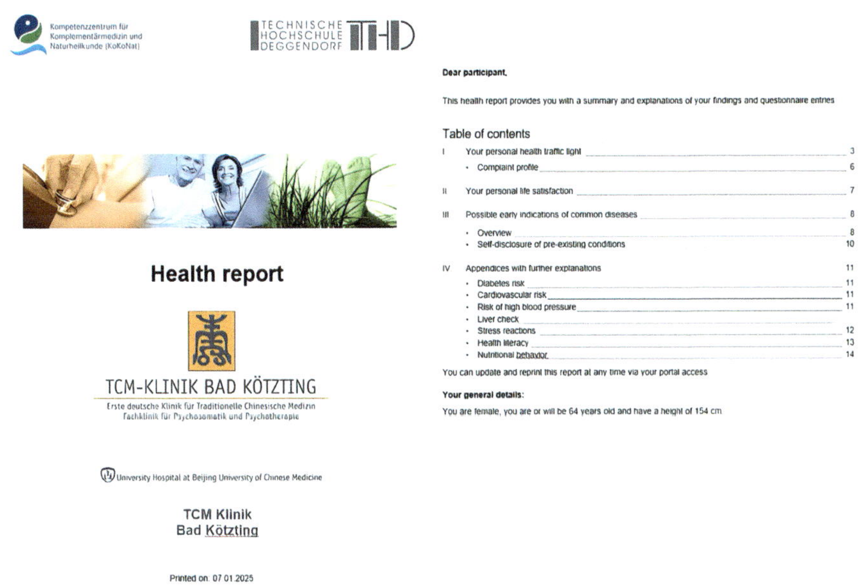

Fig. 6.3 The Health report is customized for all patients of the TCM-Klinik Bad Kötzting

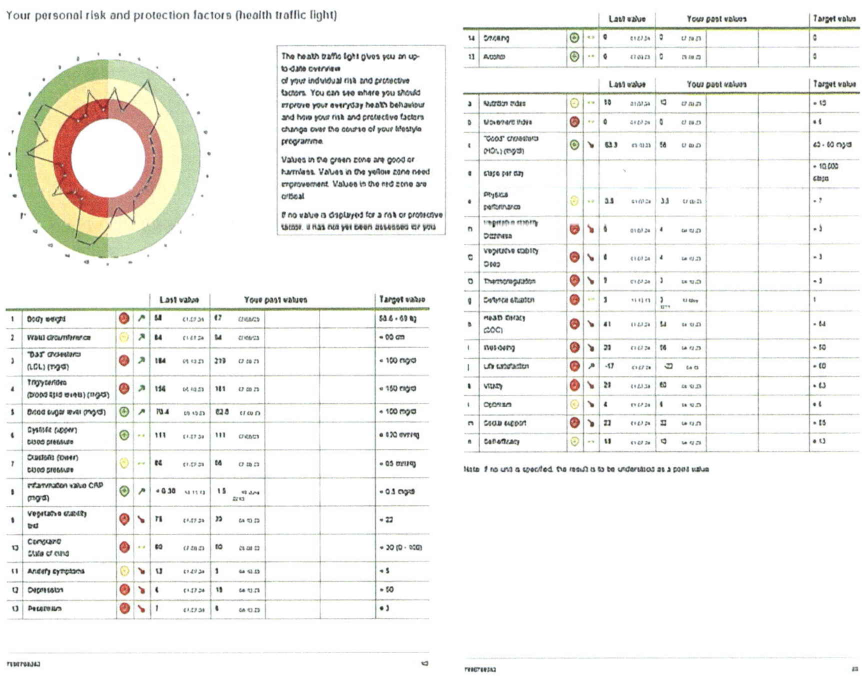

Fig. 6.4 The Health report shows a health traffic light that gives an up-to-date overview about individual risk and protective factors

6.6 Feature for Displaying the History of Patient Treatment

Another feature for recording the diagnostic and therapeutic procedures of a hospital patient is an overview display on the PROFI page of the VITERIO portal. Here, all procedures are automatically summarized in an overview (Fig. 6.5).

No	Date		
22	11.10.2023	Tongue	Teeth marks, bluish tongue colour, tongue colour spots, thin coating, whiter coating, location Rear third Coating stickier,
23	11.10.2023	Acupuncture points	Di11LR, Di14LR, Di15LR, Dü9LR, Bl60L, Ni3L, Ni4L, Gb29R, Gb30R, Gb34LR, Gb40L,
24	10 October 2023	Secondary diagnosis	F32.1
25	10.10.2023	Primary diagnosis	F45.41
26	09.10.2023	TCM	Blood stasis, dampness,
27	09.10.2023	Secondary diagnosis	F51.0
28	09.10.2023	Secondary diagnosis	M20.1
29	09.10.2023	Secondary diagnosis	M79.61
30	09.10.2023	Secondary diagnosis	S86.0
31	09.10.2023	Secondary diagnosis	U08.9
32	09.10.2023	Secondary diagnosis	G93.3
33	09.10.2023	TCM medication	Mori ramulus/Sangzhi/6 g, Cinnamomi ramulus/Guizhi/6 g, Dipsaci radix/Xuduan/6 g, Achyranthis bidentatae radix/ Niuxi/6 g, Spatholobi caulis/Jixueteng/6 g, Paeoniae rubra radix/Chishao/6 g, Curcumae longae rhizoma/Jianghuang/6 g,Bombyx batryticatus (t)/Baijiangcan/6 g, Angelicae pubescentis radix/Duhuo/3 g, Notopterygii rhizoma seu radix/Qianghuo/3 g, Bambusae caulis in taeniam/Zhuru/6 g, Albiziae cortex/Hehuanpi/6 g, Astragali radix/Huangqi/6 g, Sappan lignum/Sumu/6 g
34	16 August 2022	Secondary diagnosis	M23.39
35	16 August 2022	Secondary diagnosis	S86.0
36	16 August 2022	Primary diagnosis	U07.2
37	16 August 2022	Secondary diagnosis	U08.9
38	16 August 2022	Secondary diagnosis	G93.3
39	16 August 2022	Secondary diagnosis	G47.0
40	16 August 2022	Secondary diagnosis	M79.61
41	16 August 2022	Secondary diagnosis	M20.1
42	14 August 2022	Acupuncture points	Di4LR, Di11L, Di15L, Hz7LR, Bl34L, Bl36L, Bl60L, Le3LR, Lg20,
43	12 August 2022	Secondary diagnosis	F32.1
44	12 August 2022	Primary diagnosis	F45.41
45	10 August 2022	Acupuncture points	Di4LR, Di11L, Di15L, Hz7LR, Bl34L, Bl36L, Bl60L, Le3LR, Lg20,
46	08.08.2022	Acupuncture points	Di4LR, Di11L, Di15L, Hz7LR, Bl34L, Bl36L, Bl60L, Le3LR, Lg20,
47	04.08.2022	Consultation information@zept	Quinoa fasting day (600 kcal green)
48	04.08.2022	Consultation info@zept	Millet relief day (900 kcal green)

nd3841 2/8

Fig. 6.5 Inpatient history of the patient with diagnostic and therapeutic procedures (course of treatment)

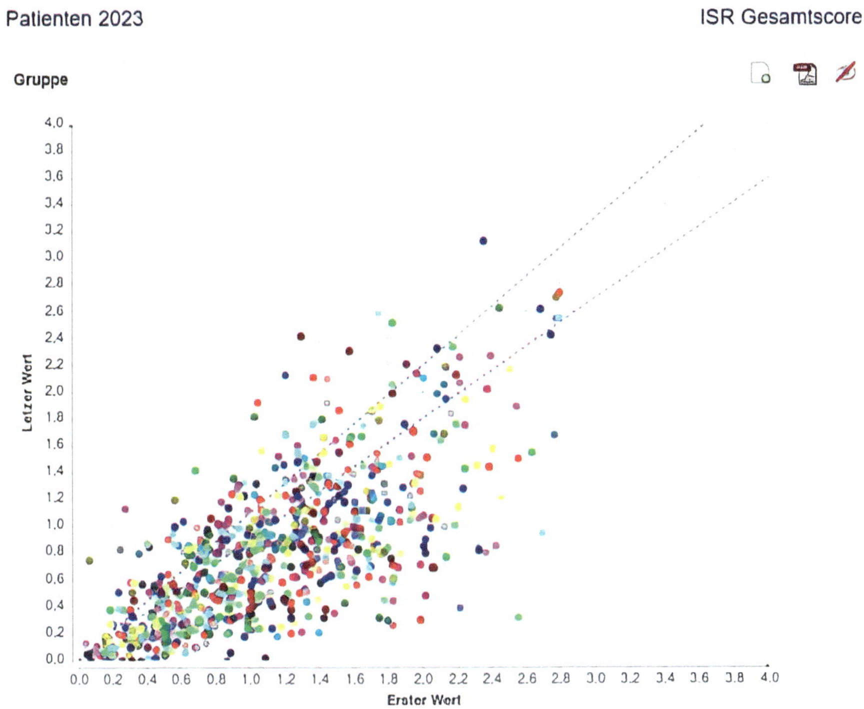

Fig. 6.6 Scatter plot of a group of patients with ISR-total scores at admission and discharge of the hospital

Therapists have access to a tool on the VITERIO web portal that allows them to compile any combination of patients and target parameters for the evaluation and progress tracking of therapy groups or patients with specific indications or hospital wards. Definable patient groups can be displayed individually or in groups of a selectable number, with specific indicators within a definable time period, in the form of various graphs.

Figure 6.6 shows a group of around 100 patients and their change in ICD-10 symptom rating (ISR) total score over time. The display shows the admission and discharge values of the patients as a diagonal line. No changes are shown on the diagonal line with a deviation of plus or minus 10%. Values below the diagonal line represent improvements, while values above it indicates deterioration in the ISR total score.

6.7 Quality Improvement Projects

6.7.1 Short Case-Report Form for Psychometrics History

The psychologists at the TCM Clinic in Bad Kötzting requested a one-page evaluation report for doctors' letters describing inpatient treatment for their patients. Figure 6.7 shows our solution, which provides an alternative to the standard case report by offering a significantly shorter, psychometrics-focused summary.

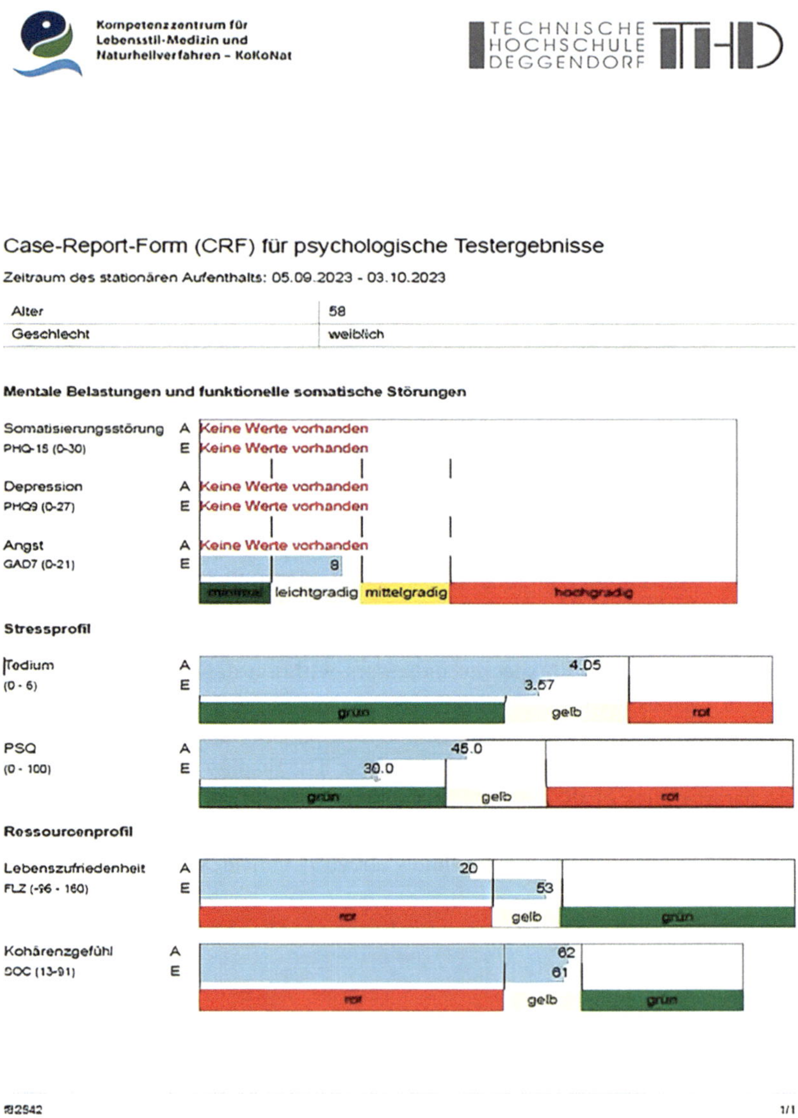

Fig. 6.7 Short psychometric report on the inpatient course of patients with evaluation

In addition, CoCoNat has decided to change the indicator concept of the evaluation. In future, the most frequently diagnosed disorders, namely somatoform disorders and depression, will be recorded and mapped using the Patient Health Questionnaire PHQ-9 and PHQ-15 instead of ICD-10 Symptom Rating (ISR).

6.7.2 Pre-admission Screening Tool as Integrated Part of VITERIO®

Another project aimed to integrate pre-admission registration and the pre-selection of patients for potential admission to the TCM Clinic in Bad Kötzting into the VITERIO health portal using the German version of the Patient Health Questionnaire (PHQ). The goal was to expand the health portal to include data on patients' overall progress from the pre-admission stage. Until now, data has been collected on paper or in a non-networked, stand-alone manner.

6.7.3 Adjustments and Improvements to the IHM Lifestyle Programme SINOCUR in Inpatient and Outpatient Settings

Inpatient Setting
During the pandemic, group-based training sessions were significantly reduced. This had a particularly negative impact on the IHM lifestyle programme and the psychoeducation component of the programme. For this reason, the teaching units for the IHM programme were reformed and relocated to the SINOCUR Prevention Centre, and thus to the outpatient section of the clinic. These larger patient groups, which have regular, sequential teaching sessions, have been very well received by inpatients and will become the standard in future.

The IHM lifestyle program SINOCUR is taught in at least 10 different focus training sessions. These include two training units introducing the VITERIO web portal, three nutrition training sessions with general and TCM-based recommendations, one practical and theoretical unit on exercise, an introduction to and in-depth study of qigong, various self-help techniques from Kneipp and TCM, and a learning unit on stress management with several focus areas.

Outpatient Setting
To provide an alternative to costly one-year lifestyle programmes, a two-hour screening and consultation programme called 'IHM-Health Invest SINOCUR' (2–2.5 h of health investment) has been designed for spa guests and residents of the region (Fig. 6.7). This offer is also aimed at companies, whose employees can be invited to the SINOCUR Prevention Centre in medium-to-large groups for a 'Health Day'.

Development of a Strategic Concept for IHM-Health Invest SINOCUR

- Application and recruitment of defined target groups (e.g. burnout, cardiovascular metabolism, sleep disorders, dementia, osteoarthritis, back pain and fibromyalgia) through individual risk perception using risk algorithms in the form of digital questionnaires and written feedback reports.
- Active registration of participants in the Prevention Centre via online registration, email or telephone, due to interest in the measure or for an information event.
- Participation in the IHM- Health Invest programme involving the recording of health data, VNS analysis, and an individual questionnaire assessment with a health report and an individual consultation.
- Health offers for the post-Invest phase related to the indications.

In addition to targeted screening tools, a so-called health passport for the Bad Kötzting spa town is also to be developed. This is intended to enable everyone to access the screening through low-threshold media offerings, such as business cards and QR codes in restaurant menus, for example. A draft can be seen in Figs. 6.8 and 6.9.

IHM-Health Invest is to be offered to both groups and individuals.

The various screening tools for spa guests, interested citizens, companies or patients, along with their corresponding QR codes, are summarized in Fig. 6.10. Unlike the health passport, which covers multiple areas, these screening tools can be used to query specific areas such as stress, sleep and diabetes mellitus.

6.7.4 Establishing of Core-Team Meetings

Core team meetings will be established approximately every two weeks, with a 'journal club' and 'feedback topics' from implementation practice. The management is carried out under the CoCoNat of the DIT.

6.8 Current and Relevant Examples of Evidence from Clinical Research (PubMed, 02.11.2025)—State of Efficacy

If we compile the relevant literature on the most important areas of indication in connection with individual therapies, as well as the overall field of Traditional Chinese Medicine and Complementary Medicine as a whole, this will provide an initial overview of the current state of scientific knowledge in this field.

The literature search was conducted in PubMed using the filter settings 'Meta-analysis, systematic reviews, and randomized clinical trials (RCTs)'. The search period was from 1990 to 2025.

The search terms used were 'Traditional Chinese Medicine, acupuncture, Chinese herbal medicine, TCM medicines, qigong' and 'lifestyle medicine,

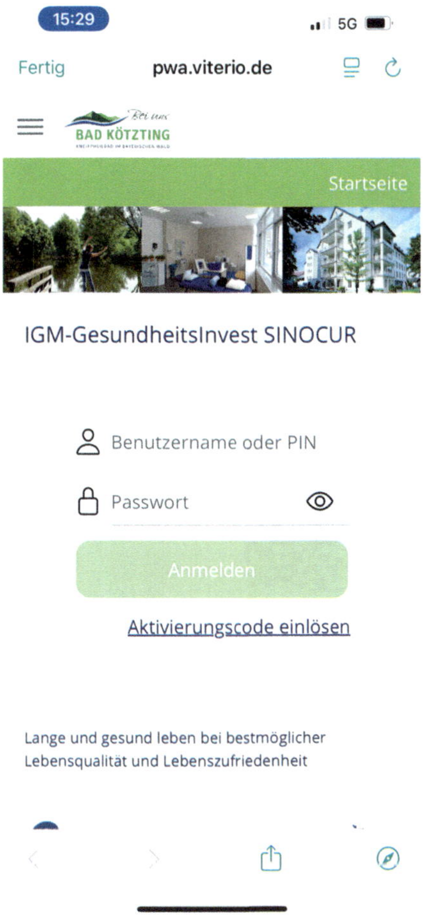

Fig. 6.8 IHM-Health Invest SINOCUR (=IGM-GesundheitsInvest)

mind–body medicine, relaxation therapy, herbal medicine, yoga therapy, osteopathic medicine, homeopathy and anthroposophic medicine' (Fig. 6.11).

This outlines the key areas of complementary and integrative medicine in keywords. Taking into account the filters relating to the exclusive consideration of existing randomized controlled trials (RCTs), meta-analyses and systematic reviews reveals a surprising state of scientific knowledge. Even as an initial inventory, the mere number of 66,280 PubMed hits is striking. Traditional Chinese medicine tops the list of identified studies with 14,974 hits. Acupuncture, a subset of TCM subject to certain limitations, is a popular area of research, accounting for 10,151 hits.

The herbal medicine category yields almost the same number of results, with 14,167 hits. Mind-body medicine ranks third with 10,547 hits. The aforementioned acupuncture (10,151) is followed by lifestyle medicine (6938) and relaxation techniques (5071).

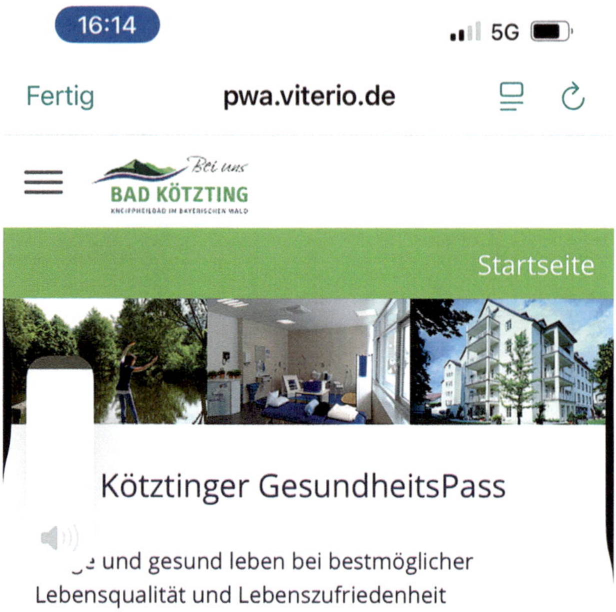

Kompetenzzentrum für Lebensstil-Medizin und Naturheilverfahren – KoKoNat

Fig. 6.9 Health Passport Bad Kötzting for spa guests and residents

Of the four types of therapy—yoga, manual medicine, homeopathy and anthroposophy—the first two have been the subject of the most research, with 2344 and 1544 publications respectively. Anthroposophic medicine has the least supporting evidence, which is mainly based on the RCT technique.

The TCM-Klinik Bad Kötzting is approved as a psychosomatic medicine hospital within the statutory health insurance system. Currently, there is no separate category in Germany for clinics that specialize in specific types of therapy.

This classification affects both the selection of patients referred to the clinic, as well as the quality structures that must be demonstrated, such as staff qualifications and available equipment. Another fundamental problem is that psychotherapy disciplines do not have any 'hard', objective outcome parameters such as laboratory

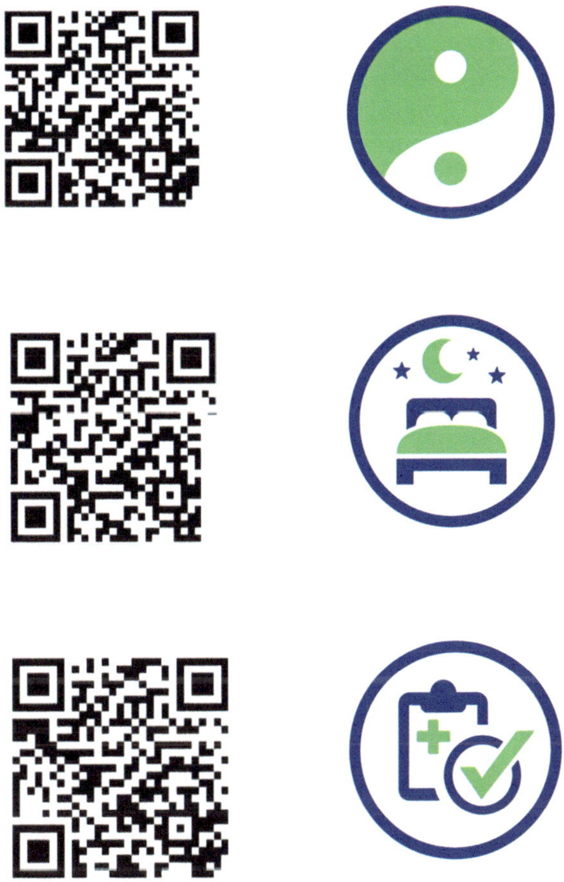

Fig. 6.10 Different screening tools for stress, sleep and diabetes mellitus

values that can be used to determine the success of therapy. This special methodological position also applies to complementary methods used in this area of indication. Blinding problems or a lack of patient or therapy controls often mean that psychotherapy and complementary medicine frequently have to use less restrictive methods of evaluation. However, this does not mean that there is no scientific basis in higher-quality clinical studies for either area.

Evidence-based medicine is a key aspect of clinical practice. For this reason, the state of evidence for inpatient psychotherapy and psychosomatics should first be briefly summarized. The application of TCM and its individual components in relation to psychosomatic indications and lifestyle medicine should then be outlined and compared.

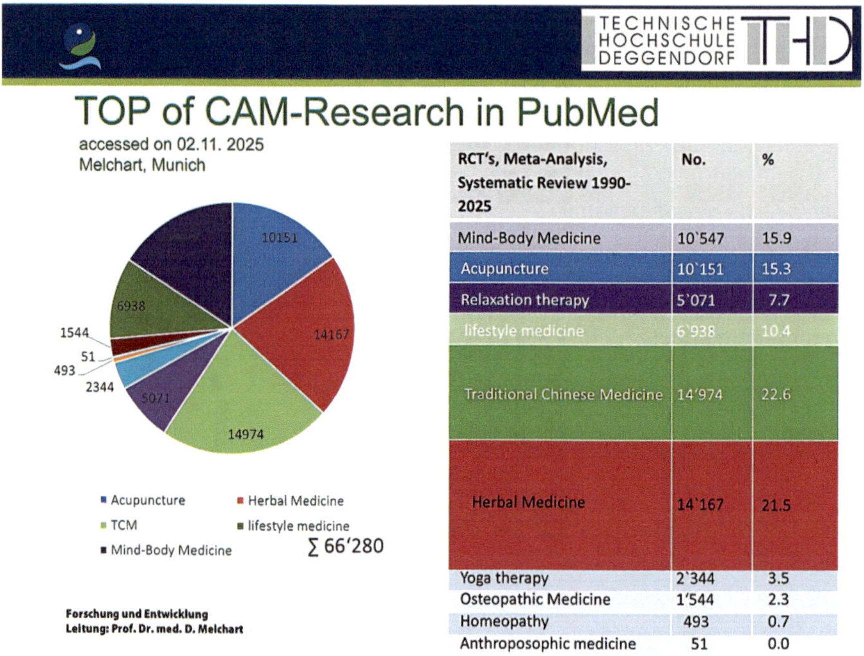

Fig. 6.11 Top of Complementary Medicine Research in PubMed; accessed on 02.11.2025; filter only RCT's, Meta-Analysis and Systematic Reviews between 1990 and 2025

6.8.1 State of Evidence for Psychotherapy and Psychosomatic Medicine

In addition to medication, three forms of treatment are recognized within a psychosomatic hospital, as defined in the German Psychotherapy Guideline.

These are:

- Psychodynamic methods (analytical and depth psychology psychotherapy)
- Behavioural therapy (behavioural activation and cognitive therapy)
- Systemic therapy, which focuses on the social context

More than one million people receive psychotherapy for depression and anxiety each year as part of the IAPT (Improving Access to Psychological Therapies) program in the UK. Two out of three patients feel better after treatment (Wakefield S. et al. 2021). The systematic review [1] identified $N = 60$ studies, with $N = 47$ studies suitable for meta-analysis. The primary meta-analysis showed large *pre-post treatment effect sizes for depression* ($d = 0.87$, 95% CI [0.78–0.96], $p < .0001$) and anxiety ($d = 0.88$, 95% CI [0.79–0.97], $p < .0001$), and *a moderate effect on functional impairment* ($d = 0.55$, 95% CI [0.48–0.61], $p < .0001$). The results are by no means better than the own effect sizes presented in the previous chapter. However, the same problems exist with regard to relapse prevention and a reduction in drop-out. Another study by von Brachel et al. (2019) shows similar effect sizes for cognitive behavioural therapy in outpatient psychotherapy. Pre- to post-treatment *effect sizes ranged from 0.63 to 0.75,* while pre-treatment to *follow-up effect sizes ranged from 0.75 to 0.92,* depending on the measurement parameter [2].

Between 17% and 29% of patients experienced a clinically significant change at post-treatment, and between 24% and 42% at follow-up. However, *about a quarter of the patients did not respond sufficiently to therapy*, neither concerning short-term nor long-term effects.

Notably, the follow-up results were even better than the post-treatment results, indicating further improvement. Similar improvements in therapy can also be observed in our own follow-up studies. However, according to Lambert and Bergin (1994), therapeutic success in psychotherapy does not primarily depend on individual procedures, but rather on the patient's experience of illness, their own lay aetiology, their expectations of treatment, and their openness to psychotherapy [3]. This is once again demonstrated by our own data regarding patients' positive treatment expectations and openness to TCM treatments and the achievable treatment outcome.

A closer analysis of the evidence for behavioural therapy measures in relation to somatization disorders reveals only moderate effect sizes in the area of pain and somatization, with $d = 0.54$ *to* $d = 0.32$. The results of intensive behavioural therapy for these patients are better in the area of fatigue symptoms, with an average effect size of $d = 0.87$ [4].

Publications on Psychotherapy

1. Wakefield S, Kellett S, Simmonds-Buckley M, Stockton D, Bradbury A, Delgadillo J. Improving Access to Psychological Therapies (IAPT) in the United Kingdom: A systematic review and meta-analysis of 10-years of practice-based evidence. Br J Clin Psychol. 2021 Mar;60(1):1–37. doi: https://doi.org/10.1111/bjc.12259. Epub 2020 Jun 23. PMID: 32578231 .
2. von Brachel R, Hirschfeld G, Berner A, Willutzki U, Teismann T, Cwik JC, Velten J, Schulte D, Margraf J. Long-Term Effectiveness of Cognitive Behavioral Therapy in Routine Outpatient Care: A 5- to 20-Year Follow-Up Study. Psychother Psychosom. 2019;88(4):225–235. doi: https://doi.org/10.1159/000500188. Epub 2019 May 23. PMID: 31121580 .
3. Lambert, M. J., & Bergin, A. E. The effectiveness of psychotherapy. In A. E. Bergin & S. L. Garfield (Eds.), Handbook of psychotherapy and behavior change 1994 (4th ed., pp. 143–189). John Wiley & Sons. https://psycnet.apa.org/record/1994-97069-004.
4. Leaviss J, Davis S, Ren S, Hamilton J, Scope A, Booth A, Sutton A, Parry G, Buszewicz M, Moss-Morris R, White P. Behavioural modification interventions for medically unexplained symptoms in primary care: systematic reviews and

economic evaluation. Health Technol Assess. 2020 Sep;24(46):1–490. doi: https://doi.org/10.3310/hta24460. PMID: 32975190 ; PMCID: PMC7548871.

The following section will analyse the literature on the evidence for TCM for specific TCM methods in relation to indications that are relevant to the TCM-Klinik Bad Kötzting. Given the scope of the existing literature, this analysis is bound to be incomplete and biased.

6.8.2 The Current State of the Evidence Base for Acupuncture in the Treatment of Pain

On 3 November 2025, a review of the clinical evidence for acupuncture in the PubMed database, using the search criteria 'acupuncture' and 'pain', as well as 'meta-analyses', 'systematic reviews' and 'RCTs', shows that there **are 3661 results**. The search period was from 1990 until 3 November 2025. The following important and recent publications clearly demonstrate the substantial body of evidence in favour of using acupuncture in general pain therapy and in special issues like somatic symptom disorder, low back pain, radiculopathies, and headaches.

The publication by Stubbs et al. (2025) demonstrates the importance of recognizing and treating pain in patients with mental health conditions. It highlights the frequency with which pain occurs alongside mental illness. An umbrella review of over 957,000 individuals with mental health conditions revealed that, on average, acupuncture combined with standard medication had a larger effect size ($d = -1.06$, 95% CI −1.65 to −0.47), compared to cognitive behavioural therapy, which had a smaller effect size (SMD = 0.27, 95% CI −0.08 to 0.61) [1].

The clinical effects of acupuncture have a particularly nonspecific effect on patients through a combination of pain and stress reduction, muscle relaxation, and neurovegetative equilibration. There are a variety of mechanisms of action that are not yet fully understood, but important starting points, such as signal transduction, are neurophysiologically comprehensible. The work of Lai et al. (2019) provides a good overview of this topic [2].

Unlike most of the RCT studies and review articles cited below, the outdated Cochrane working group came to a much more sceptical conclusion in its 2020 publication about the effectiveness of acupuncture in treating chronic non-specific low back pain [23]. According to the guidelines of the American College of Physicians (ACP) and the 2021 publication by Urits et al., acupuncture is still considered a primary treatment for managing non-pharmacological care in patients with low back pain [24].

The latest statement from April 2021 by the Scientific Committee of the National Institute for Health and Care Excellence (NICE) in England recognizes acupuncture as an effective, albeit short-term, therapy primarily for reducing chronic pain and improving quality of life [25]. This is the first time NICE has issued such a recommendation (1B.C). This recommendation is based on thirteen RCTs involving around 1000 patients. It has also been positively included in the guidelines for pain management in Scotland.

The work of Li et al. (2020) shows that, in most studies, at least 5 weeks of acupuncture treatment are necessary to achieve an 80% reduction in pain [26]. However, a meta-analysis by Vickers et al. (2018) of high-quality studies involving 29,827 patients demonstrated that sustained pain relief can be achieved through acupuncture, with this relief still present after one year (although the original effect strength had reduced by around 15%) [27].

However, this limitation applies to all medical procedures. If they are discontinued, the effect ceases. The only method that demonstrates a long-term effect in the treatment of chronic back pain is active movement. The medical concept of the TCM clinic also relies on this combination. Often, active movement training and stabilization are only possible thanks to the pain reduction provided by acupuncture.

1. Stubbs B, Ma R, Solmi M, Veronese N, Van Damme T, Romano E, Stewart R, Mossaheb N, López-Gil JF, Firth J, Vancampfort D. Chronic pain in mental disorders: An umbrella review of the prevalence, risk factors, and treatments across 957,168 people with mental disorders and 16,606,910 controls. Eur Psychiatry. 2025 Aug 12;68(1):e113. doi: https://doi.org/10.1192/j.eurpsy.2025.10074. PMID: 40790851 ; PMCID: PMC12438992.

   Conclusion: This review confirms chronic pain CP as a significant comorbidity in mental disorders. Clinicians should prioritize routine pain screening and multimodal treatments. Researchers need longitudinal studies with standardized assessments to clarify causality and improve interventions. Taken together, this work highlights an urgent need for integrated psychiatric care approaches, emphasizing that addressing CP could enhance mental health outcomes and overall patient well-being.
2. Lai HC, Chang QY, Hsieh CL. Signal Transduction Pathways of Acupuncture for Treating Some Nervous System Diseases. Evid Based Complement Alternat Med. 2019 Jul 11;2019:2909632. doi: https://doi.org/10.1155/2019/2909632. PMID: 31379957 ; PMCID: PMC6657648.

   Acupuncture affects synaptic plasticity, causes an increase in neurotrophic factors, and results in neuroprotection, cell proliferation, antiapoptosis, antioxidant activity, anti-inflammation, and maintenance of the blood-brain barrier.
3. Zhao F, Wang W, Feng X, Li J, Gang W, Jing X, Chen H, Liang Y. Effect of acupuncture on somatic symptom disorder: a systematic review and meta-analysis. Front Med (Lausanne). 2025 Oct 1;12:1625230. doi: https://doi.org/10.3389/fmed.2025.1625230. PMID: 41103694 ; PMCID: PMC12521258.

   Conclusion: Our findings indicated potential added benefits of acupuncture combined with SSRI/SNRI for SSD-related anxiety, although effects on pain were inconsistent. High-quality RCTs with larger sample sizes are required to confirm acupuncture's efficacy and safety for SSD.
4. Jixing G, Changchun JI, Chaoju X, Xiang R, Zhangyin S, Yu X, Rongni Z, Qiangqiang QU, Youpeng D, Jinsheng Y. Various acupuncture therapies for

managing nonspecific low back pain: a network Meta-analysis. J Tradit Chin Med. 2025 Oct;45(5):954–962. doi: https://doi.org/10.19852/j.cnki.jtcm.2025.05.002. PMID: 41015793 ; PMCID: PMC12453989.

Conclusion: Bloodletting was the most effective treatment for relieving pain, and scraping therapy was the most effective treatment for improving dysfunction. Warm acupuncture was the preferred treatment for cold and wet NLBP. However, further high-quality clinical studies are needed for validation.

5. DeBar LL, Wellman RD, Justice M, Avins AL, Beyrouty M, Eng CM, Herman PM, Nielsen A, Pressman A, Stone KL, Teets RY, Cook AJ. Acupuncture for Chronic Low Back Pain in Older Adults: A Randomized Clinical Trial. JAMA Netw Open. 2025 Sep 2;8(9):e2531348. doi: https://doi.org/10.1001/jamanetworkopen.2025.31348. PMID: 40938602 ; PMCID: PMC12432643.

   Conclusion: The findings of this randomized clinical trial of older adults with chronic low back pain (CLBP) suggest that acupuncture needling provided greater improvements in back pain-related disability at 6 months and at 12 months compared with Usual Medical Care alone. These findings support acupuncture needling as an effective and safe treatment option for older adults with CLBP.

6. Wan R, Zheng Q, Zeng X, Luo Y, Sun L, Chen S, Luo F, Zhang Y, Zhu Z, Chen X, Zhao Y, Li Y. Differential placebo effect of sham acupuncture for chronic pain: a network meta-analysis of randomized controlled trials. BMC Complement Med Ther. 2025 Sep 1;25(1):323. doi: https://doi.org/10.1186/s12906-025-05055-x. PMID: 40890765 ; PMCID: PMC12403578.

   Conclusion: The placebo effect of sham acupuncture is significant, among which the no penetration (acupoint or nonacupoint) groups exhibited the lowest placebo effect. Nevertheless, further head-to-head trials are warranted to obtain direct evidence.

7. Zhao S, Yang J. Network meta-analysis of tuina or acupuncture in combination with adjunctive therapy for cervical spondylotic radiculopathy. Front Neurol. 2025 Aug 8;16:1612024. doi: https://doi.org/10.3389/fneur.2025.1612024. PMID: 40860976 ; PMCID: PMC12370718.

   Conclusion: Needling + warm needle acupuncture, warm needle acupuncture + auricular acupuncture, and warm needle acupuncture + conventional therapy may better alleviate symptoms in patients with cervical spondylotic radiculopathy CSR. However, more well-designed multicentre, large-sample RCTs are needed to further analyse the findings from this study.

8. Wang Z, Zhao C, Li M, Zhang L, Diao J, Wu Y, Yang T, Shi M, Lei Y, Wang Y, Li M, Bian Y, Zhou Y, Xu H. Efficacy and Safety of External Therapies of Traditional Chinese Medicine in Patients with Knee Osteoarthritis: A Systematic Review and Network Meta-Analysis. Rejuvenation Res. 2025 Oct;28(5):248–262. doi: https://doi.org/10.1089/rej.2025.0039. Epub 2025 Jun 13. PMID: 40511477 .

   The results of the network meta-analysis revealed that in terms of improving Visual Analog Scale (VAS) and Western Ontario and McMaster Universities Osteoarthritis Index (WOMAC) function scores, each external therapy was better than conventional medicine. Electroacupuncture may be the most effective intervention in improving the VAS score and TNF-α level. Moxibustion resulted in the greatest improvement in WOMAC function and IL-6 levels. The most effective interventions for reducing WOMAC pain scores were the manual needle knife, followed by electroacupuncture and Tuina therapy (SUCRA = 82.9%, 79.0%, and 71.4%, respectively). Warming acupuncture dominantly increased Lysholm scores. The safety results showed that the three safest interventions were the sham intervention, Tuina therapy, and moxibustion (SUCRA = 90.6%, 83.1%, and 68.8%, respectively). Silver needle had the best comprehensive effect. Electroacupuncture has the best effect on improving pain symptoms, and moxibustion can be prioritized when functional limitations are the main symptoms.

9. Teng Z, Zhu J, Li K, Tong T, Li W, Chu H, Sun P. Efficacy and safety of acupuncture as an adjuvant therapy for osteoporosis: a systematic review and meta-analysis of randomized controlled trials. Front Endocrinol (Lausanne). 2025 May 9;16:1561344. doi: https://doi.org/10.3389/fendo.2025.1561344. PMID: 40416525 ; PMCID: PMC12098033.

   Acupuncture demonstrates efficacy and safety as an OP adjuvant therapy. Current evidence is limited by regional bias and methodological heterogeneity. Multicentre, large-sample RCTs are needed to standardize protocols and validate long-term therapeutic efficacy.

10. Deng B, Xu T, Deng Z, Jiang Y, Li L, Liang W, Zhang Y, Wang H, Xu Y, Chen G. Efficacy of acupuncture-related therapy for postmenopausal osteoporosis: a systematic review and network meta-analysis based on randomized controlled trials. Front Med (Lausanne). 2025 Apr 9;12:1483819. doi: https://doi.org/10.3389/fmed.2025.1483819. PMID: 40270507 ; PMCID: PMC12015985.

    The results suggest that several acupuncture-related therapies, either alone or in conjunction with CWM, outperform CWM alone and may be regarded as an alternative or supplementary therapy to PMOP, though higher-quality trials are needed.

11. Wu Q, Fan L, Wu D, Gao H, Han D, Hu H, Qian L. Determining the efficacy and safety of acupuncture for the treatment of menstrual migraine: an updated systematic review and meta-analysis. Front Neurol. 2025 Sep 17;16:1673321. doi: https://doi.org/10.3389/fneur.2025.1673321. PMID: 41041685 ; PMCID: PMC12484189.

    Conclusion: Findings suggest that acupuncture for MM produced the most notable reductions in migraine severity. Nevertheless, the GRADE assessment indicated low overall certainty of the evidence, with considerable heterogeneity present in multiple pooled analyses.

12. Tu J, Shi G, Yan S, et al. Acupuncture vs Sham Acupuncture for Chronic Sciatica From Herniated Disk: A Randomized Clinical Trial. JAMA Intern Med. Published online October 14, 2024. doi: https://doi.org/10.1001/jamainternmed.2024.5463

    Among other things, this study led to the American Medicare covering the costs of 12 acupuncture treatments for sciatic pain.

13. Zhao L, Sun M, Yin Z, Cui J, Wang R, Ji L, Geng G, Chen J, Cai D, Liu Q, Zheng H, Liang F. Long-Term Effects of Individualized Acupuncture for Chronic Neck Pain: A Randomized Controlled Trial. Ann Intern Med. 2024 Oct;177(10):1330–1338. doi: https://doi.org/10.7326/M23-2425. Epub 2024 Sep 3. PMID: 39222507 .

Conclusion: Individualized acupuncture interventions using high- or low-sensitivity acupuncture points were more effective in reducing Chronic Neck Pain than Sham Acupoints and Waiting List control groups sustained through 24 weeks, but the magnitude of relative improvement did not reach a minimal clinically important difference.

14. Wang Y, Lu W, Wang Y, Chen W, Zhao H. Efficacy of different acupuncture-related therapies for tension-type headache: a systematic review and network meta-analysis. Front Neurol. 2024 Dec 5;15:1481715. doi: https://doi.org/10.3389/fneur.2024.1481715. PMID: 39703352 ; PMCID: PMC11655348.

Conclusion: This comprehensive analysis of 21 acupuncture and related therapies demonstrates that Electro Acupuncture is the most effective in reducing headache frequency and shortening headache duration, while EA + Cupping Therapy and Manual Acupuncture + Western Medicine are the optimal therapies for enhancing responder rate and reducing pain intensity, respectively. However, clinical decisions should be individualized based on the specific needs of each patient.

15. Tao, QF, Huang, YB, Yuan, L. et al. Acupuncture versus tricyclic antidepressants in the prophylactic treatment of tension-type headaches: an indirect treatment comparison meta-analysis. J Headache Pain 25, 67 (2024). https://doi.org/10.1186/s10194-024-01776-5.

Conclusion: Acupuncture had similar effect as TCAs in reducing headache frequency of TTH, and acupuncture had a lower adverse events rate than amitriptyline, as shown by very low certainty of evidence.

16. Yu H, Wang D, Verville L, Southerst D, Bussières A, Gross DP, Pereira P, Mior S, Tricco AC, Cedraschi C, Brunton G, Nordin M, Shearer HM, Wong JJ, Connell G, Myrtos D, da Silva-Oolup S, Young JJ, Funabashi M, Romanelli A, Lee JGB, Stuber K, Guist B, Muñoz Laguna J, Hofstetter L, Murnaghan K, Hincapié CA, Cancelliere C. Systematic Review to Inform a World Health Organization (WHO) Clinical Practice Guideline: Benefits and Harms of Needling Therapies for Chronic Primary Low Back Pain in Adults. J Occup Rehabil. 2023 Dec;33(4):661–672. doi: https://doi.org/10.1007/s10926-023-10125-3. Epub 2023 Nov 22. PMID: 37991648 ; PMCID: PMC10684627.

Conclusion: Based on low to very low certainty evidence, adults with CPLBP experienced some benefits in pain, functioning, or HRQoL with NT; however, evidence showed little to no differences for other outcomes.

17. Giovanardi CM, Gonzalez-Lorenzo M, Poini A, Marchi E, Culcasi A, Ursini F, Faldini C, Di Martino A, Mazzanti U, Campesato E, Matrà A, Cevoli S, Benedetti MG. Acupuncture as an alternative or in addition to conventional treatment for chronic non-specific low back pain: A systematic review and

meta-analysis. Integr Med Res. 2023 Sep;12(3):100972. doi: https://doi.org/10.1016/j.imr.2023.100972. Epub 2023 Jul 7. PMID: 37637183 ; PMCID: PMC10448023.

Conclusions: We are uncertain whether acupuncture is more effective and safer than CT. In the comparisons without estimates' imprecision, acupuncture showed promising results. Acupuncture could be an option based on patients' preferences.

18. Li R, Chen L, Ren Y, Huang J, Xu Y, Lin X, Zhen R. Efficacy and safety of acupuncture for pregnancy-related low back pain: A systematic review and meta-analysis. Heliyon. 2023 Jul 25;9(8):e18439. doi: https://doi.org/10.1016/j.heliyon.2023.e18439. PMID: 37593601 ; PMCID: PMC10427988.
19. Liu H, Li YP, Hou MJ, Huang WJ, Chen XL, Gao Z, Jiang Z. Effect of trigger point acupuncture on pain and functional activity in patients with chronic non-specific low back pain: a randomized controlled trial. Acupunct Med. 2023 Jun;41(3):130–141. doi: https://doi.org/10.1177/09645284221107685. Epub 2023 Feb 9. PMID: 36760118 .
20. Kim G, Kim D, Moon H, Yoon DE, Lee S, Ko SJ, Kim B, Chae Y, Lee IS. Acupuncture and Acupoints for Low Back Pain: Systematic Review and Meta-Analysis. Am J Chin Med. 2023;51(2):223–247. doi: https://doi.org/10.1142/S0192415X23500131. Epub 2022 Dec 31. PMID: 36585839 .
21. Rybicka M, Gąsowski J, Przeklasa-Muszyńska A, Dobrogowski J, Wierzbicka J, Hui KK, Ptasnik S, Kocot-Kępska M. NADA Ear Acupuncture and Medical Acupuncture for Pain- and Health-Related Quality of Life among Older Patients with Chronic Nonspecific Low Back Pain: A Prospective Clinical Trial. Brain Sci. 2024 Feb 23;14(3):205. doi: https://doi.org/10.3390/brainsci14030205. PMID: 38539594 ; PMCID: PMC10968796.

    Conclusion: The outcomes of this study suggest that both MA Medical Acupuncture and NADA National Acupuncture Detoxification Association ear acupuncture could be a valuable and personalized component of a comprehensive approach to managing chronic nonspecific LBP in older patients. Incorporation of MA and NADA ear acupuncture into the clinical management of chronic nonspecific LBP in elderly patients has the potential to reduce pain intensity and improve the overall quality of life of affected individuals. However, further studies are needed to confirm our findings.
22. Jamali Dastjerdi M, Azadvari M, Kordafshari G, Zhao BX, Adel-Mehraban MS, Alipour R, Karimi M, Kazemi AH, Sourani A, Vafaie Sefti A. Comparative efficacy of acupuncture, venesection, and physical therapy on chronic low back pain outcomes: a randomized clinical trial. Ann Med Surg (Lond). 2024 Mar 18;86(5):2729–2738. doi: https://doi.org/10.1097/MS9.0000000000001944. PMID: 38694293 ; PMCID: PMC11060228.

    Conclusion: Considering the pain and functional scores, both acupuncture and venesection can reproduce reliable results. Acupuncture and venesection both have sustained effects on pain and daily function of the patients even after treatment termination, while physical therapy had more relapse in pain and functional limitations.

23. Mu J, Furlan AD, Lam WY, Hsu MY, Ning Z, Lao L. Acupuncture for chronic nonspecific low back pain. Cochrane Database Syst Rev. 2020 Dec 11;12(12):CD013814. doi: https://doi.org/10.1002/14651858.CD013814. PMID: 33306198 ; PMCID: PMC8095030.

Authors' conclusions: *We found that acupuncture may not play a more clinically meaningful role than sham in relieving pain immediately after treatment or in improving quality of life in the short term, and acupuncture possibly did not improve back function compared to sham in the immediate term. However, acupuncture was more effective than no treatment in improving pain and function in the immediate term. Trials with usual care as the control showed acupuncture may not reduce pain clinically, but the therapy may improve function immediately after sessions as well as physical but not mental quality of life in the short term. The evidence was downgraded to moderate to very low-certainty considering most of studies had high risk of bias, inconsistency, and small sample size introducing imprecision.* ***The decision to use acupuncture to treat chronic low back pain might depend on the availability, cost and patient's preferences.***

24. Urits I, Wang JK, Yancey K, Mousa M, Jung JW, Berger AA, Shehata IM, Elhassan A, Kaye AD, Viswanath O. Acupuncture for the Management of Low Back Pain. Curr Pain Headache Rep. 2021 Jan 14;25(1):2. doi: https://doi.org/10.1007/s11916-020-00919-y. PMID: 33443607 .

Chronic LBP is more typically defined by its chronicity with pain persisting > 12 weeks in duration. Conventional treatment for chronic LBP includes both pharmacologic and non-pharmacologic options. First-line pharmacologic therapy involves the use of NSAIDs, then SNRI/TCA/skeletal muscle relaxants, and antiepileptics. Surgery is usually not recommended for chronic non-specific LBP patients. According to the 2016 CDC Guidelines for Prescribing Opioids for Chronic Pain and the 2017 American College of Physicians (ACP) clinical practice guidelines for chronic pain, non-pharmacologic interventions, acupuncture can be a first-line treatment for patients suffering from chronic low back pain. Many studies have been done, and most show promising results for acupuncture as an alternative treatment for low back pain.

25. NICE Guideline NG 193. National Institute for Health and Care Excellence. Evidence review for acupuncture for chronic primary pain. Chronic pain (primary and secondary) in over 16s: assessment of all chronic pain and management of chronic primary pain.2021. ISBN: 978-1-4731-4066-0 . Available: https://www.nice.org.uk/guidance/ng193/evidence/g-acupuncture-for-chronic-primary-pain-pdf-9071987012

The committee considered the overall benefit of acupuncture, particularly for reducing pain and improving quality of life, in combination with the lack of harm, other than discontinuation from the therapy. The committee agreed that although there was some uncertainty within some of the outcomes (with a small proportion of outcomes crossing the line of no effect), there was generally a benefit of acupuncture seen within the evidence when compared to both usual care and sham. The committee considered that the evidence base was large enough to justify a recommendation and therefore agreed to recommend the use of acupuncture in clinical practice for people with chronic primary pain. The committee also noted that acupuncture is recommended in the NICE guideline for headaches (CG150) for prophylactic treatment of chronic tension-type headache, where there was also evidence of benefit of acupuncture compared to sham.

26. Li C, Pei Q, Chen Y, Luo X, Yang N, Li TT, Ding J, Wang Y. The response-time relationship and covariate effects of acupuncture for chronic pain: A systematic review and model-based longitudinal meta-analysis. Eur J Pain. 2020 Oct;24(9):1653–1665. doi: https://doi.org/10.1002/ejp.1617. Epub 2020 Jul 31. PMID: 32533885 .

    Seventy-seven randomized clinical trials involved chronic shoulder, neck, knee and low back pain were included. The response-time analysis suggested that the treatment duration of acupuncture will be 5 weeks or more to achieve 80% of maximum analgesic effect. Higher analgesic effect was related to higher baseline pain intensity and pain location of neck, shoulder and knee. The absolute maximum analgesic effects of sham acupuncture and conventional therapy were 22.6 and 15.8 points at a 0–100 NRS scale. The absolute effect of true acupuncture was 26.1 points for low back pain (relative effect of 3.5 and 9.4 points to sham and conventional therapy), 34.9 points for other pain body locations (relative effect of 12.3 and 19.1 points to sham and conventional therapy), in patients with a baseline pain intensity of 60 points.

27. Vickers AJ, Vertosick EA, Lewith G, MacPherson H, Foster NE, Sherman KJ, Irnich D, Witt CM, Linde K; Acupuncture Trialists' Collaboration. Acupuncture for Chronic Pain: Update of an Individual Patient Data Meta-Analysis. J Pain. 2018 May;19(5):455–474. doi: https://doi.org/10.1016/j.jpain.2017.11.005. Epub 2017 Dec 2. PMID: 29198932 ; PMCID: PMC5927830.

    Data received for a total of 20,827 patients from 39 trials. Acupuncture was superior to sham as well as no acupuncture control for each pain condition (all P < .001) with differences between groups close to.5 SDs compared with no acupuncture control and close to.2 SDs compared with sham. We also found clear evidence that the effects of acupuncture persist over time with only a small decrease, approximately 15%, in treatment effect at 1 year. Acupuncture is effective for the treatment of chronic musculoskeletal, headache, and osteoarthritis pain. Treatment effects of acupuncture persist over time and cannot be explained solely in terms of placebo effects. Referral for a course of acupuncture treatment is a reasonable option for a patient with chronic pain.

28. Wu X, Li S, Wu M. Advances in Electroacupuncture for Treatment of Knee Osteoarthritis: Mechanisms, Efficacy, and Future Directions. J Pain Res. 2025 Sep 30;18:5083–5108. doi: https://doi.org/10.2147/JPR.S543346. PMID: 41050143 ; PMCID: PMC12495921.

    Growing evidence suggests that EA not only reduces pain and enhances joint mobility but also modulates diverse biological processes, such as neuroendocrine signalling, inflammatory cascades, cartilage metabolism, and local hemodynamics. Mechanistically, EA acts through multi-target mechanisms, including suppression of pro-inflammatory mediators, promotion of anti-inflammatory and chondroprotective factors, and regulation of critical signalling pathways such as NF-κB, MAPK, and Wnt/β-catenin. Additionally, EA engages central and peripheral neuromodulatory systems involving opioid, serotonergic, and cannabinoid receptors, underpinning its analgesic properties.

6.8.3 The Current State of the Evidence Base for Acupuncture in the Treatment of Depression (Anxiety)

A total of n = 827 results were found under the above filter settings and time in PubMed.

1. Jang A, Wenninger M, Lee H, Zheng S. Acupuncture for Anxiety: A Systematic Review and Meta-Analysis of Randomized Controlled Trials. J Clin Psychol. 2025 Dec 29. doi: https://doi.org/10.1002/jclp.70079. Epub ahead of print. PMID: 41460176.
2. Han X, Gao Y, Yin X, Zhang Z, Lao L, Chen Q, Xu S. The mechanism of electroacupuncture for depression on basic research: a systematic review. Chin Med. 2021 Jan 13;16(1):10. doi: https://doi.org/10.1186/s13020-020-00421-y. Erratum in: Chin Med. 2021 Feb 10;16(1):20. doi: https://doi.org/10.1186/s13020-021-00430-5. PMID: 33436036; PMCID: PMC7805231.

   Conclusions: This review reveals that the mechanisms underlying the effect of acupuncture involve multiple pathways and targets, suggesting that acupuncture is a wholistic treatment for people rather than for diseases. Our findings also explain why acupuncture can treat various disorders in addition to depression.

   Treatment of depression by Electroacupuncture involves multiple therapeutic mechanisms, including inhibition of HPA axis hyperactivity and inflammation, regulation of neuropeptides and neurotransmitters, modulation of the expression of particular genes, restoration of hippocampal synaptic, increased expression of BDNF, and regulation of several signalling pathways.
3. Ma J, Yin X, Cui K, Wang J, Li W, Xu S. Mechanisms of acupuncture in treating depression: a review. Chin Med. 2025 Mar 3;20(1):29. doi: https://doi.org/10.1186/s13020-025-01080-7. PMID: 40033393; PMCID: PMC11877828.

   Results: By analysing the effect of acupuncture on rodent model of depression, the mechanism of acupuncture against depression was explored. In general, several acupuncture methods, mainly based on electroacupuncture (EA), regulate the levels of 5-hydroxytryptamine (5-HT), glutamic acid (Glu) and dopamine (DA), regulate the calcium signalling pathway, increase the expression of synaptic protein, promote mitochondrial repair and reduce oxidative stress, and enhance synaptic plasticity.
4. Liao HY, Satyanarayanan SK, Lin YW, Su KP. Clinical efficacy and immune effects of acupuncture in patients with comorbid chronic pain and major depression disorder: A double-blinded, randomized controlled crossover study. Brain

Behav Immun. 2023 May;110:339–347. doi: https://doi.org/10.1016/j.bbi.2023.03.016. Epub 2023 Mar 21. PMID: 36948325

5. Li J, Zhang K, Zhao T, Huang W, Hou R, Wang S, Zhao M, Guo Y. Acupressure for depression: A systematic review and meta-analysis. Asian J Psychiatr. 2024 Feb;92:103884. doi: https://doi.org/10.1016/j.ajp.2023.103884. Epub 2023 Dec 23. PMID: 38171225 .

   Research has demonstrated that acupuncture exerts diverse physiological effects in animal models of depression, encompassing modulation of the brain, serum, and brain-gut axis. These effects are attributed to various mechanisms, including anti-inflammatory and anti-oxidative actions, promotion of neuronal plasticity, neuroprotection, neurotrophic effects, modulation of neurotransmitters, regulation of endocrine and immune functions, and modulation of cell signal pathways. Currently, the therapeutic mechanism of acupuncture involves the engagement of multiple targets, pathways, and bidirectional regulation.

6. Ding X, Zhao F, Zhu M, Wang Q, Wei S, Xue J, Li Z. A systematic review and meta-analysis of interventions to reduce perceived stress in breast cancer patients. Complement Ther Clin Pract. 2024 Feb;54:101803. doi: https://doi.org/10.1016/j.ctcp.2023.101803. Epub 2023 Dec 19. PMID: 38159534 .
7. Sun B, Cao X, Xin M, Guan R. Treatment of Depression with Acupuncture Based on Pathophysiological Mechanism. Int J Gen Med. 2024 Jan 31;17:347–357. doi: https://doi.org/10.2147/IJGM.S448031. PMID: 38314195 ; PMCID: PMC10838506.
8. Kong L, Ren J, Fang S, Li Y, Wu Z, Zhou X, Hao Q, Fang M, Zhang YQ. Effects of traditional Chinese mind-body exercises for patients with chronic fatigue syndrome: A systematic review and meta-analysis. J Glob Health. 2023 Nov 24;13:04157. doi: https://doi.org/10.7189/jogh.13.04157. PMID: 37994837 ; PMCID: PMC10666566.
9. Hwang SI, Yoon YJ, Sung SH, Cho SJ, Park JK. Acupuncture Treatment for Emotional Problems in Women with Infertility: A Systematic Review and Meta-Analysis. Healthcare (Basel). 2023 Oct 10;11(20):2704. doi: https://doi.org/10.3390/healthcare11202704. PMID: 37893778 ; PMCID: PMC10606758.
10. Tan C, Qiao M, Ma Y, Luo Y, Fang J, Yang Y. The efficacy and safety of transcutaneous auricular vagus nerve stimulation in the treatment of depressive disorder: A systematic review and meta-analysis of randomized controlled trials. J Affect Disord. 2023 Sep 15;337:37–49. doi: https://doi.org/10.1016/j.jad.2023.05.048. Epub 2023 May 23. PMID: 37230264 .
11. Li X, Wang Y, Wu L, Zhao X, Zhu T. Acupuncture for tumor-related depression: a systematic review and meta- analysis. Front Oncol. 2023 Aug 8;13:1198286. doi: https://doi.org/10.3389/fonc.2023.1198286. PMID: 37614513 ; PMCID: PMC10442935.
12. Cai W, Wei XF, Zhang JR, Hu C, Shen WD. Does acupuncture treatment have satisfactory clinical efficacy for late-life depression? A systematic review and meta-analysis. Geriatr Nurs. 2023 May–Jun;51:215–221. doi: https://doi.org/10.1016/j.gerinurse.2023.03.008. Epub 2023 Apr 2. PMID: 37015141 .

13. Liao HY, Satyanarayanan SK, Lin YW, Su KP. Clinical efficacy and immune effects of acupuncture in patients with comorbid chronic pain and major depression disorder: A double-blinded, randomized controlled crossover study. Brain Behav Immun. 2023 May;110:339–347. doi: https://doi.org/10.1016/j.bbi.2023.03.016. Epub 2023 Mar 21. PMID: 36948325 .
14. Wang T, Tan JB, Yao LQ, Huilin Cheng, Zhao I, Eliseeva S, Polotan MJ. Effects of somatic acupoint stimulation on anxiety and depression in cancer patients: An updated systematic review of randomized controlled trials. Complement Ther Clin Pract. 2023 May;51:101735. doi: https://doi.org/10.1016/j.ctcp.2023.101735. Epub 2023 Feb 13. PMID: 36812735 .
15. Mao Q, Wang Y, Xu S, Wu D, Huang G, Li Z, Jiao L, Chi Z. Research hotspots and frontiers in non-specific low back pain: a bibliometric analysis. Front Neurol. 2024 Oct 30;15:1464048. doi: https://doi.org/10.3389/fneur.2024.1464048. PMID: 39539665 ; PMCID: PMC11557401.

    Conclusion: This article summarizes the current research status of NSLBP (non-specific low back pain) and predicts future research hotspots and frontiers. In recent years, adolescents have become a high-risk group for NSLBP. Pain neuroscience education, motor control, spinal manipulative therapy, and acupuncture are effective means to treat NSLBP. Biomechanics and trunk muscles as entry points are effective ideas for the treatment of NSLBP. Furthermore, anxiety, neck pain, non-specific musculoskeletal pain, fibromyalgia, and musculoskeletal disorders are diseases that are closely related to NSLBP. In the future, attention should be paid to the design of research plans, increasing the research intensity of randomized controlled trials, strengthening follow-up, and the timely updating of guidelines, which will result in higher quality and high-level scientific evidence for research on NSLBP.
16. Zhao FY, Zheng Z, Fu QQ, Conduit R, Xu H, Wang HR, Huang YL, Jiang T, Zhang WJ, Kennedy GA. Acupuncture for comorbid depression and insomnia in perimenopause: A feasibility patient-assessor-blinded, randomized, and sham-controlled clinical trial. Front Public Health. 2023 Feb 6;11:1120567. doi: https://doi.org/10.3389/fpubh.2023.1120567. PMID: 36815166 ; PMCID: PMC9939459.

    Conclusion: Acupuncture is safe and can contribute to clinically relevant improvements in comorbid PMD and PMI, with satisfactory short-and medium-term effects. Whether the anti-depressive benefit of acupuncture is specific or non-specific remains to be determined. No evidence was found for any longer-term benefit of acupuncture compared to sham at 16 weeks. Further research is required to elucidate mechanisms underlying the short to medium-term effects of acupuncture.
17. Lam Ching W, Li HJ, Guo J, Yao L, Chau J, Lo S, Yuen CS, Ng BFL, Chau-Leung Yu E, Bian Z, Lau AY, Zhong LL. Acupuncture for post-stroke depression: a systematic review and network meta-analysis. BMC Psychiatry. 2023 May 4;23(1):314. doi: https://doi.org/10.1186/s12888-023-04749-1. PMID: 37143014 ; PMCID: PMC10161596.

Conclusions: The results of this study indicate that AC alone or combined with other therapies appears to be effective in improving depression symptoms of stroke survivors. Moreover, in comparison to WM, AC alone or plus RTMS, TCM, TCM with WM, or WM, were more effective in improving depression symptoms of PSD. Also, AC with RTMS seems to be the most effective with the highest probability.

6.8.4 The Current State of the Evidence Base for Chinese Herbal Medicine in the Treatment of Depression (Anxiety)

A PubMed search for clinical studies on herbal medicines from 1990 to 14 November 2025 yields 4829 results. Narrowing the search to Chinese herbal medicine leaves 2067 publications. Applying the meta-analysis, randomized controlled trial (RCT) and systematic review filters leaves 325 hits.

1. Jang A, Wenninger M, Lee H, Zheng S. Acupuncture for Anxiety: A Systematic Review and Meta-Analysis of Randomized Controlled Trials. J Clin Psychol. 2025 Dec 29. doi: https://doi.org/10.1002/jclp.70079. Epub ahead of print. PMID: 41460176 .
2. Yang S, Xu Y, Peng W, Han D, Feng F, Wang Z, Gu C, Zhou X, He H. Chinese herbal medicine for symptoms of depression and anxiety in chronic obstructive pulmonary disease: A systematic review and meta-analysis. Complement Ther Clin Pract. 2021 Nov;45:101470. doi: https://doi.org/10.1016/j.ctcp.2021.101470. Epub 2021 Aug 4. PMID: 34375807 .

   Conclusion: The evidence verified the efficacy and safety of CHM on relieving depression and anxiety in COPD. However, further large-scale and rigorously designed studies are urgently warranted to strengthen the evidence.
3. Wang Y, Shi YH, Xu Z, Fu H, Zeng H, Zheng GQ. Efficacy and safety of Chinese herbal medicine for depression: A systematic review and meta-analysis of randomized controlled trials. J Psychiatr Res. 2019 Oct;117:74–91. doi: https://doi.org/10.1016/j.jpsychires.2019.07.003. Epub 2019 Jul 15. PMID: 31326751 .

   Conclusion: The findings of present systematic review, at least to a certain extent, provided supporting evidence for the routine use of CHM for depression.
4. Xie Z, Lu J, Zhang X, Jia H, Zhang Y. Efficacy of Chinese herbal medicine in the treatment of anxiety and depression in male sexual dysfunction: a systematic review and meta-analysis. Sex Med. 2025 Jul 10;13(3):qfaf048. doi: https://doi.org/10.1093/sexmed/qfaf048. PMID: 40641608 ; PMCID: PMC12240729.

   Conclusions: Our findings provide the first robust evidence that CHM significantly alleviates anxiety and depression in MSD patients, while concurrently improving core MSD symptoms, such as PE and ED.
5. Dang C, Wang Q, Li Q, Xiong Y, Lu Y. Chinese herbal medicines for the treatment of depression: a systematic review and network meta-analysis. Front

Pharmacol. 2024 Apr 3;15:1295564. doi: https://doi.org/10.3389/fphar.2024.1295564. PMID: 38633609 ; PMCID: PMC11021639.

Results: A total of 198 RCTs involving 8923 patients were analysed, assessing 17 Chinese herbal medicines. Surface Under the Cumulative Ranking results indicated that the top three treatments with the best response rate were possibly Guipiwan, Ease Pill, and Chaihu Jia Longgu Muli Decoction; the top three treatments on the reduction of HAMD scores were Chai Hu Shu Gan San, Xingnao Jieyu Decoction, and Xiaoyao Powder; and the top three treatments with the lowest adverse effects rates were Xiaoyao Powder, Alprazolam, and Xingnao Jieyu Decoction. Interestingly, commonly used synthetic drugs such as Fluoxetine, Escitalopram, Amitriptyline, Sertraline, Flupentixol and Melitracen, and Venlafaxine, not only ***appeared to be less effective*** *than specific Chinese herbal medicines (Gan Mai Da Zao Decoction, Chaihu Jia Longgu Muli Decoction, Chai Hu Shu Gan San, Danzhi-Xiaoyao-San, and Xingnao Jieyu Decoction), but they were also related to substantially higher risk of adverse events.*

Conclusion: Our findings elucidate the promising therapeutic potential of Chinese herbal medicines as viable alternatives in the treatment of depression, with certain herbs demonstrating enhanced efficacy and safety profiles. The outcomes of this study advocate for the integration of these alternative modalities into contemporary depression management paradigms. However, it underscores the necessity for larger, methodologically robust trials to further validate and refine these preliminary findings.

6. Li QF, Lu WT, Zhang Q, Zhao YD, Wu CY, Zhou HF. Proprietary Medicines Containing Bupleurum chinense DC. (Chaihu) for Depression: Network Meta-Analysis and Network Pharmacology Prediction. Front Pharmacol. 2022 Apr 6;13:773537. doi: https://doi.org/10.3389/fphar.2022.773537. PMID: 35462897 ; PMCID: PMC9019785.

   Conclusion: This is the very first systematic review and network meta-analysis evaluating different oral proprietary Chinese medicines containing Chaihu in depressive disorder. This study suggested that the combination of proprietary Chinese medicines containing Chaihu with antidepressants was generally better than antidepressant treatment. The incidence of adverse reactions with antidepressants alone was higher than that with proprietary Chinese medicines containing Chaihu alone or in combination with antidepressants. DZXY + SNRI showed significantly better results in efficacy, HAMD scores, and safety. The antidepressant effect of DZXY may be related to its regulation of neuroinflammation and apoptosis.

7. Ran S, Peng R, Guo Q, Cui J, Chen G, Wang Z. Bupleurum in Treatment of Depression Disorder: A Comprehensive Review. Pharmaceuticals (Basel). 2024 Apr 16;17(4):512. doi: https://doi.org/10.3390/ph17040512. PMID: 38675471 ; PMCID: PMC11054835.

   *Results: This review highlights various antidepressant ingredients isolated from Bupleurum, including s***aikosaponin A, saikosaponin D, rutin, puerarin***, and quercetin, each with distinct mechanisms of action. Additionally, Chinese* *herb prescriptions and extracts containing Bupleurum, such as Chaihu Shugansan, Xiaoyaosan, and Sinisan, are also included due to their demonstrated antidepressant effects.* ***This review reveals that these Bupleurum compounds exhibit antidepressant effects through the regulation of neurotransmitter mechanisms (such as 5-HT and DA), the NMDA (N-methyl-D-aspartate) system, brain-derived neurotrophic factor (BDNF), and other intracellular signalling pathways.***

8. Bai C, Wang J, Wang Y, Liu H, Li J, Wang S, Bai Z, Guo R. Exploration of the mechanism of Traditional Chinese Medicine for anxiety and depression in patients with diarrheal irritable bowel syndrome based on network pharmacology and meta-analysis. Front Pharmacol. 2024 May 21;15:1404738. doi: https://doi.org/10.3389/fphar.2024.1404738. PMID: 38835657 ; PMCID: PMC11148253.

   Conclusion: Chinese herbal medicine (CHM) offers a promising and safe treatment approach for patients dealing with diarrheal irritable bowel syndrome (IBS-D) accompanied by anxiety and depression; thus, indicating its potential for practical implementation. The most active metabolites of CHM could simultaneously act on the pathological targets of IBS-D, anxiety, and depression. The diverse scope of CHM's therapeutic role includes various aspects and objectives, underscoring its potential for broad utilization.

9. Wang B, Teng Y, Li Y, Lai S, Wu Y, Chen S, Li T, Han X, Zhou H, Wang Y, Lu Z, Li H, Ding Y, Ma L, Zhao M, Wang X. Evidence and Characteristics of Traditional Chinese Medicine for Coronary Heart Disease Patients With Anxiety or Depression: A Meta-Analysis and Systematic Review. Front Pharmacol. 2022 May 5;13:854292. doi: https://doi.org/10.3389/fphar.2022.854292. PMID: 35600859 ; PMCID: PMC9117623.

   Conclusion: CHM (Chinese herbal medicine) exhibited an obvious efficacy in treating CHD (coronary heart disease) patients with anxiety or depression, especially for improving the symptom of angina pectoris. The most active compounds of CHM could simultaneously act on the pathological targets of CHD, anxiety, and depression. Multiple effective components and multiple targets were the advantages of CHM compared with WM.

10. Fan L, Zeng P, Wang X, Mo X, Ma Q, Zhou X, Yuan N, Liu Y, Xue Z, Huang J, Li X, Ding J, Chen J. Xiaoyao Pills, a Chinese patent medicine, treats mild and moderate depression: A randomized clinical trial combined with DNA methylation analysis. Phytomedicine. 2024 Jul 25;130:155660. doi: https://doi.org/10.1016/j.phymed.2024.155660. Epub 2024 Apr 20. PMID: 38815407 .

    Conclusions: Our study provides new insights into the epigenetic mechanism underlying depression and the therapeutic effects of XYP Xiaoyao pills, along with an experimental basis for using XYP in the treatment of depression.

11. Li B, Xu M, Wang Y, Feng L, Xing H, Zhang K. Gut microbiota: A new target for traditional Chinese medicine in the treatment of depression. J Ethnopharmacol. 2023 Mar 1;303:116038. doi: https://doi.org/10.1016/j.jep.2022.116038. Epub 2022 Dec 15. PMID: 36529248 .

Conclusion: This review summarized the anti-depression effects of TCM on the gut microbiota, providing evidence that TCMs are safe and effective in the treatment of depression and may provide a new therapeutic approach.

12. Li M, Chen Z, Liu Z, Zhang N, Liu J, Wang H, Wang W, Liang Y, Chen J, Liu Z, Li Y, Zhai S. Twelve Chinese herbal preparations for the treatment of depression or depressive symptoms in cancer patients: a systematic review and meta-analysis of randomized controlled trials. BMC Complement Altern Med. 2019 Jan 23;19(1):28. doi: https://doi.org/10.1186/s12906-019-2441-8. PMID: 30674300 ; PMCID: PMC6345004.

    Conclusions: According to the investigation of the twelve herbal preparations, the CHM intervention appears to alleviate depressive symptoms in cancer patients, either alone or combined with antidepressants or psychological treatments. However, a high risk of bias and high heterogeneity made the mean estimates uncertain. Well-designed trials with comprehensive and transparent reporting are warranted in the future.

13. Chen C, Yin Q, Tian J, Gao X, Qin X, Du G, Zhou Y. Studies on the potential link between antidepressant effect of Xiaoyao San and its pharmacological activity of hepatoprotection based on multi-platform metabolomics. J Ethnopharmacol. 2020 Mar 1;249:112432. doi: https://doi.org/10.1016/j.jep.2019.112432. Epub 2019 Nov 29. PMID: 31790818 .

    Results: In traditional Chinese medicine (TCM) theory, depression is considered to be 'liver qi stagnation', and relieving 'liver qi stagnation' is regarded as an effective method for treating depression. Xiaoyao San (XYS) is a well-known TCM formula for the treatment of depression by relieving 'liver qi stagnation'. This formula consists of Radix Paeoniae Alba (Paeonia lactiflora Pall.), Radix Bupleuri (Bupleurum chinense DC.), Poria (Poria cocos (Schw.) Wolf), Rhizoma Atractylodis Macrocephalae (Atractylodes macrocephala Koidz.), Radix Angelicae Sinensis (Angelica sinensis (Oliv.) Diels), Radix Glycyrrhizae (Glycyrrhiza uralensis Fisch.), Rhizoma Zingiberis Recens (Zingiber officinale Roscoe) and Herba Menthae Haplocalycis (Mentha haplocalyx Briq.). XYS could significantly improve the depressive and liver injury symptoms induced by CUMS (chronic unpredictable mild stress). The metabolomics results indicate that the regulation of glutamine and glutamate metabolism to maintain the balance of ammonia and promote energy metabolism is a potential junction between the antidepressant and hepatoprotective effects of XYS.

14. Sun Y, Xu X, Zhang J, Chen Y. Treatment of depression with Chai Hu Shu Gan San: a systematic review and meta-analysis of 42 randomized controlled trials. BMC Complement Altern Med. 2018 Feb 17;18(1):66. doi: https://doi.org/10.1186/s12906-018-2130-z. PMID: 29454341 ; PMCID: PMC5816377.
15. Yan L, Xu X, He Z, Wang S, Zhao L, Qiu J, Wang D, Gong Z, Qiu X, Huang H. Antidepressant-Like Effects and Cognitive Enhancement of Coadministration of Chaihu Shugan San and Fluoxetine: Dependent on the BDNF-ERK-CREB Signaling Pathway in the Hippocampus and Frontal Cortex. Biomed Res Int. 2020 Feb 22;2020:2794263. doi: https://doi.org/10.1155/2020/2794263. PMID: 32185198 ; PMCID: PMC7060874.

16. Meng P, Han Y, Yang Q, Yang H, Zhu Q, Lin X, Zhang X, Zhao H, Liu Z, Liu J, Tang L, Luo W, Wang Y. Xiaoyao Kangai Jieyu Fang, a Chinese Herbal Formulation, Ameliorates Cancer-Related Depression Concurrent with Breast Cancer in Mice via Promoting Hippocampal Synaptic Plasticity. Evid Based Complement Alternat Med. 2018 Nov 18;2018:3967642. doi: https://doi.org/10.1155/2018/3967642. PMID: 30581482 ; PMCID: PMC6276466.
17. Chen C, Yin Q, Tian J, Gao X, Qin X, Du G, Zhou Y. Studies on the Changes of Pharmacokinetics Behaviors of Phytochemicals and the Influence on Endogenous Metabolites After the Combination of Radix Bupleuri and Radix Paeoniae Alba Based on Multi-Component Pharmacokinetics and Metabolomics. Front Pharmacol. 2021 Mar 8;12:630970. doi: https://doi.org/10.3389/fphar.2021.630970. PMID: 33762950 ; PMCID: PMC7982521
18. Yu M, Jia HM, Zhang T, Shang H, Zhang HW, Ma LY, Zou ZM. Gut Microbiota is the Key to the Antidepressant Effect of Chaihu-Shu-Gan-San. Metabolites. 2020 Feb 10;10(2):63. doi: https://doi.org/10.3390/metabo10020063. PMID: 32050718 ; PMCID: PMC7074034.

6.8.5 The Current State of the Evidence Base for Acupuncture in the Treatment of Somatic Symptom Disorder and Insomnia

A total of $n = 8$ and $n = 364$ results were found under the above filter settings and time in PubMed.

1. Zhao F, Wang W, Feng X, Li J, Gang W, Jing X, Chen H, Liang Y. Effect of acupuncture on somatic symptom disorder: a systematic review and meta-analysis. Front Med (Lausanne). 2025 Oct 1;12:1625230. doi: https://doi.org/10.3389/fmed.2025.1625230. PMID: 41103694 ; PMCID: PMC12521258.

   Conclusion: Our findings indicated potential added benefits of acupuncture combined with SSRI/SNRI for SSD-related anxiety, although effects on pain were inconsistent. High-quality RCTs with larger sample sizes are required to confirm acupuncture's efficacy and safety for SSD.
2. Boluda-Verdú I, Catalá-López F. Efectividad y coste-efectividad de intervenciones no farmacológicas para trastornos somáticos funcionales: revisión sistemática de metaanálisis y evaluaciones económicas [Effectiveness and cost-effectiveness of non-pharmacological interventions for functional somatic disorders: systematic review of meta-analyses and economic evaluations]. Gac Sanit. 2025;39 Suppl 1:102457. Spanish. doi: https://doi.org/10.1016/j.gaceta.2025.102457. Epub 2025 Mar 6. PMID: 40055062 .

   Conclusions: The evidence on the effectiveness and cost-effectiveness of non-pharmacological interventions for functional somatic disorders should be interpreted with caution since the majority of the systematic reviews were of low or critically low methodological quality, and with a high level of uncertainty in the case of economic evaluations. The diversity of definitions of the diagnosis and interventions makes it difficult to generalize these results.

3. Paterson C, Taylor RS, Griffiths P, Britten N, Rugg S, Bridges J, McCallum B, Kite G; CACTUS study team. Acupuncture for 'frequent attenders' with medically unexplained symptoms: a randomised controlled trial (CACTUS study). Br J Gen Pract. 2011 Jun;61(587):e295-305. doi: https://doi.org/10.3399/bjgp11X572689. PMID: 21801508 ; PMCID: PMC3103692.

   Conclusion: The addition of 12 sessions of five-element acupuncture to usual care resulted in improved health status and well-being that was sustained for 12 months.
4. Kim SA, Lee SH, Kim JH, van den Noort M, Bosch P, Won T, Yeo S, Lim S. Efficacy of Acupuncture for Insomnia: A Systematic Review and Meta-Analysis. Am J Chin Med. 2021;49(5):1135–1150. doi: https://doi.org/10.1142/S0192415X21500543. Epub 2021 May 27. PMID: 34049475 .

   Results: These results suggest that insomnia patients may experience significant improvement in symptoms after more than three weeks of acupuncture treatment compared to pharmacological treatments.
5. Yu Y, Li X, Zhu Z, Wang Y, Xi Q, Qiu J, Xu Y, Liang R, Guo Y, Zhang M. Acupuncture for chronic insomnia disorder: a systematic review with meta-analysis and trial sequential analysis. Front Neurol. 2025 Apr 30;16:1541276. doi: https://doi.org/10.3389/fneur.2025.1541276. PMID: 40371085 ; PMCID: PMC12074954.

   Conclusion: Compared with sham acupuncture, acupuncture is effective in improving sleep quality in patients with chronic insomnia disorder. However, whether acupuncture improves patients' objective sleep indices compared to sham acupuncture is uncertain and more high-quality clinical trial evidence is needed to validate this.
6. Zhao FY, Kennedy GA, Spencer SJ, Conduit R, Zhang WJ, Fu QQ, Zheng Z. The Role of Acupuncture in the Management of Insomnia as a Major or Residual Symptom Among Patients With Active or Previous Depression: A Systematic Review and Meta-Analysis. Front Psychiatry. 2022 Apr 15;13:863134. doi: https://doi.org/10.3389/fpsyt.2022.863134. PMID: 35492706 ; PMCID: PMC9051249.

   Conclusions: There is a low to moderate level of evidence supporting acupuncture as a safe and effective remedy alternative to or adjuvant to conventional pharmacotherapy (antidepressant and/or hypnotic) in improving insomnia and other depression symptoms among patients with active depression. Furthermore, the patients' complaint of disrupted sleep continuity is most likely to benefit from acupuncture. The benefit of acupuncture on residual insomnia associated with previous or partially remitted depression is limited. Future acupuncture studies need to consider applying optimal dosage and addressing deficiencies in trial quality.
7. Lam Ching W, Li HJ, Guo J, Yao L, Chau J, Lo S, Yuen CS, Ng BFL, Chau-Leung Yu E, Bian Z, Lau AY, Zhong LL. Acupuncture for post-stroke depression: a systematic review and network meta-analysis. BMC Psychiatry. 2023

May 4;23(1):314. doi: https://doi.org/10.1186/s12888-023-04749-1. PMID: 37143014 ; PMCID: PMC10161596.

Conclusions: The results of this study indicate that AC alone or combined with other therapies appears to be effective in improving depression symptoms of stroke survivors. Moreover, in comparison to WM, AC alone or plus RTMS, TCM, TCM with WM, or WM, were more effective in improving depression symptoms of PSD. Also, AC with RTMS seems to be the most effective with the highest probability.

8. Liu P, Li L, Xu D, Xin S, Hu N, Li C. Acupuncture for cancer-related insomnia: systematic review and meta-analysis of randomised controlled trials. BMJ Support Palliat Care. 2024 Nov 20;14(4):378–391. doi: https://doi.org/10.1136/spcare-2024-005051. PMID: 39384192

   Conclusion: The change in PSQI and ISI scores showed that acupuncture moderately improved insomnia in patients with cancer. Acupuncture is safe and effective, enabling subsequent clinical treatments.

9. Liu X, Xu N, Wang S, Jia Q. Efficacy of electroacupuncture for insomnia in cancer patients: a systematic review and meta-analysis. Front Neurol. 2025 Feb 10;16:1512052. doi: https://doi.org/10.3389/fneur.2025.1512052. PMID: 39995786 ; PMCID: PMC11847688.

   Conclusion: Electroacupuncture has shown promising potential in treating cancer-related insomnia by increasing total sleep time and reducing sleep disturbances. However, additional high-quality studies are necessary to validate these findings.

10. Yan L, Wang X, Liu X, Cai J, Zhang Z, Yang B. An analysis of electroacupuncture as adjunctive treatment for insomnia: a new perspective targeting GABA-mediated microbiome-gut-brain axis. Front Neurol. 2025 Apr 30;16:1504316. doi: https://doi.org/10.3389/fneur.2025.1504316. PMID: 40371088 ; PMCID: PMC12077820.

    Insomnia is a prevalent psychiatric disorder that significantly impacts mental and physical health. Emerging evidence suggests that gut microbiota, particularly γ-aminobutyric acid (GABA) producing bacteria, plays a critical role in the microbiome-gut-brain axis (MGBA), influencing sleep and mental states. Electroacupuncture (EA) has been shown to have favourable anti-insomnia effects. This research protocol outlines a randomized controlled trial (RCT) designed to investigate the efficacy of EA in modulating GABA levels via the MGBA to alleviate insomnia.

11. Wang X, Yan L, Zhang X, Liu X, Yang B. Electroacupuncture as adjunctive therapy for insomnia via targeting the GABAergic microbiota-gut-brain axis: a mini review. Front Psychiatry. 2025 Jul 18;16:1613408. doi: https://doi.org/10.3389/fpsyt.2025.1613408. PMID: 40756316 ; PMCID: PMC12313576.

    Insomnia, affecting up to 30% of adults (typically 18–65 years), is characterized by GABAergic dysfunction and hyperarousal. This mini-review establishes three pivotal advances in insomnia therapeutics: Firstly, it is demonstrated that microbiota-gut-brain axis (MGBA) dysregulation is mechanistically central to insomnia, directly linking gut dysbiosis to vagal, hypothalamic-pituitary-adrenal (HPA), and γ-aminobutyric acid (GABA) axis dysfunction and neuroinflammation. Secondly, ***the present study documents the unique multitarget effects of electroacupuncture (EA), which have been shown to simultaneously normalize HPA axis activity, enrich GABA-producing microbiota, improve the vagal tone, and suppress neuroimmune activation.*** *The aforementioned effects collectively resolve insomnia's multifactorial aetiology. Thirdly, clinical evidence confirms the sustained efficacy of EA to be comparable to that of hypnotics, yet with superior safety and durability. EA redefines therapeutic frameworks by integrating biological and neural interventions that are inaccessible to single-target approaches.*

12. Li Z, Yin S, Feng J, Gao X, Yang Q, Zhu F. Acupuncture combined with Chinese herbal medicine in the treatment of perimenopausal insomnia: A systematic review and meta-analysis. Medicine (Baltimore). 2023 Nov 10;102(45):e35942. doi: https://doi.org/10.1097/MD.0000000000035942. PMID: 37960761 ; PMCID: PMC10637479.

    Conclusion: The current analysis results show that acupuncture combined with Chinese medicine seems to have a more positive effect than Western medicine alone in improving sleep and FSHF in PMI patients, but no difference has been found in improving E2 and LH. This study provides a basis for acupuncture combined with Chinese medicine to treat PMI. However, due to the higher risk of evaluation in included studies, more rigorous randomized controlled trials and higher quality studies are needed to validate the included studies.

6.8.6 The Current State of the Evidence Base for Lifestyle Medicine in the Treatment of Mental Illness

Searching for the keyword 'lifestyle medicine' yields 6987 results, whereas searching for 'lifestyle interventions' yields 17,348.

1. Maurus I, Wagner S, Spaeth J, Vogel A, Muenz S, Seitz V, von Philipsborn P, Solmi M, Firth J, Stubbs B, Vancampfort D, Hallgren M, Kurimay T, Gerber M, Correll CU, Gaebel W, Möller HJ, Schmitt A, Hasan A, Falkai P. EPA guidance on lifestyle interventions for adults with severe mental illness: A meta-review of the evidence. Eur Psychiatry. 2024 Dec 10;67(1):e80. doi: https://doi.org/10.1192/j.eurpsy.2024.1766. PMID: 39655999 ; PMCID: PMC11733621.

    Recommendation Grade A: Lifestyle interventions that combine behaviour change techniques, dietary modifications, and physical activity should be offered to individuals with ***SMI (severe mental illness) for reducing weight and other metabolic syndrome components, as well as depressive and anxiety symptoms.***
2. Teasdale SB, Machaczek KK, Marx W, Eaton M, Chapman J, Milton A, Oyeyemi AL, Pelupessy DC, Schuch FB, Gatera G, Ahmed HU, Diatri H, Jidda IM, Gutiérrez-Peláez M, Elshazly M, Fugu MA, Grinko N, Indu PS, Oo SS, Balasubramanian S, Deenik J, Vancampfort D, Stubbs B, Matthews E, Ward PB, Curtis J, Hassan L, Cortese S, Gilbody S; Lancet Psychiatry Physical Health

Commission Consortium; Firth J, Rosenbaum S. Implementing lifestyle interventions in mental health care: third report of the Lancet Psychiatry Physical Health Commission. Lancet Psychiatry. 2025 Sep;12(9):700–722. doi: https://doi.org/10.1016/S2215-0366(25)00170-1. PMID: 40812962 .

The physical health disparities experienced by people who live with mental illness are well documented. This population group has cardiometabolic risks and diseases at rates 1·4–2·0 times higher than people without mental illness, and physical health conditions are responsible for 70% of the deaths of people with severe mental illness. They are the major drivers of the 13–15 year reduction in life expectancy that is found in individuals with mental illness, compared with those without mental illness.

3. Kunugi H. Depression and lifestyle: Focusing on nutrition, exercise, and their possible relevance to molecular mechanisms. Psychiatry Clin Neurosci. 2023 Aug;77(8):420–433. doi: https://doi.org/10.1111/pcn.13551. Epub 2023 Apr 25. PMID: 36992617 ; PMCID: PMC11488618.

   There is accumulating evidence at the meta-analysis level for interventions to modify these lifestyle habits in the protection and treatment of depressive disorder. Main biological mechanisms of the link between lifestyle factors and depression include monoamine imbalance, inflammation, altered stress response, oxidative stress, and dysfunction of brain-derived neurotrophic factor, although other players such as insulin, leptin, and orexin also play a role.

4. Heissel A, Heinen D, Brokmeier LL, Skarabis N, Kangas M, Vancampfort D, Stubbs B, Firth J, Ward PB, Rosenbaum S, Hallgren M, Schuch F. Exercise as medicine for depressive symptoms? A systematic review and meta-analysis with meta-regression. Br J Sports Med. 2023 Aug;57(16):1049–1057. doi: https://doi.org/10.1136/bjsports-2022-106282. Epub 2023 Feb 1. PMID: 36731907 ; PMCID: PMC10423472.

   Conclusion: Exercise is efficacious in treating depression and depressive symptoms and should be offered as an evidence-based treatment option focusing on supervised and group exercise with moderate intensity and aerobic exercise regimes. The small sample sizes of many trials and high heterogeneity in methods should be considered when interpreting the results.

5. Kunugi H. Depression and lifestyle: Focusing on nutrition, exercise, and their possible relevance to molecular mechanisms. Psychiatry Clin Neurosci. 2023 Aug;77(8):420–433. doi: https://doi.org/10.1111/pcn.13551. Epub 2023 Apr 25. PMID: 36992617 ; PMCID: PMC11488618.

   Main biological mechanisms of the link between lifestyle factors and depression include monoamine imbalance, inflammation, altered stress response, oxidative stress, and dysfunction of brain-derived neurotrophic factor, although other players such as insulin, leptin, and orexin also play a role. To increase resilience to modern stress and ameliorate depression through modification of lifestyle habits, a list of 30 recommended interventions is presented.

6. Gallardo-Alfaro L, Bibiloni MDM, Mascaró CM, Montemayor S, Ruiz-Canela M, Salas-Salvadó J, Corella D, Fitó M, Romaguera D, Vioque J, Alonso-Gómez ÁM, Wärnberg J, Martínez JA, Serra-Majem L, Estruch R, Fernández-García JC, Lapetra J, Pintó X, García Ríos A, Bueno-Cavanillas A, Gaforio JJ, Matía-Martín P, Daimiel L, Micó-Pérez RM, Vidal J, Vázquez C, Ros E, Fernandez-Lázaro CI, Becerra-Tomás N, Gimenez-Alba IM, Zomeño MD, Konieczna J, Compañ-Gabucio L, Tojal-Sierra L, Pérez-López J, Zulet MÁ, Casañas-Quintana T, Castro-Barquero S, Gómez-Pérez AM, Santos-Lozano JM, Galera A, Basterra-Gortari FJ, Basora J, Saiz C, Pérez-Vega KA, Galmés-Panadés AM, Tercero-Maciá C, Sorto-Sánchez C, Sayón-Orea C, García-Gavilán J, Muñoz-Martínez J, Tur JA. Leisure-Time Physical Activity, Sedentary Behaviour and Diet Quality are Associated with Metabolic Syndrome Severity: The PREDIMED-Plus Study. Nutrients. 2020 Apr 7;12(4):1013. doi: https://doi.org/10.3390/nu12041013. PMID: 32272653 ; PMCID: PMC7230557.

   Participants with highest MetSSS showed higher values of cardiovascular risk factors (except for total cholesterol and LDL cholesterol), depression risk, sedentary and TV viewing time, and lower moderate and vigorous leisure-time physical activity (LTPA). Highest MetSSS participants tended to a pro-inflammatory dietary pattern and tended to lower MD adherence. In addition, they showed lower carbohydrate and nut intake and higher intake of protein, saturated and trans fatty acids, cholesterol, iodine, sodium, red and processed meat products, other oils different from olive oil and spirit alcoholic drinks.

7. Ruan J, Chen S, Liang J, Ho FYY, Cheung T, Ho JYS, Chan WC, Chen H, Au DCW, Lee RWY, Mak YW, Yeung WF. Traditional Chinese medicine-based integrated health interventions for depression: A systematic review and meta-analysis. J Clin Nurs. 2023 Sep;32(17–18):5632–5651. doi: https://doi.org/10.1111/jocn.16666. Epub 2023 Mar 22. PMID: 36946424 .

   Results: Eighteen RCTs with a total of 1448 depressed participants were included. Healthcare providers, mainly nurses (14 studies), implemented TCM-based integrated health interventions. The pooled results showed that TCM-based integrated health interventions had larger effects on reducing depressive symptoms (15 studies; standardized mean difference = −2.05; 95% CI: −2.74, −1.37; p < .00001) compared with usual care at posttreatment but showed no significant difference contrasted to cognitive behavioural therapy (two studies, p = .31). However, the overall evidence was low.

   Conclusions: The meta-analysis results indicated that TCM-based integrated health interventions were effective in reducing depression. However, the results should be interpreted with caution because of the low quality of the included studies. Future RCTs with rigorous designs should be conducted to provide robust evidence of the efficacy of TCM-based integrated health interventions in treating depression.

6.9 Recent References on Acupuncture for Depression

1. Zhao H, Zhang Y, Cui H, Tang L, Gao Y, Tang C, Shen W. Efficacy and Influencing Factors of Acupuncture in Major Depressive Disorder: A Systematic Review and Exploratory Network Meta-Analysis. CNS Spectr. 2026 Mar 2:1–33. https://doi.org/10.1017/S1092852926100868. Epub ahead of print. PMID: 41769707

   Conclusion: Acupuncture demonstrates significant efficacy in alleviating depressive symptoms, with treatment outcomes being modulated by acupuncture dosage, acupuncture modalities, treatment course, treatment frequency, and needle retention time. Critical parameters for optimal efficacy appear to include higher treatment dosage (30 sessions), treatment courses exceeding 6 weeks, treatment frequency of three times a week, needle retention times of 20–30 minutes, and EA application.
2. Wang Y, Wu PT, Penpat I, Zeng FC, Lu Q, Hu ZH. Acupuncture on 5-hydroxytryptamine levels and clinical outcomes in depression: A systematic review and meta-analysis of randomized controlled trials. World J Psychiatry. 2026 Feb 19;16(2):113049. https://doi.org/10.5498/wjp.v16.i2.113049. PMID: 41641205 ; PMCID: PMC12865452

   Conclusion: The efficacy of traditional acupuncture improving symptoms, sleep, and anxiety and alleviating antidepressant side effects is highly encouraging. However, the low quality of the included studies warrants cautious interpretation.
3. Cui F. A Meta-analysis of Acupuncture's Improvement of Mood Disorders, Pain and Quality of Life in Migraine Patients. Altern Ther Health Med. 2024 Nov;30(11):304–311. PMID: 38430159 .

   Conclusion: Acupuncture and moxibustion in improving the SAS and SDS scores of migraine patients were similar to Western medication and sham acupuncture, but they were more effective in reducing VAS score, MSQ score, headache days, and headache score than sham acupuncture and Western medication treatments. However, due to the limited number of studies included in this research, more high-quality randomized controlled trials are still needed to further strengthen the evidence base in evidence-based medicine.
4. Li Z, Feng J, Yin S, Chen X, Yang Q, Gao X, Che D, Zhou L, Yan H, Zhong Y, Zhu F. Effects of acupuncture on mental health of migraine patients: a systematic review and meta-analysis. BMC Complement Med Ther. 2023 Aug 4;23(1):278. https://doi.org/10.1186/s12906-023-04103-8. PMID: 37542321 ; PMCID: PMC10401757

   Conclusion: The present results suggest that, compared with Western medicine and sham acupuncture, acupuncture seems to be able to effectively improve anxiety and depression in migraine patients. And it may be more effective in improving SF36-mental health, VAS, and MSQ than sham acupuncture or Western medicine. The results of this study need to be verified by higher-quality RCTs.

5. Kuang HJ, Yang HS, Feng YX, Tang H, Fan Q, Xu YQ, Cui S, Musil R, Luxenburger H, Zhang YX, Zhao H, Zhang YQ. Efficacy and safety of acupuncture therapies for adult patients with mild and moderate major depressive disorder: A systematic review and meta-analysis. J Integr Med. 2025 Sep;23(5):471–491. https://doi.org/10.1016/j.joim.2025.06.008. Epub 2025 Jun 30. PMID: 40744847 .

Conclusion: Acupuncture therapy may provide antidepressant effects and relieve insomnia with mild adverse effects for adult patients with mild and moderate MDD.

6. Tan Y, Duan R, Wen C. Efficacy of acupuncture for depression: a systematic review and meta-analysis. Front Neurosci. 2024 Apr 30;18:1347651. https://doi.org/10.3389/fnins.2024.1347651. PMID: 38745939 ; PMCID: PMC11091333

Conclusion: Acupuncture, when compared to conventional pharmacotherapy, exhibits significant efficacy as a standalone treatment after 4 weeks of intervention, with fewer side effects and adverse reactions. However, further investigation is needed to determine the most effective acupoints and appropriate types of acupuncture techniques for treating depression.

7. Yang L, Zhang Q, Wen M, Li S, Lu A, Li K, Peng C, Chen J. Clinical evidence for acupuncture-assisted treatment of depression: A systematic review and meta-analysis with meta-regression. Gen Hosp Psychiatry. 2025 Nov-Dec;97:64–71. https://doi.org/10.1016/j.genhosppsych.2025.09.002. Epub 2025 Sep 15. PMID: 41033107 .

Conclusion: This systematic review and meta-analysis demonstrate the efficacy of acupuncture interventions for depression, suggesting it as a viable evidence-based treatment option. However, the high heterogeneity of the studies, the presence of publication bias, and the lack of sham acupuncture controls in many studies limit the strength of these conclusions.

8. Jiang H, Ma R, Huang Y, Li X, Hao Y. Efficacy of acupuncture versus sham acupuncture on generalized anxiety disorder: a meta-analysis of randomized controlled trials. Front Neurol. 2025 Nov 12;16:1682400. https://doi.org/10.3389/fneur.2025.1682400. PMID: 41312341 ; PMCID: PMC12646924.

Conclusion: Acupuncture is more effective than sham acupuncture in alleviating anxiety symptoms and improving sleep and mood in patients with GAD, though effect sizes are modest, and evidence certainty varies. These findings support acupuncture as a potential non-pharmacological option for GAD, yet further high-quality trials are needed to standardize protocols and clarify mechanisms.

9. Jiang J, Ji B, Jin W, Zhang P, Chen H, Cong W, Jin X, Li L. Clinical Efficacy and Therapeutic Mechanism of Acupuncture in the Treatment of Adolescent Depression. J Integr Neurosci. 2025 Sep 23;24(9):38071. https://doi.org/10.31083/JIN38071. PMID: 41074408 .

Conclusions: Acupuncture improves adolescents' depressive mood and sleep quality and alleviates somatic symptoms by modulating neurotransmitter levels and brain activity.

10. Si Y, Ma W, Zhang Q, Zhang Y, An J, Zhang M, Fu Y, Yu Y, Zhang H, Fang Y, Zhang D. Investigating acupuncture therapy in depression: mechanisms of synaptic plasticity regulation. Neuroscience. 2025 Jul 23;579:284–301. https://doi.org/10.1016/j.neuroscience.2025.06.005. Epub 2025 Jun 10. PMID: 40506009

Conclusions: Acupuncture synergistically modulates the neuro-immune-microbiome multidimensional network and integrates crosstalk among key pathways such as CREB, thereby systemically restoring synaptic plasticity. This multi-dimensional integrative mechanism likely underlies its therapeutic superiority over single-target antidepressants. This review aims to elucidate how acupuncture restores cerebral synaptic plasticity by rectifying depression-related systemic dysfunctions and signalling pathway abnormalities, which will advance our understanding of its regulatory potential in depression treatment and inform the development of precision therapeutic strategies.

11. Wu Z, Lv F, Shao S, Chen Y, Weng N, Xia Y. Recent advances in traditional Chinese medicine-mediated regulation of microglial metabolic reprogramming in neurological disease therapy. J Ethnopharmacol. 2026 May 10;362:121355. https://doi.org/10.1016/j.jep.2026.121355. Epub 2026 Feb 10. PMID: 41679362 .

Conclusion: TCM restores microglial metabolic homeostasis, enhancing M2 polarization and neuroprotection. These findings highlight TCM's potential for developing metabolism-immunity dual-target interventions for neurological diseases. Further research is needed to elucidate acupuncture's mechanisms and effects on microglial metabolism.

6.10 Recent Publications on Lifestyle Interventions and Mental Illness

1. Jones M, Schwenn PE, Metse AP, Watkins A, Hermens DF, Driver C. Improving mental health during crisis: Outcomes from the EMERALD online lifestyle medicine and coaching program. Soc Sci Med. 2026 May;397:119131. https://doi.org/10.1016/j.socscimed.2026.119131. Epub 2026 Feb 26. PMID: 41785656 .

Conclusions: These findings support the benefits of online mental health coaching and lifestyle medicine interventions for improving psychological well-being during periods of elevated need.

2. Norton J, Jaussent I, Edouard E, Boubert L, Mura T, Akbaraly T. Unhealthy lifestyle factors and the risk of incident depressive symptomatology in older adults: Findings from the Three-City study. J Affect Disord. 2026 Apr 15;399:121125. https://doi.org/10.1016/j.jad.2025.121125. Epub 2026 Jan 5. PMID: 41494545 .

Conclusions: The risk of DepS onset increased hand-in-hand with the number of unhealthy lifestyle factors. Interventions targeting unhealthy lifestyles, and in particular sleep disturbances, smoking, and social isolation, could have a substantial public health impact on reducing late-onset depression.

3. Dong C, Chen H, Li Y, Sun Y, Pan Y, Xu Q, Sun H. Patterns of Health-Risk Behaviours and Their Associations With Anxiety and Depression Among Chinese Young Adults by Gender: A Latent Class Analysis. Psychol Rep. 2026 Apr;129(2):1222–1248. https://doi.org/10.1177/00332941241258922. Epub 2024 Jun 6. PMID: 38842056 .

   Conclusions: Lower anxiety levels (odds ratio [OR]: 0.892; 95% confidence interval [CI]: 0.823-0.966) and greater depression levels (OR: 1.074; 95% CI: 1.008-1.143) were associated with a sedentary lifestyle, substance use, and unhealthy diet class only in female young adults compared with a sedentary-only class. These findings underscore the need for the implementation of targeted interventions based on gender differences.

4. Zhang Y, Zhao P, Lou H, Zhang W, Zhang C, Liao J, Zhou H, Sun H. A healthy lifestyle is associated with lower risk of depression in type 2 diabetes, irrespective of genetic susceptibility: A UK biobank cohort study. J Affect Disord. 2026 Mar 20;405:121657. https://doi.org/10.1016/j.jad.2026.121657. Epub ahead of print. PMID: 41866049 .

   Conclusions: A composite healthy lifestyle was significantly associated with a lower risk of depression in individuals with type 2 diabetes, showing a clear dose–response relationship that was independent of genetic susceptibility.

5. Ding L, Zhang H, Wang X, Ma M, Kong W. Association between different sedentary types and risk of depression: A systematic review and dose-response meta-analysis. J Affect Disord. 2026 Mar 15;397:120860. https://doi.org/10.1016/j.jad.2025.120860. Epub 2025 Dec 7. PMID: 41365442 .

   Conclusions: Prolonged daily sedentary behaviour (particularly, passive screen, or TV exposure) may increase future depression risk, with adolescents and females being more susceptible. Limiting passive sedentary behaviour to <4 h/day and TV viewing to <6.75 h/day could represent pragmatic preventive targets.

6. Marx W, Manger SH, Blencowe M, Murray G, Ho FY, Lawn S, Blumenthal JA, Schuch F, Stubbs B, Ruusunen A, Desyibelew HD, Dinan TG, Jacka F, Ravindran A, Berk M, O'Neil A. Clinical guidelines for the use of lifestyle-based mental health care in major depressive disorder: World Federation of Societies for Biological Psychiatry (WFSBP) and Australasian Society of Lifestyle Medicine (ASLM) taskforce. World J Biol Psychiatry. 2023 Jun;24(5):333–386. https://doi.org/10.1080/15622975.2022.2112074. Epub 2022 Oct 6. PMID: 36202135 ; PMCID: PMC10972571.

   Conclusions: Lifestyle-based interventions are recommended as a foundational component of mental health care in clinical practice for adults with major depressive disorder, where other evidence-based therapies can be added or used in combination. The findings and recommendations of these guidelines support the need for further research to address existing gaps in efficacy and implementation research, especially for emerging lifestyle-based approaches (e.g. green space, loneliness, and social support interventions) where data are limited. Further work is also needed to develop innovative approaches for delivery and models of care and to support the training of health professionals regarding lifestyle-based mental healthcare.

6.11 Own Publications Since the Beginning of the TCM-Klinik Bad Kötzting

6.11.1 Books

1. Dai Jingzhang, Wang Jing, Ma Shuhui, Yan Yangyang, Zhao Jing, Li Yuanyuan, Qi Xiaohuan, Xiong Hang, Zhang Jiawei, Chen Lu. Theorien und Anwendungen von Yin und Yang, den Fünf Elementen, den Funktionskreisen sowie den Haupt- und Netzleitbahnen. 1st ed., Beijing: China Press of Traditional Chinese Medicine; 2023
2. Dai Jingzhang, Wang Jing, Ma Shuhui, Yan Yangyang, Zhao Jing, Li Yuanyuan, Qi Xiaohuan, Xiong Hang, Zhang Jiawei, Chen Lu. Theorien und Anwendungen von Yin und Yang, den Fünf Elementen, den Funktionskreisen sowie den Haupt- und Netzleitbahnen. 1st ed. Beijing: China Press of Traditional Chinese Medicine; 2023
3. Dai Jingzhang, Zhao Jinxi, Yu Guoyong, Zhang yong, He Xiulan, Ma Shuhui, Zhao Jing Yuan Hongwei, Liu Zhnebo, Wei Dongfang. Traditionelle chinesische Medizin—Alte Gesundheitsweisheit. 1st ed. Beijing: China Press of Traditional Chinese Medicine; 2021
4. Melchart D, Dai J, Staudinger A. Evaluation der Patientenversorgung in der Chinesischen Medizin. 1st ed. Bad Kötzting: Verlag systemische Medizin; 2021
5. Melchart D, Dai J. Chinesisch-Deutsches Zentrum für Traditionelle Chinesische Medizin (Bad Kötzting) Klinikbericht 2017/8. 1.st. ed. Beijing: China Press of Traditional Chinese Medicine; 2020
6. She J, Li H-J, Sang BS (Chinese editors), Melchart D, Hempen CH, Engelhardt U. (German editors). Übersetzung der internationalen Standardnomenklatur der chinesischen Medizin in Chinesisch-Deutsch. 1st ed. Beijing: People`s Medical Publishing House (PMPH); 2017
7. Wagner H, Bauer R, Melchart D, Xiao P-G (eds). Chromatographic Fingerprint Analysis of Herbal Medicines. Volume 5,1st ed. Wien, New York: Springer; 2017
8. Wagner H, Bauer R, Melchart D, Xiao P-G (eds). Chromatographic Fingerprint Analysis of Herbal Medicines Volume 4, 1st ed. Wien, New York; Springer; 2016
9. Wagner H, Bauer R, Melchart D, Xiao P-G (eds). Chromatographic Fingerprint Analysis of Herbal Medicines Volume 3, 1st ed. Wien, New York: Springer; 2015
10. Melchart D. Staudinger A. (eds) TCM-Klinik Bad Kötzting 20 Jahre wissenschaftliche Evaluation der Traditionellen Chinesischen Medizin und Klinikbericht. 1st ed., Bad Kötzting: Verlag systemische Medizin; 2011
11. Wagner H, Bauer R, Melchart D, Xiao P-G (eds). Chromatographic Fingerprint Analysis of Herbal Medicines., Volume 2, 1st ed. Wien, New York: Springer; 2011

12. Wagner H, Bauer R, Melchart D, Xiao P-G (eds). Chromatographic Fingerprint Analysis of Herbal Medicines., Volume 1, 1st ed. Wien, New York: Springer; 2011

6.11.2 Original Papers

1. Melchart D, Wühr E, Bachmeier B, Jötten LI. Individual Health Management (IHM) for Stress-A Randomised Controlled Trial (TALENT II Study). Healthcare (Basel). 2025 Dec 4;13(23):3181. doi: https://doi.org/10.3390/healthcare13233181. PMID: 41373397 ; PMCID: PMC12692462.
2. Dai, J. Stationäre Behandlung des Post-Covid- und chronischen Erschöpfungssyndroms. Dtsch Z Akupunkt 2025, 68;1:14–15. https://doi.org/10.1007/s42212-024-00716-3
3. LI Y Y, XIONG H, MA S H, et al. Clinical observation on acupuncture for 80 patients with abdominal obesity in Germany: based on the theory of unblocking and regulating the Belt Vessel. J Acupunct Tuina Sci, 2023,21,2:137–141 DOI: https://doi.org/10.1007/s11726-022-1333-5
4. Melchart D. Quo Vadis TCM?—From the Long Road of Traditional Chinese Medicine to Scientific Acknowledgement. Journal Club Complement Med Res 2021;28:387–393. doi: https://doi.org/10.1159/000519063resp. https://www.karger.com/Article/Pdf/519063
5. Melchart D. A Joint Statement for "Tighter Regulation" of Traditional Chinese Medicine Issued by the Federation of European Academies of Medicine (FEAM) and the European Academies' Science Advisory Council (EASAC): Scare Stories or Obstruction of Access? Complement Med Res. 2020;27(1):3–5. doi: https://doi.org/10.1159/000505479. Epub 2020 Jan 22. PMID: 31968335 .
6. Xiong H, Ma SH, Li YY, Dai JZ Clinical Observation on the Treatment of Insomnia in Germany with Deficiency of Heart and Spleen by the Ear Bean Therapy. World Journal of integrated traditional and western medicine 2020;6,9:7–11.
7. Xiong H, Ma SH, Li YY, Dai JZ Treatment of acupuncture and decoction for 120 German patients with depression. Modern Chinese Clinical Medicine, 2020, 27,6:21–26
8. Melchart D, Fischer V, Dai J, Hager S, Dersch L, Bachmeier BE. Multimodal Treatment of Patients with Mental Symptom Load: A Pre-Post Comparison. J Clin Med. 2019 Oct 3;8(10):1610. doi: https://doi.org/10.3390/jcm8101610. PMID: 31623396 ; PMCID: PMC6832432.
9. Yuan H, Dai JZ Present status and strategy of the development of TCM in Germany in the policy of One Belt One Road. World Journal of Integrated Traditional and Western Medicine. 2019, 14,2:282–286
10. Ma SH Praktische Deutsch-chinesische Gespräche der TCM-Klinik. 1.st Ed. Beijing: China Press of Traditional Chinese Medicine; 2019
11. Bachmeier BE, Melchart D. Therapeutic Effects of Curcumin-From Traditional Past to Present and Future Clinical Applications. Int J Mol Sci.

2019 Aug 1;20(15):3757. doi: https://doi.org/10.3390/ijms20153757. PMID: 31374813 ; PMCID: PMC6695654.

12. Bachmeier BE, Wühr E, Wifling K, Melchart D. Participant satisfaction with a comprehensive lifestyle counselling Program for health promotion, disease prevention and patient education. 2019; Health Edu Care,4:1–8. doi: https://doi.org/10.15761/HEC.1000153. Please refer to the PDF at: https://www.researchgate.net/publication/340081739_Participant_satisfaction_with_a_comprehensive_lifestyle_counselling_Program_for_health_promotion_disease_prevention_and_patient_education_Abbreviations_IHM_Individual_Health_Management_PRO_patient_rep#fullTextFileContent
13. Melchart D, Bachmeier BE, Hager St Case Report of a Phototoxic Reaction after Application of a Footbath with Herbal Traditional Chinese Medicine (TCM) Nursing and Health Care 2018; 4: 13–16–3877 doi: https://doi.org/10.33805/2573-3877.130. Please refer to the PDF at: https://edelweisspublications.com/articles/29/341/Case-Report-of-a-Phototoxic-Reaction-after-Application-of-a-Footbath-with-Herbal-Traditional-Chinese-Medicine-(TCM)
14. Melchart D, Wühr E, Wifling K, Bachmeier BE. The TALENT II study: a randomized controlled trial assessing the impact of an individual health management (IHM) on stress reduction. BMC Public Health. 2018 Jul 4;18(1):823. doi: https://doi.org/10.1186/s12889-018-5756-3. PMID: 29973165 ; PMCID: PMC6030744.
15. Melchart D, Bachmeier BE comprehensive lifestyle intervention pro gram “Individual Health Management” (IHM)—An exemplar for complementary medicine J Transl Sci, 2018 doi: https://doi.org/10.15761/JTS.1000221 Volume 4(3): 1–3
16. Melchart D, Eustachi A, Gronwald S, Wühr E, Wifling K, Bachmeier BE Introduction of a web portal for an Individual Health Management and observational health data sciences. Patient Relat Outcome Meas. 2018 Jun 21;9:183–196. doi:10.2147/PROM.S157410 . eCollection 2018
17. Ma SH, Dai JZ. Necessity and connotation of humanistic education in clinical teaching of Chinese medicine. Education of Chinese Medicine, 2018,37,4:34–36.
18. Ma SH, Dai JZ, Discussion of Five Views in the Inner Canon of Huangdi. Chinese Journal of Basic Medicine in Traditional Chinese Medicine. 2018, 24,4:429–430.
19. Ma SH, Dai JZ. Discussion on Treatment of Fibromyalgia Syndrome with Combination of Syndrome and Disease. World Chinese Medicine. 2018, 13,3:781–784.
20. Ma SH, Zhao Li, Cai Ch. et al. Clinical observation of fibromyalgia symptom with acupuncture at mainly back-shu points combined with Chinese herbal medicine in 136 cases. Modern Chinese Clinical Medicine, 2018, 25,2:11–13.
21. Rolf Teschke, Dieter Melchart, Tran Dang Xuan Hormesis and dose-responses in herbal traditional Chinese medicine (TCM) alone are insufficient solving

real clinical TCM challenges and associated herbal quality issues Longhua Chin Med 2018;1:3 https://doi.org/10.21037/lcm.2018.03.01

22. Bachmeier BE, Killian PH, Melchart D. The Role of Curcumin in Prevention and Management of und Disease. Int J Mol Sci. 2018 Jun 9;19(6). pii: E1716. doi: https://doi.org/10.3390/ijms19061716. Review
23. Melchart D. From Complementary to Integrative Medicine and Health: Do We Need a Change in Nomenclature? Complement Med Res. 2018;25(2):76–78. doi: https://doi.org/10.1159/000488623. Epub 2018 Apr 17.
24. Melchart D, Hager S, Albrecht S, Dai J, Weidenhammer W, Teschke R. Herbal Traditional Chinese Medicine and suspected liver injury: A prospective study. World J of Hepatol 2017,18,9;29:1141–1157. doi: https://doi.org/10.4254/wjh.v9.i29.1141.
25. Melchart D, Löw P, Wühr E, Kehl V, Weidenhammer W Effects of a tailored lifestyle self-management intervention (TALENT) study on weight reduction: a randomized controlled trial. Diabetes Metab Syndr Obes 2017,19;10:235–245. doi: https://doi.org/10.2147/DMSO.S135572. eCollection 2017.
26. Melchart D, Wühr E, Doerfler W, Eustachi A, Wellenhofer-Li Y, Weidenhammer W. Preliminary outcome data of a Sino-European-PreventionProgram (SEPP) in individuals with perceived stress. J Prev Med Healthc 2017,1;1:1003.
27. Melchart D, Wühr E, Weidenhammer W High and Low Responder in a Comprehensive Lifestyle Program for Weight Loss—Secondary Analysis of a Randomized Controlled Trial. Complement Med Res 2017, 24;4:232–239. doi: https://doi.org/10.1159/000475663. Epub 2017 Jul
28. Dai JZ, Ma SH. Reflections and Enlightenment on International Cooperation and Service of Traditional Chinese Medicine, Guiding Journal of Traditional Chinese Medicine and Pharmacology, 2017, 23,27:1–6.
29. Eustachi A, Melchart D. Studie: Säure-Basen-Messung bei gesunden Probanden mittels venöser Blut-Titration. Zaenmagazin 2017, 9; 4:39–43.
30. Melchart D First-Page Preview. Journal Club. Complement Med Res 2017;24:8–13 https://doi.org/10.1159/000457327
31. Melchart D Journal Club, Complementary Medicine—Commentary; Complement Med Res 2017;24:76–81 DOI: https://doi.org/10.1159/000474491- Liu C, Fan H, Li Y, Xiao X: Research Advances on Hepatotoxicity of Herbal Medicines in China. Biomed Res Int 2016;2016:7150391.
32. Melchart D, Hager S, Dai J, Weidenhammer W. Quality Control and Complication Screening Programme of Chinese Medicinal Drugs at the First German Hospital of Traditional Chinese Medicine—A Retrospective Analysis. Forsch Komplementmed 2016;23:21–28, DOI: https://doi.org/10.1159/000444983.
33. Wagner H, Bauer R, Melchart D. New Analytical Monographs on TCM Herbal Drugs for Quality Proof. Forsch Komplementmed 2016;23:16–20, DOI: https://doi.org/10.1159/000444730.

34. Weidenhammer W, Melchart D. Quality Profiling at the TCM Hospital Bad Kötzting –Examples from an Ongoing Systematic Patient Documentation. Forsch Komplementmed 2016;23:8–15, DOI: https://doi.org/10.1159/000445009.
35. Melchart D, Eustachi A, Wellenhofer-Li Y, Doerfler 'W, Bohnes E. Individual Health Management—A Comprehensive Lifestyle Councelling Programme for Health Promotion, Disease Prevention and Patient Education. Forsch Komplementmed 2016;23:30–35.
36. Eustachi A, Doerfler W, Melchart D. Komplementärmedizin in der Onkologie—Evidenz und praxisorientierte Vorgehensweise. Deutsche Zeitschrift für Onkologie 2015; 47(04): 148–154.
37. Melchart D, Doerfler W, Eustachi A, Wellenhofer-Li Y, Weidenhammer W. The Talent study: a multicentre randomized controlled trial assessing the impact of a 'tailored lifestyle self-management intervention' (talent) on weight reduction. BMC Obesity 2015; 2:38.
38. Melchart D, Bohnes E, Doerfler W, Eustachi A, Herrmann T, Wellenhofer-Li Y. Kompetenztraining für Patienten. Das naturheilkundliche Tumorbegleitprogramm des KoKoNat der TU München. Deutsche Zeitschrift für Onkologie 2014;46(04): 158–162
39. Dai JZ, Ma SH. The present situation and thinking of Chinese medicine education in Germany. Education of Chinese Medicine, 2013, 32,3:61–63.
40. Melchart D, Bohnes E, Doerfler W, Eustachi A, Wellenhofer-Li Y. Das Individuelle Gesundheits-Management (IGM) als umfassendes Lebensstil-Programm. Erfahrungsheilkunde 2012;61(6):327–333 DOI: https://doi.org/10.1055/s-0032-1314724; view publication at: https://www.thieme-connect.com/products/ejournals/abstract/10.1055/s-0032-1314724
41. Angermayr L, Melchart D, Linde K. Multifactorial Lifestyle Interventions in the Primary and Secondary Prevention of Cardiovascular Disease and Type 2 Diabetes Mellitus—A Systematic Review of Randomized Controlled Trials. Ann Behav Med 2010;40:49–64.
42. Weidenhammer W, Bornschein S, Zilker T, Eyer F, Melchart D, Hausteiner C. Predictors of treatment outcomes after removal of amalgam fillings: associations between subjective symptoms, psychometric variables and mercury levels. Community Dent Oral Epidemiol 2010; 37: 1–10.
43. Wang J, Zhao J, Dai JZ et al. Immediate curative effect of needling singly in Jing point in patient with migraine. Modern Chinese Clinical Medicine, 2010, 17,6:14–16.
44. Koch P, Schilling J, Läubli M, Mitscherlich F, Melchart D, Bellucci S. Health technology assessment in Switzerland. Intl.J. of Technology Assessment in Health Care. 2009, 25 (Suppl 1):174–177
45. Weidenhammer W, Melchart D. Welche Hinweise geben die Studien der Modellvorhaben auf eine qualitativ gute Akupunktur? Teilergebnisse eines komplexen Evaluationsprogamms PEP-AC. Dt. Ztschr f Akup 2009;52(3):11–17.

46. Weidenhammer W, Hausteiner C, Zilker T, Melchart D, Bornschein S. Does a specific dental amalgam syndrome exist? A comparative study. Acta Odont Scand 2009;67(4):233–239.
47. Hoppe A, Weidenhammer W, Wagenpfeil S, Melchart D, Linde K. Correlations of headache diary parameters, quality of life and disability scales. Headache 2009;49:868–878.
48. Li Y, Linde K, Dai J, Zhang J, Hager S, Saller R, Melchart D. Zur Reliabilität der Beschreibung morphologischer Merkmale in der traditionellen chinesischen Zungendiagnostik. Forsch Komplementärmed. 2009;16:98–104.
49. Dai JZ, Wang J, Guo J et al. Clinical observation of 396 primary fibromyalgia syndrome cases treated with traditional Chinese medicine, Journal of Beijing University of Chinese Medicine, 2009, 32,4:278–279.
50. Eustachi A, Pajtler H, Linde K, Melchart D, Weidenhammer W. Patients of an interdisciplinary cancer treatment centre: use of, knowledge about, and demand for CAM treatment options. Integr Cancer Ther. 2009;8:56–62.
51. Weidenhammer W, Streng A, Melchart D, Linde K. Unerwünschte Wirkungen und Komplikationen bei Akupunkturbehandlung. Dt. Ztschr f Akup 2008;51:6–14.
52. Melchart D, Vogt S, Köhler W, Streng A, Weidenhammer W, Kremers L, Hickel R, Felgenhauer N, Zilker T, Wühr E, Halbach S. Treatment of health complaints attributed to amalgam. J Dent Res 2008;87:349–353.
53. Melchart D, Wessel A, Brand R, Hager S, Weidenhammer W. Profiling quality of care for patients with chronic headache in three different German hospitals—a case study BMC Health Services Research 2008, 8:13 (doi: https://doi.org/10.1186/1472-6963-8-13).
54. Melchart D, Köhler W, Linde K, Zilker T, Kremers L, Saller R, Halbach S. Biomonitoring of mercury in patients with complaints attributed dental amalgam, healthy amalgam bearers, and amalgam-free subjects: a diagnostic study. Clin Toxicol 2008;46:133–140.
55. Bäcker M, Grossman P, Schneider J, Michalsen A, Knoblauch N, Tan L, Niggemeyer C, Linde K, Melchart D, Dobos GJ. Acupuncture in migraine—investigation of autonomic effects. Clin J Pain 2008;24:106–115.
56. Halbach S, Vogt S, Köhler W, Felgenhauer N, Welzl G, Kremers L, Zilker T, Melchart D. Blood and urine mercury levels in adult amalgam patients of a randomized controlled trial: Interaction of Hg species in erythrocytes. Environ Res 2008;107:69–78.
57. Weidenhammer W, Streng A, Linde K, Hoppe A, Melchart D. Acupuncture for chronic pain within the research program of 10 German Health Insurance Funds—Basic results from an observational study. Complement Ther Med 2007;15:238–246.
58. Weidenhammer W, Wessel A, Melchart D. Qualitätsprofil einer Rehabilitationsfachklinik für Naturheilverfahren—Teil 2: Patienten- und Ergebnisprofil. Forsch Komplementärmed 2007;14:335–345.
59. Melchart D, Wessel A, Wunderlich S. Qualitätsprofil einer Rehabilitationsfachklinik für Naturheilverfahren—Teil 1: Struktur,

Qualitätssicherung und Interventionen. Forsch Komplementärmed 2007;14:281–288.
60. Brinkhaus B, Witt CM, Jena S, Linde K, Streng A, Hummelsberger J, Irnich D, Hammes M, Pach D, Melchart D, Willich SN. Physician and treatment characteristics in a randomised multicentre trial of acupuncture in patients with osteoarthritis of the knee. Complement Ther Med 2007;15:180–189.
61. Linde K, Streng A, Hoppe A, Weidenhammer W, Wagenpfeil S, Melchart D. Randomized trial vs. observational study of acupuncture for migraine found that patients characteristics differed but outcomes were similar. J Clin Epidemiol 2007;60:280–287.
62. Weidenhammer W, Linde K, Streng A, Hoppe A, Melchart D. Acupuncture for chronic low back pain in routine care: a multicenter observational study. Clin J Pain 2007 23:128–135.
63. Linde K, Witt CM, Streng A, Weidenhammer W, Wagenpfeil S, Brinkhaus B, Willich SN, Melchart D. The impact of patients expectations on outcomes in four randomized controlled trials of acupuncture in patients with chronic pain. Pain 2007;128:264–271.
64. Köhler W, Linde K, Halbach S, Zilker T, Kremers L, Saller R, Melchart D. Prognos in the diagnosis of amalgam hypersensitivity—a diagnostic case-control study. Forsch Komplementärmed 2007;14:18–24.
65. Linde K, Streng A, Hoppe A, Jürgens S, Weidenhammer W, Melchart D. The programme for the evaluation of patient care with acupuncture (PEP-Ac)—a project sponsored by ten German social health insurance funds. Acup Med 2006;24 (suppl):S25–32.
66. Streng A, Linde K, Hoppe A, Pfaffenrath V, Hammes M, Wagenpfeil S, Weidenhammer W, Melchart D. Effectiveness and tolerability of acupuncture compared with metoprolol in migraine prophylaxis. Headache 2006;46:1492–1502.
67. Weidenhammer W, Wessel A, Hutter A, Melchart D, Schröder A. Das chronische Erschöpfungssyndrom in der naturheilkundlichen Rehabilitation—Prädiktoren des Behandlungsergebnisses. Rehabilitation 2006; 45:299–308.
68. Brinkhaus B, Witt CM, Jena S, Linde K, Streng A, Irnich D, Hummelsberger J, Hammes M, Pach D, Melchart D, Willich SN. Interventions and physician characteristics in a randomized multicenter trial of acupuncture in patients with low-back pain. J Altern Complement Med 2006;12:649–57.
69. Streng A, Linde K, Hoppe A, Jürgens S, Melchart D, Weidenhammer W. Befragung der am „Modellvorhaben der Ersatzkassen" teilnehmenden Akupunkturärzte zur Struktur- und Prozessqualität. Dt Ztschr Akupunktur 2006;49 (3):18–25.
70. Melchart D, Streng A, Hoppe A, Weidenhammer W, Linde K. Akupunktur bei chronischen Schmerzen—Schlusswort. Deutsches Ärzteblatt 2006;103:A1749–1750.
71. Linde K, Streng A, Hoppe A, Brinkhaus B, Witt CM, Hammes M, Irnich D, Hummelsberger J, Williche SN, Melchart D. Treatment in a randomized

multicenter trial of acupuncture for migraine (ART Migraine). Forsch Komplementärmed 2006;13:101–108.
72. Melchart D, Ihbe-Heffinger A, Leps B, von Schilling C, Linde K. Acupuncture and acupressure for the prevention of chemotherapy-induced nausea—a randomised cross-over pilot study. Support Care Cancer 2006;14:878–882.
73. Weidenhammer W, Menz G, Streng A, Linde K, Melchart D. Akupunktur bei chronischen Schmerzpatienten. Behandlungsergebnisse—Rolle des Akupunkteurs. Schmerz 2006;20:418–432.
74. Brinkhaus B, Witt CM, Jena S, Linde K, Streng A, Wagenpfeil S, Irnich D, Walther HU, Melchart D, Willich SN. Acupuncture in patients with chronic low back pain: a randomized controlled trial. Arch Intern Med 2006;166:450–457.
75. Melchart D, Weidenhammer W, Streng A, Hoppe A, Pfaffenrath V, Linde K. Acupuncture for chronic headaches—an epidemiological study. Headache 2006;46:632–641.
76. Melchart D, Streng A, Hoppe A, Jürgens S, Weidenhammer W, Linde K. Akupunktur bei chronischen Schmerzen. Ergebnisse aus dem Modellvorhaben der Ersatzkassen. Deutsches Ärzteblatt 2006;103:A187–A195.
77. Linde K, Weidenhammer W, Streng A, Hoppe A, Melchart D. Acupuncture for osteoarthritic pain: an observational study in routine care. Rheumatology 2006;45:222–227.
78. Melchart D, Streng A, Hoppe A, Brinkhaus B, Becker-Witt C, Hammes M, Irnich D, Hummelsberger J, Willich SN, Linde K. The acupuncture randomised trial (ART) for tension-type headache—details of the treatment. Acup Med 2005;23:157–165.
79. Linde K, Barrett B, Wölkart K, Bauer R, Melchart D. Echinacea bei Erkältungen—eine systematische Übersicht der randomisierten klinischen Studien. Zeitschr Phytother 2005;26 (Supplement 3):S12.
80. Melchart D, Streng A, Hoppe A, Brinkhaus B, Witt C, Wagenpfeil S, Pfaffenrath V, Hammes M, Hummelsberger J, Irnich D, Weidenhammer W, Willich SN, Linde K. Acupuncture in patients with tension-type headache—a randomised trial. BMJ 2005;331: 376–379. (längere online-Version doi: https://doi.org/10.1136/bmj.38512.405440.8F)
81. Witt C, Brinkhaus B, Jena S, Linde K, Streng S, Wagenpfeil S, Hummelsberger J, Walther HU, Melchart D, Willich SN. Acupuncture in patients with osteoarthritis of the knee—a randomised trial. Lancet 2005;366:136–143.
82. Linde K, Streng A, Jürgens S, Hoppe A, Brinkhaus B, Witt C, Wagenpfeil S, Pfaffenrath V, Hammes MG, Weidenhammer W, Willich SN, Melchart D. Acupuncture for patients with migraine. A randomized controlled trial. JAMA 2005;293:2118–2125.
83. Weidenhammer W, Streng A, Jürgens S, Hoppe A, Linde K, Melchart D. Aufbau, Realisierung und Datenübersicht einer Beobachtungsstudie im Rahmen des Programms zur Evaluation der Patientenversorgung mit

Akupunktur (PEP-AK) des Modellvorhabens der Ersatzkassen. Gesundheitswesen 2005;67:264–273.
84. Dai JZ, Wang H, Wang R et al. Comprehensive Treatment of 197 Cases of Primary Fibromyalgia Syndrome with Chinese Medicine. Modern Chinese Clinical Medicine, 2005, 12,5:19–21.
85. Melchart D. et al. Programm zur Evaluation Komplementärmedizin (PEK) Abschlussbericht 2005 https://www.bag.admin.ch/dam/de/sd-web/f1B9h3KShqDA/programm-evaluation-komplementaermedizin-pek.pdf.
86. Melzer J, Melchart D, Saller R. Entwicklung der Ordnungstherapie durch Bircher-Benner in der Naturheilkunde im 20. Jahrhundert. Forsch Komplementärmed Klass Naturheilkd 2004;11:293–303.
87. Melchart D, Hager S, Hager U, Liao J, Weidenhammer W, Linde K. Treatment of patients with chronic headaches in a hospital for traditional Chinese medicine in Germany. A randomised, waiting list controlled trial. Complement Ther Med 2004;12:71–78.
88. Melchart D, Streng A, Reitmayr S, Hoppe A, Weidenhammer W, Linde K. Programm zur Evaluation der Patientenversorgung mit Akupunktur (PEP-AC)—Die wissenschaftliche Begleitung des Modellvorhabens der Ersatzkassen. Z ärztl Fortbild Qual Gesundhwes 2004;98:471–472.
89. Weidenhammer W, Linde K, Melchart D. Treatment outcomes in patients with migraine: an ex-post facto comparison of two in-patient facilities. Forsch Komplementärmed Klass Naturheilkd 2004;11 (suppl 1):30–35.
90. Melchart D, Weidenhammer W, Streng A, Reitmayr S, Hoppe A, Ernst E, Linde K. Prospective investigation of adverse effects of acupuncture in 97 733 patients. Arch Intern Med 2004;164:104–105.
91. Halbach S, Vogt S, Köhler W, Felgenhauer N, Kremers L, Melchart D, Zilker T. Relationships between dose and concentrations of total and inorganic mercury in blood and urine of amalgam patients. Environmental Sciences 2003;10:71–81.
92. Weidenhammer W, Streng A, Reitmayr S, Hoppe A, Aigner C, Linde K, Melchart D. Acupuncture for chronic low back pain, osteoarthritic pain and headache: a prospective observational study in routine care. FACT 2003;8:554.
93. Melchart D, Linde K, Streng A, Reitmayr S, Hoppe A, Brinkhaus B, Becker-Witt C, Wagenpfeil S, Pfaffenrath V, Hammes M, Willich SN, Weidenhammer W. Acupuncture Randomized Trials (ART) in patients with migraine or tension-type headache—design and protocols. Forsch Komplementärmed Klass Naturheilkd 2003;10:179–184.
94. Brinkhaus B, Becker-Witt C, Jena S, Linde K, Streng A, Wagenpfeil S, Irnich D, Hummelsberger J, Melchart D, Willich SN. Acupuncture Randomized Trials (ART) in patients with chronic low back pain and osteoarthritis of the knee—design and protocols. Forsch Komplementärmed Klass Naturheilkd 2003;10:185–191.
95. Weidenhammer W, Streng A, Reitmayr S, Hoppe A, Linde K, Melchart D. A large observational study on acupuncture for chronic pain in Germany—preliminary results. FACT 2003;8:159.

96. Linde K, ter Riet G, Hondras M, Melchart D, Willich S.N. Characteristics and quality of systematic reviews of acupuncture, herbal medicines, and homeopathy. Forsch Komplementärmed Klass Naturheilkd 2003;10:88–94.
97. Linde K, ter Riet G, Hondras M, Vickers A, Saller R, Melchart D; Cochrane Complementary Medicine Field. Systematic reviews of herbal medicines--an annotated bibliography. Forsch Komplementarmed Klass Naturheilkd. 2003 Apr;10 Suppl 1:17–27. doi: https://doi.org/10.1159/000071688. PMID: 12808358 .
98. Melchart D, Weidenhammer W, Linde K, Saller R. „Quality profiling“ for complementary medicine: The example of a hospital for traditional Chinese medicine. Journal of Alternative and Complementary Medicine. 2003;9:193–206.
99. Melchart D, Thormaehlen J, Hager S, Liao J, Linde K, Weidenhammer W. Acupuncture versus placebo versus sumatriptan for early treatment of migraine attacks: a randomized controlled trial. J Intern Med 2003;253:181–188.
100. Weidenhammer W, Holzwarth R, Wunderlich S, Melchart D, Dobos G. Effekte einer stationären Rehabilitationsmaßnahme auf Kontrollüberzeugungen und Verhalten der Patienten im Bereich Gesundheit. Praxis Klin Verhaltensmed Rehab 2002;59:235–243.
101. Melchart D, Saller R. Programm zur Evaluation der Patientenversorgung (PEP) mit Naturheilverfahren/Komplementärmedizin—Ergebnisqualität in der stationären Versorgung. Perfusion 2002;15:102–112.
102. Melchart D, Thormaehlen J, Hager S, Liao J, Linde K, Weidenhammer W. Randomisierte klinische Studie zur Überprüfung der Wirksamkeit von traditioneller chinesischer Medizin im Vergleich zu subcutan appliziertem Sumatriptan und medikamentöser Placebotherapie als Frühbehandlung von Patienten im Initialstadium eines akuten Migräneanfalls. Der Schmerz 2002;16 (suppl 1):S52.
103. Weidenhammer W, Streng A, Reitmayr S, Hoppe A, Linde K, Melchart D. Das Modellvorhaben Akupunktur der Ersatzkassen. Ein Zwischenbericht zu den Ergebnissen der Beobachtungsstudie. Dt Ztschr f Akup 2002;45:183–192.
104. Melchart D, Linde K, Weidenhammer W, Streng A, Reitmayr S. Patient Care Evaluation Program for Acupuncture (PEPAC). FACT 2002;7:100.
105. Michalsen A, Weidenhammer W, Melchart D, Langhorst J, Saja J, Dobos G. Kurzzeitiges Fasten in der Behandlung von chronischen Schmerz- und Erschöpfungssyndromen—Verträglichkeit und Nebenwirkungen mit und ohne begleitende Mineralstoffergänzung. Forsch Komplementärmed Klass Naturheilkd 2002;9:221–227.
106. Melchart D, Steger HG, Linde K, Makarian K, Hatahet Z, Brenke R, Saller R. Integrating patient preferences in clinical trial: a pilot study of acupuncture versus midazolam for gastroscopy. J Alt Complement Med 2002;3:265–274.
107. Linde K, Melchart D, Mulrow CD, Berner M. St John’s wort and depression (letter). JAMA 2002;288:447–448.

108. Melchart D, Clemm C, Weber B, Draczynski T, Worku F, Linde K, Weidenhammer W, Wagner H, Saller R. Polysaccharides from Echinacea purpurea herba cell cultures to counteract undesired effects of chemotherapy—a pilot study. Phytother Res 2002;16:138–142.
109. Linde K, Scholz M, Melchart D, Willich SN. Should systematic reviews include non-randomized and uncontrolled studies? The case of acupuncture for chronic headache. Journal of Clinical Epidemiology 2002;55: 77–85.
110. Linde K, Melchart D, Willich S. Beschreibung der Therapie in klinischen Studien zur Akupunktur bei chronischen Kopfschmerzen. Deutsche Zeitschrift für Akupunktur 2001;44: 8–14.
111. Linde K, Jonas WB, Melchart D, Willich S. The methodological quality of randomized controlled trials of homeopathy, herbal medicines and acupuncture. International Journal of Epidemiology 2001;30: 526–531.
112. Melchart D, Gehring, T. Gesundheitsbewusstsein und Krankheitsverständnis im Wandel: Konsequenzen für die Patientenversorgung. Forschende Komplementärmedizin und Klassische Naturheilkunde 2001;8: 90–97.
113. Melchart D, Wagner H, Hager S, Saller R, Ernst E. Quality assurance and evaluation of Chinese medicine in Germany. Alternative Therapies in Health and Medicine 2001;7: 24.
114. Melchart D, Weidenhammer W, Pollok-Müller A, Brand J, Brand R, Saller R. Ergebnisqualität bei der Behandlung chronischer Kopfschmerzpatienten in einer Migräneklinik. Forschende Komplementärmedizin und Klassische Naturheilkunde 2001;8: 218–226.
115. Thormaehlen J, Melchart D, Weidenhammer W. Utilization of complementary and alternative medicine and the resulting satisfaction among inpatients and outpatients in Germany. Alternative Therapies in Health and Medicine 2001;7:33.
116. Linde K, Vickers A, Hondras M, ter Riet G, Thormählen J, Berman B, Melchart D. Systematic reviews of complementary therapies—an annotated bibliography. Part I: Acupuncture. BMC Complementary and Alternative Medicine 2001;1: Dokument 3.
117. Linde K, ter Riet G, Hondras M, Vickers A, Saller R, Melchart D. Systematic reviews of complementary therapies—an annotated bibliography. Part 2: Herbal medicine. BMC Complementary and Alternative Medicine 2001;1: 5.
118. Linde K, Hondras M, Vickers A, ter Riet G, Melchart D. Systematic reviews of complementary therapies—an annotated bibliography. Part 3: Homeopathy. BMC Complementary and Alternative Medicine 2001;1: Dokument 4.
119. Melchart D, Linde K, Fischer P, Berman B, White A, Vickers A, Allais G. Acupuncture for idiopathic headache (Cochrane Review). The Cochrane Library, Issue 2, 2001. Oxford: Update Software.
120. Melchart D, Weidenhammer W, Thormählen J, Gehring T, Saller R. Qualitätsmanagement mit Forschungsbegleitung. Ein pragmatisches Konzept zur Evaluation und Optimierung von Naturheilverfahren im Rahmen eines Klinik- und Praxisverbundes. Zeitschrift für ärztliche Fortbildung und Qualitätssicherung 2000;94: 751–757.

121. Linde K, Scholz M, Ramirez G, Clausius N, Melchart D, Jonas WB. Impact of study quality on outcome in placebo-controlled trials of homeopathy. Journal of Clinical Epidemiology 1999;52: 631–636.
122. Melchart D, Linde K, Hager S, Kaesmayr J, Shaw D, Bauer R, Weidenhammer W. Monitoring of liver enzymes in patients treatet with traditional Chinese drugs. Complementary Therapies in Medicine 1999;7: 208–216.
123. Melchart D, Linde K, Weidenhammer W, Hager S, Liao JZ, Bauer R, Wagner H. Use of traditional drugs in a hospital of Chinese medicine in Germany. Pharmacoepidemiology and Drug Safety 1999;8:115–120.
124. Melchart D, Weidenhammer W, Hager S, Shaw D, Bauer R. Liver enzyme elevations in patients treated with traditional chinese medicine. JAMA 1999;282: 28–29.
125. Melchart D, Linde K, Fischer P, White A, Allais G, Vickers A, Berman B. Acupuncture for recurrent headaches: a systematic review of randomized controlled trials. Cephalalgia 1999;19: 779–786.
126. Melchart D. Strukturiertes Gesundheitstraining als naturheilkundliche Ordnungstherapie. Prävention 1999;22: 46–49.
127. Melchart D, Kaesmayr J, Hager S, Liao J, Weidenhammer W. Randomisierte klinische Studie zur Überprüfung der Wirksamkeit von traditioneller chinesischer Akupunktur im Vergleich zu s.c. appliziertem Sumatriptan (5-HT1-Rezeptor-Agonist) und medikamentöser Plazebotherapie als Frühbehandlung (Anfallskupierung von Patienten im Initialstadium eines akuten Migräneanfalles). AKU 1999;27: 104–105.
128. Melchart D, Gaisbauer M, Weidenhammer W, Heigl F. Stationäre naturheilkundliche Behandlung der Neurodermitis. Eine prospektive Beobachtungsstudie mit katamnestischer Patientenbefragung soll den Stellenwert der naturheilkundlichen Basiskonzepte bei der Behandlung des atopischen Ekzems verdeutlichen. Zeitschrift für Dermatologie 1999;185: 17–23.
129. Michalsen A, Löer D, Melchart D, Dobos G. Veränderungen der Kurzzeit-Herzfrequenzvariabilität bei Hyperthermiebehandlung mit Infrarot-A-Ganzkörperbestrahlung. Forschende Komplementärmedizin 1999;6: 212–215.
130. Mitzdorf U, Beck K, Horton-Hausknecht J, Weidenhammer W, Kindermann A, Takács M, Astor G, Melchart D. Why do patients seek treatment in hospitals of complementary medicine? Journal of Alternative and Complementary Medicine 1999;5: 463–473.
131. Linde K, Melchart D. Randomized controlled trials of individualized homeopathy: a state-of-the-art review. Journal of Alternative and Complementary Medicine 1998;4: 371–388.
132. Melchart D, Walther E, Linde K, Brandmaier R, Lersch C. Echinacea root extracts for the prevention of upper respiratory tract infections. A double-blind, placebo-controlled randomized trial. Archives of Family Medicine 1998;7: 541–545.

133. Melchart D, Wühr E, Weidenhammer W, Kremers L. A multicenter survey of amalgam fillings and subjective complaints in non-selected patients in the dental practice. European Journal of Oral Sciences 1998;106: 770–777.
134. Melchart D, Gaisbauer M, Brenke R, Riker U, Liao JZ, Hager S, Linde K, Weidenhammer W. Beobachtungsstudien im Rahmen eines naturheilkundlichen Klinikverbunds. Teil I: Methoden und Übersicht der Ergebnisse in den beteiligten Kliniken. Forschende Komplementärmedizin 1998;5: 18–25.
135. Melchart D, Hager S, Liao JZ, Linde K, Weidenhammer W. Beobachtungsstudien im Rahmen eines naturheilkundlichen Klinikverbunds. Teil II: Detaillierte Ergebnisse der Klinik für Traditionelle Chinesische Medizin Kötzting. Forschende Komplementärmedizin 1998;5: 81–86.
136. Melchart D, Hager S, Liao JZ, Weidenhammer W. Beobachtungsstudien im Rahmen eines naturheilkundlichen Klinikverbunds. Teil III: Zwischenergebnisse der diagnosespezifischen Dokumentation Migräne in der Klinik für Traditionelle Chinesische Medizin Kötzting. Forschende Komplementärmedizin 1998;5: 132–135.
137. Melchart D, Weidenhammer W, Linde K. Beobachtungsstudien im Rahmen eines naturheilkundlichen Klinikverbunds. Teil IV: Methodische Aspekte, Diskussion und Empfehlungen. Forschende Komplementärmedizin 1998;5: 184–189.
138. Melchart D, Hager S, Weidenhammer W, Liao JZ, Söllner C, Linde K. Tolerance of and compliance with traditional drug therapy among patients in a hospital for Chinese medicine in Germany. International Journal of Risk and Saftey in Medicine 1998;11: 61–64.
139. Melchart D, Hager S, Weidenhammer W, Liao JZ, Liu Y, Linde K. Die Erhebung von “Nebenwirkungen” und Begleitsymptomen bei Akupunkturbehandlung—eine Pilotstudie. AKU 1998;26: 87–92.
140. Weidenhammer W, Melchart D, Hager S. Stabilität der Erfassung von Lebensqualität im Vorfeld einer stationären Einweisung bei Patienten mit chronischen Erkrankungen. Zeitschrift für medizinische Psychologie 1998;7: 68–74.
141. Linde K, Melchart D, Weidenhammer W. Randomisierte klinische Studien in der Komplementärmedizin—mehr Schaden als Nutzen? Forschende Komplementärmedizin 1997;4: 169–173.
142. Linde K, Clausius N, Ramirez G, Melchart D, Eitel F, Hedges LV, Jonas WB. Are the clinical effects of homoeopathy placebo effects? A meta-analysis of placebo-controlled trials. Lancet 1997;350: 834–843.
143. Melchart D, Weidenhammer W, Hager S, Gehrke A. Verlaufsuntersuchung stationärer Patienten mit Migräne und chronischen bewegungsabhängigen Schmerzen unter naturheilkundlicher Behandlung—ein Vergleich zweier Messmethoden. Physikalische Medizin, Rehabilitationsmedizin und Kurortmedizin 1997;7: 261–268.

144. Melchart D, Linde K, Liao JZ, Hager S, Weidenhammer W. Systematic clinical auditing in complementary medicine: rationale, concept, and a pilot study. Alternative Therapies in Halth and Medicine 1997;3: 33–39.
145. Melchart D, Worku F, Draczynski T, Linde K, Weidenhammer W, Wagner H. Randomisierte placebokontrollierte Doppelblindstudie zur Überprüfung immunmodulierender Effekte eines Thymushydrolysates bei gesunden Probanden. Forschende Komplementärmedizin 1997;4: 219–223.
146. Linde K, Worku F, Stör W, Wiesner-Zechmeister M, Pothmann R, Weinschütz T, Melchart D. Randomized clinical trials of acupuncture for asthma—a systematic review. Forschende Komplementärmedizin 1996;3: 148–155.
147. Linde K, Ramirez G, Mulrow CD, Pauls A, Weidenhammer W, Melchart D. St John's wort for depression—an overview and meta-analysis of randomised clinical trials. British Medical Journal 1996;313: 253–258.
148. Melchart D, Weidenhammer W, Linde K. Scientific quality management in a network of clinics using complementary medicine. Complementary Therapies in Medicine 1996;4: 163–168.
149. Melchart D, Linde K, Liao X, Hager S. Herbal treatment in a hospital for traditional chinese medicine in Germany. Phytomedicine 1996;3 (Suppl.1): SL-128.
150. Melchart D, Wühr E, Lechner J, Weidenhammer W. Strukturdatenerhebung in der Internationalen Gesellschaft für Ganzheitliche Zahn-Medizin. Forsch Komplementärmed 1996;3:21–24.
151. Söllner C, Melchart D, Liao X, Hager S. Risk monitoring in a hospital for traditional chinese medicine in Germany. Phytomedicine 1996;3 (Suppl.1): SL-129.
152. Melchart D, Linde K, Worku F, Sarkady L, Holzmann M, Jurcic K et al. Results of five randomized studies on the immunomodulatory activity of preparations of Echinacea. J Altern Complement Med 1995; 1:145–160.
153. Melchart D, Linde K, Weidenhammer W, Worku F, Wagner H. The integration of natural healing procedures into research and teaching at german universities. Altern Ther Health Med 1995; 1:30–33.
154. Melchart D, Weidenhammer W, Perkuhn K. Zur Situation der ärztlichen Weiterbildung in Naturheilverfahren: Beispiele europäischer Länder und eines Qualitätssicherungsprojekts. Forsch Komplementärmed 1995; 2:203–210.
155. Linde K, Melchart D, Brandmaier R, Eitel F. Critical evaluation of papers reviewing controlled clinical trials in homoeopathy. Br Homeopath J 1994; 83:167–173.
156. Linde K, Jonas WB, Melchart D, Worku F, Wagner H, Eitel F. Critical review and meta-analysis of serial agitated dilutions in experimental toxicology. Hum Exp Toxicol 1994; 13:481–492.
157. Linde K, Melchart D. Die Cochrane Collaboration—systematische Übersichtsarbeiten randomisierter klinischer Studien. Forsch Komplementärmed 1994; 1:152–153.

158. Linde K, Melchart D, Jonas WB. Durchführung und Interpretation systematischer Übersichtsarbeiten kontrollierter Studien in der Komplementärmedizin. Forsch Komplementärmed 1994; 1:8–16.
159. Linde K, Melchart D, Brandmaier R, Eitel F. Übersichtsarbeiten: Das Beispiel Homöopathie. Dtsch Ärztebl 1994; 91:A-108–A-112.
160. Linde K, Melchart D, Jonas WB, Hornung J. Ways to enhance the quality and acceptance of clinical and laboratory studies in homoeopathy. Br Homeopath J 1994; 83:3–7.
161. Melchart D, Linde K, Worku F, Bauer R, Wagner H. Immunmodulation mit Echinacea-haltigen Arzneimitteln—eine kriteriengestützte Analyse der kontrollierten klinische Studien. Forsch Komplementärmed 1994; 1:26–36.
162. Melchart D, Linde K, Worku F, Bauer R, Wagner H. Immunomodulation with Echinacea—a systematic review of controlled clinical trials. Phytomedicine 1994; 1:245–254.
163. Melchart D, Weidenhammer W, Miller R, Sebisch M, Gaisbauer M, Gadomski M. Qualitätssicherung der ärztlichen Weiterbildung im Bereich Naturheilverfahren—eine nationale und internationale Aufgabe. Forsch Komplementärmed 1994; 1:42–50.
164. Melchart D. Qualitätssicherung im Bereich Naturheilverfahren. Forsch Komplementärmed 1994; 1:207.
165. Melchart D, Linde K, Miller R, Polonius D. Qualitätssicherungsvorhaben "Naturheilverfahren" im Rahmen des Klinikverbundes "Münchener Modell". Forsch Komplementärmed 1994; 1:128–137.
166. Melchart D, Worku F, Linde K, Wagner H. The university project Münchener Modell for the integration of naturopathy into research and teaching at the Ludwig-Maximilians- University in Munich. Complement Ther Med 1994; 2:147–153.
167. Baar HA, Brand J, Doenicke A, Melchart D, Luben V, Tryba M et al. Treatment of acute migraine with subcutaneous GR43175 in West Germany. Cephalalgia 1989; 9(suppl.):83 87.
168. Doenicke A, Melchart D, Bayliss EM. Effective improvement of symptoms in patients with acute migraine by GR43175 administered in dispersible tablets. Cephalalgia 1989; 9 (suppl.):89–92.
169. Jurcic K, Melchart D, Holzmann M, Martin P, Bauer R, Doenicke A et al. Zwei Probandenstuidien zur Stimulierung der Granulozytenphagozytose durch Echinacea-Extrakt-haltige Präparate. Z Phytother 1989; 10:67–70.

References

1. Melchart D, Löw P, Wühr E, Kehl V, Weidenhammer W. Effects of a tailored lifestyle self-management intervention (TALENT) study on weight reduction: a randomized controlled trial. Diabetes Metab Syndr Obes. 2017;10:235–45. https://doi.org/10.2147/DMSO.S135572. PMID: 28684917 ; PMCID: PMC5484507.
2. Means B, Toyama Y, Murphy R, Bakia M. The effectiveness of online and blended learning: a meta-analysis of the empirical literature. Teach Coll Rec. 2013;115(3):1–48.

3. Al-Badri M, Kilroy CL, Shahar JI. In-person and virtual multidisciplinary intensive lifestyle interventions are equally effective in patients with type 2 diabetes and obesity. Ther Adv Endocrinol Metab. 2022:13. https://doi.org/10.1177/20420188221093220.
4. Melchart D, Bachmeier BE. The comprehensive lifestyle intervention programme "Individual Health Management" (IHM)—an exemplar for complementary medicine. J Transl Sci. 2018;4(3):1–3. https://doi.org/10.15761/JTS.1000221.
5. Becker P. Mental health and behavioural control. An integrative personality theory and its clinical application. Göttingen: Hogrefe; 1995.
6. Boessmann U, Peseschkian N. Workbook positive order therapy. Stuttgart: Hippokrates Verlag; 1995.
7. Berking M. Training emotional competencies. 4th ed. Heidelberg/Berlin: Springer; 2017.
8. Ellis A. Reason and emotion in psychotherapy. Secaucus: Citadel Press; 1977.
9. Melchart D, Doerfler W, Eustachi A, Wellenhofer-Li Y, Weidenhammer W. The Talent study: a multicentre randomised controlled trial assessing the impact of a 'tailored lifestyle self-management intervention' (talent) on weight reduction. BMC Obesity. 2015;2:38.
10. Melchart D, Wühr E, Weidenhammer W. High and low responder in a comprehensive lifestyle programme for weight loss—secondary analysis of a randomised controlled trial. Complement Med Res. 2017;24(4):232–9. https://doi.org/10.1159/000475663. Epub 2017 July.
11. Singh N, Stewart RAH, Benatar JR. Intensity and duration of lifestyle interventions for long-term weight loss and association with mortality: a meta-analysis of randomised trials. BMJ Open. 2019;9(8):e029966. https://doi.org/10.1136/bmjopen-2019-029966. PMID: 31427335 ; PMCID: PMC6701694.
12. Wagner H, Bauer R, Melchart D, Xiao P-G, editors. Chromatographic fingerprint analysis of herbal medicines, vol. 5. 1st ed. Wien/New York: Springer; 2017.
13. Wagner H, Bauer R, Melchart D, Xiao P-G, editors. Chromatographic fingerprint analysis of herbal medicines, vol. 4. 1st ed. Wien/New York: Springer; 2016.
14. Wagner H, Bauer R, Melchart D, Xiao P-G, editors. Chromatographic fingerprint analysis of herbal medicines, vol. 3. 1st ed. Wien/New York: Springer; 2015.
15. Wagner H, Bauer R, Melchart D, Xiao P-G, editors. Chromatographic fingerprint analysis of herbal medicines, vol. 2. 1st ed. Wien/New York: Springer; 2011.
16. Wagner H, Bauer R, Melchart D, Xiao P-G, editors. Chromatographic fingerprint analysis of herbal medicines, vol. 1. 1st ed. Wien/New York: Springer; 2011.

Summary and Conclusion of the Patient Care Evaluation Programme (PEP) TCM-Klinik Bad Kötzting—Clinic Report 2025

7

Dieter Melchart and Lara Isabel Jötten

The 2025 Clinic Report details the patient care provided by TCM-Klinik Bad Kötzting in 2023, with a follow-up period extending to at least 6 months in 2024. A routine pre-post inpatient observation study was statistically evaluated using RStudio version 2023.12.0, a statistical programming language.

The book begins with an overview of the Patient Care Evaluation Program (PEP). This program provides important information for decisions relating to the clinic made by patients, physicians, health insurance companies, and politicians. This is achieved by describing various quality and evaluation levels. It also highlights the hospital's scientific activities and the ongoing work of the science mentors.

The clinic's structural profile provides an overview of its organisational and content-related conditions and concepts, and its working methods. The clinic's multimodal medical concept, incorporating Western medicine, traditional Chinese medicine, lifestyle medicine, and psychosomatic medicine, illustrates the associated complexity and effort. The principles of the diagnostic and therapeutic approach of TCM and a detailed description of the most important individual TCM measures are explained. The 81-bed facility is one of Bavaria's contract hospitals, meaning it has a care contract with the state's health insurance funds and is listed in the Bavarian hospital plan.

D. Melchart (✉)
Former Head of Competence Centre for Lifestyle Medicine and Naturopathy (CoCoNat), Member of the Faculty of Applied Healthcare Sciences, Deggendorf Institute of Technology (DIT), Deggendorf, Germany
e-mail: dieter.melchart@th-deg.de

L. I. Jötten
Faculty of Applied Healthcare Sciences, Deggendorf Institute of Technology (DIT), Competence Centre for Lifestyle Medicine and Naturopathy, Bad Kötzting, Germany
e-mail: lara.joetten@th-deg.de

D. Melchart et al. (eds.), *TCM-Klinik Bad Kötzting*,
https://doi.org/10.1007/978-3-032-23307-3_7

In 2023, more than 1666 people were interested in inpatient treatment. Of these, 1211 received a recommendation for inpatient admission, with 825 patients being admitted to the hospital—corresponding to an occupancy rate of 79%. The previous year, the clinic had an inpatient occupancy rate of only 730 patients due to the coronavirus pandemic. Seventy-six per cent of clients were referred by general practitioners, internists, and psychiatrists. 94% of documented patients in 2023 had statutory health insurance, primarily with TKK (27.7%), AOK Bayern (24.2%), or Barmer (5.3%). The average length of hospital stay in 2023 was 27 days (SD = 2.4).

The structural profile also describes the clinic's most important organisational and communication processes. The clinic's facilities, staff, and local medical partners, who are available for special diagnostic investigations or emergencies, are introduced.

The patient profile shows that 79.4% (n = 655) of the 825 patients are female, with a mean age of 55.1 years (SD = 11.6) for both sexes. Patients had suffered from their main complaint for an average of 10.3 years (SD = 11.0). Of these patients, 58.6% (n = 415) reported progression, i.e. a worsening of symptoms since the onset of the disease. Overall, 71.9% of patients reported receiving psychotherapy, 37.8% of whom were receiving acute treatment at the time of the survey. Just under half of those who had received psychotherapy (43.8%) had received between 26 and 160 h of therapy. Most patients had attended outpatient treatment several times in the past year (67.6% more than three visits). Most of these visits were unsuccessful or only partially successful. 18.1% of patients reported being hospitalised for their main complaint in the past year. Of the 516-working people, 83.7% had been unable to work in the 6 months prior to attending the TCM clinic. On average, they had 76.39 (SD = 74.17) days of incapacity to work. On admission to the clinic, patients mainly complained of a deterioration in their self-esteem (70.3%) and their relationship with their own body (69.9%) because of their illness. Most patients considered stress (75.8%), work and stressful life events (both 72.0%) to be the main causes of their complaints.

Considering all main and secondary diagnoses, including the mental health diagnoses of the ICD-10-F chapter, somatoform disorders (F45) were the most prevalent, accounting for 42.0% of cases. This was followed by recurrent depressive disorder (F33; 20.5%), non-organic sleep disorders (F51; 10.9%), depressive episodes (F32; 7.0%), and reactions to severe stress and adjustment disorders (F43; 6.2%). Compared to previous years, there has been a significant increase in the number of patients with depression (27.5% vs. 22.5%). Focusing solely on the primary mental health diagnoses, somatoform disorders (62.3%) and recurrent depression (25.1%) emerge as the most prevalent in the ICD-10-F chapter. The most frequent somatic diagnoses were "chronic back pain (M54)" (n = 496), "other diseases of the brain (G93)" (n = 410), "other diseases of soft tissues (M79)" (n = 266), and "sleep disorders (G47)" (n = 236). The TCM syndrome diagnoses documented by Chinese physicians mainly show "general stasis", followed by "liver qi stagnation" and "spleen qi deficiency" or combinations of these syndromes.

Patients' psychosomatic distress is recorded and assessed as part of the Patient Evaluation Programme (PEP), which is a comprehensive initial and follow-up assessment of various indicators. The intensity of symptoms is recorded on a numerical rating scale (from 0 = not present to 100 = extremely severe) and, after the patient's primary assessment, is converted into data on a visual analogue scale (VAS). This shows an average mental and physical pain and stress intensity of 71.16 (SD = 18.95) points on admission. The ICD symptom rating instrument (ISR) is used to identify and measure the type and intensity of psychological distress experienced by patients for all diagnoses. Depressive syndrome is the most common. 58.9% of all patients report moderate to severe symptoms on admission. This finding is supported by measurement of the WHO-5 Wellbeing Index, which indicates an average distress intensity of 28.78 (SD = 19.95) out of a maximum of 100 points, which is associated with "mild depression". Generalised anxiety disorders are also prevalent, with an average score of 10.36 (SD = 4.81) on the Generalised Anxiety Disorder Scale-7 (GAD-7) questionnaire, indicating an average anxiety symptom range. The Tedium test indicates an average critical stress level of 4.24 (SD = 0.94). The exhaustion sub-score shows the highest value. Similar values are found in the PSQ (Perceived Stress Questionnaire), with an average score of 57.63 (SD = 18.07) and a notable tension sub-score. Elevated values on the motor level in the 3-level stress test are also consistent with this. A self-developed questionnaire comprising 42 individual items was used to assess common functional somatic stress disorders. In addition to the frequency and intensity of the individual symptoms, the various functional and organ systems affected by the complaints are recorded and calculated in an index. Musculoskeletal and gastrointestinal symptoms are focal points of functional physical complaints.

A special feature of the patient profile is the in-depth analysis of risk and protective health factors. This is due to complementary medicine's general orientation towards salutogenesis, and towards lifestyle medicine and psychoeducation. The aim is to educate people to strengthen their own physical and mental resources for maintaining health, and to recognise and reduce individual risks. Self-awareness training and the "self-dating" of attitudes, feelings, and behaviour in everyday life using web-based techniques play a central role. Targeted training to develop basic psychosocial and cognitive skills requires the initial identification and assessment of one's own protective factors and mental health resources, with the aim of strengthening and changing them in everyday life in the long term. The assessment of psychosocial resources includes life satisfaction (FLZ), sense of coherence (SOC), well-being (5-Wellbeing Index), vitality (SF36), self-efficacy, optimism (SWOP), and social support (SSS). Physical health protective factors include basic physiological functions that can be measured and trained. These include breathing, nutrition, exercise, sleep, thermoregulation, and cardiovascular functions. Life satisfaction (FLZ) is one of the most important protective factors for human health and is therefore used to introduce resource training. The overall score of 24.15 (SD = 34.92) is clearly in the critical range for all patients. By way of comparison, the average "normal value" for life satisfaction (FLZ) in the general German population is over 61 points. The greatest limitation is found in the sub-dimension "health", which patients primarily interpret in physical terms. Physical resource training therefore focuses on healthy exercise and nutrition. Recent literature highlights the growing importance of exercise in preventing and treating mental health issues such as depression and anxiety. Combining daily exercise with mindfulness-based Qi Gong exercises has been shown to be more effective than promoting exercise alone.

Exercise is also essential for reducing cardiometabolic risk in psychosomatic patients, since the long-term use of psychotropic drugs often increases this risk. Our own analyses show that 27.0% (n = 167) of patients already meet the criteria for metabolic syndrome. Additionally, the Fatty Liver Index (FLI) indicates possible fatty liver disease in older men, with a mean value of 50.10 (SD = 29.21).

The clinic's intervention profile indicates that all patients are offered individual psychological counselling and therapy groups during their stay. The aim is to introduce and guide patients through the psychotherapeutic process. The focus is on addressing conflicts arising from biographical life events and post-traumatic stress disorder and reducing stress through emotional clarification and cognitive restructuring. Chinese doctors give each patient an average of five prescriptions for Chinese medicine. Each prescription contains an average of 13 individual medicines, at a quantity of approximately 8.5 g per traditional Chinese medicine (TCM). The prescriptions are in the form of decoctions. An increasing number of publications report the specific antidepressant effects of individual Chinese herbs, such as Bupleurum chinense DC (Chaihu), or combinations of herbs. These findings are supported by modern pharmacological and clinical studies. Each individual TCM substance is assigned a specific therapeutic effect. These active principles and single drugs are coded and can therefore be statistically evaluated in terms of their frequency. The most prescribed drugs were Astragali radix and Angelicae sinensis radix.

The intervention profile describes overall 83,955 documented acupuncture points. The most frequently used acupoints are GV (Governing Vessel) 20, LI (Large Intestine) 4, and ST (Stomach Meridian) 36. In addition, all patients receive an average of ten acupuncture sessions, covering approximately eleven acupuncture points per treatment. Acupuncture is a recognised method of pain management which reduces levels of pain and neurovegetative arousal. There are numerous studies, in particular, on the successful treatment of chronic back pain, sciatica, fibromyalgia, and other pain conditions. The specific antidepressant effects of acupuncture are also being discussed and supported by clinical studies (see the publications section).

The clinic's outcome profile presents information on patient satisfaction and the benefits and side effects of care. Across all diagnoses, 36.8% of patients rated their overall symptoms as "no longer present" or "significantly reduced" at discharge, compared to 41.1% at 6 months. At discharge, 45% of patients rated their symptoms as "somewhat less", compared to 33.3% at follow-up. The remainder (12% vs. 16.2%) rated their complaints as unchanged between discharge and follow-up or worse in 6.2% vs. 9.4% of cases. When the main complaint is measured using the VAS, and only patients for whom admission, discharge, and follow-up values are available are evaluated (n = 618), there is a reduction in complaint severity between admission and discharge, from 70.68 (SD = 19.08) to 45.36 (SD = 21.86), and at follow-up, to 47.44 (SD = 24.27). This progression corresponds to strong treatment effects ($d = 1.23$ vs. $d = 1.06$), which, according to Cohen, start at d-values of 0.8. When comparing changes in the ICD symptom rating (ISR) at different time points, the ISR total score shows a mean affective symptom burden of 1.14 (SD = 0.59) versus 0.82 (SD = 0.55) versus 0.78 (SD = 0.55). Considering only the complete datasets of 603 patients, the mean effect sizes between the survey periods are $d = 0.58$ vs. $d = 0.63$. The strongest clinical effect is found in the depression subdimension of the ISR, with $d = 0.98$ vs. $d = 0.82$. In the area of anxiety disorders, the Generalised Anxiety Disorder (GAD) questionnaire shows significantly large effect sizes of $d = 0.98$ at discharge and $d = 0.75$ at follow-up. To estimate the bias in the outcome data due to the loss of approximately 25% of the follow-up data, the last value carried forward (LOCF) method was used for the entire sample. Comparing the severity of the original chief complaint surveyed at discharge with the severity of the chief complaint at follow-up shows slight differences, with slight deterioration from discharge to follow-up. There were no significant differences between the follow-up results with and without imputation (LOCF).

Overall, treatment success was rated as "good" or "very good" by 64.9% of patients at discharge and 72.4% at follow-up. For 31.8% vs. 24.4% of patients, the overall success was only "fair", and for 3.3% vs. 3.2%, there was "no treatment success". When asked to rate the elements of therapy that had helped them most, acupuncture, TCM drugs, tuina, and qigong were rated the highest. While 62.9% of patients reported being employed at the time of the initial survey, this figure fell to 58.7% in the follow-up survey. Of these patients, 83.7% reported being unable to work for up to 6 months prior to hospitalisation. At the follow-up survey, the proportion of those unable to work fell to 52.7%. The median number of sick leave days decreased from 30 to 20. The mean number of sick leave days decreased from 76.39 (SD = 74.17) to 72.11 (SD = 94.32). The success of the treatment is also reflected in the reduction in post-hospital medication use. Some 54.6% of patients reported a reduction in conventional medication use after their hospital stay (33.8% significantly less and 20.8% slightly less). At discharge, the health portal asks questions about possible adverse drug reactions (ADRs) using freehand documentation, which 50.2% of patients (i.e. 414 cases) commented on. In most cases, these were gastrointestinal symptoms caused by Chinese medicines, which are usually bitter tasting. There is a significant correlation ($p = .023$) between reporting adverse therapeutic effects (ATEs) and assessing treatment success, although the effect size is small ($d = .16$). This suggests that "side effects" or "adverse events" associated with treatment are only minimally associated with poorer ratings of overall treatment success. As part of the clinic's Complication Screening Programme (CSP), liver enzyme levels are regularly monitored in all patients at baseline and at the end of treatment. Recording baseline and follow-up alanine aminotransferase (ALT) and alkaline phosphatase (AP) levels is important for clinically assessing liver injury. To make the laboratory values easier to understand, they are expressed as multiples of the upper limit of normal (ULN) (2 to more than 5 times). Liver injury is present if the ALT value is ≥5xULN or the AP value is ≥2xULN. There were no suspected cases in the TCM hospital in 2023.

The supplementary report presents the results for the main psychiatric diagnoses (F45, F32/F33) and somatic indications (M54/M53/M79/G43/G47).

For somatoform disorders (F45), the clinical picture of somatoform disorders is characterised by persistent negative thoughts, feelings, and dysfunctional behaviours associated with somatic symptoms. These patients often experience long-term chronicity and develop comorbid depression and anxiety. Patients with a primary diagnosis of F45 showed clinically significant improvements in their main complaints (as measured by the VAS scale), with high effect sizes ($d = 1.09$) at discharge and ($d = 1.11$) at follow-up. At discharge, 14.9% of patients rated their overall success as "very good" and 50.1% as "good". When asked, "From today's point of view, was the treatment worthwhile?", 40.5% answered "very worthwhile" and 54.4% answered "partly worthwhile". At the follow-up examination, the overall result was rated even better, with 53.8% saying it was "very worthwhile" and 39.6% saying it was "worthwhile". As stress-induced hyperalgesia exacerbates the clinical picture, reducing stress levels is beneficial from a therapeutic point of view. Measurement of self-perceived stress using the PSQ (Perceived Stress Questionnaire) shows that this was achieved for many patients. The effect size was $d = 0.97$ at discharge and $d = 0.57$ at follow-up. Strong measures of change were also observed in the indicators for well-being ($d = 1.17$ vs. $d = 0.73$), vitality ($d = 0.93$ vs. $d = 0.71$), ISR depression ($d = 0.96$ vs. $d = 0.80$), GAD anxiety ($d = 0.94$ vs. $d = 0.74$), and the psycho-vegetative complaint complex ($d = 0.87$ vs. $d = 0.78$).

Depression-related diagnostic groups F32 and F33 show high effect sizes in the VAS (0–100) measurement, with $d = 1.35$ at discharge and $d = 1.16$ at follow-up. Half of all patients with primary depression also report pain. Patients with primary pain and comorbid depression can also be included. At discharge, 15% of depression patients rated the success of their treatment as "very good" and 48.4% as "good", while at follow-up, these figures were 24.5% and 49%, respectively. When asked, "From today's point of view, was the treatment worthwhile?", 45.1% of patients answered "very worthwhile" and 47.6% answered "worthwhile" at discharge. In the follow-up survey, these figures were 55.2% and 39.1%, respectively. The effect sizes achieved in the ISR depression subscale were $d = 1.02$ at discharge and $d = 0.93$, 6 months later. The other outcome indicators for this group of patients are as follows: GAD anxiety ($d = 1.09$ vs. $d = 0.80$), well-being ($d = 1.16$ vs. $d = 0.78$), vitality ($d = 0.97$ vs. $d = 0.81$), PSQ ($d = 1.07$ vs. $d = 0.80$), life satisfaction (health sub-dimension, $d = 0.67$ vs. $d = 0.68$), and PSQI daily sleepiness ($d = 0.83$ vs. $d = 0.51$).

When we compare our data on the effectiveness of inpatient psychosomatic therapy treatments with the results of two meta-analyses, we find that the effect sizes achieved at the TCM clinic are sometimes higher than the pre-post effect sizes achieved in inpatient rehabilitation ($d = 0.51$) and hospital treatment ($d = 0.73$).

The most common principal somatic diagnosis is chronic back pain (M54). This also includes M53, "other diseases of the spine", with cervico-brachial syndromes being the most common. Back pain or other spinal conditions were diagnosed in 425 of the 825 patients during their inpatient stay. Of these, approximately 33.2% were localised in the lumbar region, while around 43.7% were localised in the cervical region. The assessment of change in symptoms according to the VAS scale reveals remarkably high effect sizes for both indications: M54 ($d = 1.29$ vs. $d = 1.12$) and M53 ($d = 1.41$ vs. $d = 1.20$). Fourteen per cent of patients with back pain rated the overall success as "very good", while 49.6% rated it as "good". Among M53 patients, 11.7% rated it as "very good", while 54.5% rated it as "good".

Strong effect sizes were again found for measures of affective parameters, such as anxiety and depression: GAD anxiety (d = 0.96 vs. $d = 0.71$) and ISR depression ($d = 0.95$ vs. $d = 0.75$). Well-being ($d = 1.14$ vs. $d = 0.68$), vitality ($d = 0.90$ vs. $d = 0.70$), self-perceived stress (PSQ: $d = 0.96$ vs. $d = 0.60$), and the sleep subdimensions sleep quality ($d = 0.51$ vs. $d = 0.49$) and daytime sleepiness ($d = 0.85$ vs. $d = 0.56$) also improved.

Indications of fibromyalgia (M79) and pain in the extremities and joints (M25) also showed high effect sizes for the main complaint at discharge (M79: $d = -1.25$; M25: $d = -1.41$) and at follow-up (M79: $d = 0.103$; M25: $d = 1.13$).

Overall, the treatment results for chronic pain patients demonstrate targeted optimisation of psychosocial risk factors. This explains the positive outcomes for patients with musculoskeletal pain.

Other indications, such as chronic headaches (G43 and G44), show similarly effective treatment results. Patients with tension or other headache syndromes (G44) achieved extremely high VAS effect sizes of $d = -1.35$ at discharge and follow-up ($d = -1.22$). For migraine (G43), the effect sizes are $d = 1.07$ vs. $d = 1.05$. Clinically relevant reductions were also found for psycho-vegetative complaints ($d = 0.97$ vs. d = 0.94), self-perceived stress (PSQ: $d = 1.10$ vs. $d = 0.65$), ISR depression ($d = 0.98$ vs. $d = 0.77$), and GAD anxiety ($d = 0.95$ vs. $d = 0.72$).

Finally, patients with sleep disorders (G47) benefit from positive change scores, with a global reduction in symptoms of $d = 1.29$ vs. $d = 1.16$. At discharge, 11.3% of these patients rated their improvement as "very good", 53.8% as "good", 30.8% as "moderate", and 4.0% as "not successful". Six months later, these ratings had improved to 23.1% "very good", 48.7% "good", 24.1% "moderate", and 4.1% "no success". The results of the Pittsburgh Sleep Quality Index (PSQI) show significant medium-range effects for the three domains of sleep efficiency, sleep quality, and daytime sleepiness ($d = 0.54$, $d = 0.65$, $d = 0.53$) at follow-up. The exception was the use of sleeping pills, which was comparable at follow-up to the use before admission.

As an evaluation and quality assurance profile, this clinic report contains a sample of the individual case reports and health reports generated for each patient by the TCM health portal for doctors and patients. For the model project IHM Lifestyle Programme Sinocur with AOK Bayern, an application was submitted to the Bavarian Medical Service for recognition as an "Intensive Lifestyle Intervention (ILI)" for the indication obesity grade I and II as an additional rehabilitation service according to §43 SGB-V. Planned improvement projects include the development of a mobile version of the health portal, optimisation of the indicator concept, and a reorganisation of the lectures on psychoeducation and lifestyle medicine. Another section of the evaluation and quality assurance profile presents important publications relating to specific TCM methods and indications. It also presents the clinic's own publications since its inception. Examining the vast amount of literature on traditional Chinese medicine and its components reveals a surprising number of over 14,000 results in the PubMed database when searching for controlled randomised studies, meta-analyses, or systematic reviews. Nevertheless, critics often wrongly point to the poor quality of clinical TCM studies. They frequently do so unfairly. The likelihood hypothesis is the well-described phenomenon of assessing studies of non-rational treatment methods less favourably than would be necessary when comparing conventional medicine. There needs to be more intensive discussion on this issue.

With this report, the TCM-Klinik Bad Kötzting, its management, and the entire Chinese German staff fully meet the transparency and evaluation requirements for an international medical-scientific hospital.

Batch number: 10183654

Printed by Printforce, the Netherlands